PUBLIC HEALTH YEARBOOK 2012

HEALTH AND HUMAN DEVELOPMENT

JOAV MERRICK - SERIES EDITOR

NATIONAL INSTITUTE OF CHILD HEALTH
AND HUMAN DEVELOPMENT,
MINISTRY OF SOCIAL AFFAIRS, JERUSALEM

Adolescent Behavior Research:
International Perspectives
Joav Merrick and Hatim A. Omar (Editors)
2007. ISBN: 1-60021-649-8

Complementary Medicine Systems:
Comparison and Integration
Karl W. Kratky
2008. ISBN: 978-1-60456-475-4 (Hardcover)
2008. ISBN: 978-1-61122-433-7 (E-book)

Pain in Children and Youth
Patricia Schofield and Joav Merrick
(Editors)
2008. ISBN: 978-1-60456-951-3 (Hardcover)
2008. ISBN: 978-1-61470-496-6 (E-book)

Alcohol-Related Cognitive Disorders:
Research and Clinical Perspectives
Leo Sher, Isack Kandel and Joav Merrick
(Editors)
2009. ISBN: 978-1-60741-730-9 (Hardcover)
2009. ISBN: 978-1-60876-623-9 (E-book)

Challenges in Adolescent Health:
An Australian Perspective
David Bennett, Susan Towns,
Elizabeth Elliott
and Joav Merrick (Editors)
2009. ISBN: 978-1-60741-616-6 (Hardcover)
2009. ISBN: 978-1-61668-240-8 (E-book)

Children and Pain
Patricia Schofield and Joav Merrick
(Editors)
2009. ISBN: 978-1-60876-020-6 (Hardcover)
2009. ISBN: 978-1-61728-183-9 (E-book)

Living on the Edge: The Mythical,
Spiritual, and Philosophical
Roots of Social Marginality
Joseph Goodbread
2009. ISBN: 978-1-60741-162-8 (Hardcover)
2013. ISBN: 978-1-61122-986-8 (Softcover)
2011. ISBN: 978-1-61470-192-7 (E-book)

Obesity and Adolescence:
A Public Health Concern
Hatim A. Omar, Donald E. Greydanus,
Dilip R. Patel and Joav Merrick (Editors)
2009. ISBN: 978-1-60692-821-9 (Hardcover)
2009. ISBN: 978-1-61470-465-2 (E-book)

Poverty and Children:
A Public Health Concern
Alexis Lieberman and Joav Merrick (Editors)
2009. ISBN: 978-1-60741-140-6 (Hardcover)
2009. ISBN: 978-1-61470-601-4 (E-book)

Bone and Brain Metastases:
Advances in Research and Treatment
Arjun Sahgal, Edward Chow
and Joav Merrick (Editors)
2010. ISBN: 978-1-61668-365-8 (Hardcover)
2010. ISBN: 978-1-61728-085-6 (E-book)

Chance Action and Therapy:
The Playful Way of Changing
Uri Wernik
2010. ISBN: 978-1-60876-393-1 (Hardcover)
2011. ISBN: 978-1-61122-987-5 (Softcover)
2011. ISBN: 978-1-61209-874-6 (E-book)

**Positive Youth Development:
Implementation of a Youth Program
in a Chinese Context**
*Daniel T.L Shek, Hing Keung Ma
and Joav Merrick (Editors)*
2011. ISBN: 978-1-61668-230-9 (Hardcover)

**Principles of Holistic Psychiatry:
A Textbook on Holistic Medicine
for Mental Disorders**
Soren Ventegodt and Joav Merrick
2011. ISBN: 978-1-61761-940-3 (Hardcover)
2011. ISBN: 978-1-61122-263-0 (E-book)

Public Health Yearbook 2009
Joav Merrick (Editor)
2011. ISBN: 978-1-61668-911-7 (Hardcover)
2011. ISBN: 978-1-62417-365-3 (E-book)

**Rural Child Health:
International Aspects**
Erica Bell and Joav Merrick (Editors)
2011. ISBN: 978-1-60876-357-3 (Hardcover)
2011. ISBN: 978-1-61324-005-2 (E-book)

**Rural Medical Education:
Practical Strategies**
*Erica Bell, Craig Zimitat and Joav Merrick
(Editors)*
2011. ISBN: 978-1-61122-649-2 (Hardcover)
2011. ISBN: 978-1-61209-476-2 (E-book)

**Self-Management and the Health Care
Consumer**
Peter William Harvey
2011. ISBN: 978-1-61761-796-6 (Hardcover)
2011. ISBN: 978-1-61122-214-2 (E-book)

Sexology from a Holistic Point of View
Soren Ventegodt and Joav Merrick
2011. ISBN: 978-1-61761-859-8 (Hardcover)
2011. ISBN: 978-1-61122-262-3 (E-book)

**Social and Cultural Psychiatry
Experience from the Caribbean Region**
*Hari D. Maharajh and Joav Merrick
(Editors)*
2011. ISBN: 978-1-61668-506-5 (Hardcover)
2010. ISBN: 978-1-61728-088-7 (E-book)

**The Dance of Sleeping and Eating
among Adolescents:
Normal and Pathological Perspectives**
Yael Latzer and Orna Tzischinsky (Editors)
2011. ISBN: 978-1-61209-710-7 (Hardcover)
2011. ISBN: 978-1-62417-366-0 (E-book)

**Understanding Eating Disorders:
Integrating Culture,
Psychology and Biology**
*Yael Latzer, Joav Merrick and Daniel Stein
(Editors)*
2011. ISBN: 978-1-61728-298-0 (Hardcover)
2011. ISBN: 978-1-61470-976-3 (Softcover)
2011. ISBN: 978-1-61942-054-0 (E-book)

**Adolescence and Chronic Illness.
A Public Health Concern**
*Hatim Omar, Donald E. Greydanus,
Dilip R. Patel
and Joav Merrick (Editors)*
2012. ISBN: 978-1-60876-628-4 (Hardcover)
2010. ISBN: 978-1-61761-482-8 (E-book)

**AIDS and Tuberculosis: Public
Health Aspects**
Daniel Chemtob and Joav Merrick (Editors)
2012. ISBN: 978-1-62081-382-9 (Softcover)
2012. ISBN: 978-1-62081-406-2 (E-book)

Alternative Medicine Yearbook 2010
Joav Merrick (Editor)
2012. ISBN: 978-1-62100-132-4 (Hardcover)
2011. ISBN: 978-1-62100-210-9 (E-book)

HEALTH AND HUMAN DEVELOPMENT

PUBLIC HEALTH YEARBOOK 2012

JOAV MERRICK
EDITOR

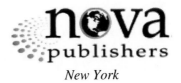

New York

For permission to use material from this book please contact us:
Telephone 631-231-7269; Fax 631-231-8175
Web Site: http://www.novapublishers.com

NOTICE TO THE READER

The Publisher has taken reasonable care in the preparation of this book, but makes no expressed or implied warranty of any kind and assumes no responsibility for any errors or omissions. No liability is assumed for incidental or consequential damages in connection with or arising out of information contained in this book. The Publisher shall not be liable for any special, consequential, or exemplary damages resulting, in whole or in part, from the readers' use of, or reliance upon, this material. Any parts of this book based on government reports are so indicated and copyright is claimed for those parts to the extent applicable to compilations of such works.

Independent verification should be sought for any data, advice or recommendations contained in this book. In addition, no responsibility is assumed by the publisher for any injury and/or damage to persons or property arising from any methods, products, instructions, ideas or otherwise contained in this publication.

This publication is designed to provide accurate and authoritative information with regard to the subject matter covered herein. It is sold with the clear understanding that the Publisher is not engaged in rendering legal or any other professional services. If legal or any other expert assistance is required, the services of a competent person should be sought. FROM A DECLARATION OF PARTICIPANTS JOINTLY ADOPTED BY A COMMITTEE OF THE AMERICAN BAR ASSOCIATION AND A COMMITTEE OF PUBLISHERS.

Additional color graphics may be available in the e-book version of this book.

Library of Congress Cataloging-in-Publication Data

ISBN: 978-1-62808-078-0

Published by Nova Science Publishers, Inc. † New York

CONTENTS

INTRODUCTION

Joav Merrick[*], MD, MMedSci, DMSc[1,2,3,4]

[1] National Institute of Child Health and Human Development
[2] Health Services, Office of the Medical Director, Division for Intellectual and Developmental Disabilities, Ministry of Social Affairs and Social Services, Jerusalem
[3] Department of Pediatrics, Hadassah-Hebrew University Medical Center, Mount Scopus Campus, Jerusalem, Israel
[4] Kentucky Children's Hospital, University of Kentucky, Lexington, United States

In this Public Health Yearbook 2012 we will touch upon several public health topics like burns, infant mortality, maltreatment, tropical pediatics, building community capacity and HIV research.

Tropical medicine is a branch of medicine focusing on disorders usually found in subtropical and tropical areas of the world. Tropical pediatrics is a branch of tropical medicine focusing on children in these areas. The current process of global warming and the widespread issue of international travel are bringing these conditions to many places of the globe. Section two highlights selective concepts of tropical pediatrics that are of importance to clinicians caring for children and adolescents. This section is dedicated to clinicians around the world, who care for these precious patients growing up in remote corners of globe. It should always be remembered that sometimes these issues become important to civilized corners of the world as well.

Advances in science, innovations in business, and technological development in the last century and the continued rapid pace of change in these areas have created an environment, where the world today in the twenty-first century knows few boundaries. Health care is a field that has been enhanced and able to expand as a result of progress in these diverse yet integrated areas. However, for all of the improvement that new drugs, health care re-organization and focused delivery, and accessible electronic medical records, for example, can afford many of the "haves" in society, there still remains a significant segment of the population in the industrialized world, and certainly in developing countries, who comprise

[*] Correspondence: Professor Joav Merrick, MD, MMedSci, DMSc, Medical Director, Health Services, Division for Intellectual and Developmental Disabilities, Ministry of Social Affairs, POBox 1260, IL-91012 Jerusalem, Israel. E-mail: jmerrick@zahav.net.il.

the "have nots" and do not benefit from this progress. This disparity in health among populations across the globe has existed for decades despite our advances in health care and will be discussed in section three. In this section it will be discussed what we, as public health academicians and practitioners have learned when partnering with minority and immigrant community members to help them address persistent public health issues that affect them and their families on a daily basis. These are lessons that need to be shared so disadvantaged populations can build their capacity to address and solve persistent public health problems in their communities. Every segment of the population, regardless of where they live, deserves to enjoy the health care and public health advances of the last century and the rapid improvements currently occurring. It is our hope that these lessons will help to decrease the global prevalence of health disparities that are grounded in complex public health issues.

In the last section the chapters represent a small cross-section of some of the types of approaches that contemporary social scientists are taking in their efforts to minimize the harms resulting from HIV and AIDS. These chapters represent the utilization of a variety of methodologies, focus on a variety of "at risk" population groups, and advocate a variety of things that might be done from a social science perspective to help curtail the adverse effects of HIV. These articles do not represent social science efforts against HIV as a whole. Rather, they comprise a smattering of different approaches currently underway–a small portion of a much greater whole. Taken as a group, however, they do illustrate one thing quite clearly: Social scientists are working hard to understand HIV and to figure out ways to reduce the harms brought about by HIV infection.

SECTION ONE - PUBLIC HEALTH

In: Public Health Yearbook 2012
Editor: Joav Merrick

ISBN: 978-1-62808-078-0
© 2013 Nova Science Publishers, Inc.

Chapter 1

ON SCENE FIRST AID AND EMERGENCY CARE FOR BURN VICTIMS

William HC Tiong, MD, MRCS, MB BCh[*]

Department of Plastic and Reconstructive Surgery,
Beaumont-Connolly Hospital, Dublin, Ireland

ABSTRACT

Burn injury is damage to the skin or other body parts caused by extreme heat, flame, or contact with heated objects or chemicals. In United Kingdom (UK), it accounted for 175,000 emergency department attendances and 15,000 admissions. A further 250,000 burn patients were managed in the community by general practitioners or other healthcare professionals. A survey in 1998 showed that up to 58% of UK ambulance services had no specific treatment policy for burn patients. In Ireland and Australia, only 23% and 39% respectively, had employed the correct first aid burn management in studies conducted on their primary careers. Early burn management, both on scene and upon arrival to the hospital, are important to reduce the potential morbidity and mortality of burn victims. The initial management of burn, from removal of patients from zone of incident to the topical administration of cool water, has been shown to significantly reduce the extent of injury of burn patients. Further critical and timely assessment and management of these patients, pre-hospital and on arrival to emergency department, improve their chances of survival through adequate airway management and resuscitation. The need for emergency surgical procedure from emergency department to operating theatre should also be instituted when warranted without delay. Here, we review the pathophysiological rationale and evidence of practice behind each of these steps, from the first aid burn treatment to their assessment and resuscitation, and finally emergency procedure, together with their ancillary treatment, in practice.

Keywords: First aid, emergency burn care, inhalation injury, burn referral criteria, burn resuscitation

---

[*] Correspondence: Mr. William HC Tiong, MD, MRCS, MB BCh, Department of Plastic and Reconstructive Surgery, Beaumont-Connolly Hospital, Dublin, Ireland. Email: willhct@yahoo.com

INTRODUCTION

Burn injury is damage to the skin or other body parts caused by extreme heat, flame, or contact with heated objects or chemicals. The World Health Organization estimated that 322000 people die each year from fire related burns with >95% of these occurred in developing countries [1]. The mortality rates were much greater at both ends of the age spectrum. Thirty-eight percent of all burn deaths were due to multiple organ failure and only 4.1% were due to burn wound sepsis [2]. The biggest factor in burn mortality was inhalation injury with increased mortality to 26.3% in the 6.5% of burn patients admitted with inhalation injury [2].

In United Kingdom (UK), burns accounted for 175,000 emergency department attendances and 13000 admissions, and a further 250,000 patient were managed in the community by general practitioners and allied professionals [3]. Although recent data from Burn Repository in USA showed significant improvement of overall burns mortality, there are still many areas that can be improved especially in the early stage of burns treatment to optimize chances of survival and outcome [2]. A survey in 1998 showed that up to 58% of UK ambulance services had no specific treatment policy for burn patients [4]. In Ireland and Australia, only 23% and 39% respectively, had employed the correct first aid burn management in studies conducted on their primary carers [5,6]. Equally, a review of the management of minor burns within the emergency departments of hospitals in Ontario, Canada, showed that 70% of responding physicians would not measure the extent of the burn area when making an assessment, whereas 45% failed to discuss analgesic requirements [7]. Based on these data, there is still much room to improve in the basic care of burn victims.

PATHOPHYSIOLOGY OF BURNS

Burn from thermal source inflicts damage through various mechanisms, both locally and systemically, through direct injury and reactive physiology. The natural functions of skin are to act as a barrier to bacteria and prevention of water loss through its epidermal layer. The deeper, dermal layer provides mechanical strength and integrity through its abundant connective tissue composition, and nourishment to epidermal and dermal layers through myriad of vascular plexuses. The dermal layer is also the home to many dermal appendages such as sweat glands and hair follicles, which houses regenerative epidermal cells that are capable of replenishing injured skin. When such functions of skin are compromised, attending physician should institute treatments that will minimize the injury and compensate its deficits through adequate first aid and resuscitation. Early burns management is one of the most important determinant factor in reducing the potential morbidity and mortality of burn victims. In USA, approximately 75% of severe burn deaths occur on scene or during initial transport [8].

The pathophysiology of thermal burn injury is related to the initial distribution of heat within the skin with its severity dependent upon the temperature of the source of insult and the duration of contact [9]. On a cellular level, the initial response to thermal injury involves direct heat-induced protein denaturation and cell death. This is followed by inflammation and ischemia-induced injury, which resulted in burn of varying skin depth. Because skin is a good insulator, most burns generally involve only the epidermis or part of the dermis. Only with prolonged exposure do burn encompasses the entire dermis or extend beneath the dermis into subcutaneous tissue such as fat, muscle, and bone. However, similar extent of burn can also occur with short exposure to an object of high temperature. For instance, a thermal blistering injury can occur after 5 minutes of exposure to water at 48.9 °C (120 °F) or after just 1 second of exposure to water at 68 °C (155°F).

The depth of burn is a dynamic process, as popularly described by Jackson [10]. The histopathology of burn consists of three concentric zones with the zone of coagulation being the area closest to the heat source. The tissue in this zone is either entirely necrotic or undergoes severe denaturation of proteins and forms an eschar. The injury in this zone is irreversible. Just below this is the zone of stasis, where there is only modest denaturation of macromolecules but characterized by hypoperfusion of tissue due to significant edema and stasis. This is attributed to capillary leak and cell membrane disruption in this zone. Beneath the zone of stasis is an area of hyperemia, where blood flow gradually increases, becoming particularly prominent by about 7 days after the injury [11]. Although tissue in the zones of stasis and hyperemia are at risk for necrosis, they are potentially salvageable given optimal intervention that preserves perfusion of these zones [10]. Conversely, a burn that appears superficial may become deeper over a period of 48 to 72 h, with the zone of stasis becoming necrotic in the face of suboptimal treatment [12]. This is especially likely to happen if the burn wound becomes infected or poorly perfused. Adequate fluid resuscitation is essential to maintain tissue perfusion in this dynamic zone [13,14].

In addition to primary tissue loss due to local protein denaturation and tissue necrosis in burn, this is rapidly followed by activation of toxic inflammatory mediators, especially in the perfused subsurface [12]. The release of vasoactive mediators translates local edema into both local and systemic fluid shifts that exacerbate hypoperfusion in vulnerable tissue, specifically in the zones of stasis and hyperemia [12-15]. Oxidants and proteases further damage skin and capillary endothelial cells, potentiating ischemic tissue necrosis [12-15]. When the burn exceeds 20% of the patient's body surface, the local tissue response becomes systemic with potential hazardous effect on distant tissues and organs [16-18]. Sequelae such as edema and altered perfusion promote progression of injury beyond the degree of initial necrotic area through worsening fluid regulation and systemic inflammatory responses [12-15]. Activation of complement and coagulation systems causes thrombosis and release of histamine and bradykinin, leading to an increase in capillary leak and interstitial edema in distant organs and soft tissue [16]. Secondary interstitial edema and organ dysfunction from bacterial overgrowth within the eschar can then result in systemic infection. Activation of the pro-inflammatory cascade and the counter-regulatory anti-inflammatory reaction then lead to immune dysfunction [16]. This increases patient's susceptibility to sepsis and multiple organ failure. The systemic response to burn also leads to a hypermetabolic state, doubling normal physiologic cardiac output over the first 48 h post-burn [19]. This is mediated by hugely increased level of catecholamines, prostaglandins, glucagons, and glucocorticoids, resulting in skeletal muscle catabolism, immune deficiency, lipolysis, reduced bone mineralization, and reduced linear growth. These systemic metabolic changes in the burn patients may continue for up to a year after injury. Therefore, mitigating factors in early treatment to decrease these effects, which include adequate first aid and resuscitation, early excision of burn and grafting, control of sepsis, supplemented nutrition through high-carbohydrate or high-protein diet, and the use of anabolic agents, need to be instituted as early as appropriate.

THE FIRST AID AND PRE-HOSPITAL CARE

All emergencies started on scene, at the site of incident. Emergency care should therefore, includes first aid, pre-hospital and en route care before actual arrival to emergency department. The first aid is emergency care or treatment given before regular medical aid can be obtained, and it serves to provide analgesia and halt the progression of burn. Walker et al. [20] summarized the consensus of the first aid management and pre-hospital care for burn victims to serve as a reminder for the carer as to the priorities in caring for burn victims (Table 1).

Historically, first aid in burns treatment ranges from the use of natural to traditional or folk remedies over the centuries, to more recent recommendation from regulatory bodies based on clinical studies. The concept of 'first aid' was believed to be initially described by the Prussian surgeon (Surgeon General) Friedrich Von Esmarch (AD 1823–1908), with his work on 'Erste hilfe' first translated from German to English in 1882 [21]. Modern first aid concept, as a set of trained drills and skills, dated only from the late nineteenth century [22].

The use of cold water as first aid for burn has the greatest volume of supporting literature in comparison to other therapies, and it has been a popular treatment throughout history. Early literature as far back as Galen (AD 129–199), Rhazes (AD 852–923), and Ibn Sina (980–1037) can be found to have used cooled or cold water for burn [23]. In 1969, St John Ambulance first aid manual advocated irrigation of burn wound with cold water even though no duration was specified [24]. More recent studies by Rose among others indicated that treatment with cold water decreased pain and mortality by reducing damage to tissues [25-32]. Other reports subversive to the use of cooled water concerned the lack of clear guidelines on the temperature of the coolant, duration of application and the effect of delay between burn injury and onset of cooling [33].

Table 1. Consensus on first aid management of burn

SAFE approach	• Shout or call for help • Assess the scene for dangers to rescuer or victim • Free or remove from danger • Evaluate the casualty
Stop burning process	• Stop burning process by allowing patient to roll on the ground, use of blanket, water or fire extinguisher • Remove clothing and accessories unless adherent to the patient. Remove any jewelry, which may become constrictive • Bring all clothing articles to the hospital for examination
Cool burn	• Irrigate the burn area for up to 20 minutes with cool running tap water [178] • Ice and very cold water should be avoided • Place a cold wet towel over area of small burn (<5%) on top of polyvinylchloride film (e.g. Clingfilm) dressing • Caution on hypothermia especially in children
Dress burn and victim	• Polyvinylchloride film dressing to keep burn area clean and help in pain relief • Use small sheet of dressings rather than large circumferential wrapping to avoid constricting effect • Alternatively use water gel dressings to cool and dress [20] • Wrap the patient in blankets or a duvet to keep warm

Studies conducted by Cuttle et al. showed that the immediate use of 2-15 °C running cold water for 20 min duration can increase healing by limiting the depth of burns, and promoted re-epithelialization over the first 2 weeks post-burn with decreased scarring at 6 weeks [34,35]. This benefit was noticeable in treatment for as little as 10 min duration with maximum benefit observed at 3 h even in cases where the onset of treatment was delayed by up to 30 min to 1 h [33,35].

Cold water reduces the extent of burn injury by cooling the tissue below the damaging temperature and subsequently assist burn healing by preventing cells from undergoing progressive necrosis 24–48 h after burn in the zone of stasis [10,25,36]. It causes a decrease in cell metabolism, which allow the compromised cells to survive a hypoxic wound environment, stabilize the vasculature by decreasing capillary leakage, increasing dermal perfusion and re-establishing blood flow, and dampens the inflammatory response to facilitate cell survival in the burn wound. Over the years, ice application has also been described to confer benefit in burn treatment [37,38]. Modern first aid recommendations however, advise that ice deepens or worsens burn injury [39]. It also increases the risk of hypothermia especially in children or patients with large body surface area burn as demonstrated by Ofeigsson's experiments [25]. Because of the perceived potential for hypothermia after cold treatment, some researchers advocated treating burn wound with lukewarm or body temperature water [40].

Warm water as first aid burn treatment was popular in the late 1800s to early 1900s. It was recommended that burned limbs should be soaked in body temperature water of 36.9 °C (98.4 °F) until suitable dressings could be found [41-43]. This was to decrease pain, and also prevent shock and infection. It was believed that the application of heat in smaller doses restores the tissue to normal. However, it was also recognized as early as 1899 that further heat application to burn simply causes more harm [44].

Other substances used for first aid burn treatment by native cultures are aloe vera and tea tree oil. Aloe vera has been shown to improve treatment of first and second degree burns in a clinical review by Maenthaisong et al. [45]. It significantly shortens the wound healing time by modulating collagen response and inhibits the inflammatory process in the healing wound [46-49]. There are several hydrogel products on the first aid market based on tea tree oil such as Water-Jel®, Burnshield®, Burnaid® and Burnfree®. These products are recommended as first aid for burns, and have been adopted by Australian ambulance and paramedic services. They contain ≥90% water and melaleuca oil in a proprietary gel. To date, there is limited evidence that these products are beneficial for burn treatment, although they are reported to soothe the burn [50,51]. Their effects were attributed to their anti-inflammatory, antibacterial and antifungal properties [52-54].

Several other oils have also been recommended for first aid treatment of burn, namely lavender and thyme oil [55,56]. There are some evidence that oils, especially those derived from plants, may act as antioxidants and either directly or indirectly scavenge oxygen-derived free radicals [57,58]. One study has demonstrated that lavender oil possesses local anaesthetic, antibacterial, and antifungal properties, which makes it effective in healing wounds including burns [55,59]. Thyme oil, from the herb thyme is used in Turkey as an excellent remedy for the treatment of burns and has been shown to also have antibacterial, antifungal and antioxidant properties [56, 60]. Other oils and creams used over the years to protect against excessive burn wound exposure to air were painted grease or butter, almond or cod-liver oil, olive oil, salad oil, castor oil or carron oil, linseed, lamp oil, or carbolic acid or thymol oil soaked cotton wool dressing, and Vaseline® or lanoline cream [21,41,43,61]. Most other common household liquids have also been used as first aid to treat burn. There are reports in the literature of treatment with toothpaste, soy sauce, eggs, honey, ink, and traditional African wound treatments such as leaves, mud, burned snail shell, a mixture of urine and mud, and cow dung [62-67]. Many of these folk remedies are based on the idea that air should be excluded from a burn as quickly as possible.

ASSESSMENT UPON ARRIVAL ± REFERRAL

Most minor burns can be managed by general practitioner in primary care, but complex and major burns warrant a specialist and skilled multidisciplinary approach to optimize clinical outcome. Upon arrival to emergency department, the first decision is whether a burn can be managed at the local facility or should be transferred to a designated burns center. Table 2 outlines the criteria for referral to specialized burns center [68].

Table 2. Criteria for referral to specialized burns center

- If 10-40 years old: ≥15% total body surface area (TBSA) partial thickness burn or ≥5% TBSA full thickness burn
- If <10 or >40 years old: ≥10% TBSA burns
- Special area burns involving face, hands, feet and/or perineum, genitals, joints
- Circumferential burns
- In extremes of age
- Polytrauma
- Significant co-morbid disorder
- If surgical management indicated (deep partial thickness, full thickness burns)
- Electrical burns

Other factors to consider include the presence of inhalational injury, adequate pain relief, home circumstances, nutritional requirement and continuity of care of the patient at home or in primary setting. If in doubt of adequate access to the necessary meticulous burn care, the burn patient should be referred to burns center. Because burn wound evolves over several days, it should be re-evaluated within 3 to 5 days [12,69]. Evaluation should confirm that the burn wound is healing, and no risk of joint contracture or infection. Even small area burn that take more than 14 days to heal need to be referred to specialized center [68]. Although it is possible to successfully treat the majority of partial thickness burns in the general hospital or community setting, full thickness burns should always be referred [70]. It is also advisable to refer to specialized burns center if the primary physician anticipates a potential need for physical or occupational therapy for their burn patient. Any failure to foresee such need is detrimental to the patient's recovery.

EARLY BURN MANAGEMENT IN HOSPITAL

Annually in the United Kingdom, around 175000 people attend emergency departments with burns from various causes [3]. Of patients referred to the hospital, some 16000 are admitted, and about 1000 patients need active fluid resuscitation [68,71]. The number of burn related deaths average 300 a year [68]. All major burns should be managed initially according to the guidelines of the American College of Surgeons Committee on Trauma and the Advanced Trauma Life Support (ATLS) manual [72-74]. The survival data analysis from 1665 burns patients from the Massachusetts General Hospital identified three risk factors for death: age over 60 years, more than 40% total body surface area (TBSA) burn, and inhalation injury [75]. Table 3 outlines the principles of emergency burn care as outlined in Emergency Management of Severe Burns (EMSB) course [69,72].

Table 3. Emergency management of severe burns (EMSB)

Airway	• Humidified oxygen (O_2) at 8L/min (40%) ± Bronchodilators
	• 100% O_2 supplement if suspecting CO poisoning (COHb ≥15% or altered level of consciousness suspicious of CO poisoning). If a patient has an isolated burn injury that is small and when no inhalation injury is suspected O_2 may not be necessary
	• Arterial blood gas (ABG) and other bloods (as indicated)
	• Intubation as indicated
Burn assessment	• TBSA
	• Depth
Circulation and resuscitation	• Parkland formula 4ml/kg/%TBSA burn (first ½ in the first 8 h from the time of incident and second ½ in the next 16 h) if large burn (≥15% TBSA adult, ≥10% TBSA child)
	• Holliday-Segar formula for maintenance fluid (4ml/kg/h for the first 10kg, 2ml/kg/h for the second 10kg, 1ml/kg/h for subsequent kg of body weight) in children
	• Two 16G IV cannulas but the cannulation itself should not unnecessarily delay the transfer time. This should be limited to two attempts only
	• Ideally warm resuscitation fluid used
	• Urinary catheterisation if ≥20% TBSA adult and ≥15% TBSA children. Urine output maintain ≥0.5ml/kg/h for adult, ≥1.0ml/kg/h if child >1 year old or <30kg, and ≥2.0ml/kg/h if <1 year old
	• Reassessment every 15-30 min
	• Fluid boluses of 5-10ml/kg in 15-20 min and/or increase the next hour fluids to 150% of calculated volume if necessary
Dire or emergency surgical procedure	• Escharotomy
	• Fasciotomy

A) Assessment and parallel management of immediately life-threatening injuries

Approximately 10% of all burns present with concomitant trauma [76]. These should be suspected, diagnosed, and managed following the guidelines of ATLS [73]. An important point to note is that in the emergency situation, attending surgeon should institute the steps in ATLS in parallel, often with the assistance of other medical personnel.

I) Airway

I. Inhalation injury

Inhalation injury is the most frequent cause of death in burns patients [77,78]. It is a greater contributor to overall morbidity or mortality than either percentage of body surface area affected or age. It has been reported recently that the presence of inhalation injury increased burn mortality by 20% [77]. Children and the elderly are especially vulnerable due to their limited physiologic reserve. Aggressive diagnosis and early prophylactic intubation can be life saving. All patients with facial burn or burn in an enclosed space should be assessed by an anesthetist, and the need for early intubation ascertained before transfer to a specialized burn center [79].

The clinical diagnosis of inhalation injury has traditionally rested upon high index of clinical suspicions, and a group of clinical observations [80]. The clinical warning signs observed include facial burns, singed nasal vibrissae, and a history of burn in enclosed space. Other tell-tale signs which should not be overlooked are changes in voice quality, hoarse brassy cough, croup-like breathing, productive cough with or without carbonaceous sputum (sputum containing soot), inspiratory stridor, and respiratory difficulty with flaring of alar nasae, tracheal tug and rib retraction [80-82]. Hypoxia, rales, rhonchi and wheezes are seldom present on admission, occurring only in those with the most severe injury and implying an extremely poor prognosis [83].

Chest radiograph taken on admission for the diagnosis of inhalation injury is generally of little value in immediate burn assessment [84]. It does however, provide a good baseline investigation for evaluation of progress as almost two-thirds of patients with inhalation injury develop focal or diffuse infiltrates or pulmonary edema within 5–10 days of injury [84]. Fiberoptic bronchoscopy is the current standard in diagnosing inhalation injury [81, 82]. It identifies upper airway injury through observation of soot, charring, mucosal necrosis and airway edema. A positive or negative finding on upper airway injury however, does not reflect on the possibility of lung parenchymal injury [82,85]. To evaluate lung parenchyma damage, Xenon scanning has been utilized to demonstrate areas of the decreased alveolar gas washout, which identifies sites of small airway obstruction caused by edema or fibrin cast formation [86].

Acute upper airway or supraglottic injury occurs in approximately ⅕ to ⅓ of hospitalized burn patients with inhalation injury and is a major hazard because of the possibility of rapid progression from mild pharyngeal edema to complete upper airway obstruction [87]. It is usually the clinical consequence of direct thermal insult to the upper airway as well as chemical irritation, especially during the first 12 h of injury [69]. The worsening of upper airway obstruction is marked by supraglottic structures edema with obliteration of the aryepiglotic folds, arytenoid eminences, and interarytenoid areas, which prolapse to occlude the airway [88]. Whenever a supraglottic injury is suspected, the most experienced anesthetist in airway management should perform endotracheal intubation. Securing the endotracheal tube can become increasingly difficult if not carried out immediately due to the rapid swelling that occurs within the next 72 h [89]. Acute upper airway obstruction is also exacerbated by systemic capillary leak, bronchospasm from aerosolized irritants, and decreased lung and chest wall compliances due to swelling or burn to the chest wall [90-94]. Although upper airway edema usually resolves in 2 to 3 days, it can continue to worsen and patient intubated for supraglottic injury should be monitored closely. Extreme care should continue be taken if these patients are extubated over the next 48 to 72 hours [79].

The pathophysiologic changes in the parenchyma of the lungs that are associated with inhalation injury are not the result of direct thermal injury. The damage to lung parenchyma or infraglottic injury is caused by the incomplete products of combustion which causes lower airways chemical tracheobronchitis and bronchospasms [95]. The small airway becomes occluded with sloughed from endobronchial debris and loss of ciliary clearance mechanism. Occluded segments of the lung causes increased intrapulmonary dead space and difficulty in gaseous exchange from intrapulmonary shunting, and interstitial and alveolar flooding. This predisposes the patient to serious infection of the already denuded tracheobronchial tree and poorly compliant pulmonary parenchyma over the next few days of admission [90-94].

Many toxic gases in house or industrial fire are hazardous to the lung parenchyma, in particular, the aldehydes and oxides of sulphur and nitrogen [96, 97]. The sulfates, phosphates, and chlorides derivatives are acidic and induce rapid pulmonary edema, as well as systemic acidosis. Burning polyvinylchloride (PVC's) yields at least 75 potentially toxic compounds, including hydrochloric acid and carbon monoxide [98]. Patients with pre-existing reactive airway diseases are particularly vulnerable to irritative gaseous exposure.

The treatment for inhalation injury demands vigorous pulmonary toilet and ventilatory support to limit rapid lung deterioration. Airway clearance techniques are an essential component of respiratory management of patients with inhalation injury and it demands the involvement of respiratory therapists, nurses and physicians who play a central role in its clinical management [99]. Bronchial hygiene therapy employs several modalities such as therapeutic coughing, chest physiotherapy, early ambulation, airway suctioning, therapeutic bronchoscopy and pharmacologic agents to achieve adequate respiratory clearance [100-107].

Among the pharmaceuticals employed are bronchodilators and mucolytics. Bronchodilators have been employed with good outcome in many cases [108,109]. Most of them act on the biochemical mechanism, which controls bronchial muscle tone. Aerosolized sympathomimetics are effective in relaxing bronchial muscle tone and stimulating mucociliary clearance. Racemic epinephrine is used as an aerosolized topical vasoconstrictor, bronchodilator, and secretion bond breaker [100]. Beta antagonists such as salbutamol may assist with exacerbation of reactive airway disease, which is very common due to the inhalation of toxins and particulate debris [109]. Water, employed as a diluent for racemic epinephrine, lowers both the adhesive and cohesive forces of the retained endobronchial secretions, thus serving as a bond-breaking vehicle [100].

II. Carbon monoxide poisoning

Combustion of carbon in an oxygen-deficient environment results in the production of carbon monoxide [98,110]. Carbon monoxide is an invisible and odourless gas with nearly 200 times greater affinity for haemoglobin than oxygen. It competes with oxygen binding sites on the haemoglobin to form carboxyhemoglobin (COHb) and thus, reduces haemoglobin oxygen carrying capacity. The deprivation of oxygen at the tissue level is made worse by a concomitant leftward shift of the oxyhemoglobin dissociation curve. Because of its high affinity for haemoglobin, only a minimum level of carbon monoxide present in fires in enclosed space can cause significant carbon monoxide poisoning. Clinical findings of headache, nausea, and behavioral disturbances occur only at COHb level above 30% [95]. The pathognomonic cherry red skin discoloration is unreliable as a sign of carbon monoxide poisoning as it only occurs at COHb level above 40% [95]. Carbon monoxide poisoning can be evaluated by measurement of serum COHb [95]. The level however, is a poor indicator of poisoning since most burn patients are placed on 100% oxygen (O_2) on scene and upon arrival to emergency department [111]. The time from injury to measurement is very important because it takes 4-5 h for levels to fall by ½ while patients breathe room air, and less than 1 h on 100% O_2 [95]. Clark et. al. has developed a nomogram to estimate the original level of COHb at the time of extrication from the fire, based both on time from extrication and O_2 concentration delivered between time of extrication and time to first blood gas [111].

Normal COHb levels are generally <3% but can rise to 10-15% in heavy smokers. Levels <10% are generally not considered harmful to a healthy person but can be deleterious in those with cardiovascular disease. As levels increase to >15%, symptoms such as headache and lethargy become common. At ≥30%, these symptoms are supervened by dizziness, nausea, and impaired vision, and unconsciousness develops at levels between 40% and 50%. Carbon monoxide poisoning at ≥60% is frequently associated with death.

Carbon monoxide can dissociate from hemoglobin, with the speed of dissociation determined by arterial oxygen content. Carboxyhemoglobin has a half-life of approximately 5 h in room air, reduced to 1 h in 100% O_2, and further reduced at hyperbaric levels of O_2 at 3 atmospheres to approximately ½ h [95,112]. Therefore, all suspected or significant exposure to carbon monoxide should be treated with administration of 100% O_2 continued for several half-lives, either by facemask or by following endotracheal intubation.

The use of hyperbaric O_2 in the treatment of carbon monoxide poisoning is controversial [112,113]. Physiologically, the rationale is clear as the half-life of COHb is reduced by almost 90% at 3 atmospheres compared with room air but a recent meta-analysis failed to support the use of hyperbaric O_2 therapy as a beneficial standard practice [114]. When considered against the backdrop of transferring a critically ill patient to a poorly accessible hyperbaric oxygen chamber and without a clear benefit of treatment, it is hard to justify its usage in common practice.

II) Burn assessment

Burn should be gently cleaned and debrided on initial assessment to determine its depth. The European working party of burn specialists recommended cleaning burn with soap and water or disinfectant to remove loose skin, including open blisters [115]. The raised epidermis of bullae should be removed or deroofed, followed by excision of sloughed tissue. All blisters should be deroofed apart from the isolated lax blisters of <1 cm^2 [116]. Although the clinical evidence for 'deroofing' of blisters is poor, without 'deroofing' burn depth cannot be adequately examined.

I. Burn size

Burn size assessment is an important exercise during early burn management as it determines the amount of fluid, which the burn patient requires. There are a few commonly accepted methods to estimate the percentage of TBSA burn, with some more practical than others in their use in emergency department or specialized burns center. The initial assessment of burn size should be performed with a standardized Lund and Browder chart (Figure 1) [117]. It takes into account changes in body surface area with age and growth, therefore making it very useful across all age groups. It also has good interobserver agreement. Whilst Lund and Browder chart gives more accurate TBSA burn estimation, its use in pre-hospital setting is uncommon and they are not, therefore, as widely used in non-specialized center. The simpler Wallace's rule of nines is helpful for rapid assessment but less accurate (Figure 2) [117]. It tends to overestimate the percentage of TBSA burn by about 3%. It is taken to be the current standard technique for assessing burn area in pre-hospital setting, and hence the tool that most management decisions are based on.

Another method of burn assessment is based on the palm being taken as a gauge of 1% TBSA. But studies of body surface area have shown that the adult palm with fingers corresponds to 0.8% of TBSA in adults and 1% in children [118]. This method is useful for estimating small burns (<15%) or large burns (>85%). In very large burns, the burnt area can also be quickly calculated by estimating the area of uninjured skin and subtracting it from 100 [119].

More recently, a serial halving method has been described [120]. This latter technique is effective in burn size estimation in pre-hospital assessment due to its rapidity and ease of use. The approach is based on serial halves of >50%, <50%, 25–50%, or <25% [120]. When compared with rule of nines, it allows management decisions to be made that are equivalent to those that would have been made using the rule of nines. This is particularly valuable in pre-hospital assessment, where a key end point is appropriate disposal to further care. However, it is advocated that the serial halving method only be used as an initial assessment tool or with conjunction with other existing methods.

II. Burn depth

Quantifying the depth of burn is an important initial step in the treatment of burn as the attending surgeon weighs on the decision for resuscitation, transfer, and surgical debridement [121]. A common mistake in burn depth assessment in the inexperienced is inclusion of erythema. Only de-epithelialized area should be included in burn assessment calculation. Although it is ideal to assess burn depth accurately in emergency situation, the distinction between superficial and deep partial dermal burns is not always precise and burn wound may not be homogeneous with respect to depth. Clinical estimation of burn depth is often a subjective process with independent blinded comparison among experienced surgeons showed only 60-80% concurrence [122]. Fortunately, a detailed formal depth assessment is not necessary for partial thickness burn, as the distinction between superficial and deep partial thickness dermal burns is based largely on their healing times. Under normal circumstances, superficial partial thickness dermal burns do not require surgery and heal within 10–14 days by epithelialisation without scarring [115, 123]. Deep partial and full thickness dermal burns take longer to heal and are likely to scar. Deep partial thickness dermal burn requires excision and skin grafting. A retrospective cohort study by Cubison et. al. examined 337 children with up to a five year follow-up found hypertrophic scarring occurred in less than 20% of superficial scalds that healed within 21 days but in up to 90% of burns that took 30 days or more to heal [123]. In order to achieve good aesthetic outcomes, all partial thickness dermal burns that have not healed by 10-14 days should be referred to a specialized burns center [115].

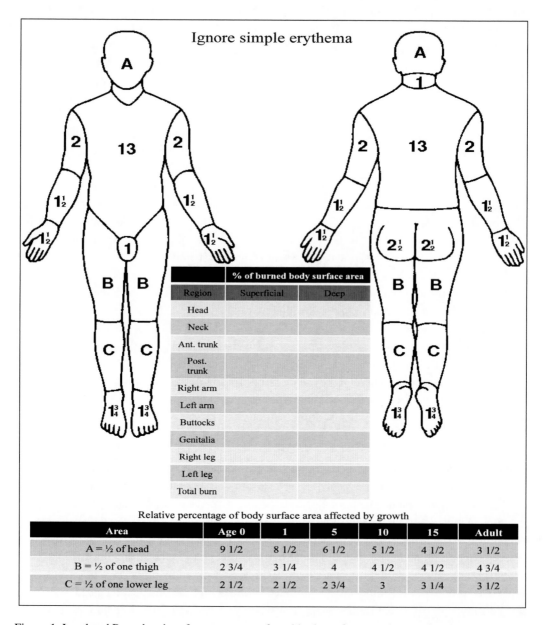

	% of burned body surface area	
Region	Superficial	Deep
Head		
Neck		
Ant. trunk		
Post. trunk		
Right arm		
Left arm		
Buttocks		
Genitalia		
Right leg		
Left leg		
Total burn		

Relative percentage of body surface area affected by growth

Area	Age 0	1	5	10	15	Adult
A = ½ of head	9 1/2	8 1/2	6 1/2	5 1/2	4 1/2	3 1/2
B = ½ of one thigh	2 3/4	3 1/4	4	4 1/2	4 1/2	4 3/4
C = ½ of one lower leg	2 1/2	2 1/2	2 3/4	3	3 1/4	3 1/2

Figure 1. Lund and Browder chart for percentage of total body surface area burn estimation.

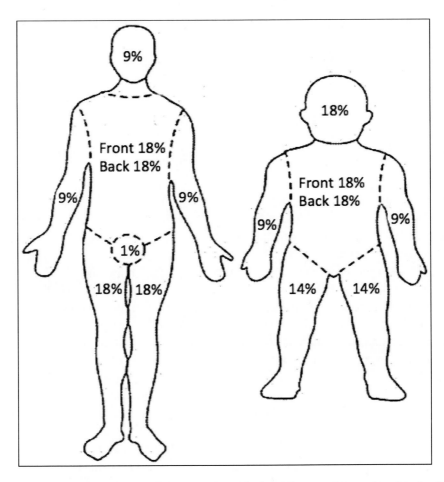

Figure 2. Wallace's rule of nines for percentage of total body surface area burn estimation. In children, the head and neck account for 18% and lower limbs 14% each. Note that for every year above one year old, the head decreases by about 1% and each lower limb gain about 0.5%. The adult proportion will be attained at 10 years old.

In superficial partial thickness dermal burns, the layer of necrosis occupies only the upper (papillary) dermis, with normal underlying reticular dermis. Clinically, such burns are pink or red, may have blistering, are painful, and have a good blood supply. These are usually managed conservatively without excision and grafting. In contrast, in deep partial thickness dermal burns, the layer of necrosis extends into the reticular dermis, with the zone of stasis extending deep into the dermis. Clinically, these burns tend to be less red with poor blood flow. Table 4 summarizes the key characteristic of various burn depth appearances as outlines in EMSB course [69]. It is important to be aware that burn wounds are dynamic and need reassessment in the first 24-72 hours because the depth can increase especially if inadequately treated or infected [69]. There have been various methods described to improve the accuracy of burn depth assessment but the high outlay costs for these equipments preclude their use outside specialized burns centers [122, 124, 125].

Table 4. The key clinical characteristics that distinguish different level of burn depth

Depth of burn	Color	Blisters	Capillary refill	Sensation	Healing
Superficial	Red	No	Present	Present	Yes
Superficial partial thickness dermal	Pale pink	Small	Present	Painful	Yes
Deep partial thickness dermal	Dark pink or blotchy red	+ / −	Absent	Absent	No
Full thickness dermal	White	No	Absent	Absent	No

III) Circulation and resuscitation

Thermal burn injuries pose a significant local and systemic insult. The presence of burn is associated with significant fluid loss due to the damage and loss of protective keratin layer of the skin and their systemic reactive changes. Effective fluid resuscitation remains the cornerstone of management in major burns. It is widely accepted that one of the principal factors responsible for the reduction in mortality from acute burn is the introduction of fluid resuscitation. In the UK, expert consensus recommends that fluid resuscitation be initiated in all children with ≥10% TBSA burns and in adults with ≥15% TBSA burns (Table 3) [14 78]. Fluid replacement should also be started on scene for burn >25% TBSA and/or if time to hospital is more than one hour from the time of injury. Children who had fluid resuscitation within 2 h had a lower incidence of sepsis, renal failure, and overall mortality [14, 69].

Over the years, several formulas based on body weight and area burnt, estimate volume requirements for the first 24 h. Although none is ideal, the Parkland formula and its variations are the most commonly used (Table 3) [126]. The aims are to maintain vital organ perfusion and tissue perfusion to the zone of stasis to prevent extension of tissue necrosis. Although multiple studies have reported the inadequacy of standard fluid resuscitation formula, with needs routinely exceeding the calculated requirements, this is likely due to variations in body mass index, accuracy of the calculated size of burn, and differences in mechanical ventilation [127-129]. It may also be that none of the present protocols are ideal because simply that different protocol suit different patient in different situation.

The preferred resuscitation fluid varies greatly. This is reflected by the evolving protocols for resuscitation from the plasma infusions of the 1940s to crystalloid resuscitation using the Parkland formula-guided Hartmann's infusion today [130-132]. There is no robust scientific evidence to support the adoption of one particular protocol over the others. Many believe that resuscitation fluids should be isotonic for the first 24 h, and then colloid added after 24 h, when capillary integrity returns [126, 133, 134]. Although in theory, the addition of colloids in burn resuscitation may decrease total volume requirement, randomized controlled trials are still needed to evaluate its full benefits [135]. A recent Cochrane meta-analysis of 65 randomized controlled trials of trauma, burns, and post-surgery patients found no evidence that colloid resuscitation reduces mortality more effectively than crystalloids [136]. Currently, the most popular type of fluid is crystalloid Hartmann's solution, which effectively treats hypovolemia and extracellular sodium deficits [126, 133]. Many burn centers continue to add colloid after the first 12 h for large burns [137]. Sodium chloride solution (0.9%) should be avoided because it causes hyperchloremic metabolic acidosis [138]. A recent survey of burns centers in USA and Canada revealed that 78% of centers used the Parkland formula to estimate resuscitation fluid volumes and that Ringer's lactate (similar to Hartmann's solution) was the most popular type of fluid used [133]. In UK and Ireland, the estimated resuscitation volumes were also calculated using the Parkland formula in 76% of units, and Hartmann's solution remained the most widely used [126]. Minor burns (<15-20% TBSA) need 150% of normal maintenance intravenous fluids [139-141]. Approximately half of the centers did not routinely change the type of intravenous fluid administered after the initial period of resuscitation [126]. Resuscitations were discontinued after 24 h in 35% of centers and after 36 h in 30% of centers [126].

Resuscitation starts from the time of injury, and thus any delay in presentation or transfer to the hospital or specialized burns center should be taken into account, and fluid infusion rate calculated accordingly. The goal of resuscitation is to achieve enough volume to ensure end organ perfusion while avoiding intra-compartmental edema and joint stiffness. Care should also be taken not to over-infuse small, frail, elderly patients with a history of cardiac failure. Resuscitation formulas are only guidelines, and the volume must be titrated against monitored physiological parameters such as urine output, lactate, base excess, peripheral temperature, blood pressure, and heart rate [142, 143]. In UK, it is recommended that adults with burn >20% TBSA and >15% TBSA in children requires burn resuscitation monitored with urinary catheter for adequate urine output (Table 3) [69]. Patients with pre-existing conditions that may affect the correlation between volume and urine output require invasive monitoring for circulatory end points such as mean arterial blood pressure, central venous pressure, and if a pulmonary artery catheter is placed, pulmonary artery wedge pressure [128, 142, 143]. Central venous pressure or pulmonary capillary wedge pressure should be considered in patients with known myocardial dysfunction, age greater than 65 years, severe inhalation injury, or fluid requirements greater than 150% of that predicted by the Parkland formula [140].

IV) Dire or emergency surgical procedure

Any deep partial thickness or full thickness dermal burns that encompass or almost encompass a region of the body can form a tight tourniquet as a result of eschar formation which limits tissue elasticity and excursion [69]. On initial examination, there may be no signs of compromise, but with the development of edema from the burn injury and fluid resuscitation, problems will eventually be compounded through the combination of external splintage and internal structural compression. As edema in the region continues to worsen, this tourniquet effect is enhanced. In the extremities, it will deprive the limbs of blood supply by the circumferential banding of eschar. Any burns involving extremities must be checked for circumferential burn and compartment syndrome [69]. The release of a restricting eschar and sometimes, fasciotomy will improve perfusion of distal extremity.

As the resuscitation continues, chest and abdominal walls may also become edematous. This causes constriction to the trunk by the existing eschars, which makes ventilation more difficult especially in patients with an already compromised, direct pulmonary injury. Ventilation insufficiency is due to the presence of burn eschar on the chest, forming a tight cuirass that restricts movement of the chest wall. These truncal constrictions require rapid and complete escharotomies to allow the underlying viable tissue to springs through the eschar and facilitate respiratory excursion. Often, circumferential burn of the neck, especially in children, can worsen respiratory embarrassment due to unyielding eschar that externally compresses and obstructs the airway. Escharotomy to the neck will be helpful in reducing the tight collar eschar and therefore, decrease the pressure exerted on the trachea. The elevated intra-abdominal pressure reduces the excursion of the diaphragm causing diminished functional reserve capacity of the lung. Raised abdominal compartment syndrome also has a negative impact on splanchnic, renal, and limb perfusion.

Theoretically, escharotomy should be a painless procedure, requiring no anaesthesia. However, it is rare for a burn to be full thickness in its entirety without areas of partial thickness loss that are exquisitely painful. Escharotomy bleed profusely and therefore, need to be performed in a monitored environment equipped with electrocautery and conscious sedation [76]. For this reason, it is good practice to infiltrate the proposed line of incision with a solution of 0.5% lidocaine with 1:200,000 epinephrine (maximum dose of 7 mg/kg), leaving it for at least 10 min before incising. The addition of hyalase (1500 iU per 50 ml) to the solution will improve penetration of the eschar. The incision should extend into normal tissue in both extent and depth, with the healthy tissue bulging through the release, forcing the eschar apart. Fasciotomy may also need to be undertaken in patients with deep burn, or those caused by high voltage current.

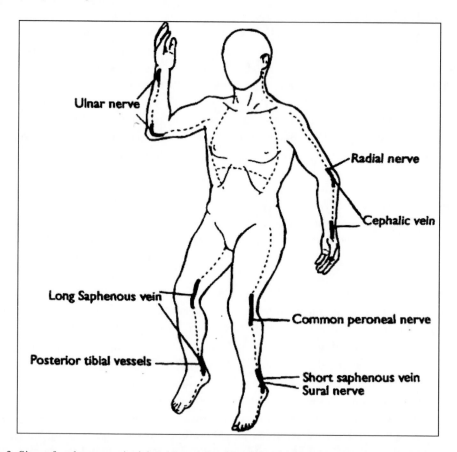

Figure 3. Sites of escharotomy incision (dotted lines) with particular attention over areas where vital nerves and vessels (thick lines) are adjacent to the site of incisions.

Fasciotomy for release of edematous muscle should be performed in controlled environment such as in operating room to allow for appropriate visualization of the anatomy [76]. Although escharotomy may be needed to avert respiratory distress or vascular compromise of the limbs from constriction in full thickness circumferential burns involving the neck, chest, abdomen, or limbs, a proportion of patients will have no signs of any compromise to circulation or ventilation. In these cases, escharotomies should be performed prophylactically if they are to be transported any distance without ability for regular monitoring or to act on new onset clinical findings. In the limbs, prophylactic escharotomy was proven to be beneficial [100]. Whilst the value in the fingers is controversial, a controlled study demonstrated a statistically significant number of phalanges were salvaged in circumferentially burned fingers with early escharotomy [144].

Care should be taken in the placement of incisions for escharotomy to insure adequate release and to avoid damaging vital structures such as nerves and vessels. The concept and techniques for escharotomy and fasciotomy have been well described by Burd et. al. based on the fundamentals of decompression [145]. Figure 3 illustrates in brief, the position of escharotomy incisions as taught in EMSB course in UK [69].

B) Analgesia

The pain threshold temperature for skin is 42 °C [20]. Control of burn pain must begin upon initiation of medical care. As previously indicated, analgesia is best accomplished by cooling and covering the burned area [4]. Once intravenous access is gained and resuscitation started, intravenous opioids should be administered. Intravenous morphine is the first line of acute pain management in burns (Table 3). Its effect is immediate with peak analgesia at 10 min. The recommended intravenous dose for adult is 1–2 mg repeated every 3–5 min, and 20 mcg/kg repeated every 3–5 min in children above one year old [146]. The opioid dose occasionally exceeds the standard weight-based recommendations and is necessary to achieve adequate pain control. Intravenous opioids can be titrated to make the adult patient more comfortable and should be accompanied by an antiemetic. There is no evidence that opioid addiction occurs more often in burn patients than in other populations requiring opioids for acute pain (approximately 1 in 3000) [147]. Oral opioids can also be administered in adults if no intravenous access available. Entonox should only be used when these options are unavailable as it is difficult to administer, has varying efficacy, and decreases the oxygen delivery. It is typically self-administered by an awake, cooperative patient via a mouthpiece or face mask in a concentration of 50% nitrous oxide and 50% oxygen [148]. In children, intranasal diamorphine is another alternative option that may be considered [149, 150].

C) Antibiotic use

The use of systemic prophylaxis antibiotic in burn is controversial. In the acute setting, Ravat et. al., through their review recommended that systemic antibiotic prophylaxis could be used in patients needing invasive surgery but not in those for dressing changes. They recommended oxacillin or cloxacillin (30 mg/kg) or first generation cephalosporin (30 mg/kg) to target methicillin-sensitive Staphyllococcus. In case of allergy, clindamycin should be used (10 mg/kg) [151]. Another recent systematic review and meta-analysis by Avni et. al. reported that systemic antibiotic prophylaxis, given for 4 to 14 days after admission, cut all-cause in-hospital mortality by 46% [152]. But the authors cautioned that none of those findings are definitive as the overall methodological quality of the studies were poor. Other available data from adult, paediatric and mixed population studies had demonstrated that systemic antibiotic prophylaxis in burn patients has no role in the prevention of bacterial infections [153-160]. There has also been a paucity of evidence on the relevance of post-operative antibiotic use in the management of paediatric burn and with the lack of support of the role of prophylactic antibiotic in the surgical management of paediatric burn, there is diminishing role for peri-operative antibiotic use [153, 155, 156, 161-163]. Peri-operative antibiotic prophylaxis had not been shown to decrease the incidence of graft or donor site infection [164]. There has been significant evidence that antibiotic therapy prescribed to prevent infection of burned skin did not actually prevent it and even facilitated the emergence of multi-resistant bacteria [159]. It is likely that diffusion of antibiotic in the burned skin is questionable and cannot achieve bactericidal concentrations so that bacteria can grow and develop resistances. The compromise to skin barrier and the overgrowth of bacteria in the burn eschar leading to sepsis have led to a high rate of antibiotic resistance in common organisms.

On the other hand, early application of burn with topical antimicrobial has been shown to decrease the bacterial overgrowth and incidence of burn wound sepsis. Topical antimicrobials also keep the wound moist and control pain. Local burn wounds management with topical agents has a well documented efficiency in both preventing and treating burn infections [165]. Current treatment regimens include silver sulfadiazine, Bactroban, or Sulfamylon in conjunction with daily cleaning and debridement. Its use however, is no substitute for a timely surgical intervention. Without eventual surgery, the benefit of topical antimicrobial preparations on mortality is only minor on burns less than 40% TBSA [166].

Patients who show signs of sepsis should receive a complete work-up, with a special focus on the most commonly encountered bacteria in burn centers, including Staphylococcus aureus, enterococci and Pseudomonas aeruginosa [167, 168]. Diagnosis of infection in burn patients is not easy because clinical and biological infection criteria are poorly relevant, especially in larger burn patients. Clinical parameters such as hyperthermia, hyperleukocytosis and increased C-reactive proteins can be part of physiological reactions to large thermal insult. A major burn triggers a systemic inflammatory response syndrome (SIRS), which mimics usual clinical and biological signs of infection [169]. Children with significant burn can often have moderate fever in the absence of infection and in this circumstances, administration of broad-spectrum antibiotic is not appropriate and may ultimately worsen outcomes in previously uninfected children [162, 163]. On the other hand, there is also insufficient data to show judicious use of antibiotics in febrile paediatric victims being unacceptable. As long as the infection is not documented, antibiotic therapy is empiric. Therefore, broad-spectrum antibiotics should be chosen for maximum efficacy. In established burn wounds sepsis, targeted antibiotic usage is helpful to eradicate the bacteraemia or septicaemia, and reduces mortality rates [163].

TRANSFER

There are a number of published guidelines and requirements concerning the transport of the critically ill and injured [170, 171]. These should be used in devising local policies with the inclusion of specific requirements of burn patients as laid down in EMSB course [172]. Of primary importance is the need to avoid any delay in the transfer of someone with burn injury to a place of definitive care. All treatment should be carried out with the aim of reducing on scene times and delivering the patient to the appropriate treatment center. This should be the nearest appropriate emergency department, unless local protocols allow direct transfer to a specialized burns center. The use of retrieval teams and/or aeromedical transfer needs to be balanced in each case. Communication with the recipient hospital should give essential information only such as age, sex, incident time and mechanism, ABC problems, relevant treatment received and expected time of arrival [3, 173-177]. Important issues to also consider when transporting children with serious burn include maintenance of body temperature, fluid administration if transport time >1 h, accurate documentation, notification of family, and identification of the child's legal custodian. In some cases, the possibility of non-accidental injury should also be borne in one's mind. It is recommended by the National Burn Centre Response Committee (NBCRC) in UK that all complex burns referred for admission reach the specialized burns center within 6 h of injury across the British Isles and within 4 h of injury if referred from an urban site [3]. A failure to achieve these targets should be regarded as a critical incident and the reasons investigated.

CONCLUSION

Care to the burn victims by healthcare professionals begins on scene with first aid before arrival to the emergency department. Emergency burn management during transport and on arrival to hospital should follow guidelines as set up by Advanced Trauma Life Support (ATLS) and Emergency Management of Severe Burns (EMSB) to optimize patients' outcome. Criteria for referral and transfer for severely burn patients to specialized burns center should be adhered to allow satisfactory emergency care with its ancillary procedures. Many healthcare professionals continue to require continuous education to facilitate adequacy of their performance in caring for these patients. Awareness and emphasis of prompt first aid care to burns and their subsequent referral to specialized burns center should continue to be part of healthcare professionals continuous medical education in the general hospital and primary care setting. The ever-evolving field of emergency care for burns requires primary care physicians' active participation in providing first line service to the general public. The importance of adequate emergency burn care and contributions made by primary healthcare professionals in the management of burns cannot be overemphasized as they are vital gatekeepers to the outnumbered, specialized burns centers in the world.

REFERENCES

[1]   Facts about injuries: Burns. Accessed 2011 Jun 01. URL: http://www.who.int/violence_injury_ prevention/publications/other_injury/en/burns_factsheet

[2]   Miller SF, Bessey PQ, Schurr MJ, Browning SM, Jeng JC, Caruso DM, Gomez M, Latenser BA, Lentz CW, Saffle JR, et al. National Burn Repository 2005: A ten-year review. J Burn Care Res 2006;27:411-36.

[3]   National Burn Care Review Committee Report. Standards and Strategy for Burn Care 2001. Accessed 2011 Jun 01. URL: http://www.specialisedservices.nhs.uk

[4]   Allison K. The UK pre-hospital management of burn patients: current practice and the need for a standard approach. Burns 2002;28:135-42.

[5]   O'Neill AC, Purcell E, Jones D, Pasha N, McCann J, Regan P. Inadequacies in the first aid management of burns presenting to plastic surgery services. Ir Med J 2005;98:15-6.

[6]   Rea S, Kuthubutheen J, Fowler B, Wood F. Burn first aid in Western Australia--do healthcare workers have the knowledge? Burns 2005;31:1029-34.

[7]   Bezuhly M, Gomez M, Fish JS. Emergency department management of minor burn injuries in Ontario, Canada. Burns 2004;30:160-4.

[8]   Orgill DP. Excision and skin grafting of thermal burns. New Engl J Med 2009;360:893-901.

[9]   Moritz AR, Henriques FC. Studies of thermal injury: II. The relative importance of time and surface temperature in the causation of cutaneous burns. Am J Pathol 1947;23:695-720.

[10]   Jackson DM. The diagnosis of the depth of burning. Br J Surg 1953; 40:588-96.

[11]   Despa F, Orgill DP, Neuwalder J, Lee RC. The relative thermal stability of tissue macromolecules and cellular structure in burn injury. Burns 2005;31:568-77.

[12]   Kao CC, Garner WL. Acute Burns. Plastic Reconstruct Surg 2000;101:2482-93.

[13]   Kim DE, Phillips TM, Jeng JC, Rizzo AG, Roth RT, Stanford JL, et al. Microvascular assessment of burn depth conversion during varying resuscitation conditions. J Burn Care Rehabil 2001;22:406-16.

[14]   Barrow RE, Jeschke MG, Herndon DN. Early fluid resuscitation improves outcomes in severely burned children. Resuscitation 2000;45:91-6.

[15]   Ward PA, Till GO. Pathophysiologic events related to thermal injury of skin. J Trauma 1990;30:S75-9.

[16]   Schwacha MG. Macrophages and post-burn immune dysfunction. Burns 2003;29:1-14.

[17]   Youn YK, LaLonde C, Demling R. The role of mediators in the response to thermal injury. World Journal Surg 1992;16:30-6.

[18]   Demling RH, Niehaus G, Perea A, Will JA. Effect of burn-induced hypoproteinemia on pulmonary transvascular fluid filtration rate. Surgery 1979; 85:339-43.

[19]   Yu YM, Tompkins RG, Ryan CM, Young VR. The metabolic basis of the increase of the increase in energy expenditure in severely burned patients. J Parenteral Enteral Nutr 1999;23:160-8.

[20]   Walker A, Baumber R, Robson B. Pre-hospital management of burns by the UK fire service. Emerg Med J 2005;22:205-8.

[21]   Esmarch F. First aid to the injured. Five ambulance lectures, 1st ed. London: Smith Elder, 1882.

[22]   Pearn J. The earliest days of first aid. BMJ 1994;309:1718-20.

[23]   Majno G. The healing hand: Man and wound in the ancient world, 1st ed. Cambridge, MA: Harvard University Press, 1991.

[24]   First Aid. Manual of St John Ambulance Association, 8th rev ed. London Dorling Kindersley, 2006.

[25]   Ofeigsson OJ. Water cooling: First-aid treatment for scalds and burns. Surgery 1965;57:391-400.

[26]   Rose H. Initial cold water treatment for burns. Northwest Med 1936;35:267-70.

[27]   Brown CR, Price PB, Reynolds LE. Effects of local chilling in the treatment of burns. Surg Forum 1956;6:85-7.

[28]   King TC, Zimmerman JM, Price PB. Effect of immediate short-term cooling on extensive burns. Surg Forum 1962;13:487-8.

[29]   King TC, Price PB. Surface cooling following extensive burns. JAMA 1963;183:677-8.

[30]   Poy NG, Williams HB, Woolhouse FM. The alteration of mortality rates in burned rats using early excision, homografting and hypothermia, alone and in Combination. Plastic Reconstruct Surg 1965;35:198-206.

[31]   Shulman AG. Ice water as primary treatment of burns. Simple method of emergency treatment of burns to alleviate pain, reduce sequelae, and hasten healing. JAMA 1960;173:1916-9.

[32]   Ofeigsson O. Observations and experiments on the immediate cold-water treatment for burns and scalds. Br J Plast Surg 1959;12:104-19.

[33]   Venter TH, Karpelowsky JS, Rode H. Cooling of the burn wound: The ideal temperature of the coolant. Burns 2007;33:917-22.

[34]   Cuttle L, Kempf M, Kravchuk O, Phillips GE, Mill J, Wang XQ, Kimble RM. The optimal temperature of first aid treatment for partial thickness burn injuries. Wound Repair Regeneration 2008, 16:626-634.

[35]   Cuttle L, Kempf M, Liu PY, Kravchuk O, Kimble RM. The optimal duration and delay of first aid treatment for deep partial thickness burn injuries. Burns 2010;36:673-9.

[36] Zimmerman TJ. Thermally induced dermal injury: a review of pathophysiologic events and therapeutic intervention. J Burn Care Rehabil 1984; 5:193-201.

[37] Blocker TGJr, Eade GG, Lewis SR, Jacobson HS, Grant DA, Bennett JE. Evaluation of a semi-open method in the management of severe burns after the acute phase. Tex Med 1960;56:402-8.

[38] Iung OS, Wade FV. The treatment of burns with ice water, phisohex, and partial hypothermia. Industr Med Surg 1963; 32:365-70.

[39] Sawada Y, Urushidate S, Yotsuyanagi T, Ishita K. Is prolonged and excessive cooling of a scalded wound effective? Burns 1997;23:55-8.

[40] Ofeigsson OJ. First-aid treatment of scalds and burns by water cooling. Postgrad Med 1961;30:330-8.

[41] Cantlie J: First aid to the injured. London: St John Ambulance Assoc, 1901.

[42] Mason C. A complete handbook for the sanitary troops of the US Army and Navy and National Guard and Naval Militia, 4th ed. New York: William Wood, 1918.

[43] Martin J. Ambulance lectures, 1st ed. London: JA Churchill, 1886.

[44] Shepherd P. First aid to the injured. London: St John Ambulance Assoc, 1899.

[45] Maenthaisong R, Chaiyakunapruk N, Niruntraporn S, Kongkaew C. The efficacy of aloe vera used for burn wound healing: A systematic review. Burns 2007; 33:713-8.

[46] Chithra P, Sajithlal GB, Chandrakasan G: Influence of aloe vera on collagen turnover in healing of dermal wounds in rats. Indian J Exp Biol 1998;36:896-901.

[47] Chithra P, Sajithlal GB, Chandrakasan G. Influence of aloe vera on collagen characteristics in healing dermal wounds in rats. Mol Cell Biochem 1998;181:71-6.

[48] Chithra P, Sajithlal GB, Chandrakasan G. Influence of aloe vera on the healing of dermal wounds in diabetic rats. J Ethnopharmacol 1998;59:195-201.

[49] Duansak D, Somboonwong J, Patumraj S. Effects of aloe vera on leukocyte adhesion and TNF-alpha and IL-6 levels in burn wounded rats. Clin Hemorheol Microcirc 2003; 29:239-46.

[50] Jandera V, Hudson DA, de Wet PM, Innes PM, Rode H. Cooling the burn wound: evaluation of different modalites. Burns 2000;26:265-70.

[51] Cuttle L, Kempf M, Kravchuk O, George N, Liu PY, Chang HE, Mill J, Wang XQ, Kimble RM. The efficacy of aloe vera, tea tree oil and saliva as first aid treatment for partial thickness burn injuries. Burns 2008;34:1176-82.

[52] Brand C, Ferrante A, Prager RH, Riley TV, Carson CF, Finlay-Jones JJ, Hart PH. The water-soluble components of the essential oil of Melaleuca alternifolia (tea tree oil) suppress the production of superoxide by human monocytes, but not neutrophils, activated in vitro. Inflamm Res 2001;50:213-9.

[53] Caldefie-Chezet F, Guerry M, Chalchat JC, Fusillier C, Vasson MP, Guillot J. Anti-inflammatory effects of Melaleuca alternifolia essential oil on human polymorphonuclear neutrophils and monocytes. Free Radic Res2004;38:805-11.

[54] Koh KJ, Pearce AL, Marshman G, Finlay-Jones JJ, Hart PH. Tea tree oil reduces histamine-induced skin inflammation. Br J Dermatol 2002;147:1212-7.

[55] Cavanagh HM, Wilkinson JM. Biological activities of lavender essential oil. Phytother Res 2002;16:301-8.

[56] Dursun N, Liman N, Ozyazgan I, Gunes I, Saraymen R. Role of thymus oil in burn wound healing. J Burn Care Rehabil 2003;24:395-9.

[57] Dammak I, Boudaya S, Abdallah FB, Hamida T, Attia H. Date seed oil inhibits hydrogen peroxide-induced oxidative stress in normal human epidermal melanocytes. Connect Tissue Res 2009;50:330-5.

[58] Dammak I, Abdallah FB, Boudaya S, Besbes S, Keskes L, El Gaied A, Turki H, Attia H, Hentati B. Date seed oil limit oxidative injuries induced by hydrogen peroxide in human skin organ culture. BioFactors 2007;29:137-45.

[59] Ghelardini C, Galeotti N, Salvatore G, Mazzanti G. Local anaesthetic activity of the essential oil of Lavandula angustifolia. Planta Med 1999;65:700-3.

[60] Karaman S, Digrak M, Ravid U, Ilcim A. Antibacterial and antifungal activity of the essential oils of Thymus revolutus Celak from Turkey. J Ethnopharmacol 2001;76:183-6.

[61] Shepherd P. First aid to the injured: A pocket aide-memoire (compiled for the instruction of the troops in Zululand). London: St John Ambulance Assoc, 1879.

[62] Johnson D, Coleman DJ. Ink used as first aid treatment of a scald. Burns 2000;26:507-8.

[63]   Tse T, Poon CH, Tse KH, Tsui TK, Ayyappan T, Burd A. Paediatric burn prevention: an epidemiological approach. Burns 2006;32:229-34.

[64]   Rea S, Wood F. Minor burn injuries in adults presenting to the regional burns unit in Western Australia: a prospective descriptive study. Burns 2005;31:1035-40.

[65]   Rawlins JM, Khan AA, Shenton AF, Sharpe DT. Epidemiology and outcome analysis of 208 children with burns attending an emergency department. Pediatr Emerg Care 2007;23:289-93.

[66]   Chipp E, Walton J, Gorman DF, Moiemen NS. A 1 year study of burn injuries in a British Emergency Department. Burns 2008;34:516-20.

[67]   Forjuoh SN, Guyer B, Smith GS. Childhood burns in Ghana: epidemiological characteristics and home-based treatment. Burns 1995;21:24-8.

[68]   National Burn Care Review Report Appendix 2: National Burn Injury Referral Guidelines. Accessed Jun 01. URL: http://www.britishburnassociation.org/referral

[69]   Emergency management of severe burns course manual, UK version. Manchester: Wythenshawe Hospital, British Burn Assoc, 2008.

[70]   Johnson RM, Richard R. Partial-thickness burns: identification and management. Adv Skin Wound Care 2003;16:178-88.

[71]   Wilkinson E. The epidemiology of burns in secondary care, in a population of 2.6 million people. Burns 1998;24:139-43.

[72]   Emergency management of severe burns course manual. Sydney, Australian and New Zealand Burn Association (ANZBA), 1996.

[73]   Advanced trauma life support for doctors (ATLS). Chicago, IL: Am Coll Surgeons, 1997.

[74]   American College of Surgeons Committee on Trauma: Resources of Optimal Care of the Injured Patient. Chicago, IL: Am Coll Surgeons, 1993.

[75]   Ryan CM, Schoenfeld DA, Thorpe WP, Sheridan RL, Cassem EH, Tompkins RG. Objective estimates of the probability of death from burn injuries. N Engl JMed 1998;338:362-6.

[76]   Wong L, Spence RJ. Escharotomy and fasciotomy of the burned upper extremity. Hand Clin 2000;16:165-174.

[77]   Smith DL, Cairns BA, Ramadan F, Dalston JS, Fakhry SM, Rutledge R, Meyer AA, Peterson HD. Effect of inhalation injury, burn size, and age on mortality: a study of 1447 consecutive burn patients. J Trauma 1994;37:655-9.

[78]   Thompson PB, Herndon DN, Traber DL, Abston S. Effect on mortality of inhalation injury. J Trauma 1986;26:163-5.

[79]   Rabinowitz PM, Siegel MD. Acute inhalation injury. Clin Chest Med 2002;23:707-15.

[80]   Moylan JA, Chan CK. Inhalation injury--an increasing problem. Ann Surg 1978;188:34-7.

[81]   Wanner A, Cutchavaree A. Early recognition of upper airway obstruction following smoke inhalation. Am Rev Respir Dis 1973;108:1421-3.

[82]   Moylan JA, Adib K, Birnbaum M. Fiberoptic bronchoscopy following thermal injury. Surg Gynecol Obstet 1975;140:541-3.

[83]   Stone HH, Martin JD, Jr. Pulmonary injury associated with thermal burns. Surg Gynecol Obstet 1969;129:1242-6.

[84]   Putman CE, Loke J, Matthay RA, Ravin CE. Radiographic manifestations of acute smoke inhalation. Am J Roentgenol 1977;129:865-70.

[85]   Hunt JL, Agee RN, Pruitt BA, Jr. Fiberoptic bronchoscopy in acute inhalation injury. J Trauma 1975;15:641-9.

[86]   Moylan JA, Jr., Wilmore DW, Mouton DE, Pruitt BA, Jr. Early diagnosis of inhalation injury using 133 xenon lung scan. Ann Surg 1972;176:477-84.

[87]   Haponik EF, Meyers DA, Munster AM, Smith PL, Britt EJ, Wise RA, Bleecker ER. Acute upper airway injury in burn patients. Serial changes of flow-volume curves and nasopharyngoscopy. Am Rev Respir Dis 1987;135:360-6.

[88]   Haponik EF, Munster AM, Wise RA, Smith PL, Meyers DA, Britt EJ, Bleecker ER. Upper airway function in burn patients. Correlation of flow-volume curves and nasopharyngoscopy. Am Rev Respir Dis 1984;129:251-7.

[89]   Helvig B, Mlcak R, Nichols RJ, Jr. Anchoring endotracheal tubes on patients with facial burns. Review from Shriners Burns Institute, Galveston, Texas. J Burn Care Rehabil 1987;8:236-7.

[90]   Head JM. Inhalation injury in burns. Am JSurg 1980;139:508-512.

[91]   Walker HL, McLeod CG, Jr., McManus WF. Experimental inhalation injury in the goat. J Trauma 1981;21:962-4.

[92]   Venus B, Matsuda T, Copiozo JB, Mathru M. Prophylactic intubation and continuous positive airway pressure in the management of inhalation injury in burn victims. Crit Care Med 1981;9:519-23.

[93]   Nieman GF, Clark WR, Jr., Wax SD, Webb SR. The effect of smoke inhalation on pulmonary surfactant. Ann Surg 1980;191:171-81.

[94]   Robinson NB, Hudson LD, Robertson HT, Thorning DR, Carrico CJ, Heimbach DM. Ventilation and perfusion alterations after smoke inhalation injury. Surgery 1981;90:352-63.

[95]   Zikria BA, Budd DC, Floch F, Ferrer JM. What is clinical smoke poisoning? Ann Surg 1975;181:151-6.

[96]   Dowell AR, Kilburn KH, Pratt PC. Short-term exposure to nitrogen dioxide. Effects on pulmonary ultrastructure, compliance, and the surfactant system. Arch Intern Med 1971;128:74-80.

[97]   Prien T, Traber LD, Herndon DN, Stothert JC, Jr., Lubbesmeyer HJ, Traber DL. Pulmonary edema with smoke inhalation, undetected by indicator-dilution technique. J Appl Physiol 1987;63:907-11.

[98]   Einhorn IN. Physiological and toxicological aspects of smoke produced during the combustion of polymeric materials. Environ Health Perspect 1975;11:163-89.

[99]   Haponik EF. Smoke Inhalation Injury: Some priorities for respiratory care professionals. Irving, TX: Daedalus, I, 1992.

[100]   Herndon DN. Inhalation Injury. In: Herndorn, DN, ed. Total burn care. 2nd ed. Philadelphia, PA: WB Saunders, 2002.

[101]   Landa JF, Kwoka MA, Chapman GA, Brito M, Sackner MA. Effects of suctioning on mucociliary transport. Chest 1980;77:202-7.

[102]   Oldenburg FA, Jr., Dolovich MB, Montgomery JM, Newhouse MT. Effects of postural drainage, exercise, and cough on mucus clearance in chronic bronchitis. Am Rev Respir Dis 1979;120:739-45.

[103]   Marini JJ, Pierson DJ, Hudson LD. Acute lobar atelectasis: a prospective comparison of fiberoptic bronchoscopy and respiratory therapy. Am Rev Respir Dis 1979;119:971-8.

[104]   Hirsch SR, Zastrow JE, Kory RC. Sputum liquefying agents: a comparative in vitro evaluation. J Lab Clin Med 1969;74:346-53.

[105]   Brown M, Desai M, Traber LD, Herndon DN, Traber DL. Dimethylsulfoxide with heparin in the treatment of smoke inhalation injury. J Burn Care Rehabil 1988;9:22-5.

[106]   Desai MH, Mlcak R, Richardson J, Nichols R, Herndon DN. Reduction in mortality in pediatric patients with inhalation injury with aerosolized heparin/N-acetylcystine [correction of acetylcystine] therapy. J Burn Care Rehabil 1998;19:210-2.

[107]   Wanner A, Zighelboim A, Sackner MA. Nasopharyngeal airway: a facilitated access to the trachea. For nasotracheal suction, bedside bronchofiberscopy, and selective bronchography. Ann Intern Med 1971;75:593-5.

[108]   Ogura H, Saitoh D, Johnson AA, Mason AD, Jr., Pruitt BA, Jr., Cioffi WG, Jr. The effect of inhaled nitric oxide on pulmonary ventilation-perfusion matching following smoke inhalation injury. J Trauma 1994;37:893-8.

[109]   Manocha S, Gordon AC, Salehifar E, Groshaus H, Walley KR, Russell JA. Inhaled beta-2 agonist salbutamol and acute lung injury: an association with improvement in acute lung injury. Crit Care 2006;10:R12.

[110]   Traber DL, Hawkins HK, Enkhbaatar P, Cox RA, Schmalstieg FC, Zwischenberger JB, Traber LD. The role of the bronchial circulation in the acute lung injury resulting from burn and smoke inhalation. Pulm Pharmacol Ther 2007;20:163-6.

[111]   Clark CJ, Campbell D, Reid WH. Blood carboxyhaemoglobin and cyanide levels in fire survivors. Lancet 1981;1:1332-5.

[112]   Weaver LK, Hopkins RO, Chan KJ, Churchill S, Elliott CG, Clemmer TP, Orme JF, Jr., Thomas FO, Morris AH. Hyperbaric oxygen for acute carbon monoxide poisoning. New Engl J Med 2002;347:1057-67.

[113] Juurlink DN, Buckley NA, Stanbrook MB, Isbister GK, Bennett M, McGuigan MA. Hyperbaric oxygen for carbon monoxide poisoning. Cochrane Database Syst Rev 2005:CD002041.

[114] Buckley NA, Juurlink DN, Isbister G, Bennett MH, Lavonas EJ. Hyperbaric oxygen for carbon monoxide poisoning. Cochrane Database Syst Rev 2011:CD002041.

[115] Alsbjorn B, Gilbert P, Hartmann B, Kazmierski M, Monstrey S, Palao R, Roberto MA, Van Trier A, Voinchet V. Guidelines for the management of partial-thickness burns in a general hospital or community setting--recommendations of a European working party. Burns 2007;33:155-60.

[116] Hudspith J, Rayatt S. First aid and treatment of minor burns. BMJ 2004;328:1487-9.

[117] Wachtel TL, Berry CC, Wachtel EE, Frank HA. The inter-rater reliability of estimating the size of burns from various burn area chart drawings. Burns 2000;26:156-70.

[118] Jose RM, Roy DK, Vidyadharan R, Erdmann M. Burns area estimation-an error perpetuated. Burns 2004;30:481-2.

[119] Hettiaratchy S, Papini R. Initial management of a major burn: II--assessment and resuscitation. BMJ 2004;329:101-3.

[120] Smith JJ, Malyon AD, Scerri GV, Burge TS. A comparison of serial halving and the rule of nines as a pre-hospital assessment tool in burns. Br JPlast Surg 2005;58:957-67.

[121] Cone JB. What's new in general surgery: burns and metabolism. J Am Coll Surg 2005;200:607-15.

[122] La Hei ER, Holland AJ, Martin HC. Laser Doppler imaging of paediatric burns: burn wound outcome can be predicted independent of clinical examination. Burns 2006;32:550-3.

[123] Cubison TC, Pape SA, Parkhouse N. Evidence for the link between healing time and the development of hypertrophic scars (HTS) in paediatric burns due to scald injury. Burns 2006;32:992-9.

[124] McGill DJ, Sorensen K, MacKay IR, Taggart I, Watson SB. Assessment of burn depth: a prospective, blinded comparison of laser Doppler imaging and videomicroscopy. Burns 2007;33:833-42.

[125] Renkielska A, Nowakowski A, Kaczmarek M, Ruminski J. Burn depths evaluation based on active dynamic IR thermal imaging--a preliminary study. Burns 2006;32:867-75.

[126] Baker RH, Akhavani MA, Jallali N. Resuscitation of thermal injuries in the United Kingdom and Ireland. J Plast Reconstr Aesthet Surg 2007;60:682-5.

[127] Engrav LH, Colescott PL, Kemalyan N, Heimbach DM, Gibran NS, Solem LD, Dimick AR, Gamelli RL, Lentz CW. A biopsy of the use of the Baxter formula to resuscitate burns or do we do it like Charlie did it? J Burn Care Rehabil 2000;21:91-5.

[128] Holm C. Resuscitation in shock associated with burns. Tradition or evidence-based medicine? Resuscitation 2000;44:157-64.

[129] Mitra B, Fitzgerald M, Cameron P, Cleland H. Fluid resuscitation in major burns. ANZ JSurg 2006;76:35-8.

[130] Muir I. The use of the Mount Vernon formula in the treatment of burn shock. Intensive Care Med 1981;7:49-53.

[131] Baxter C. Fluid resuscitation, burn percentage, and physiologic age. J Trauma 1979;19:864-5.

[132] Baxter C. Guidelines for fluid resuscitation. J Trauma 1981;21:687-889.

[133] Fakhry SM, Alexander J, Smith D, Meyer AA, Peterson HD. Regional and institutional variation in burn care. J Burn Care Rehabil 1995;16:85-90.

[134] Boldt J, Papsdorf M. Fluid management in burn patients: results from a European survey-more questions than answers. Burns 2008;34:328-38.

[135] Pham TN, Cancio LC, Gibran NS. American Burn Association practice guidelines burn shock resuscitation. J Burn Care Res 2008;29:257-66.

[136] Perel P, Roberts I. Colloids versus crystalloids for fluid resuscitation in critically ill patients. Cochrane Database Syst Rev 2011;3:CD000567.

[137] Wharton SM, Khanna A. Current attitudes to burns resuscitation in the UK. Burns 2001;27:183-4.

[138] Ho AM, Karmakar MK, Contardi LH, Ng SS, Hewson JR. Excessive use of normal saline in managing traumatized patients in shock: a preventable contributor to acidosis. J Trauma 2001;51:173-7.

[139] Cartotto RC, Innes M, Musgrave MA, Gomez M, Cooper AB. How well does the Parkland formula estimate actual fluid resuscitation volumes? J Burn Care Rehabil 2002;23:258-65.

[140] Yowler CJ, Fratianne RB. Current status of burn resuscitation. Clin Plast Surg 2000;27:1-10.

[141] Sheridan RL. Burn care: results of technical and organizational progress. JAMA 2003;290:719-22.

[142] Baxter CR. Fluid volume and electrolyte changes of the early postburn period. Clin Plast Surg 1974;1:693-703.

[143] Baxter CR. Problems and complications of burn shock resuscitation. Surg Clin North Am 1978;58:1313-22.

[144] Salisbury RE, Taylor JW, Levine NS. Evaluation of digital escharotomy in burned hands. Plast Reconstr Surg 1976;58:440-3.

[145] Burd A, Noronha FV, Ahmed K, Chan JY, Ayyappan T, Ying SY, Pang P. Decompression not escharotomy in acute burns. Burns 2006;32:284-92.

[146] Richardson P, Mustard L. The management of pain in the burns unit. Burns 2009;35:921-36.

[147] Porter J, Jick H. Addiction rare in patients treated with narcotics. The New Engl J Med 1980;302:123.

[148] Filkins S, Cosgrave P, Marvin J. Self-administered anesthetic: a method of pain control. J Burn Care Rehabil 1981;3:3.

[149] Wilson JA, Kendall JM, Cornelius P. Intranasal diamorphine for paediatric analgesia: assessment of safety and efficacy. J Accid Emerg Med 1997;14:70-2.

[150] Kendall JM, Reeves BC, Latter VS. Multicentre randomised controlled trial of nasal diamorphine for analgesia in children and teenagers with clinical fractures. BMJ 2001;322:261-5.

[151] Ravat F, Le-Floch R, Vinsonneau C, Ainaud P, Bertin-Maghit M, Carsin H, Perro G. Antibiotics and the burn patient. Burns 2011;37:16-26.

[152] Avni T, Levcovich A, Ad-El DD, Leibovici L, Paul M. Prophylactic antibiotics for burns patients: systematic review and meta-analysis. BMJ 2010;340:241.

[153] Alexander JW, MacMillan BG, Law EJ, Krummel R. Prophylactic antibiotics as an adjunct for skin grafting in clean reconstructive surgery following burn injury. J Trauma 1982;22:687-90.

[154] Bang RL, Gang RK, Sanyal SC, Mokaddas EM, Lari AR. Beta-haemolytic Streptococcus infection in burns. Burns 1999;25:242-6.

[155] Timmons MJ. Are systemic prophylactic antibiotics necessary for burns? Ann R Coll Surg Engl1983;65:80-2.

[156] Boss WK, Brand DA, Acampora D, Barese S, Frazier WH. Effectiveness of prophylactic antibiotics in the outpatient treatment of burns. J Trauma 1985;25:224-7.

[157] Steer JA, Papini RP, Wilson AP, McGrouther DA, Nakhla LS, Parkhouse N. Randomized placebo-controlled trial of teicoplanin in the antibiotic prophylaxis of infection following manipulation of burn wounds. Br JSurg 1997;84:848-53.

[158] Ergun O, Celik A, Ergun G, Ozok G. Prophylactic antibiotic use in pediatric burn units. Eur J Pediatr Surg 2004;14:422-6.

[159] Ugburo AO, Atoyebi OA, Oyeneyin JO, Sowemimo GO. An evaluation of the role of systemic antibiotic prophylaxis in the control of burn wound infection at the Lagos University Teaching Hospital. Burns 2004;30:43-8.

[160] Rashid A, Brown AP, Khan K. On the use of prophylactic antibiotics in prevention of toxic shock syndrome. Burns 2005;31:981-5.

[161] Herndon DN, Barrow RE, Rutan RL, Rutan TC, Desai MH, Abston S. A comparison of conservative versus early excision. Therapies in severely burned patients. Ann Surg 1989;209:547-552.

[162] Parish RA, Novack AH, Heimbach DM, Engrav LR. Fever as a predictor of infection in burned children. J Trauma 1987;27:69-71.

[163] Sheridan RL. Infections in critically ill paediatric burn patients. Semin Pediatr Infect Dis 2000;11:25-34.

[164] Rodgers GL, Fisher MC, Lo A, Cresswell A, Long SS. Study of antibiotic prophylaxis during burn wound debridement in children. J Burn Care Rehabil 1997;18:342-6.

[165] Herndon D. Treatment of infection in burns. In: Total burn care. 2nd ed. London, WB Saunders, 2002.

[166] Brown TP, Cancio LC, McManus AT, Mason AD, Jr. Survival benefit conferred by topical antimicrobial preparations in burn patients: a historical perspective. J Trauma 2004;56:863-6.

[167] Brusselaers N, Monstrey S, Snoeij T, Vandijck D, Lizy C, Hoste E, Lauwaert S, Colpaert K, Vandekerckhove L, Vogelaers D, Blot S. Morbidity and mortality of bloodstream infections in patients with severe burn injury. Am J Crit Care 2010;19:e81-7.

[168] Rafla K, Tredget EE. Infection control in the burn unit. Burns 2011;37:5-15.

[169] Jeschke MG, Mlcak RP, Finnerty CC, Norbury WB, Gauglitz GG, Kulp GA, Herndon DN. Burn size determines the inflammatory and hypermetabolic response. Crit Care 2007;11:R90.

[170] Wallace PG, Ridley SA. ABC of intensive care. Transport of critically ill patients. BMJ 1999;319:368-71.

[171] Kortbeek JB, Al Turki SA, Ali J, Antoine JA, Bouillon B, Brasel K, Brenneman F, Brink PR, Brohi K, Burris D, et al. Advanced trauma life support, 8th edition, the evidence for change. J Trauma 2008;64:1638-50.

[172] Stone CA, Pape SA. Evolution of the Emergency Management of Severe Burns (EMSB) course in the UK. Burns 1999;25:262-4.

[173] Cummings G, O'Keefe G. Scene disposition and mode of transport following rural trauma: a prospective cohort study comparing patient costs. J Emerg Med 2000;18:349-54.

[174] Baack BR, Smoot EC, 3rd, Kucan JO, Riseman L, Noak JF. Helicopter transport of the patient with acute burns. J Burn Care Rehabil 1991;12:229-33.

[175] Palmer JH, Sutherland AB. Problems associated with transfer of patients to a regional burns unit. Injury 1987;18:250-7.

[176] Nakae H, Wada H. Characteristics of burn patients transported by ambulance to treatment facilities in Akita Prefecture, Japan. Burns 2002;28:73-9.

[177] Slater H, O'Mara MS, Goldfarb IW. Helicopter transportation of burn patients. Burns 2002;28:70-2.

[178] Yuan J, Wu C, Holland AJ, Harvey JG, Martin HC, La Hei ER, Arbuckle S, Godfrey TC. Assessment of cooling on an acute scald burn injury in a porcine model. J Burn Care Res 2007;28:514-20.

Submitted: June 29, 2011. *Revised:* August 20, 2011.
Accepted: August 30, 2011.

In: Public Health Yearbook 2012
Editor: Joav Merrick

ISBN: 978-1-62808-078-0
© 2013 Nova Science Publishers, Inc.

Chapter 2

A COMMENT ON INFANT MORTALITY RATE IN INDIA

Nilanjan Patra, PhD, MPhil, MSc, BSc[*]

Centre for Economic Studies and Planning, School of Social Sciences,
Jawaharlal Nehru University, New Delhi, India

ABSTRACT

Infant mortality rate (IMR) is taken as a key indicator of child health and the well-being of a society. In India, both the National Family Health Survey (NFHS) and the Sample Registration System (SRS) published by Registrar General of India (RGI) provide reliable data on population and demographic indicators. In this comment it is shown that the IMR differs in these two surveys and after discussing the difference in sampling techniques of these surveys, it is argued for a standardisation of data source for IMR calculation.

Keywords: Infant mortality rate, surveys, India

INTRODUCTION

This review uses unit-level record (individual recoded data file) from the National Family Health Survey (NFHS)-III (2005-06), NFHS-II (1998-99), and NFHS-I (1992-93) conducted in India. 'NFHS-III collected information from a nationally representative sample of 109,041 households, 124,385 women age 15-49 and, 74,369 men age 15-54. The NFHS-III sample covered 99 percent of India's population living in all 29 states' (1: xxix). 'The NFHS-II survey covered a representative sample of more than 90,000 eligible women age 15-49 from 26 states that comprise more than 99 percent of India's population' (2: xiii). The NFHS-I survey covered a representative sample of 89,777 ever-married women age 13-49 from 24 states and the National Capital Territory of Delhi, which comprise 99 percent of the total

---

[*] Correspondence: Nilanjan Patra, Centre for Economic Studies and Planning, School of Social Sciences, Jawaharlal Nehru University, New Delhi-110067, India. E-mail: nilanjanpatra@gmail.com

population of India (3: xix). It is worth to note that NFHS-II (1998-99), the second round of the series, is regarded as a 'storehouse of demographic and health data in India' (4).

To compare with NFHS data, we use data from the Sample Registration System (SRS) published by the Registrar General of India (RGI), Government of India (5-7). With a view to generate reliable and continuous data on these indicators, RGI initiated the scheme of sample registration of births and deaths in India popularly known as SRS in 1964-65 on a pilot basis and on full scale since 1969-70. The SRS since then has been providing data on a regular basis. The SRS is a large scale demographic survey for providing reliable annual estimates. The sample size of these data are based on the preceding census frame and covered over 6,000,000 people living in more than 903,300 households. The revision of SRS sampling frame is undertaken in every ten years based on the results of latest census. While changing the sample, modifications in the sampling design, wider representation of population, overcoming the limitations in the existing scheme, meeting the additional requirements are taken into account. To fulfil its objective of monitoring the changes in vital indicators, the SRS sampling units are retained for about 10 years, making it a panel household survey. The first replacement (of sampling units) was carried out in 1977-78, then in 1983-85, in 1993-95 and the last being in 2004. Whereas the replacement of samples in earlier years was undertaken in phases spread over 2-3 years, the replacement in 2004 was done at one go within a year. In 1992, the overall sample at the national level comprised 6022 (4176 rural and 1846 urban) sample units, each comprising nearly 150 households and about a 1,000 population. The overall sample at the national level rose to 6671 (4436 rural and 2235 urban) and 7597 (4433 rural and 3164 urban) sample units in SRS-1998 and SRS-2005 data.

DIFFERENCE IN SAMPLING TECHNIQUES

NFHS

A uniform sample design adopted in each state is a systematic, stratified sample of households, with two-stages in rural areas and three-stages in urban areas. The rural and urban samples within states were drawn separately and, to the extent possible, sample allocation was proportional to the size of the rural-urban populations. In each state, the rural sample was selected in two-stage stratified random sampling, with the selection of Primary Sampling Units (PSU), which are villages, with probability proportional to population size (PPS) at the first stage, followed by the random selection of households within each PSU at the second stage. Villages were stratified prior to selection on the basis of several variables. The first level of stratification was geographic, with districts being subdivided into contiguous regions according to their geographical characteristics. Within each of these regions, villages were further stratified using some of the following variables: village size, distance from the nearest town, proportion of non-agricultural worker, proportion of the population belonging to scheduled castes/ scheduled tribes, and female literacy. Female literacy was often used for implicit stratification (i.e., the villages were ordered prior to selection according to the proportion of females who were literate). PSUs were selected systematically with PPS. The households to be interviewed were selected from the household lists using systematic sampling with equal probability. On an average, 30 households were selected for interviewing in each selected PSU.

In urban areas, a three-stage stratified random sampling procedure was followed. All cities and towns were subdivided into three strata: a) self-selecting cities (i.e., cities with a population large enough to be selected with certainty), b) towns that are district headquarters, and c) other towns. Within each stratum, the cities/ towns were arranged according to the same kind of geographic stratification used in the rural areas. In self-selecting cities, the sample was selected according to a two-stage sample design: selection of the required number of urban blocks, followed by selection of households in each of the selected blocks. For district headquarters and other towns, a three-stage sample design was used: selection of towns with PPS, followed by selection of two census blocks per selected town, followed by selection of households from each selected block. On an average 20 households per block was selected systematically. The maximum level of error was 10 prse (percentage relative standard error) for infant mortality rate.

SRS

The RGI, since 1969-70, has been conducting a continuous demographic survey known as the SRS in the randomly selected sample units (village/ segment of a village in rural areas and census enumeration block (CEB) in urban areas) spread across the country to provide reliable unbiased annual estimates of fertility, mortality and other advanced indicators at the state and national level using 17 kinds of forms. To capture change in the age structure, marital status, literacy and other demographic variables, the SRS sample is replaced every ten years based on the latest census frame. On an average, this accounted for nearly 20–25 births and 9 deaths annually per unit. SRS is a dual record system wherein a resident part-time enumerator continuously records births and deaths in each household within the sample unit every month. A full-time SRS supervisor thereafter independently collects the vital events along with other related details for each of the preceding two six-month periods during the calendar year. The two sets of figures are matched. Partially matched/un-matched events are re-verified in the field to get an unduplicated count of events.

The sample design adopted for SRS is a uni-stage stratified simple random sample without replacement. In rural areas, each district within a state has been divided into two strata, viz., strata-I- villages with population less than or equal to 1500 and strata-II- villages with population more than 1500. In order to cover the village by one part-time enumerator, villages belonging to the second strata were segmented into two or more segments of equal size. A simple random sample of villages and segments has been selected from each of the two strata, without replacement in each state/ union territory.

In urban areas, six stratification has been done on the basis of population of the towns/ cities. (The towns/ cities were grouped into five classes, viz., a) towns with population below 20,000, b) towns with population of 20,000 or more but less than 50,000, c) towns with population of 50,000 and more but less than 100,000, d) towns with population of 100,000 or more but less than 500,000, e) cities with population of 500,000 or more but less than 1,000,000, and f) each city with population 1,000,000 or more, treated as a separate stratum). The sampling unit in urban area is a CEB. The sample CEB within each substratum was selected at random with equal probability. A simple random sample of these enumeration blocks have been selected within each sub-strata without replacement from each of the size classes of towns/cities in each state/union territory.

The earlier sample was based on the reliability of birth rate at the state level, whereas the 2004 sample is estimated using IMR and reliability at natural division level (natural divisions are National Sample Survey (NSS) classified group of contiguous administrative districts with distinct geographical and other natural characteristics). The infant mortality is the decisive indicator for estimation of sample size at natural division, the ultimate level for estimation and dissemination of indicators for rural areas. The permissible level of error has been taken as 10 prse (percentage relative standard error) at natural division level for rural areas and 10 prse at state level for urban areas, with respect to major states having population more than 10 million as per Census 2001. For minor states, 15 prse has been fixed at the total state level.

A COMMON HEALTH INDICATOR:
INFANT MORTALITY RATE

Infant mortality rate (IMR) is taken as a proxy for child health conditions. The IMR is an important measure of the well-being of infants, children, and pregnant women because it is associated with a variety of factors, such as maternal health, quality and access to medical care, socioeconomic conditions, and public health practices (8). IMR is the number of infants dying under one year of age in a year in a given geographical region per thousand live births in the same year and geographical region. IMR is treated as the most sensitive and commonly used indicator of general health and medical facilities available in a community as well as of the social and economic development of a population. The causes of infant mortality are 'strongly correlated to those structural factors, like economic development, general living conditions, social wellbeing, and the quality of the environment that affect the health of entire populations' (9). If mortality conditions improve, the IMR is immediately affected. Many health experts see the IMR as a sentinel indicator of child health and the well-being of a society over time. IMR also reflects the general standard of living of the people and effectiveness of interventions for improving maternal and child health in a country (10). Changes in specific health interventions affect IMR more rapidly and directly (10). The 2005 United Nations' Human Development Report states: 'no indicator captures the divergence in human development opportunity more powerfully than child mortality'(11).

IMR is calculated as a probability measure only after adjusting for year of birth and year of death (12). The direct method uses data collected on birth histories of women of childbearing age and produces the probability of dying before age one for children born alive, among women of childbearing age, during five year periods before the survey (0-4, 5-9, etc.). Direct methods require each child's date of birth, survival status, and date or age at death. This information is typically found in vital registration systems and in household surveys that collect complete birth histories from women of childbearing age. Birth histories include a series of detailed questions about each child a woman has given birth to during her lifetime, including the date the child was born, whether the child is still alive, and if not, the age at death.

State-wise IMRs are computed from the unit-level record for the major sixteen states of India for five-year period preceding the survey for both boys and girls separately as well as for all children. The IMRs by state and gender taken from three rounds of NFHS data is provided in table 1. The IMRs by state and gender from the three SRS rounds corresponding to the three NFHS rounds is shown in table 2.

Table 1. IMR by State and Gender in three NFHS Rounds

	Total			Boy			Girl		
Number of infant deaths under one year of age per thousand live births for the five-year period preceding the survey by selected states	NFHS-I (1988-92)	NFHS-II (1994-98)	NFHS-III (2001-05)	NFHS-I (1988-92)	NFHS-II (1994-98)	NFHS-III (2001-05)	NFHS-I (1988-92)	NFHS-II (1994-98)	NFHS-III (2001-05)
India	**78.5**	**67.6**	**57.0**	**81.1**	**68.1**	**56.3**	**76.2**	**67.3**	**57.7**
Haryana	73.3	56.8	41.7	64.9	59.4	42.4	82.5	53.6	40.9
H.P.	55.8	34.4	**36.1**	64.6	37.2	36.1	45.8	31.2	**36.1**
Punjab	53.7	**57.1**	41.7	57.5	50.3	39.1	49.5	**65.0**	45.3
Rajasthan	72.6	**80.4**	65.3	66.3	**76.4**	54.5	79.7	**84.8**	77.4
M.P.$	85.2	**86.1**	69.5	91.1	86.6	64.4	79.2	**85.6**	74.8
U.P.$	99.9	86.7	72.7	99.4	85.2	70.3	100.5	88.4	75.3
Bihar$	89.2	72.9	61.7	92.4	76.8	58.7	86.0	68.8	65.2
Orissa	112.1	81.0	64.7	123.6	83.6	71.4	99.4	78.2	57.6
W.B.	75.3	48.7	48.0	70.3	53.8	**56.0**	80.6	43.0	39.7
Assam	88.7	69.5	66.1	95.6	75.2	68.8	82.0	63.1	63.3
Gujarat	68.7	62.6	49.7	62.0	**69.5**	46.8	75.6	55.2	52.9
Maharashtra	50.5	43.7	37.5	57.7	43.7	38.4	42.6	**43.7**	36.5
Andhra P.	70.4	65.8	53.5	77.1	64.5	54.8	63.5	**67.3**	52.0
Karnataka	65.4	51.5	43.2	71.6	52.3	47.0	58.8	50.6	39.0
Kerala	23.8	16.3	15.3	25.6	21.9	16.6	22.0	8.8	**12.0**
Tamil Nadu	67.7	48.2	30.4	79.9	43.3	27.7	56.7	53.2	33.2

Note: $: For 1992 and 1998, MP includes Chhattisgarh, UP includes Uttarakhand and Bihar includes Jharkhand.. For states, an increase in IMR from the previous time-period is marked in bold in table 1 and 2.

From table 1 and 2, it is clear that the IMR estimate from both NFHS and SRS for all-India has declined over time. So is the case for most of the sixteen major states. Kerala is the only state that witnessed a rise in IMR for girl children between 1998 and 2005 which is evident from both NFHS and SRS data. Rajasthan is the only state that witnessed a rise in IMR rate in NFHS-II for both boys and girls. Punjab, Madhya Pradesh (in NFHS-II) and Himachal Pradesh (in NFHS-III) are the states where an increase in IMR for all children is actually due to rise in girl children's IMR.

Table 2. IMR by State and Gender in three SRS Rounds

Number of infant deaths under one year of age per thousand live births in a year in a given geographical region

	Total			Boy			Girl		
	SRS-1992	SRS-1998	SRS-2005	SRS-1992	SRS-1998	SRS-2005	SRS-1992	SRS-1998	SRS-2005
India	**79***	**72***	**58**	**79***	**70***	**56**	**80***	**73***	**61**
Haryana	75	70	60	73	61	51	78	**81**	70
H.P.	67	**68**	49	67	60	47	66	**77**	51
Punjab	56	54	44	54	53	41	60	56	48
Rajasthan	90	83	68	88	83	64	92	84	72
M.P.$	104	98	76	109	99	72	98	97	79
U.P. $	98	85	73	92	79	71	105	93	75
Bihar$	73	67	61	71	67	60	74	66	62
Orissa	115	98	75	114	98	74	116	97	77
W.B.	65	53	38	67	59	38	62	48	39
Assam	82	76	68	86	85	66	78	67	69
Gujarat	67	64	54	66	63	52	69	66	55
Maharashtra	59	49	36	61	42	34	57	56	37
Andhra Pr.	71	66	57	73	65	56	68	68	58
Karnataka	73	58	50	77	61	48	67	56	51
Kerala	17	16	14	21	18	14	12	13	**15**
Tamil Nadu	58	53	37	58	48	35	59	58	39

Source: RGI (5,6,7). Note: *: excluding J & K.

Table 3. State-wise Difference in IMR between NFHS and SRS for All Children

	(NFHS-I)- (SRS-1992)	(NFHS-II) - (SRS-1998)	(NFHS-III) - (SRS-2005)
Haryana	-1.7	**-13.2**	**-18.3**
H.P.	**-11.2**	**-33.6**	**-12.9**
Punjab	-2.3	3.1	-2.3
Rajasthan	**-17.4**	-2.6	-2.7
M.P.$	**-18.8**	**-11.9**	-6.5
U.P. $	1.9	1.7	-0.3
Bihar$	**16.2**	5.9	0.7
Orissa	-2.9	**-17**	**-10.3**
W.B.	**10.3**	-4.3	**10**
Assam	6.7	-6.5	-1.9
Gujarat	1.7	-1.4	-4.3
Maharashtra	-8.5	-5.3	1.5
Andhra Pr.	-0.6	-0.2	-3.5
Karnataka	-7.6	-6.5	-6.8
Kerala	6.8	0.3	1.3
Tamil Nadu	**9.7**	-4.8	-6.6

Table 4. State-wise Difference in IMR between NFHS and SRS for Girl Children

	(NFHS-I)- (SRS-1992)	(NFHS-II) - (SRS-1998)	(NFHS-III) - (SRS-2005)
Haryana	4.5	**-27.4**	**-29.1**
H.P.	**-20.2**	**-45.8**	**-14.9**
Punjab	**-10.5**	**9.0**	-2.7
Rajasthan	**-12.3**	0.8	5.4
M.P.$	**-18.8**	**-11.4**	-4.2
U.P. $	-4.5	-4.6	0.3
Bihar$	12	2.8	3.2
Orissa	**-16.6**	**-18.8**	**-19.4**
W.B.	**18.6**	-5	0.7
Assam	4	-3.9	-5.7
Gujarat	6.6	**-10.8**	-2.1
Maharashtra	**-14.4**	**-12.3**	-0.5
Andhra Pr.	-4.5	-0.7	-6
Karnataka	**-8.2**	-5.4	**-12**
Kerala	**10**	-4.2	-3
Tamil Nadu	-2.3	-4.8	-5.8

In Maharashtra and Andhra Pradesh (in NFHS-II), there is an increase in girl children's IMR without any corresponding rise in all children's IMR. However, the two states of Gujarat (NFHS-II) and West Bengal (NFHS-III) witnessed a rise in IMR for boys without any such increase in IMR for all children.

As IMR from NFHS data is calculated for the five-year period preceding the survey, we would expect that IMR from NFHS will be higher than the corresponding IMR from SRS annual data (as generally, IMR declines over time). State-wise difference in IMR for all children between NFHS and SRS is shown in table 3. Only for West Bengal and Bihar, the IMR estimate from NFHS is higher than that of SRS. But NFHS gives a consistently lower estimate than SRS for Rajasthan, Haryana, Himachal Pradesh, Madhya Pradesh, Orissa and Karnataka. State-wise difference in IMR for girl children between NFHS and SRS is shown in table 4. Again, NFHS gives a consistently lower IMR estimate than SRS for Haryana, Himachal Pradesh, Madhya Pradesh, Orissa, Maharashtra and Karnataka.

DISCUSSION

The IMR estimates for all children are more or less consistent (i.e., difference is low) in both sets of data for the states of Kerala, Uttar Pradesh, Andhra Pradesh, Gujarat and Punjab. However, there are states for which difference in IMR estimates from NFHS and SRS is huge. For example, in 1992 there are six states where the gap is of 10 or more with Madhya Pradesh having the highest gap of 19. In 1998, there are four states with a gap of 10 or more with Himachal Pradesh displaying the highest gap of 34. The number of states with a gap of 10 or more remains the same four with the highest gap of 18 witnessed in Haryana in 2005.

The picture is more revealing when we look at the difference in IMR estimates from NFHS and SRS for girl children only. Here we do not have a single state that gives closely consistent estimate from the two data sets. In 1992, there are nine states (out of sixteen major states) where the gap is 10 or more with Himachal Pradesh exhibiting the highest gap of 20. Himachal Pradesh remains the state with highest gap of 46 in 1998 and during this period there are six states with a gap of 10 or more. The number of states with a gap of 10 or more, decreased slightly to four with the highest gap of 29 registered by Haryana in 2005.

These wide-spread gaps in the state-wise IMR estimates given by NFHS and SRS data raise serious questions on the relative as well as absolute reliability of these widely used data. There is no rule of thumb by which one can be chosen over the other. In general, we can say that NFHS gives a lower IMR estimate than the SRS (as it is evident from table 3 and 4, for most of the selected states). The difference in the estimates of IMR may have cropped up due to the difference in sampling techniques in the two data sets. As NFHS estimate is based on the last five years recall on mortality, child deaths may be under-reported as the mothers are often interviewed in front of older women of the household (e.g., mother-in-law).

Such a divergence in the IMR estimates from the NFHS and SRS can also create confusion in the government policy areas. Policies based on one data might be conflicting with the policies based on the other. Health financing or health infrastructure development based on one of the data sets might be biased if the policy makers use one benchmark rather than the other. As poverty measures are calculated from NSS data, there is also a need for standardisation of source from which IMR should be calculated.

ACKNOWLEDGMENTS

I am grateful to Prof. Jayati Ghosh and Prof. KR Nayar for their valuable comments. All remaining errors, if any, will solely be my responsibility.

REFERENCES

[1] International Institure Population Science. Measure DHS+ and ORC Macro. National family health survey (NFHS-3), 2005-06: India, Vol-1. Mumbai, India: Int Inst Populat Sci, 2007.

[2] International Institure Population Science. National family health survey (NFHS-2), 1998-99: India. Mumbai, India: Int Inst Populat Sci, 2000.

[3] International Institure Population Science. National family health survey (NFHS-1), 1992-93: India. Mumbai, India: Int Inst Populat Sci, 1995.

[4] Rajan SI, James KS. Second national family health survey: Emerging issues. Econ Polit Weekly 2004;Feb 14:647-51.

[5] RGI. Statistical report. Sample Registration System, Registrar General of India, GoI. various years.

[6] RGI. Compendium of India's fertility and mortality indicators 1971-97. RGI, GoI, 1999.

[7] Sample Registration System. Accessed 2011 Jun 15. URL: http://censusindia.gov.in/Vital_Statistics/SRS/Sample_Registration_System.aspx

[8] Definition of infant mortality. Accessed 2011 Jun 15. URL: http://www.medterms.com/script/main/art.asp?rticlekey=3967

[9] Reidpath D, Allotey P. Infant mortality rate as an indicator of population health. J Epidemiol Commun Health 2003;57:344-6.

[10] Singh B. IMR in India: Still a long way to go. Indian J Pediatr 2007; 74:454.

[11] UNDP. Human development report 2005. New York: United Nations. 2005:4.

[12] Ram F, Shekhar C, Mohanty SK. Human development: Strengthening district level vital statistics in India. Mumbai: International Institure Population Science, 2005.

Submitted: June 25, 2011. *Revised:* August 20, 2011.
Accepted: August 31, 2011.

In: Public Health Yearbook 2012
Editor: Joav Merrick

Chapter 3

CHILDHOOD MALTREATMENT AND HIV RISK-TAKING AMONG MEN USING THE INTERNET SPECIFICALLY TO FIND PARTNERS FOR UNPROTECTED SEX

Hugh Klein[*], *PhD and David Tilley*[**], *MS*

[*]Kensington Research Institute, Silver Spring, Maryland, and Prevention Sciences Research Center, Morgan State University, Baltimore, Maryland, USA
[**]Department of Community and Family Health, University of South Florida, Tampa, Florida, USA

ABSTRACT

Using a Syndemics Theory conceptual model, this study examines the relationship between childhood maltreatment experiences and involvement in HIV risk taking in a sample of adult men who actively seek partners for unprotected sex via the Internet. Methods: The study was based on a national random sample of 332 men who have sex with men (MSM), who use the Internet to seek men with whom they can engage in unprotected sex. Data collection was conducted via telephone interviews between January 2008 and May 2009. Structural equation analysis was undertaken to examine the specific nature of the relationships involved in understanding HIV risk practices. Results: Childhood maltreatment experiences were not found to be related directly to involvement in HIV risk taking in adulthood. Childhood maltreatment, particularly in the form of emotional neglect, was found to be an important variable in the overall structural equation. Its effect on HIV risk taking was indirect, operating principally by having a negative impact upon self-esteem, which in turn had a negative effect on attitudes toward condom use, which in turn were related strongly and directly to risk taking. Conclusions: Childhood maltreatment experiences are relevant to understanding HIV risk practices among MSM in adulthood, but the relationship is not as simple as usually conceptualized.

[*] Correspondence: Hugh Klein, PhD, Kensington Research Institute, 401 Schuyler Road, Silver Spring, Maryland 20910, USA. E-mail: hughk@aol.com (primary) or hughkhughk@yahoo.com (secondary)

Rather, childhood maltreatment appears to impact risk taking indirectly, through its effects on mental health functioning, which in turn affects risk-related attitudes.

Keywords: Childhood maltreatment, HIV risk, men who have sex with men (MSM)

INTRODUCTION

Childhood maltreatment, whether in the form of sexual abuse, physical abuse, emotional abuse, or neglect, has been linked with a wide variety of adverse outcomes in adulthood. These include mental health problems (e.g., depression, anxiety, post-traumatic stress disorder, attempted suicide, history of substance abuse) (1), HIV risk behaviors (2,3) and obesity (4). This has been true for a number of populations, including men who have sex with men (3,5), heterosexual men (6), lesbians (4), and heterosexual women (2), indicating that the effects of early-life maltreatment are far-reaching and long-lasting.

Sexual abuse experiences have been linked with a greater risk for practicing risky sex later in life in men who have sex with men (MSM), specifically because of the effect of these experiences on men's psychological health. Childhood sexual abuse was discussed as a precursor to adulthood involvement in HIV risk-taking in Fields, Malebranche, and Feist-Price's (7) research on African American MSM. Catania and colleagues (8: 925) noted that childhood sexual abuse "contributes to the ongoing HIV epidemic among MSM by distorting or undermining critical motivational, coping, and interpersonal factors that, in turn, influence adult sexual risk behavior." Dorais' (5) qualitative study of childhood sexual abuse and HIV risk taking among MSM revealed the former to be associated with an inability to assert oneself with regard to one's sexual safety and a greater tendency toward sexual compulsivity. In their bi-coastal study of HIV-positive MSM, O'Leary, Purcell, Remien, and Gomez (9) reported a link between childhood sexual abuse and engaging in unprotected anal intercourse with serodiscordant partners. In a study of gay and bisexual men attending a midwestern gay pride festival, childhood sexual abuse was found to be related to the likelihood of being HIV-positive, having exchanged sex for money, and the use of sex-related drugs, but not to the practice of unprotected sex (10). In another study of men attending a different city's gay pride festival (11), childhood sexual abuse was found to be related to a history of exchanging sex for drugs and/or money, but not to unprotected anal intercourse. Saewyc and colleagues (12) studied adolescents located in the Pacific Northwest, and concluded that sexual victimization contributed to greater overall HIV risk behavior involvement (based on a composite scale measuring seven different HIV risk practices) among the gay and bisexual students in their sample. Rosario, Schrimshaw, and Hunter (13) also based their work on gay and bisexual adolescents and young adults, and found that childhood sexual abuse was related to having a larger number of sex partners, which in turn was related to a greater likelihood of engaging in unprotected anal sex.

In contrast to the preceding, the present authors find it noteworthy that studies examining the effects of other types of childhood maltreatment (e.g., physical abuse, emotional abuse, emotional neglect, physical neglect) on HIV risk taking are very scarce in the published literature. One noteworthy exception is the research conducted by Paul, Catania, Pollack, and Stall (14) on the topic of physical abuse. These authors found that parent-child physical abuse, one component of what they termed "adverse familial experiences," was a mediating factor for six sexual risk factors, including having unprotected sex with a non-primary partner and having unprotected sex with a serodiscordant partner. Much more needs to be learned and reported regarding the effects that childhood physical abuse has on HIV risk-taking later in life, and on the effects that other types of childhood maltreatment have on subsequent involvement in risky practices.

Contemporary thinking on the relationship between childhood maltreatment experiences and HIV risk behaviors in adulthood (primarily based on the childhood sexual abuse literature) suggests that the former influence the latter by virtue of their impact upon various aspects of mental health functioning, which in turn is related more closely to risk practices because of its temporal proximity. Rather than conceptualizing the relationship as maltreatment → HIV risk, increasingly, evidence suggests that it is better to conceptualize this relationship as maltreatment → psychological/psychosocial functioning →HIV risk.

Studies such as those conducted by Catania and colleagues (8) and Rosario, Schrimshaw, and Hunter (13) have documented just how complicated the effects of childhood maltreatment can be, particularly when trying to link them to adulthood involvement in HIV risk behaviors. Relatively few studies, however, have utilized a structural modeling approach to understand the impact that maltreatment experiences can have on subsequent mental health functioning and risk practices. This is unfortunate, as the complex nature of these interrelationships requires closer study in order to develop truer understandings of the myriad ways in which childhood sexual, physical, and emotional abuse, as well as neglect, may affect adulthood behaviors.

In the present paper, a structural approach is used to develop a better understanding of how childhood maltreatment experiences affect HIV risk involvement in adulthood in a sample of men who use the internet specifically to find other men with whom they can engage in unprotected sex. Based on previously published studies, the following conceptual model was examined:

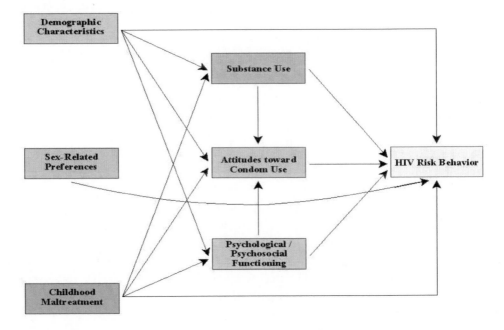

Figure 1. Conceptual model.

In this exploratory model, childhood maltreatment experiences are hypothesized to have both direct and indirect effects on men's involvement in risky practices. The indirect effects are hypothesized to operate both through the impact of maltreatment on men's psychological/psychosocial functioning, its effects on substance use/abuse, and its impact on their attitudes toward condom use. As the conceptual model shows, childhood maltreatment experiences are one of six types of influences hypothesized to affect men's HIV risk practices. The others are demographic variables (e.g., race/ethnicity, age, HIV serostatus), sex-related behavioral preferences (e.g., self-identification as a sexual "top" versus a "bottom," preferring to have sex that is "wild" or "uninhibited"), substance use/abuse, attitudes toward condom use, and psychological/psychosocial functioning (e.g., depression, self-esteem, impulsivity).

To a great extent, this conceptual model owes its intellectual origins to the notion of syndemic and to Syndemics Theory.

"Syndemic" refers to the tendency for multiple epidemics to co-occur and, for the various maladies to interact with one another, with each one worsening the effects of the others (15,16). Walkup et al. (17) noted that health problems may be construed as syndemic when two or more conditions/afflictions are linked in such a manner that they interact synergistically, with each contributing to an excess burden of disease in a particular population. It is noteworthy that their work also addresses the syndemic of HIV, substance abuse, and mental illness.

A good example of how conditions may become syndemic is offered by Romero-Daza, Weeks and Singer (18) in their study of street prostitution.

The authors wrote:

> streetwalkers' continuous exposure to violence, both as victims and as witnesses, often leaves them suffering from major emotional trauma. In the absence of adequate support services, women who have been victimized may turn to drug use in an attempt to deal with the harsh realities of their daily lives. In turn, the need for drugs, coupled with a lack of educational and employment opportunities, may lead women into prostitution. Life on the street increases women's risk for physical, emotional, and sexual abuse as well as their risk for HIV/AIDS. Exposure to traumatic experiences deepens the dependence on drugs, completing a vicious cycle of violence, substance abuse, and AIDS risk (pp. 233–234)

Stall and colleagues (19) applied Syndemics Theory to urban MSM's risk for acquiring HIV and focused on the intertwined epidemics of substance abuse, depression, childhood sexual abuse (CSA), and intimate partner violence (IPV). They found that the presence of the co-occurring epidemics increased the likelihood that MSM had engaged in unprotected sex and increased their likelihood of being HIV-positive. A number of authors, particularly during the past few years, have written about syndemics and Syndemics Theory as they apply to sexual risk taking and the HIV epidemic (16,18,20–22), including specific mention of the applicability of the concept and theory to men who have sex with men (21).

Using the conceptual model shown above, the present study represents an effort to examine the role that childhood maltreatment experiences play in the HIV risk syndemic faced by one population of men who are at particularly great risk of contracting HIV–namely, MSM who use the internet in search of partners for unprotected sex.

The main research questions examined in this exploratory analysis are as follows: (1) How prevalent are experiences with neglect, sexual abuse, physical abuse, and emotional abuse in this population? (2) How, if at all, are these experiences related to men's involvement in HIV risk taking? (3) How, if at all, does childhood maltreatment affect men's psychological/psychosocial functioning and other factors hypothesized to be related to their HIV risk practices?

METHODS

The data reported in this paper come from The Bareback Project, a National Institute on Drug Abuse-funded study of men who use the internet specifically to find other men with whom they can engage in unprotected sex. The data were collected between January 2008 and May 2009. A total of 332 men were recruited from 16 different websites. Some of the sites catered exclusively to unprotected sex (e.g., Bareback.com, RawLoads.com) and some of them did not but made it possible for site users to identify which persons were looking for unprotected sex (e.g., Men4SexNow.com, Squirt.org). A nationwide random sample of men was derived, with random selection being based on a combination of the first letter of the person's online username, his race/ethnicity (as listed in his profile), and the day of recruitment. The study design called for an oversampling of men of color, to ensure good representation of racial minority group men in the sample and to facilitate the examination of racial differences in risk taking and risk-related preferences. Recruitment efforts were undertaken seven days a week, during all hours of the day and nighttime, variable from week to week throughout the duration of the project. This was done to maximize the representativeness of the final research sample, in recognition of the fact that different people use the internet at different times.

Depending upon the website involved, men were approached initially either via instant message or email (much more commonly via email). A brief overview of the study was provided as part of the initial approach and informed consent-related procedures, and all men were given the opportunity to ask questions about the study before deciding whether or not to participate. A website link to the project's online home page was also made available, to provide men with additional information about the project and to help them feel secure in the legitimacy of the research endeavor. Men who were interested in participating were scheduled for an interview, which was conducted as soon after they expressed an interest in taking part in the study as possible, typically within a few days. Interviews were conducted during all hours of the day and nighttime, seven days a week, based on interviewer availability and participants' preferences, to maximize convenience to the participants. All of the study's interviewers were gay or lesbian, to engender credibility with the target population and to enhance participants' comfort during the interviews.

Participation in the study entailed the completion of a one-time, confidential telephone interview covering a wide array of topics. The questionnaire was developed specifically for use in The Bareback Project, with many parts of the interview derived from standardized scales previously used and validated by other researchers. The interview covered such subjects as: degree of "outness," perceived discrimination based on sexual orientation, general health practices, HIV testing history and serostatus, sexual practices (protected and unprotected) with partners met online and offline, risk-related preferences, risk-related hypotheticals, substance use, drug-related problems, internet usage, psychological and psychosocial functioning, childhood maltreatment experiences, HIV/AIDS knowledge, and some basic demographic information. Interviews lasted an average of 69 minutes (median = 63, *s.d.* = 20.1, range = 30–210). Men who completed the interview were compensated $35 for their time. Two payment options were offered, one of which allowed men to maintain complete anonymity (PayPal) and one of which required them to provide a name and mailing address to receive payment (check). Approximately 10-15% of the men participating in the study declined the $35. Prior to implementation in the field, the research protocol was approved by the institutional review boards at Morgan State University (approval number 07/12-0145), where the principal investigator and one of the research assistants were affiliated, and George Mason University (approval number 5659), where the other research assistant was located.

Measures used

The Childhood Trauma Questionnaire (23) was used to examine childhood maltreatment experiences. Six measures, all of which asked men about their experiences prior to the age of 18, were used: sexual abuse (Cronbach's alpha = 0.93), physical abuse (Cronbach's alpha = 0.85), emotional abuse (Cronbach's alpha = 0.89), physical neglect (Cronbach's alpha = 0.71), emotional neglect (Cronbach's alpha = 0.93), and total amount of childhood maltreatment experienced (Cronbach's alpha = 0.94)

The **main outcome measure** (i.e., dependent variable) used in this particular paper indicates the percentage of sex acts that involved the use of protection. It is a continuous measure based on participants' self-reported sexual practices during the 30 days prior to interview.

Numerous measures examining demographic characteristics were examined. These included: age (dichotomous, comparing men aged 18–49 years to those aged 50+), race / ethnicity (categorical), relationship status (involved in a marital-type relationship versus not involved), educational attainment (continuous), sexual role identity (top, versatile top, versatile, versatile bottom, bottom), HIV serostatus (positive, negative, unknown), and knowing anyone currently living with AIDS (yes / no).

Four items measuring men's sex-related preferences were examined. These were: how rough they preferred their sex to be (continuous), how long they most liked their sexual sessions to last (continuous), how much they liked having sex in public venues (continuous), and how much they liked having sex that was "wild" or "uninhibited" (continuous).

The substance use / abuse domain was assessed with three measures: currently a user of illegal drugs (yes / no), number of drug problems experienced (continuous scale measure, Cronbach's alpha = 0.87), and total amount of illegal drug use reported during the preceding 30 days (continuous measure of quantity × frequency of recent use, summed across nine drug types).

Attitudes toward condom use were assessed via a 17-item scale that was found to be highly reliable (Cronbach's alpha = 0.91). Individual items were scored on a five-point Likert scale, and higher scores on the scale corresponded with attitudes that were more conducive of condom use. The scale was derived from the work of Brown (24). Only items that were relevant to MSM and their sexual practices were used, so that the scale would be applicable to the study population.

Finally, psychological and psychosocial functioning were examined. Measures examined were: self-esteem (using the Rosenberg self-esteem scale [25]; Cronbach's alpha = 0.89), depression (using the CES-D [26]); Cronbach's alpha = 0.93), concern about potential sex partners' HIV serostatus (yes / no), and perceived accuracy of HIV serostatus information provided verbally by sex partners (ordinal).

Analysis

The analysis for this research took place in several steps. Initially, bivariate analyses were conducted to examine which of the independent measures were related one-on-one to the dependent measure in question. Whenever the independent variable was dichotomous (e.g., race, sexual orientation), Student's t tests were used. Whenever the independent variable was ordinal with five or more response options or continuous in nature (e.g., extent of sexual abuse, level of self-esteem), simple regression was used to test the bivariate relationships.

Items that were found to be related either significantly ($p<.05$) or marginally ($.15>p>.05$) to the dependent measure in these bivariate analyses were entered into a multivariate equation, and then removed in stepwise fashion until a best fit model containing only statistically-significant measures remained. This approach was used for the main outcome measure (i.e., percentage of protected sex) and for each of the relevant endogenous measures (e.g., condom-related attitudes, level of self-esteem).

As a final analytical step, the relationships depicted in Figure 2 (which portrays the results of the analyses just described) were subjected to a structural equation analysis to determine whether the way the relationships depicted there is an appropriate and effective representation of the study data. SAS's PROC CALIS procedure was used to assess the overall fit of the model to the data. When conducting a structural equation analysis, several specific characteristics are examined and sought: (1) a goodness-of-fit index as close to 1.00 as possible, but no less than 0.90, (2) a Bentler-Bonett normed fit index value as close to 1.00 as possible, but no less than 0.90, (3) an overall chi-square value for the model that is statistically nonsignificant, preferably as far from attaining statistical significance as possible, and (4) a root mean square error approximation value as close to 0.00 as possible, but no greater than 0.05. If these conditions are met, then the structural relationships depicted are considered to indicate a good fit with the data.

Throughout all of the analyses, results are reported as statistically significant whenever $p<.05$.

RESULTS

In total, 332 men participated in the study. They ranged in age from 18 to 72 (mean = 43.7, s.d. = 11.2, median = 43.2). Racially, the sample is a fairly close approximation of the American population, with 74.1% being Caucasian, 9.0% each being African American and Latino, 5.1% self-identifying as biracial or multiracial, 2.4% being Asian, and 0.3% being Native American. The large majority of the men (89.5%) considered themselves to be gay; 10.2% said they were bisexual; and 0.3% self-identified as "curious." On balance, men participating in The Bareback Project were fairly well-educated. About 1 man in 7 (14.5%)

had completed no more than high school; 34.3% had some college experience without earning a college degree; 28.9% had a bachelor's degree; and 22.3% were educated beyond the bachelor's level. Slightly more than half of the men (59.0%) reported being HIV-positive; most of the rest (38.6%) were HIV-negative; and some men (2.4%) did not know about their current HIV serostatus.

Maltreatment experiences during men's formative years were quite prevalent in this study population. It should be noted that the following figures provide conservative, low-end prevalence figures because responses of "rarely" to the component items are not being counted as affirmative in the reporting of these "yes/no" childhood maltreatment summary measures. (Please note that, in computing the scale measures used in the remainder of the analyses for this paper, raw data values are summed, including the appropriate differentiations of values for the "never" and "rarely" responses.) Nearly two-thirds of the men (61.7%) gave answers indicating that they had been abused emotionally. More than half (51.1%) had been abused physically at least sometimes. More than one-quarter (25.5%) reported having been sexually abused "sometimes," "often," or "very often" before the age of 18. More than half of the men (52.0%) had been victims of emotional neglect and more than one-third (34.4%) had been physically neglected during their formative years. Overall, 80.6% of the men reported at least one of these forms of maltreatment during their childhood and/or adolescent years.

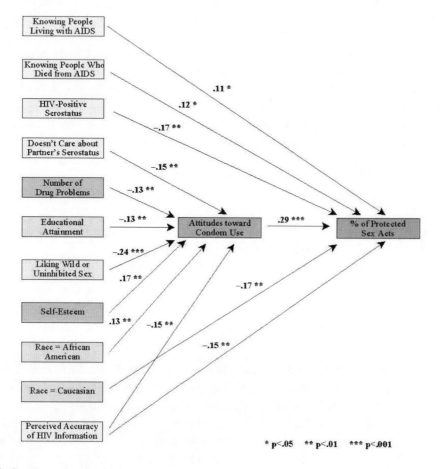

Figure 2. Condom related attitudes and protected sex.

Childhood maltreatment and HIV risk practices

Contrary to our initial research hypothesis, childhood maltreatment experiences were not found to be related to men's involvement in risky sex. This was true for sexual abuse ($p=.534$), physical abuse ($p=.568$), emotional abuse ($p=.352$), emotional neglect ($p=.433$), physical neglect ($p=.852$), and the total amount of maltreatment ($p=.666$) alike.

Childhood maltreatment and attitudes toward condom use

In the bivariate analyses, three of the six childhood maltreatment measures were found to be associated with men's attitudes toward condom use. In each instance, the more maltreatment that men experienced during their formative years, the worse their attitudes toward using condoms tended to be in adulthood. This was true with regard to emotional abuse ($F[1,327df]=5.80$, $p=.017$), emotional neglect ($F[1,327df]=8.85$, $p=.003$), and the total amount of maltreatment experienced ($F[1,327df]=4.88$, $p=.028$).

When these measures were added to the multivariate equation, however, none of them was retained as a statistically significant contributor once the effects of other measures were taken into account. As Figure 2 demonstrates, the effects of childhood maltreatment on attitudes toward condom use were secondary to those of seven other measures. Condom-related attitudes were reported by men who: were African American ($p=.008$), had a lower amount of education ($p=.009$), cared about their sex partners' HIV serostatus ($p=.004$), had a lesser preference for engaging in "wild or uninhibited" sex ($p<.001$), had fewer problems resulting from substance abuse ($p=.009$), perceived their sex partners to be less truthful about their HIV serostatus when discussing the subject with them ($p=.004$), and those who had a higher self-esteem ($p=.002$).

Childhood maltreatment and self-esteem

In the bivariate analyses, four of the six childhood maltreatment measures were found to be predictive of men's levels of self-esteem. In all four of these instances, greater maltreatment was associated with lower self-esteem. This was true with regard to emotional abuse ($F[1,327df]=24.69$, $p<.001$), emotional neglect ($F[1,327df]=36.34$, $p<.001$), physical neglect ($F[1,327df]=29.69$, $p<.001$), and the total amount of maltreatment experienced ($F[1,327df]=22.70$, $p<.001$).

As Figure 2 depicts, when these items were entered into the multivariate equation, one of them–emotional neglect–was found to contribute uniquely and significantly to the overall prediction of men's levels of self-esteem ($p<.001$). Also predictive of lower levels of self-esteem were race (specifically, not being African American, $p=.008$), lower educational attainment ($p=.009$), being under the age of 50 ($p=.047$), and being overweight ($p=.027$).

Testing the structural equation model shown in Figure 2

As a final analytical step, the results of the multivariate analyses were subjected to a structural equation analysis, to examine the totality of the relationships portrayed in Figure 2.

This analysis provided strong confirmatory support for the way that the relationships are depicted there. When conducting structural equation analysis, we want to obtain a goodness-of-fit index that is greater than 0.900. For this equation, the coefficient was 0.987. When conducting structural equation analysis, we want a Bentler-Bonett normed fit index that is greater than 0.900. For this equation, the coefficient was 0.946. In this type of analysis, we strive for an overall chi-square value for the model that is statistically nonsignificant, preferably as far from attaining statistical significance as possible. Here, it was $p=.213$. Finally, using structural equation modeling, we strive for a root mean square error approximation value as close to 0.00 as possible, but no greater than 0.050. Here, it was 0.028.

DISCUSSION

One of this study's main hypotheses was that childhood maltreatment would be related to men's involvement in HIV risk practices. To our surprise, however, in this study, childhood maltreatment had no direct effect on men's HIV risk taking. This finding stands in clear contrast to most of the published literature that shows childhood maltreatment is associated with greater HIV risk taking (5,7–14)

This is not to say, however, that childhood maltreatment is irrelevant to understanding risk in this population. As Figure 2 demonstrates, childhood maltreatment *is* important in the overall prediction of men's HIV risk behavior, but its effect was found to be indirect rather than direct. The relationship of childhood maltreatment to HIV risk behavior appears to operate in the following manner: Men's experiences of childhood maltreatment lowers their self-esteem. Lower self-esteem, in turn, alters their attitudes towards using condoms in a negative manner and that, in turn, ultimately increases their likelihood of engaging in unprotected sex. Thus, in the present study population, childhood maltreatment experiences appeared to be operating "in the background" when it comes to their influence on HIV risk taking in adulthood.

In recent years, there has been increasing support in the scientific community for the notion that childhood maltreatment experiences are complex in terms of how they affect people later in life. Although many studies (5,7–13) have suggested that childhood maltreatment has a direct effect upon risk taking, increasingly, evidence suggests that maltreatment operates through a variety of "intermediary" or "mediating" mechanisms when having long-term effects on people. Studies such as those conducted by Catania and colleagues (8) and Rosario, Schrimshaw, and Hunter (13) have documented just how complicated the effects of childhood maltreatment can be, particularly when trying to link them to adulthood involvement in HIV risk behaviors. Our findings support the main contentions of these researchers, and suggest that future research in this area would be well-advised to examine exactly how it is that childhood maltreatment leads to greater risk taking later in life. In particular, we believe that research focusing on the psychological and psychosocial effects of being maltreated, and how exactly it is that these psychological/psychosocial effects are related to subsequent risk behavior taking, would be beneficial and informative to the scientific community.

In addition to the preceding, we would also like to point out that, in this study, the single most useful, or applicable, measure of childhood maltreatment was emotional neglect. This stands in contrast to most of the previously-published studies, which generally have focused specifically on sexual abuse. In the analyses conducted in conjunction with the present research, the total amount of childhood maltreatment experienced was related to men's levels of self-esteem; but the extent to which they had been victims of emotional neglect during their formative years was related to their levels of self-esteem more closely. When one considers the types of items that comprised the emotional neglect subscale (e.g., "You felt loved" or "Someone in your family helped you feel important or special"), it makes perfect sense that men who had been emotionally neglected during their formative years would have lower self-esteem as adults since they felt isolated as a child/adolescent and did not feel that they had the love and support that society says ought to be there for them. Additionally, it stands to reason that feelings of emotional abandonment and familial betrayal—betrayal of what society tells them they should expect from members of their immediate family—will have a negative impact on a man's self-esteem. A person's self-esteem and sense of self— who he is in the world—are formed when he is young. If he grows up with a good sense of self, then that is likely to remain with him throughout his lifetime. Alternatively, if he suffered from emotional neglect and does not have that good opinion of himself, he is likely to suffer long-term consequences if he does not receive help and counseling to increase his self-esteem.

In conclusion, this study found that childhood maltreatment is important in predicting HIV risk taking in this population of high risk MSM, but not in a manner that has been shown by most other published studies. In this study, emotional neglect was the single most influential measurement of childhood maltreatment that affected HIV risk behavior. It did so by lowering men's levels of self-esteem, which in turn altered their feelings about using condoms in a negative manner, which in turn led them to be less likely to practice protected sex. Future research should attempt to replicate these findings in other populations of MSM to see if they are replicable. If so, this would indicate that HIV prevention interventionists need to address the lasting negative sequelae associated with emotional neglect in childhood— mainly low self-esteem—to interrupt the pathway between childhood emotional neglect and engaging in unprotected sex.

ACKNOWLEDGMENTS

This research was supported by a grant from the National Institute on Drug Abuse (R24-DA019805). The authors would like to acknowledge, with gratitude, the significant contribution made to the study's data collection, data entry, and data cleaning efforts by Thomas P Lambing.

REFERENCES

[1]   McCauley J, Kern DE, Kolodner K, Dill L, Schroder AF, DeChant HK, et al. Clinical characteristics of women with a history of childhood abuse: Unhealed wounds. JAMA 1997;277:1362-8.

[2]   Bensley LS, VanEenwyk J, Simmons KW. Self-reported childhood sexual and physical abuse and adult HIV-risk behaviors and heavy drinking. Am J Prev Med 2000;18:151-8.

[3]   Mimiaga MJ, Noonan E, Donnell D, Safren SA, Koenen KC, Gortmaker S, et al. Childhood sexual abuse is highly associated with HIV risk-taking behavior and infection among MSM in the EXPLORE Study. J Acquir Immune Defic Syndr 2009;51:340-8.

[4]   Smith HA, Markovic N, Danielson ME, Matthews A, Youk A, Talbott EO, Larkby C, Hughes T. Sexual abuse, sexual orientation, and obesity in women. J Womens Health 2010;19:1525-32.

[5]   Dorais M. Hazardous journey of intimacy: HIV transmission reisk behaviors of young men who are victims of past sexual abuses and who have sexual relations with men. J Homosex, 2004;48:103-24.

[6]   Schraufnagela TJ, Davis KS, George WH, Norris J. Childhood sexual abuse in males and subsequent risky sexual behavior: A potential alcohol-use pathway. Child Abuse Negl 2010;34:369-78.

[7]   Fields SD, Malebranche D, Feist-Price S. Childhood sexual abuse in black men who have sex with men: Results from three qualitative studies. Cultur Divers Ethnic Minor Psychol, 2008;14:385-90.

[8]   Catania JA, Paul J, Osmond D, Folkman S, Pollack L, Canchola J, Chang J, Nellands T. Mediators of childhood sexual abuse and high-risk sex among men-who-have-sex-with-men. Child Abuse Negl 2008;32:925-40.

[9]   O'Leary A, Purcell D, Remien RH, Gomez C. Childhood sexual abuse and sexual transmission risk behaviour among HIV-positive men who have sex with men. AIDS Care 2003:15:17-26.

[10]   Brennan DJ, Hellerstedt WL, Ross MW, Welles SL. History of childhood sexual abuse and HIV risk behaviors in homosexual and bisexual men. Am J Public Health 2007;97:1107-12.

[11]   Gore-Felton C, Kalichman SC, Brondino MJ, Benotsch EG, Cage M, DiFonzo K. Childhood sexual abuse and HIV risk among men who have sex with men: Initial test of a conceptual model. J Fam Violence 2006;21:263-70.

[12]   Saewyc E, Skay C, Richens K, Reis E, Poon C, Murphy A. Sexual orientation, sexual abuse, and HIV-risk behaviors among adolescents in the Pacific Northwest. Am J Public Health 2006;96:1104-10.

[13]   Rosario M, Schrimshaw EW, Hunter J. A model of sexual risk behaviors among young gay and bisexual men: Longitudinal associations of mental health, substance abuse, sexual abuse, and the coming-out process. AIDS Educ Prev 2006;18:444-60.

[14]   Paul JP, Catania J, Pollack L, Stall R. Understanding childhood sexual abuse as a predictor of sexual risk-taking among men who have sex with men: The Urban Men's Health Study. Child Abuse Negl 2001;25:557-84.

[15]   Singer M. Introduction to syndemics: A systems approach to public and community health. San Francisco, CA: Jossey-Bass, 2009.

[16]   Singer MC, Erickson PI, Badiane L, Diaz R, Ortiz D, Abraham T, Nicolaysen AM. Syndemics, sex and the city: Understanding sexually transmitted diseases in social and cultural context. Soc Sci Med, 2006;63:2010-21.

[17]   Walkup J, Blank MB, Gonzales JS, Safren S, Schwartz R, Brown L, et al. The impact of mental health and substance abuse factors on HIV prevention and treatment. J Acquir Immune Defic Syndr 2008; 47:s15-9.

[18]   Romero-Daza N, Weeks M, Singer M. "Nobody gives a damn if I live or die": Violence, drugs, and street-level prostitution in inner-city Hartford, Connecticut. Med Anthropol 2003;22:233-59.

[19]   Stall R, Mills T, Williamson J, Hart T. Association of co-occurring psychosocial health problems and increased vulnerability to HIV/AIDS among urban men who have sex with men. Am J Public Health 2003;93:939-42.

[20]   Gielen AC, Ghandour RM, Burke JG, Mahoney P, McDonnell KA, O'Campo P. HIV/AIDS and intimate partner violence: Intersecting women's health issues in the United States. Trauma Violence Abuse, 2007;8:178-98.

[21]   Mustanski B, Garofalo R, Herrick A, Donenberg G. Psychosocial health problems increase risk for HIV among urban young men who have sex with men: Preliminary evidence of a syndemic in need of attention. Ann Behav Med 2007;34:37-45.

[22]   Senn TE, Carey MP, Vanable PA. The intersection of violence, substance use, depression, and STDs: Testing of a syndemic pattern among patients attending an urban STD clinic. J Natl Med Assoc 2010;102:614-20.

[23]   Bernstein DP, Fink L. Childhood Trauma Questionnaire: A retrospective self-report manual. San Antonio, TX: Psychological Corporation, 1998.

[24]   Brown IS. Development of a scale to measure attitude toward the condom as a method of birth control. J Sex Res 1984;20:255-63.

[25]   Rosenberg M. Society and the adolescent self-image. Princeton, NJ: Princeton University Press, 1965.

[26]   Radloff LS. The CES-D scale: A self-report depression scale for research in the general population. Appl Psychol Meas 1977;1:385-401.

Submitted: March 12, 2011. *Revised:* April 30, 2011.
Accepted: May 07, 2011.

In: Public Health Yearbook 2012
Editor: Joav Merrick

ISBN: 978-1-62808-078-0
© 2013 Nova Science Publishers, Inc.

Chapter 4

PATIENT ACTIVATION AMONG PEOPLE WHO CONTACT CHRONIC DISEASE RELATED CONSUMER HEALTH ORGANIZATIONS

Julie H Dean[*]*, PhD, Frances M Boyle, PhD, Allyson J Mutch, PhD and Remo Ostini, PhD*

School of Population Health and Healthy Communities Research Centre,
The University of Queensland, Australia

ABSTRACT

The concept of self-management has gained prominence as health systems worldwide confront increasing rates of chronic disease. Effective self-management is associated with better health outcomes for individuals and the health system. Consumer health organizations (CHOs) are ideally placed to improve people's capacity for self-management by providing information, education and psychosocial support. However, the role of CHOs in the chronic disease self-management agenda has received little research attention. This study explores the association between people's ability to manage their health and their involvement in CHO activities. Study participants were 273 people recruited following contact with one of seven CHOs in Brisbane, Australia. The CHOs addressed diabetes, arthritis, osteoporosis, cardiovascular disease, chronic hepatitis and renal disease. Participants completed two computer-assisted telephone interviews, 4 months apart. Data were collected on patient activation and the nature and extent of CHO contact. Those with a longer history of CHO contact had significantly higher levels of patient activation and reported greater CHO involvement during the course of the study. Most (91%) engaged in some form of CHO activity, most commonly by reading printed materials (78%) and being a member of the CHO (73%). The study points to a role for CHOs in chronic disease self-management and underlines the issue of access and the importance of developing and evaluating strategies designed to reach those with greatest need.

[*] Correspondence: Julie H Dean, School of Population Health, The University of Queensland, Public Health Building, Herston Road, Herston, QLD 4006, Australia. E-mail: j.dean@sph.uq.edu.au

Keywords: Consumer health organizations, patient activation, self-management, chronic disease

INTRODUCTION

The term 'patient activation' is used to describe the extent to which people have the ability to manage their health and health care (1). Activated patients embody capabilities including knowledge, skills, beliefs and behaviours to effectively care for their health. The concept of patient activation is increasingly important given the rising prevalence of chronic disease and the growing emphasis by health systems worldwide on chronic disease self-management as one strategy to address this challenge (2-4). Evidence suggests that people with a chronic illness who are active in the management of their condition accrue benefits including increases in healthy behaviours, informed decision-making, adherence to health care decisions, containment of health care costs and better health outcomes (5-7).

Hibbard and her colleagues (1,8) conceptualized patient activation as encompassing a range of elements important in self-management that extend beyond attention to any single health behavior; such as self-efficacy, readiness to change health behaviours, development of a partnership with the health team and capacity to navigate the health system. Patient activation is seen as developmental, involving four hierarchical stages. Early in the developmental continuum are basic knowledge and beliefs about the health condition and patient role, or 'believing the active role is important.' The next step is 'having confidence and knowledge to take action.' 'Taking action' is the third stage, while the highest level of activation is maintenance of lifestyle change, particularly in the face of challenging circumstances, or 'staying the course under stress'(1). Patient activation can change over time, with research showing that gains in activation can follow a health intervention (e.g. a self-management program), and are accompanied by increasing self-care behaviours (7).

Consumer health organizations (CHOs) are broadly defined as non-profit or voluntary sector organizations that promote and represent the interests of users and/or carers (9). CHOs typically draw on the principles of self-help to provide information, education and psychosocial support, and aim to increase personal empowerment and control (10). Humphreys and Ribisl (1999) identified such organizations as an important and substantial resource to address public health problems, with three main avenues for contribution: offering accessible and effective interventions for specific problems; enhancing professionally run health promotion and health care programs; and enriching community life and building a base for public health advocacy (11). CHOs provide a variety of educational, skills training and support options relevant to the promotion of self-management, including information brochures/booklets, newsletters, links to other resources, telephone and Internet-based support, educational activities, and support groups. As such, they can accommodate a range of individual preferences and circumstances with options for low intensity participation that occurs 'at a distance' (e.g., reading the organization's newsletters) or higher intensity 'hands on' participation (e.g., volunteering with the CHO, attending regular face-to-face support meetings). CHOs offer an existing and relatively low-cost health system resource and evidence points to their benefits for people with chronic health conditions, including improvements in knowledge, mastery, coping strategies and psychosocial wellbeing (11-13). However, little is known about how people use chronic disease related CHOs or the role of such orgnisations in relation to people's capacity for chronic disease self-management. We sought to address this research gap by examining the association between patient activation and CHO involvement among people who contacted a CHO about a chronic health condition. Study participants were surveyed on two occasions, four months apart, providing a rare longitudinal perspective.

METHODS

The study involved a two-wave survey of people who contacted CHOs located in Brisbane, Australia. The CHOs provided services to people with diabetes, arthritis, osteoporosis, cardiovascular disease, chronic hepatitis or renal disease. In the main these diseases are prevalent and contribute to a large proportion of the burden of morbidity in Australia (14). All Brisbane-based CHOs addressing these conditions were invited to be involved [13 in total], with seven in a position to participate in the research. The inclusion criteria for the organizations were: private/non-government, managed by a voluntary board, non-profit distributing, formally organized and self-governing (15). Each organization identified the main avenue through which people made initial contact and this became the point of recruitment for participants into the study; for four organizations it was by telephone (Arthritis Queensland, Diabetes Australia, Hepatitis Council of Queensland, Kidney Support Network) and for three organizations it was via attendance at group activities (Ankylosing Spondylitis Group of Queensland, Arthritis Friendship Group Queensland, Heart Support Australia). Recruiting participants through one avenue over a specified time period reduced the burden to the organizations while still enabling the large majority of their contacts to be invited to participate in the study.

Participating CHOs invited eligible people who had contacted the organization between June-August 2006 to take part in a computer assisted telephone interview (CATI) conducted by The University of Queensland. Participant eligibility criteria included: aged 18 years or older, ability to complete a telephone interview, telephoning the CHO or attending a group meeting during the period of recruitment, and contacting the CHO in relation to their own health or that of a family member or friend (health professionals and others seeking general information were excluded). CHO workers recorded the age and sex of all eligible participants and the contact details of those who agreed to take part were forwarded to the research team.

Those who agreed were posted information about the project on The University of Queensland letterhead, along with a $5(AUD) supermarket voucher. Participants completed two 20-30 minute telephone interviews four months apart. Up to 10 call-backs were made in an effort to contact all eligible participants. Verbal consent was obtained and recorded by the CATI interviewer prior to commencement of the survey questionnaire. The study was approved by The University of Queensland's Behavioural and Social Sciences Ethical Review Committee.

Measures

Activation to self-manage a chronic condition was measured using the Patient Activation Measure (PAM) short form, a 13-item unidimensional, measure that assesses a person's knowledge, skill and confidence to manage their health or chronic condition (1, 8). Activation scores range from 0 to 100, with higher scores indicating a higher level of activation. Example items include 'When all is said and done, I am the person who is responsible for managing my health condition' and 'I am confident that I can maintain lifestyle changes like diet and exercise even during times of stress'. Response options were on a four-point Likert-type scale from 'agree strongly' to 'disagree strongly'. The PAM showed high reliability in the study sample with Cronbach's alpha 0.91 for the first survey and 0.90 for the second.

Measures of participation in CHO activities were developed from a review of relevant literature and our own previous research (16,17). The survey examined nine types of CHO activities available to the study participants. At the four-month interview, all were asked if they had engaged in any of the following nine activities since the previous interview: telephoned the CHO; read the CHO newsletter or other printed information; attended a CHO seminar, workshop or information session; talked with other CHO members; attended a support group or social outing; helped as a volunteer; used CHO services (e.g., exercise classes, medical aids or counselling); used CHO information to raise awareness of the condition among others; or been a member of the CHO. The nine CHO activities were examined individually and then tallied, to give each participant a score from 1-9. Standard demographic items (age, sex, country of origin, employment status, age left school and private health insurance status) as used by the Australian Bureau of Statistics (2004) were included in the survey (18). The survey questionnaire was pre-tested with CHO members and people from the wider community to confirm face and content validity.

Data analysis

SPSS 16 (SPSS for Windows, Rel 16.0, Chicago, 2007) was used for data analysis.

Summary statistics were calculated to describe the participants' socio-demographic characteristics and types of CHO activities. Associations between PAM scores and CHO activity were analyzed using t-tests and one-way ANOVA. Paired samples t-tests were used to assess changes in PAM scores across the two interviews. P values = 0.05 were considered statistically significant.

RESULTS

During the recruitment period 497 eligible people contacted the seven participating CHOs: 367 (73.8%) agreed to be contacted by the researchers and 323 completed the first interview (overall response rate 64.9%). The majority also completed the second survey (306; 94.7%). There were no statistically significant differences between respondents and non-respondents with respect to sex, age or health condition. Further, no statistically significant differences were found between those who did and did not complete the second survey for these variables or for measures of participation in CHO activities and patient activation. The following analyses focus on the 273 people who contacted a CHO in relation to their own health and completed both surveys.

The study participants were predominantly female (66.8%) with a mean age of 61.5 years (median 62, range 19-93). The majority (81.8%) were born in Australia and 61.9% were married. Just over one-quarter were in the paid workforce (29.4%) and half were retired (53.8%). Almost three-quarters (72.8%) had left school at age 16 years or younger, and 57.5% had private health insurance. The two main chronic conditions motivating CHO contact were diabetes (44.4%) and arthritis/ankylosing spondylitis (42.6%). Smaller numbers contacted for heart disease (9.4%), kidney disease or hepatitis (each 1.7%). Around one-third (31.1%) of the participants were making their first ever contact with the CHO when recruited to the study while the remainder had made contact previously: 9.3% had made their first contact less than one year ago, 24.0% from one to five years ago and 35.6% more than six years ago.

Levels of patient activation

The mean PAM score for participants at the first interview, soon after their contact with a CHO, was 67.0 (sd =15.5). Participants with a prior history of CHO contact had significantly higher activation scores than those who had contacted the CHO for the first time (68.8, sd=15.9 vs 63.1, sd=13.7, p=0.004). The mean PAM score at the second interview, four months later, was 67.8 (sd=15.0). This represented a non-significant change across the two interviews and the difference between those with and without a history of CHO contact remained statistically significant (69.3, sd=14.7 vs 64.4, sd=15.2, p=0.01).

Patient activation and participation in CHO activities

At the second interview, the 273 participants were asked whether or not they had engaged in CHO activities since the first interview four months earlier. Most (91%) reported having engaged in at least one of the nine possible CHO activities, with 26% of respondents reporting five or more activities (see table 1). Slightly less than half the respondents (46%) had initiated some form of further contact with the CHO (such as making a further telephone call, attending a CHO support group).

Less active forms of participation – reading the newsletter or other printed information produced by the CHO (78%) and being a member of the CHO (73%) – were the most commonly reported activities. Communicating information gained from the CHO with others (45%), telephoning the CHO (34%), talking with other CHO members (33%) and using CHO services and products (32%) were the next most frequently reported activities. Only a minority (11%-15%) had attended a support group, social outing, seminar or information session hosted by the CHO or helped as a volunteer.

Table 1 also shows the association between participants' PAM scores at the initial interview and their subsequent CHO activity. Overall, those who reported higher levels of CHO involvement were more activated to manage their health, with mean scores significantly higher among those who subsequently had engaged in a greater number of activities (p<0.02) and those who initiated further contact (p=0.02).

Those who read the CHO newsletter or other printed information (p=0.02), attended a CHO seminar workshop or information session (p=0.02), or were a member of the CHO (p=0.04) had significantly higher mean PAM scores at the first study interview than those who reported no involvement in these activities during the four-month study period.

Table 1. Participation in CHO activities over the 4-month study period and mean PAM score (with standard deviation) at initial study interview (n=273 survey respondents who completed both interviews)

CHO activity		n	%	Mean PAM Score (±SD)	p-value
Total number of CHO activities	*None*	25	9.2	61.68±12.85	
	1-4	177	64.8	66.29±15.06	*0.02**
	5-9	71	26.0	70.79±16.59	
Made further contact with the CHO	*Yes*	125	45.8	69.34±15.06	*0.02**
	No	148	54.2	65.09±15.56	
Telephoned the CHO	*Yes*	92	33.7	69.35±15.38	*0.08*
	No	181	66.3	65.86±15.40	
Read the CHO newsletter or other printed information	*Yes*	214	78.4	68.21±15.16	*0.02**
	No	59	21.6	62.79±15.88	
Attended a CHO seminar, workshop or information session	*Yes*	30	11.0	72.90±14.08	*0.02**
	No	243	89.0	66.32±15.49	
Talked with other CHO members	*Yes*	89	32.6	68.36±15.83	*0.33*
	No	184	67.4	66.40±15.27	
Attended a CHO support group/social outing	*Yes*	40	14.7	69.70±16.08	*0.24*
	No	233	85.3	66.58±15.33	
Helped as a volunteer	*Yes*	34	12.5	71.58±15.78	*0.07*
	No	239	87.5	66.39±15.33	
Used CHO services (e.g. counseling, exercise classes, products)	*Yes*	86	31.5	69.09±16.77	*0.14*
	No	187	68.5	66.09±14.75	
Used information from the CHO to help raise awareness among other people	*Yes*	124	45.4	67.46±15.29	*0.68*
	No	149	54.6	66.69±15.62	
Member of the CHO	*Yes*	199	72.9	68.04±15.78	*0.04**

DISCUSSION

The findings of this study demonstrate a consistent pattern of associations between patient activation and CHO involvement among people who had contacted a CHO about a chronic health condition. A longer history of CHO contact and greater engagement in CHO activities were both significantly associated with higher patient activation. Those with a history of CHO contact were more activated than those who had made their first contact with a CHO immediately before joining the study. This difference remained at the four-month follow-up. Though most participants engaged in some form of CHO activity between the two study interviews, patient activation emerged as a predictor of the extent of subsequent CHO activity: higher PAM scores were associated with the initiation of further CHO contact and engagement in a greater number of activities, especially reading the newsletter, attending a seminar, and being a member of the CHO.

To our knowledge, this is the first published study of the association between patient activation and CHO use among people with chronic illness. A key strength of the study is the recruitment of a close-to consecutive sample of CHO contacts.

A frequent criticism of research involving CHOs and other patient support groups is the self-selection of participants. We sought to address this limitation by recruiting a consecutive sample that included participants who were not necessarily committed CHO supporters, including those who made a 'one-off' phone call. Although there were occasional discontinuities in recruitment, these were due to staffing issues for CHOs and seem unlikely to have produced systematic sample bias. Caution is needed in generalizing the study findings as our sample was recruited by a small number of CHOs in a defined geographical area over a four month period and represents a 65% response rate. Despite finding no significant differences between respondents and non-respondents in relation to type of chronic condition, age or sex, it is possible there were other underlying differences between these groups. As participation in the study required people to speak English to a sufficient level to complete a telephone interview people from culturally and linguistically diverse backgrounds were under-represented. It also must be acknowledged that all data were collected by self-report and therefore subject to reporting error, including social desirability. Despite these limitations, the findings provide previously unavailable insights into the association between engagement with CHOs and patient activation. A particular strength of the study is the collection of data on two occasions to enable a prospective analysis of CHO activity in relation to patient activation and an assessment of PAM score changes over time.

Whether CHO contact led to increased patient activation or whether the observed associations reflected already higher levels of patient activation among those who contacted CHOs and participated in their activities is difficult to establish without a comparison group of people who had not contacted a CHO. Certainly our results indicate that more highly activated people have a greater propensity to engage in CHO activities. There was no change in PAM scores across the two time points, suggesting that CHO contact does not lead to greater activation. However, it is possible that a follow-up period of four months was too short to assess adequately the outcomes of an initial CHO contact. Longer exposure to a CHO might be needed to give people sufficient opportunities to engage in different activities and to gain benefits. Those participants with a longer history of CHO contact were more highly activated. Most had made their first contact at least one year ago, adding support to the possibility that benefits may accumulate over a longer time-frame than covered in this study. However, it may also be the case that those who are more highly activated are also more likely to both initiate and continue CHO contact.

People with a chronic condition frequently face challenges in adopting health-promoting behaviours (19) and a substantial majority require self-management support of some form

(20). Despite the potential role of CHOs in this regard, only a minority of people with a chronic illness ever contact such organizations (21, 22) and studies of various self-management programs show such initiatives frequently fail to reach certain groups (23). Our findings add to this knowledge by showing that people who are already activated to manage their health have a greater propensity to engage with CHOs than those whose capacity for self-management may be limited.

The study underlines the issue of access and the importance of developing and evaluating strategies designed to reach those with greatest need. Improving CHO access might be achieved by developing entry points that are effectively communicated, easily accessed, culturally sensitive and provide immediate benefit to participants (9,24). Greater integration of CHOs in formal health system structures, including referral pathways is also likely to facilitate timely and broader access (2,20,25). Further research is needed to understand the actual and potential role of CHOs in relation to chronic disease self-management especially for those who may stand to benefit most.

ACKNOWLEDGMENTS

The research reported in this paper is a project of the Australian Primary Health Care Research Institute, which is supported by a grant from the Australian Government Department of Health and Ageing. The information and opinions contained in it do not necessarily reflect the views or policy of the Australian Primary Health Care Research Institute or the Australian Government Department of Health and Ageing. The authors thank the participating consumer health organizations for their assistance with recruitment and support of the study as well as the consumers who took part in the study.

REFERENCES

[1]   Hibbard JH, Stockard J, Mahoney ER, Tusler M. Development of the Patient Activation Measure (PAM): Conceptualizing and measuring activation in patients and consumers. Health Serv Res 2004;39(4):1005-26.

[2]   Fisher EB, Brownson CA, O'Toole ML, Anwuri VV, Shetty G. Perspectives on self-management from the Diabetes initiative of the Robert Wood Johnson Foundation. Diabetes Educ 2007;33(Suppl 6):S216-S24.

[3]   Jordan JE, Osborne RH. Chronic disease self-management education programs: Challenges ahead. Med J Aust 2007;186(2):84-7.

[4]   Muir Gray JA. Self-management in chronic illness. Lancet 2004;364(9444):1467-8.

[5]   Bodenheimer T, Lorig K, Holman H, Grumbach K. Patient self-management of chronic disease in primary care. JAMA 2002;288(19):2469-75.

[6]   Lorig KR, Sobel DS, Stewart AL, Brown BW, Bandura A, Ritter P, et al. Evidence suggesting that a chronic disease self-management program can improve health status while reducing hospitalization: A randomized trial. Med Care 1999;37(1):5-14.

[7]   Hibbard JH, Mahoney ER, Stock R, Tusler M. Do increases in patient activation result in improved self-management behaviors? Health Serv Res 2007;42(4):1443-63.

[8]   Hibbard JH, Mahoney ER, Stockard J, Tusler M. Development and testing of a short form of the Patient Activation Measure. Health Serv Res 2005;40(6 part 1):1918-30.

[9]   Allsop J, Baggott R, Jones K. Health consumer groups and the national health policy process. In: Henderson S, Petersen A, eds. Consuming health. The commodification of health care. London: Routledge, 2002:48-65.

[10]   Kurtz LF. Self-help and support groups: A handbook for practitioners. Thousand Oaks: Sage, 1997.

[11]   Humphreys K, Ribisl K. The case for a partnership with self-help groups. Public Health Rep 1999;114:322-9.

[12]   Kyrouz E, Humphreys K, Loomis C. A review of research on the effectiveness of self-help mutual aid groups. In: White BJ, Madara EJ, editors. The self-help sourcebook: Your guide to community and online support groups, 7th ed. Cedar Knolls: American Self-Help Group Clearinghouse, 2002:71-85.

[13]   Grant C, Goodenough T, Harvey I, Hine C. A randomised controlled trial and economic evaluation of a referrals facilitator between primary care and the voluntary sector. BMJ 2000;320:419-23.

[14]   Begg SJ, Vos T, Barker B, Stanley L, Lopez AD. Burden of disease and injury in Australia in the new millennium: Measuring health loss from diseases, injuries and risk factors. Med J Aust 2008;188(1):36-40.

[15]   Salamon L, Anheier H. The emerging nonprofit sector: An overview. Manchester: Manchester University Press, 1996.

[16]   Boyle FM, Posner TN, Del Mar CB, McLean J, Bush RA. Self-help organisations: A qualitative study of successful collaboration with general practice. Aust J Prim Health 2003;9(2/3):75-9.

[17]   Coppa K, Boyle FM. The role of self-help groups in chronic illness management: A qualitative study. Aust J Prim Health 2003;9(2/3):68-74.

[18]   Australian Bureau of Statistics. National Health Survey and National Aboriginal and Torres Strait Islander Health Survey 2004/2005. Canberra: Australian Bureau of Statistics, 2004.

[19]   De Ridder D, Geenen R, Kuijer R, Van Middendorp H. Psychological adjustment to chronic disease. Lancet 2008;372(9634):246-55.

[20]   Jordan JE, Briggs AM, Brand CA, Osborne RH. Enhancing patient engagement in chronic disease self-management support initiatives in Australia: The need for an integrated approach. Med J Aust 2008;189(Supplement 10):S9-S13.

[21]   Ellins J, Coulter A. How engaged are people in their health care? Findings of a national telephone survey. Oxford: Picker Institute Europe, 2005.

[22]   Gucciardi E, Smith PL, DeMelo M. Use of diabetes resources in adults attending a self-management education program. Patient Educ Couns 2006;64(1-3):322-30.

[23]   Rogers A, Kennedy A, Bower P, Gardner C, Gately C, Lee V, et al. The United Kingdom Expert Patients Programme: Results and implications from a national evaluation. Med J Aust 2008;189(Suppl 10):S21-S4.

[24]   Swerissen H, Belfrage J, Weeks A, Jordan L, Walker C, Furler J, et al. A randomised control trial of a self-management program for people with a chronic illness from Vietnamese, Chinese, Italian and Greek backgrounds. Patient Educ Couns 2006;64(1-3):360-8.

[25]   Boyle F, Mutch A, Dean J, Dick M-L, Del Mar C. Consumer health organisations for people with diabetes and arthritis: Who contacts them and why? Health Soc Care Comm 2009;17(6):628-35.

Submitted: April 27, 2011. *Revised:* July 01, 2011. *Accepted:* July 25, 2011.

In: Public Health Yearbook 2012
Editor: Joav Merrick

ISBN: 978-1-62808-078-0
© 2013 Nova Science Publishers, Inc.

Chapter 5

USE OF OUTSOURCING IN ISRAELI MEDICAL CENTERS

Racheli Magnezi, PhD[*1,2], Liat Korn, PhD[1] and Haim Reuveni, MD[3]

[1]Department of Health Management, School of Health Sciences, Ariel University Center,
[2]Gertner Institute for Epidemiology and Health Policy Research, Ramat Gan and
[3]Department of Health Policy and Management, Ben Gurion University of the Negev,
Beer Sheva, Israel

ABSTRACT

Outsourcing (using external contractors to provide services) is an organizational approach that eliminates business barriers. In healthcare, outsourcing can enhance efficient, quality care. Our objective was to evaluate the use of outsourcing in Israeli hospitals. Factors that affect the decision to outsource, contracts, and funding allocated to outsourcing were compared between private and public hospitals based on a questionnaire sent to 36 administrators. We found that private hospitals invested significantly more in outsourcing than public hospitals (11–20% and 0–10%, respectively; p=0.05). Medium and large hospitals allocated approximately the same budgetary proportion to outsourcing (p=0.24). Urban hospitals allocated more to outsourcing than rural hospitals. Cost containment, flexibility, client satisfaction, and a focus on core services affected the decisions to outsource most; 75% reported that outsourcing saved costs. For private hospitals, outsourcing provided the most added value by focusing on core services, improving service, and using the provider's infrastructure. The greatest disadvantages to public hospitals were resistance to change by personnel and reliability. We concluded that outsourcing is a viable strategy for controlling costs and maintaining quality patient care. It is a well-embedded, managerial-operational strategy, globally. Expanding outsourcing to include medical and administrative services can provide novel business opportunities, enabling cost savings and competition.

Keywords: Outsourcing, private hospitals, public hospitals, Israel

---

[*] Correspondence: Racheli Magnezi, PhD, Department of Health Management, School of Health Sciences, Ariel University Center, Israel. E-mail: rachelim2@bezeqint.net

INTRODUCTION

Health care executives face an ongoing challenge of reducing costs while maintaining quality patient care. Outsourcing is one of the strategic tools healthcare executives use to meet this challenge by transferring services or operating functions to a third party that provides a partnership management (1). The use of outsourcing in the healthcare industry is increasing (2) because it enables the development of innovative services and efficient quality care (3-7). The services most frequently outsourced in the healthcare market are information technology, finance, and support services such as security, food, and training (8, 9). In some healthcare organizations, outsourcing includes medical services such as teleradiology (10, 11), emergency department, and operating service centers (6, 12) such as intensive care units with off-site patient monitoring, using closed-circuit television (13-15).

In Britain, the National Health Service (NHS) outsources healthcare services to private providers to reduce waiting times for surgery, with a high satisfaction rate (16-18). In the United States, improvement in hospital operations is the most important criterion in the decision to outsource; cost savings and improved patient satisfaction are the second and third priorities (19, 20). Additional important factors in the decision to outsource are client satisfaction, quality of service, work environment, approach of the healthcare team, and reduction of costs (21). These parameters resulted in greater patient satisfaction with external service providers than with services provided within the organization. In a random sample survey of 100 public hospitals in Greece, Moschuris and Kondylis found that reduction of costs and client satisfaction were the main reasons for using external contractors (22). Cooperation with the service provider led to considerable improvement in the quality of services. Most users were satisfied and believed that the use of outsourced services would increase (22). In Turkey, private hospitals outsource more services than public hospitals do, mainly in logistics, operations, and medical services such as laboratory and imaging (23). Hospitals in Italy are increasingly outsourcing services; however, the results do not always align with managers' expectations, especially in cost containment and efficiency (24).

Our study compared outsourcing activities in private and public hospitals in the Israeli healthcare arena. Specifically, we analyzed types of contracts, factors that affect the decision to outsource, and budgets allocated to outsourcing. Outsourcing activities were compared according to hospital size and location. We assumed that outsourcing is beneficial for all hospitals, regardless of type of ownership.

METHODS

This study was performed using a quantitative email survey sent to administrative directors of 40 hospitals in Israel in February and March 2008.

The study population included all 40 major hospitals in Israel, comprising approximately 37% of the national healthcare budget. Hospitals were categorized into for-profit (private) organizations or public hospitals, in urban or rural locations.

A questionnaire based on a previous outsourcing questionnaire for hospitals (22) was translated to Hebrew. The questionnaire focused on four parameters: the extent to which hospitals outsource services, the decision-making process when choosing a provider, the impact of outsourcing, and the future trend of outsourcing among hospitals. Questions were translated into Hebrew and back to English to verify the translation. Eight questions reflecting managerial experience were added.

Questionnaires were sent and received by email. Before sending the questionnaires, the administrative director of each hospital, was informed of the objective of the study by telephone and agreed to respond. Respondents were asked:

- To estimate the percentage of the annual hospital budget allocated to outsourcing.
- To estimate their involvement in the decision-making process regarding outsourcing, on a scale from 1 (very little) to 5 (very high).
- How the hospital becomes aware of potential outsourcing service providers.
- To assess the importance of the factors affecting the decision to use outsourcing services, on a scale from 1 (not important) to 5 (very important).
- To rate the importance of criteria for estimating contracts with external providers of services.
- To estimate the effect of outsourcing on the organization.
- To state the difficulties and obstacles that might arise in contracting with service providers.
- To state the benefits of outsourcing to the hospital.
- To state the disadvantages of outsourcing.
- To state whether outsourcing reduced expenses.
- Whether outsourcing reduced the work force and by what percentage.
- To state if they thought that the use of outsourcing would increase or decrease in their hospital over the next three years.

Statistical analysis

Data were recorded and analyzed using the SAS program and tested for reliability. The chi-square test was used to determine frequency differences between the study groups. Significance level was set at 0.05. We used Fisher's Exact Test because of the small sample size.

RESULTS

One private and three public hospitals did not answer the questionnaire and were not included in the study sample. Thus, the 36 hospital administrators (10 from private hospitals and 26 from public hospitals) who responded to the survey represent 90% of the key players in the Israeli healthcare arena.

Twenty-four (67%) were medium-sized hospitals, and 12 (33%) were large. The hospitals were distributed evenly between urban (n=19) and rural locations (n=17). The ten privately owned hospitals were all in the central region of the country.

Administrative and finance personnel had the greatest involvement in outsourcing (70%–100%) among all hospitals, compared to other hospital officials (10%–50); physicians, nursing services, and medical technicians had the least (20%–30%). In privately owned hospitals, 80% of the financial officers, 70% of the administrators, 50% of the purchase managers, and 20% of the legal advisors were involved in the outsourcing process.

Medium and large hospitals allocated approximately the same proportion of their budgets to outsourcing (p=0.24). However, privately owned hospitals invested a larger portion of their budgets in outsourcing than did public hospitals (11–20% and 0–10%, respectively; p=0.05). Urban hospitals outsourced more types of services than did rural hospitals (4–7 and 3–5, respectively), and allocated a larger portion of their budgets to it (6–15% vs. 1–5%, respectively). In comparison to rural hospitals, urban hospitals allocated relatively more (p=0.04) of their budgets to outsourcing.

In 60% of all hospitals, outsourcing contracts were longer than three years, and were for two to three years in 20%. Both private and public hospitals in urban areas found that the development of new services provided operational flexibility and improved their image. As expected, 75% of all hospitals confirmed that outsourcing reduced expenses and improved services. The main savings were in cleaning (33%), security (28%), and laundry services (14%). Reduced manpower was attributed to outsourcing by 88% of the hospitals, who used external contractors for security (33%), cleaning (45%), laundry (17%), database systems (14%), and maintenance (14%). Reductions in manpower ranged from 1–10% in about 85% of the hospitals (p < 0.01).

Private hospitals tended to outsource more services than public hospitals. Outsourcing of legal services and cafeteria services were similar (Table 1). The most significant differences were for food (p=0.0032) and laboratory services (p=0.0024).

Table 1. Outsourcing contracts among private (for-profit) and public (not-for-profit) hospitals (n=36)

| Service area | Private hospitals n=10 (%) | Public hospitals n=26 | | | Total |
		Public hospitals n=7(%)	Government hospitals n=11(%)	HMO hospitals n=8 (%)	(%)
Cleaning	6 (60)	7 (100)	6 (56)	8 (100)	21 (80.7)
Security	8 (80)	6 (86)	8 (73)	8 (100)	22 (92.3)
Laundry	9 (90)	4 (57)	6 (56)	5 (63)	15 (57.7)
Food*	7 (70)	1(14)	1 (9)	2 (25)	4 (15.4)
Cafeteria	4 (40)	5 (71)	3 (27)	5 (6%)	13 (50)
Laboratory**	6 (60)	1 (14)	0	1 (12)	2 (0.8)
Legal services	4 (40)	4 (57)	1 (9)	5 (63)	10 (38.5)
Database systems	5 (50)	3 (43)	3 (27)	4 (40)	10 (38.5)
Medical services	4 (40)	3 (43)	0	1 (12)	4(1.6)

p < 0.05, *p = 0.0032, **p = 0.0024.

Most hospitals chose one provider over another because of price (53%), meetings with consultants and experts (50%), prior experience (44%), cost containment (81%), client satisfaction (69%), focus on core services (72%), operational flexibility (75%), funding of service providers (80%), and lack of skilled workers in the field (58%). Cost containment was less of a concern for privately owned hospitals than for publicly owned hospitals (50% vs.

70–80%, respectively). Half of private hospitals stated that focusing on core services played an important role in their decision to hire external services, compared to 14.3% of public hospitals. As shown in Figure 1, cost containment (85%) and client satisfaction (73%) had the greatest impact on the decision of publicly owned hospitals to outsource, compared to privately owned hospitals (70% and 60%, respectively). Comparing private hospitals to public hospitals, the most influential factors in the decision to outsource were focusing on core services (80% vs. 69%), operational flexibility (90% vs. 69%), and improved image (40% vs. 23%), respectively.

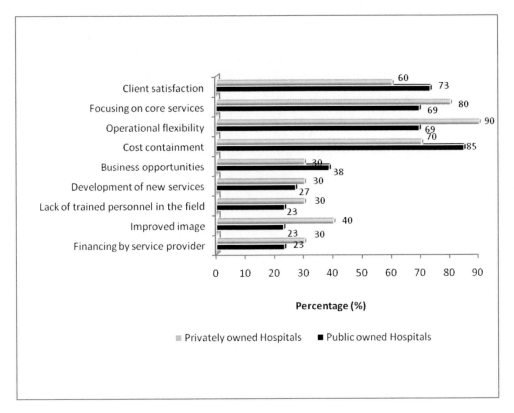

Figure 1. Factors (in %) affecting the decision to outsource among private and public hospitals (n=36).

The major advantages of outsourcing for public compared to private hospitals were financial benefits (77% vs. 30%), and increased flexibility (77% vs. 70%), respectively (Figure 2). Outsourcing was more advantageous for private hospitals in the areas of focus on core services (70% vs. 46%), improved quality of service (60% vs. 50%), decreased risks (30% vs. 19%), and using provider resources (80% vs. 27%). The biggest differences between the types of hospitals were in using the service provider's infrastructure (p=0.017) and financial benefits (p=0.017).

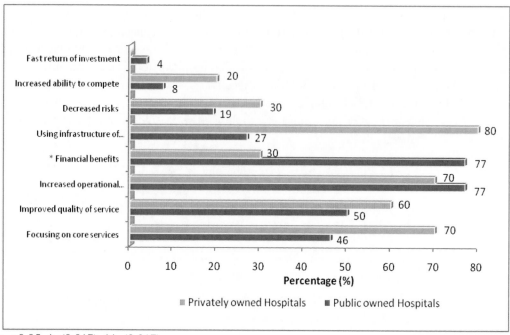

p < 0.05, *p(0.017), **p(0.017).

Figure 2. Advantages (in %) of outsourcing as perceived by private and public hospitals (n=36).

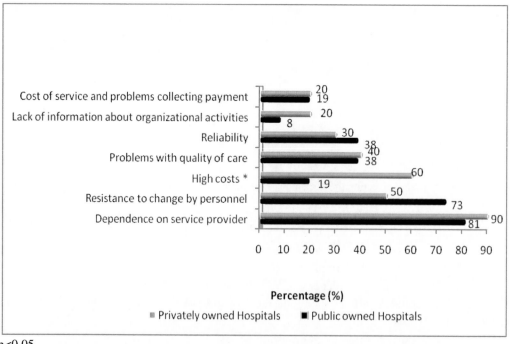

p<0.05.

Figure 3. Limitations of outsourcing as perceived by private and public hospitals (n=36).

The greatest limitations of outsourcing as perceived by private compared to public hospitals were dependence on service provider (90% vs. 81%), high costs (60% vs. 19%), and lack of information about organizational activities (20% vs. 8%), respectively (Figure 3).

DISCUSSION

Purchasing services through outsourcing is an operational strategy used by hospital managers. Our study shows that privately owned hospitals use more external contractors for medical services (laboratory, imaging, doctors, and nurses) than public hospitals do. Outsourcing is used mainly in the areas of patient food, laundry, and cafeteria services. It also eliminates work force positions and is a means of containing costs.

The greatest portion of the hospital budget in Israel compared to other hospitals worldwide is allocated to security. Due to the political situation in the Middle East, security is the most frequently outsourced service among all hospitals. Similar findings were reported in Turkey (23).

A. Outsourcing in private and public hospitals

Similar to our findings, Callahan found that privately owned hospitals use more outsourcing contactors than public hospitals do and allocate twice as much of their budgets to outsourcing (about 20% and 10%, respectively), mainly for services such as patient meals and laundry (19). Whereas public hospitals in Israel are bound by national, collective wage agreements and directives of the Ministries of Health and Finance, which require them to choose outsourcing services based primarily on price offers or tenders, private hospitals have more latitude in spending. Resistance from employee unions, which fear a loss of power when external employees are contracted, is another factor that restricts outsourcing among public hospitals.

Private hospitals tended to choose external service providers based on previous experiences and meetings with consultants and experts, while public hospitals chose external service providers based on price and meetings with consultants. Both public and private hospitals found the disadvantages of outsourcing to be dependence on external service providers, resistance of hospital personnel to change, and problems with quality of care.

B. Savings and cost containment versus client satisfaction

Budget savings and cost containment were the most important factors influencing the decision to use external contractors. Decreasing manpower is an important means of containing costs, particularly since wages and benefits comprise more than 60% of organizational budgets. The main savings from outsourcing were in operational and logistics services that are not part of the core healthcare services. Our results also showed that 75% of hospitals reported that outsourcing primarily saved costs in logistics. It was reported that hospital experience with outsourcing (mainly in radiology, laboratory services, call centers, and reduced waiting time for surgery) improved client satisfaction and increased quality, but did not necessarily save costs (19-21). Financial considerations played a significant role in selecting a provider (through price offers), and the objective was to sign long-term agreements, which required the appraisal of benefits and long-term cooperation with the service provider.

C. Budget allocation to outsourcing

Compared to large hospitals, our study showed that medium-sized hospitals allocated a greater percentage of their budgets to outsourcing. Urban hospitals tend to have a larger infrastructure, more staff and equipment, as well as more money to invest in outsourcing than rural hospitals. Because of higher budgets, urban hospitals are often willing to take more risks. In contrast, in terms of costs vs. benefits, rural hospitals rely more on contracts with an outsourcing provider because of a lack of local resources and services. However, rural hospitals are wary of outsourcing because they may become dependent on the provider. Similar findings were not reported by other studies. It is possible that smaller organizations have greater flexibility and are more open to the use of external contractors. In addition, it is possible that in less populated areas, outsourcing provides more benefit by using expert services that may be lacking in the region.

D. Decision makers and outsourcing of medical services

Private hospitals in some countries use external contractors more for medical services (laboratory, imaging, doctors, and nurses) than do public hospitals (23). Private and independent hospitals are similar in that their budgets are not controlled by the government or HMOs. It is possible that organizations that are less bound by governmental bureaucracy can be more creative in using medical outsourcing (24), with both a greater commitment and greater liability on the part of financial officers and administration.

Decision makers in public hospitals are mainly administrative directors, who are very involved in hiring external non-medical services. In private hospitals, which are more cost- and business-oriented, the Finance Departments are more involved in these decisions. In both types of hospitals, these professionals are the most influential in the decision to outsource. We found that management and legal departments are also very involved. Since finance department personnel are the key decision-makers (7) and not professional healthcare providers, fewer medical services are outsourced in both private and public hospitals.

We found that hospital location (urban vs. rural) was an independent factor that affected the decision to outsource more than did budget allocation. Most urban hospitals had a larger budget, a more diverse pool of outsourcing providers to choose from, and could take bigger financial risks when contracting for outsourcing services.

This study is limited by some of the unique features that exist in the healthcare market in Israel; it includes only 36 hospitals, of which 22% are owned by one HMO and 31% by the Ministry of Health. The number of beds per 1,000 residents is the lowest among OECD countries. Therefore, competition is mainly through the use of novel technologies, as well as outsourcing. Additional studies are needed from other OECD countries who share similar challenges in their healthcare systems to better understand the potential of using outsourcing as a tool to increase competitiveness.

PRACTICE IMPLICATIONS

Outsourcing is a viable strategy for controlling costs and maintaining quality patient care. Therefore, it is a well-embedded managerial-operational strategy among hospitals worldwide. Expanding outsourcing of medical and administrative services can provide novel business opportunities, enable competition in the healthcare area, and save costs. However, development of novel outsourcing activities presents new challenges because it will define new rules in the areas of ethics, law, and quality of healthcare services.

ACKNOWLEDGMENTS

We thank Dr Socrates J Moschuris for kindly providing us with the questionnaire published in the Journal of Health Organization and Management in 2006. We also thank Mr. Benny Rahimi and Ms. Ronit Mizrachi for their contributions to data collection. The authors have no conflicts of interest with any of the material discussed herein.

REFERENCES

[1] Roberts V. Managing strategic outsourcing in the healthcare industry. Jf Healthcare Manage 2001;46:239-49.
[2] Alper M. New trends in healthcare outsourcing. Employee Benefit Plan Review 2004;58:14-7.
[3] Smith BF. The "write" choice: a primer on outsourcing transcription services. Healthcare Finance Manager 2006;60:120-7.
[4] Billi JE, Pai CW, Spahlinger DA. Strategic outsourcing of clinical services: a model for volume-stressed academic medical centers. Health Care Manage Rev 2004;29:291-7.
[5] Dyck D. Outsourcing occupational health services: Critical elements. AAOHN Journal 2002;50:83-93.
[6] Guy RA Jr, Hill JR. 10 outsourcing myths that raise your risk. Health Care Finance Manager 2007;61:66-72.
[7] Stockamp DR. Revenue cycle outsourcing; the real costs benefits. Healthcare Financial Manager 2006;60:84-6,88,90.
[8] Romano M. Back to the basics; number of general hospitals grows for the first time in years despite slim margins, lagging reimbursements and a tight market. Modern Healthcare 2004;34:6-7,12.
[9] Lorence DP, Spink A. Healthcare information systems outsourcing. Int J Inform Manage 2004;24:131.
[10] Turner R. The scans read over the ocean. US News World Rep 2004; 137:60.
[11] Wachter RM. The "dis-location" of US medicine. The implications of medical outsourcing. N Engl J Med 2006;354:661-5.
[12] Piotrowski J. Outsiders get the call. Modern Healthcare 2004;34:49-60.
[13] Davidson, MB. More evidence to support "outsourcing" of diabetes care. Diab Care 2004;27:995.
[14] Breslow MJ, Rosenfeld BA, Doerfler M, et al. Effect of a multiple-site intensive care unit telemedicine program on clinical and economic outcomes: an alternate paradigm for intensives' staffing. Crit Care Med 2004;32:31-8.
[15] Feyrer R, Weyand M, Kunzmann U. Resource management in cardiovascular engineering: is outsourcing the solution. Perfusion 2005; 20:289-94.
[16] Brekke K, Sogard L. Public versus private health care in a national health service. Health Econ 2006;16:579-601.
[17] Dash P. New providers in UK health care. BMJ 2004;328:340-2.
[18] Dixon L, Lewis R, Rosen R, Finlayson B, Gray D. Can the NHS learn from US managed care organizations? BMJ 2004;328:223-6.

[19]   Callahan JM. 10 practical tips for successful outsourcing. Healthcare Financial Manage 2005;59:110-2,114,116.

[20]   Galloro V. Execs bullish on outsourcing. Modern Healthcare 2001;31: 64.

[21]   Magnezi R, Dankner RS, Kedem R, et al. Outsourcing primary medical care in Israeli Defense Forces: Decision-makers' versus clients' perspectives. Health Policy 2006;78:1-6.

[22]   Moschuris S J, Kondylis MN. Outsourcing in public hospitals. A Greek perspective. J Health Org Manage 2006;20:4-15.

[23]   Yigit V, Tengilimoglu D, Kisa A, et al. Outsourcing and its implications for hospital organizations in Turkey. J Health Care Finance 2007;33:86-92.

[24]   Macinati, MS. Outsourcing in the Italian National Health Service: findings from a national survey. Int J Health Plan Manage 2008;23:21-36.

Submitted: June 01, 2011. *Revised:* July 26, 2011. *Accepted:* August 05, 2011.

In: Public Health Yearbook 2012
Editor: Joav Merrick

ISBN: 978-1-62808-078-0
© 2013 Nova Science Publishers, Inc.

Chapter 6

DISPARITIES OF CHILDHOOD LIMITED ABILITIES AND SPECIAL HEALTH CARE NEEDS IN GEORGIA COMPARING WITH OTHER STATES

James H Stephens, PhD, Hani M Samawi, PhD, Gerald R Ledlow, PhD and Rohit Tyagi, MPH[*]

Jiann-Ping Hsu College Public Health, Georgia Southern University, Statesboro, Georgia, United States of America

ABSTRACT

Using data from the National Survey of Children's Health 2003, this article investigates the disparities of children with special care needs and children with limited abilities in Georgia as compared to the combined states of the United States. Asthma, ADD or ADHD, depression, behavioral or conduct problems, bone or muscle problems, diabetes, and physical impairment are the significant factors that affect children with special care needs in Georgia. However gender, age, poverty level, depression, diabetes, autism, and physical impairment are factors that affect children with special care needs in the combined US states with the state of Georgia removed. This study compared the State of Georgia to the combined U.S. states regarding special care needs and limited abilities children based on morbidities, co-morbidities and demographic and socio-economic factors. Children with asthma, ADD/ADHD, depression or anxiety problems, behavioral and conduct problems, bone, joint and muscle problems, developmental delay or physical impairment and children living in poverty are significantly more susceptible for requiring special care needs in Georgia.

Keywords: Disparities, children with limited abilities, children with special care

---

[*] Correspondence: Hani Samawi, PhD, Jiann-Ping Hsu College of Public Health, Georgia Southern University, P.O. Box 8015, Statesboro, GA 30460-8015. Phone: 912-478-1345; FAX: 912-478-5811, E-mail: hsamawi@georgiasouthern.edu.

INTRODUCTION

Children with special health care needs are a special population for health care services, economic, and policy making perspectives (1,2). The national child health survey-2003 (3) indicates that children with special needs comprise 10.64% of children in Georgia and 11.26% for United States; children with limited ability comprise 5.74% of children in Georgia as compared to 5.32% in the rest of the nation.

The federal Maternal and Child Health Bureau (4) characterize children with special health care needs are those who have or are at increased risk for a chronic physical, developmental, behavioral, or emotional condition. These children also require more health care related services as compared to children generally. They are an important population from the health care services, economic, and policy making perspectives. These children have high risk for having mental and behavioral health problems, increased bed days and school absence days, unmet health care needs and unscheduled intensive care unit admissions (4,5).

There are a variety of public health concerns related to children with special care needs and limited abilities. One is the availability and adequacy of health insurance coverage. Children with special care needs are more likely than the population of children as a whole to have insurance. Access to care is the presence of a usual source of care that families can turn to when their child is sick, as well as a personal doctor or nurse who knows the child and his or her particular needs (6). Care for children with special care needs must also be family-centered (7,8). Providers must spend enough time with the family to ensure that they have the information they need, listen to the family's concerns and be sensitive to the family's values and customs (9). Other impacts of children with special care needs are on the family's time, finances, and employment status (10,11).

The following section describes the methods used as well as the socio-demographic characteristics and medical history of children in relation to children with special care needs and children with limited ability. Results of the analysis, including the building of two logistic regression models, one for children with special care needs and the other for children with limited care, follow the methods discussion. Lastly, a conclusion discusses the results and findings in context along with a final set of recommendations.

METHODS

The total population of Georgia was about 8.2 million people in 2000 and an estimated 10 million in 2010 (Table 1) (12). The state of Georgia had about 2.2 million children in 2000.

The National Survey of Children's Health (3), served as the secondary data source for the study. The sample for Georgia is shown in Table 2. Table 2 shows that the majority of the sample is white. Some of the participants did not provide information on their racial/ethnic background, and this subgroup is identified as "Unknown" in the table.

Data for this study were obtained from the NSCH database, which contains information from all states. Data were analyzed using SAS Version 9.1(13). The Pearson Chi-square test with significant level 0.05 (14) was used to investigate association of children with limited abilities and special health care needs with socio-demographic factors, and medical conditions. Odds ratios and 95% confidence limits were calculated to assess the magnitude of observed association by socio-demographic factors, and medical conditions. To control for the effect of other factors, four multivariate logistic models are used (two for Georgia and two for the combined U.S. states with Georgia removed).

Data analysis

As indicated by (14), logistic regression is called a generalized linear model. Logistic regression usually used to predict a dichotomous dependent (response) variable such as presence/absence or success/failure. The dependent variable in logistic regression can take the value 1 with a probability of success θ, or the value 0 with probability of failure 1-θ. This type of variable is called a Bernoulli (or binary) variable.

The independent or predictor variables in logistic regression can take any form. That is, logistic regression makes no assumption about the distribution of the independent variables. They do not have to be normally distributed, linearly related or of equal variance within each group. The relationship between the predictor and response variables is not a linear function in logistic regression, instead, the logistic regression function is used, which is the logit transformation of θ:

$$\theta = \frac{e^{(\alpha+\beta_1 x_1+\beta_2 x_2+\cdots+\beta_i x_i)}}{1 + e(\alpha + \beta_1 x_1 + \beta_2 x_2 + \cdots \beta_i x_i)}$$

where α = the constant of the equation and, β = the coefficient of the predictor variables. An alternative form of the logistic regression equation is:

$$\log[\theta(x)] = \log\left[\frac{\theta(x)}{1 - \theta(x)}\right] = \alpha + \beta_1 x_1 + \beta_2 x_2 + \beta_i x_i$$

An important use of logistic regression is to correctly predict the category of outcome for individual cases using the most parsimonious model.

Stepwise regression is also used in the exploratory phase of research but it is not recommended for theory testing (15). Theory testing is the testing of a-priori theories or hypotheses of the relationships between variables. Exploratory testing makes no a-priori assumptions regarding the relationships between the variables, thus the goal is to discover relationships. Backward stepwise regression appears to be the preferred method of exploratory analyses, where the analysis begins with a full or saturated model and variables are eliminated from the model in an iterative process. The fit of the model is tested after the elimination of each variable to ensure that the model still adequately fits the data. When no more variables can be eliminated from the model, the analysis has been completed.

Logistic regression also provides knowledge of the relationships and strengths among the variables. The process by which coefficients are tested for significance for inclusion or elimination from the model involves two important techniques namely the Wald test and the Likelihood ratio test.

Table 1. 2000 populations

State	Population-All Ages			Under 18 years			Race (Total Population)			
	Total	Male	Female	Total	Male	Female	White	Black	Hispanic	Other
Georgia	8,186,453	4,027,113	4,159340	2,169,234	1,111,589	1,057,645	5,327,281	2,349,542	435,227	74,403

Source: U.S Census Bureau 2000. Total percentage might be over 100% because some people reported more than one race or ethnicity.

Table 2. National Survey of Children's Health sample

	White		African American		Multi-Racial		Other		Unknown		TOTAL	
	Male	female	Male	female	Male	female	Male	female	Male	female	Male	female
GA	629	534	243	228	19	33	28	23	54	55	973	873

A Wald test is a test of statistical significance of each coefficient (β) in the model. A Wald test calculates a Z statistic, which is:

$$Z = \frac{\hat{B}}{SE}$$

The squared value of z yields a Wald statistic with a chi-square distribution. However, several authors have identified problems with the use of the Wald statistic. The (15) warns that for large coefficients, standard error is inflated, lowering the Wald statistic (chi-square) value. As stated by (14), the likelihood-ratio test is more reliable for small sample sizes than the Wald test.

The likelihood-ratio test simply uses the ratio of the maximized value of the likelihood function for the full model (L1) over the maximized value of the likelihood function for the simpler model (L0). The likelihood-ratio test statistic equals:

$$-2\log\left(\frac{L_0}{L_1}\right) = -2[\log(L_0) - \log(L_1)] = -2(L_0 - L_1)$$

For large sample sizes, this log transformation of the likelihood functions yields a chi-squared statistic. This is the recommended test statistic to use when building a model through backward stepwise elimination. It is also important to check for the adequacy of the model fit. One of the most commonly used goodness of fit tests is the Hosmer-Lemshow test (15).

RESULTS

Table 3 shows the percentage of representation for the socio-demographic factors and medical history in relation to children with special care needs for Georgia compared to the combined states (except Georgia). This table also shows the bivariate association between the socio-demographic factors and medical history of children with special care needs.

Table 4 shows the percentage of representation for the socio-demographic factors and medical history in relation to children with limited ability for Georgia and the combined states (except Georgia). This table also shows the bivariate association between the socio-demographic factors and medical history for children with limited ability.

In Georgia, a child's gender, age, poverty level, asthma status, attention deficit disorder or attention deficit hyperactive disorder (ADD/ADHD) status, depression status or anxiety problems, behavioral or conduct problems, diabetes status, autism status and developmental delay or physical impairment are found to be significantly associated with children with special care needs. However, race and household education are found to be non-significant. In the combined states (except Georgia), a child's gender, age, race, poverty level, education level, asthma status, ADD/ADHD status, depression status or anxiety problems, behavioral or conduct problems, diabetes status, autism status, and developmental delay or physical impairment are found to be significantly associated with children with special care needs. A child's gender, age, race, poverty level, education level, asthma status, ADD/ADHD status, depression status or anxiety problems, behavioral or conduct problems, diabetes status, autism status, developmental delay or physical impairment, and special care needs are found to be significant factors affecting children with limited ability in Georgia and the combined states (except Georgia). All significant variables in Table 3 and 4 will be the basis of our model selection in addition to biologically important variables.

Table 3. Summary table for socio-demographic variables and medical history in association of children with special care needs

		Children with special care needs					
		Georgia			All states together		
		N	Percent	P-value	N	Percent	P-value
Gender	Male	123	12.60	0.0041	6678	13.03	<.0001
	Female	74	8.48		4574	9.41	
Age	0-5 yrs old	52	7.94	0.0197	2604	8.00	<.0001
	6-11 yrs old	69	12.37		4022	13.24	
	12-17 yrs old	76	11.91		4633	12.53	
Race	Hispanic	14	7.82	0.6820	1293	9.87	<.0001
	White	122	11.30		7877	11.48	
	Black	48	10.46		1054	11.62	
	Multi-racial	4	8.33		513	13.27	
	Other	5	10.00		387	9.99	
Poverty level	Household income 0-99% FPL	26	11.76	0.0078	1643	14.93	<.0001
	Household income 100-199% FPL	47	13.99		2391	12.98	
	Household income 200-399% FPL	67	13.06		3534	10.75	
	Household income 400% FPL or greater	43	7.60		2776	9.74	
Education	< High School	12	9.84	0.9501	560	12.44	0.0017
	High School	42	10.85		2426	11.70	
	>High School	142	10.68		8231	11.08	
Asthma		63	26.92	<.0001	3155	26.79	<.0001
ADD/ADHD		59	46.46	<.0001	3114	49.64	<.0001
Depression or anxiety problems		32	50.00	<.0001	2379	60.05	<.0001
Behavioral or conduct problems		47	56.63	<.0001	2592	61.07	<.0001
Bone, joint or muscle problems		30	41.67	<.0001	1591	46.24	<.0001
Diabetes		4	66.67	<.0001	248	72.30	<.0001
Autism		4	66.67	<.0001	434	89.12	<.0001
Developmental delay or Physical impairment		37	77.08	<.0001		73.36	<.0001

Table 4. Summary table for socio-demographic variables and medical history in association of children with limited ability

		Child with limited ability					
		Georgia			All states together		
		N	Percent	P-value	N	Percent	P-value
Gender	Male	68	6.94	0.0198	3136	6.09	<.0001
	Female	39	4.42		2192	4.49	
Age	0-5 yrs old	22	3.36	0.0050	1153	3.54	<.0001
	6-11 yrs old	40	7.08		1752	5.75	
	12-17 yrs old	45	6.99		2428	6.53	
Race	Hispanic	4	2.22	0.0706	619	4.71	<.0001
	White	58	5.33		3367	4.89	
	Black	36	7.83		752	8.26	
	Multi-racial	3	6.25		265	6.81	
	Other	4	8.00		245	6.31	
Poverty level	Household income 0-99% FPL	26	11.76	<.0001	1066	9.64	<.0001
	Household income 100-199% FPL	24	7.10		1224	6.63	
	Household income 200-399% FPL	34	6.60		1477	4.48	
	Household income 400% FPL or greater	13	2.28		1067	3.72	
Education	< High School	10	8.20	0.0018	350	7.75	<.0001
	High School	35	9.02		1404	6.75	
	>High School	61	4.55		3549	4.76	
Asthma		38	15.90	<.0001	1642	13.77	<.0001
ADD/ADHD		29	21.80	<.0001	1358	21.32	<.0001
Depression or anxiety problems		16	23.19	<.0001	1027	25.52	<.0001
Behavioral or conduct problems		21	24.71	<.0001	1324	30.84	<.0001
Bone, joint or muscle problems		29	39.73	<.0001	1252	36.12	<.0001
Diabetes		2	33.33	0.0036	85	24.78	<.0001
Autism		6	100.00	<.0001	359	74.33	<.0001
Developmental delay or Physical impairment		33	67.35	<.0001	1949	54.30	<.0001

Table 5. Final Model for children with special care needs for Georgia

	Analysis of Maximum Likelihood Estimates				
Parameter		DF	Estimate	Standard Error	Wald Chi-Square	P-value
Intercept		1	-3.7251	0.2878	167.5282	<.0001
Gender	Male	1	0.3221	0.2212	2.1212	0.1453
AGE_group	0-5 yrs old	1	0.0701	0.2843	0.0608	0.8052
	6-11 yrs old	1	-0.00284	0.2455	0.0001	0.9908
Asthma	Yes	1	1.5259	0.2330	42.8836	<.0001
ADD/ADHD	Yes	1	1.4703	0.3038	23.4229	<.0001
Depression or anxiety problems	Yes	1	1.2624	0.4052	9.7057	0.0018
Behavioral or conduct problems	Yes	1	1.8249	0.3556	26.3429	<.0001
Bone, joint or muscle problems	Yes	1	1.1944	0.4095	8.5062	0.0035
Diabetes	Yes	1	4.6041	1.1619	15.7017	<.0001
Developmental delay or Physical impairment	Yes	1	3.7171	0.4788	60.2739	<.0001
Poverty Levels	Household income 0-99% FPL	1	-0.00940	0.3743	0.0006	0.9800
	Household income 100-199% FPL	1	0.6510	0.2889	5.0769	0.0242
	Household income 200-399% FPL	1	0.4930	0.2646	3.4719	0.0624

Table 6. Final Model for children with special care needs for rest of combined states

	Analysis of Maximum Likelihood Estimates				
Parameter		DF	Estimate	Standard Error	Wald Chi-Square	P-value
Intercept		1	-2.8422	0.0332	7321.1052	<.0001
Dender	Male	1	0.1486	0.0292	25.9107	<.0001
Age_group	0-5 yrs old	1	-0.0560	0.0352	2.5329	0.1115
	6-11 yrs old	1	0.1221	0.0284	18.5067	<.0001
RACE	Black, non-Hispanic	1	-0.0208	0.0443	0.2195	0.6394
	Hispanic	1	-0.0810	0.0423	3.6609	0.0557
	Multi-racial, non-Hispanic	1	0.1524	0.0623	5.9821	0.0145
	Other, non-Hispanic	1	-0.1029	0.0689	2.2308	0.1353
Education	Less than high school	1	-0.0262	0.0671	0.1527	0.6959

Analysis of Maximum Likelihood Estimates					
Parameter		DF	Estimate	Standard Error	Wald Chi-Square	P-value
High school	1	-0.0928	0.0333	7.7494	0.0054

Analysis of Maximum Likelihood Estimates					
Parameter		DF	Estimate	Standard Error	Wald Chi-Square	P-value
Poverty Levels	Household income 0-99% FPL	1	0.5192	0.0464	125.4641	<.0001
	Household income 100-199% FPL	1	0.3750	0.0375	99.9989	<.0001
	Household income 200-399% FPL	1	0.1078	0.0321	11.2748	0.0008
ADD/ADHD	Yes	1	2.0000	0.0986	411.5024	<.0001
Diabetes	Yes	1	3.3290	0.1384	578.9679	<.0001
Autism	Yes	1	2.6457	0.1843	206.0601	<.0001
Developmental delay or Physical impairment	Yes	1	2.5619	0.1419	326.1623	<.0001

Model building

The model building process for variable selection is based on bivariate association between the outcome variables and possible risk factors. From Table 3 and 4, variables are selected based on the test of association which have a p-value less than 0.25.

Decisions are made based on the likelihood ratio test within the variables selection process. In the final models, all variables significant at 0.15 are selected in addition to those biologically important variables.

Table 7. Final Model for children with limited ability for Georgia

Analysis of Maximum Likelihood Estimates						
Parameter		DF	Estimate	Standard Error	Wald Chi-Square	P-value
Intercept		1	-6.6366	0.6299	110.9915	<.0001
Gender	Male	1	0.8682	0.3457	6.3085	0.0120
Age_groups	0-5 yrs old	1	-0.6190	0.4735	1.7088	0.1911
	12-17 yrs old	1	0.6121	0.3559	2.9588	0.0854
Race	Black, non-Hispanic	1	0.2317	0.3817	0.3683	0.5440
	Hispanic	1	-1.1329	0.7542	2.2566	0.1330
	Multi-racial, non-Hispanic	1	0.8259	0.9340	0.7819	0.3766
	Other, non-Hispanic	1	0.8537	0.9649	0.7828	0.3763
Education	Less than high school	1	1.6503	0.5935	7.7311	0.0054
	High school	1	0.6963	0.3915	3.1633	0.0753
Poverty Levels	Household income 0-99% FPL	1	2.3910	0.6147	15.1310	0.0001
	Household income 100-199% FPL	1	0.7445	0.5761	1.6705	0.1962
	Household income 200-399% FPL	1	1.1538	0.5013	5.2978	0.0214
Asthma	Yes	1	1.1607	0.3384	11.7627	0.0006
ADD/ADHD	Yes	1	-0.1007	0.4316	0.0545	0.8155
Depression or anxiety problems	Yes	1	0.3701	0.5334	0.4814	0.4878
Bone, joint or muscle problems	Yes	1	1.5510	0.4458	12.1016	0.0005
Diabetes	Yes	1	2.2057	1.0420	4.4806	0.0343
Developmental delay or Physical impairment	Yes	1	3.2157	0.4936	42.4385	<.0001
Mental Health Problems	Yes	1	2.4085	0.3661	43.2812	<.0001

Table 8. Final Model for children with limited ability for rest of combined states

Analysis of Maximum Likelihood Estimates						
Parameter		DF	Estimate	Standard Error	Wald Chi-Square	P-value
Intercept		1	-3.5800	0.0456	6168.6666	<.0001
Gender	Male	1	0.2978	0.0397	56.2197	<.0001
Age_groups	0-5 yrs old	1	-0.4655	0.0457	103.8614	<.0001
	6-11 yrs old	1	-0.1831	0.0365	25.1880	<.0001
Race	Black, non-Hispanic	1	0.2145	0.0497	18.6007	<.0001
	Hispanic	1	-0.3404	0.0555	37.5801	<.0001

Analysis of Maximum Likelihood Estimates						
Parameter		DF	Estimate	Standard Error	Wald Chi-Square	P-value
	Multi-racial, non-Hispanic	1	0.2278	0.0763	8.9128	0.0028
Analysis of Maximum Likelihood Estimates						
Parameter		DF	Estimate	Standard Error	Wald Chi-Square	P-value
	Other, non-Hispanic	1	0.1415	0.0794	3.1761	0.0747
Poverty	Household income 0-99% FPL	1	1.0994	0.0520	447.0583	<.0001
	Household income 100-199% FPL	1	0.6741	0.0476	200.3665	<.0001
	Household income 200-399% FPL	1	0.1999	0.0446	20.0964	<.0001
Asthma	Yes	1	0.7893	0.1085	52.9578	<.0001
Diabetes	Yes	1	1.4584	0.1491	95.7081	<.0001
Autism	Yes	1	3.6346	0.3647	99.3122	<.0001
inte1		1	0.2932	0.0720	16.5987	<.0001
inte2		1	0.4539	0.2831	2.5707	0.1089

Model building for children with special care needs

Georgia (Children with special care needs)
Eleven factors out of 13, from Table 3 for the multivariate model are found to be statistically significant in the multivariate model. However, diagnosis of the model revealed that there are some poorly fit observations (outliers) in the model. These observations may affect the fit of the model and parameter estimation. When these observation are deleted from the analysis autism status becomes insignificant. Therefore, autism is excluded from the analysis.
The Hosmer and Lemeshow Goodness of Fit test was used (15). This test gives a P-value of 0.2850 which indicates that the model is a good fit.

Combined States with Georgia Removed (Children with special care needs)
Thirteen significant factors from Table 3 for the multivariate model are found to be significant. However, the model diagnosis revealed the lack of fit in the model. This may be due to multicollinearity between variables and outliers. After dropping some collinear variables and deleting some of the outliers, the model has much better fit. In final fitted model, only 9 factors are found to be significant. The Hosmer and Lemeshow Goodness of Fit test was used. This test gives a P-value of 0.1392 which indicates that the model is a good fit.

Model building for children with limited ability

Georgia (Children with limited ability)
All 14 factors from Table 4 are found to be significant for the multivariate model. Twelve of those factors are found to significantly contribute to the multivariate model. However, diagnosis of the model revealed that there are some poorly fit observations in the model. These observations may affect the fit of the model and parameter estimation. These observations were deleted from the analysis.
The Hosmer and Lemeshow Goodness of Fit test was used. This test gives a P-value of 0.1287 which indicates that the model is a good fit.

Combined States with Georgia Removed (Children with limited ability)
Again, all 14 factors are found to be significant for the multivariate model. In the final model and after correcting for the lack of fit, 7 factors are found to be significant. Hosmer and Lemeshow Goodness of Fit test was used. This test gives a P-value of 0.3644 which indicates that the model is a good fit.

DISCUSSION

Results from the final model for Georgia compared to the rest of the combined states in the U.S. are described based on the conditional odds ratio for special care needs and limited ability children.

Asthma status, ADD/ADHD status, depression status, behavioral or conduct problems, bone or muscle problems, and developmental delay or physical impairment are found to be significantly affecting the children with special care needs in Georgia. However, in the rest of the combined states a child's gender, poverty level, education level of household, ADD/ADHD status, diabetes status, autism status, and developmental delay or physical impairment are found to be significant. A child's age and race are marginally significant for the combined states with Georgia removed.

In Georgia, Table 9 shows that conditioning on other factors in the model, the odds of a child having special care needs when he/she has asthma is 4.599 (95% CI 2.903, 7.250) times higher than those without asthma. However, in the combined states with Georgia removed, asthma has no effect on a child's propensity to have special care needs.

In Georgia conditioning on other factors in the model, the odds of a child having special care needs when he/she has attention deficit disorder or attention deficit hyperactive disorder is 4.351 (95% CI 2.379, 7.849) times higher than those without attention deficit disorder or attention deficit hyperactive disorder.

However, in the combined states with Georgia removed, conditioning on other factors in the model, the odds of a child having special care needs when he/she has attention deficit disorder or attention deficit hyperactive disorder is 7.389 (6.091, 8.965) times higher than those without attention deficit disorder or attention deficit hyperactive disorder. The odds for attention deficit disorder or attention deficit hyperactive disorder in Georgia are less as compared to the rest of the combined states.

In Georgia conditioning on other factors in the model, the odds of a child having special care needs when he/she has depression or anxiety problems is 3.534 (95% CI 1.573, 7.738) times higher than those without depression or anxiety problems. However, in the rest of the combined states, depression or anxiety problems have no impact on a child having special care needs.

In Georgia, conditioning on other factors in the model, the odds of a child having special care needs when he/she has behavioral or conduct problems is 6.202 (95% CI 3.075, 12.436) times higher than those without behavioral or conduct problems. However, in the rest of the combined states it seems to have no impact.

Table 9. Odds ratio with 95% confidence interval for child with special care needs

Factors		Georgia Odds ratio (95% CI)	Rest of Combined States Odds ratio (95% CI)
Gender	Male vs Female	1.38 (0.90, 2.14)	1.16 (1.10, 1.23)
Age	0-5 yrs old vs 12-17 yrs old	1.07 (0.61, 1.86)	0.95 (0.88, 1.01)
	6-11 yrs old vs 12-17 yrs old	1.00 (0.62, 1.61)	1.13 (1.07, 1.19)
Race	Black vs White		0.98 (0.90, 1.07)
	Hispanic vs white		0.92 (0.85, 1.00)
	Multi racial vs white		1.17 (1.03, 1.31)
	Other vs white		0.90 (0.79, 1.03)
Poverty level (Income)	0-99% FPL vs 400% FPL or greater	0.99 (0.46, 2.03)	1.68 (1.54, 1.84)
	100-199% FPL vs 400% FPL or greater	1.917 (1.09, 3.39)	1.46 (1.35, 1.57)
	200-399% FPL vs 400% FPL or greater	1.64 (0.98, 2.77)	1.11(1.05, 1.19)
Education	< High school vs > High School		0.97 (0.85, 1.11)
	High school vs > High school		0.91 (0.85, 0.97)
Asthma		4.60 (2.90, 7.25)	
ADD/ADHD		4.35 (2.38, 7.85)	7.39 (6.09, 8.97)
Depression or anxiety problems		3.53 (1.57, 7.74)	
Behavioral or conduct problems		6.20 (3.08, 12.44)	
Bone, joint or muscle problems		3.30 (1.45, 7.25)	
Diabetes		99.89 (13.09, -)	27.91 (21.37, 36.78)
Autism			14.09 (9.92, 20.46)
Developmental delay or Physical impairment		1.14 (16.77, 112.18)	12.96 (9.82, 17.13)

Also, in Georgia conditioning on other factors in the model, the odds of a child having special care needs when he/she has bone, joint or muscle problems is 3.302 (95% CI 1.448, 7.250) times higher than those without bone, joint or muscle problems. However, in the rest of the combined states, bone, joint or muscle problems have no impact.

In Georgia, conditioning on other factors in the model, the odds of a child having special care needs when he/she has diabetes is 99.892 (95% CI 13.091, >999.999) times higher than those without diabetes. However, in the rest of the combined states, conditioning on other factors in the model, the odds of a child having special care needs when he/she has diabetes is 27.910 (21.366, 36.780) times than those without diabetes. The odds of diabetes for a child having special care needs in Georgia are higher than in all of the rest of the combined states. This may be due to the fact that we have only 4 cases of children with diabetes in Georgia with special care needs. Therefore, we suggest excluding this factor from the model.

In Georgia, conditioning on other factors in the model, the odds of a child having special care needs when he/she has developmental delay or physical impairment is 41.143 (16.772, 112.181) times higher than those without developmental delay or physical impairment. However, in all the rest of the combined states, conditioning on other factors in the model, the odds of a child having special care needs when he/she has developmental delay or physical impairment is 12.960 (9.820, 17.126) times higher than those without developmental delay or physical impairment. The odds of development delay or physical impairment in Georgia is higher as compared to the rest of the combined states.

In Georgia, conditioning on other factors in the model, the odds of a child having special care needs in a family with a 100-199% federal poverty level is 1.917 (1.087, 3.388) times higher than a family with a 400% or greater federal poverty level. However, in the rest of the combined states, conditioning on other factors in the model, the odds of a child having special care needs for a family with a 100-199% federal poverty level is 1.455 (1.352, 1.566) times higher than the odds of a family with a 400% or greater federal poverty level. Other poverty levels are not significant in Georgia. These results show that poorer families are more susceptible to having a child with special care needs.

This section shows the disparities in Georgia of children with special care needs. Children with asthma, ADD/ADHD, depression or anxiety problems, behavioral and conduct problems, bone, joint and muscle problems, developmental delay or physical impairment and children living in poverty are significantly more susceptible for requiring special care needs in Georgia.

From Table 9 for the combined states with Georgia removed, conditioning on other factors in the model, the odds of a child having special care needs for males is 1.160 (1.096, 1.229) times higher than females. This shows that boys are at higher risk to have special care needs.

In the combined states with Georgia removed, conditioning on other factors in the model, the odds for a household having more than a high school education having a special care needs child is 1.098 (1.028, 1.171) times higher than the household having a high school education. These results show that educated families are more susceptible to having a child with special care needs. This may be because less educated families may be less aware about the conditions and issues associated with children needing special care.

In the combined states with Georgia removed, conditioning on other factors in the model, the odds of a child having special care needs when he/she has autism is 14.094 (9.920, 20.461) times higher than those without autism.

From Table 10 in Georgia, conditioning on other factors in the model, the odds a child has limited ability for a male child is 2.383 (1.228, 4.794) times higher than for females. Male children are more susceptible for having limited ability. However, in the rest of the combined states, conditioning on other factors in the model, the odds of a child having limited ability for a male is 1.347 (1.246, 1.456) times higher than for a female. The odds for a male child in Georgia having with limited ability are higher as compare to the rest of the combined states.

In Georgia, conditioning on other factors in the model, the odds of a child having limited ability for a family with income of 0-99% of federal poverty level is 10.925 (3.385, 38.216) times higher than the odds for a family with income of 400% or greater of federal poverty level, and the odds for a family with an income of 200-299% of federal poverty level is 3.170 (1.236, 8.986) times higher than a family with an income of 400% or greater of federal poverty level. However, in the rest of the combined states, conditioning on other factors in the model, the odds of a child having limited ability for a family with an income of 0-99% of the federal poverty level is 3.003 (2.711, 3.325) times higher than a family with an income of 400% or greater of the federal poverty level, the odds of a child having limited ability for a family with an income of 100-199% of the federal poverty level is 1.962 (1.787, 2.154) times higher than a family with an income of 400% or greater of the federal poverty level, and the odds of a child having limited ability for family with an income of 200-299% of the federal poverty level is 11.221 (1.119, 1.333) times higher than a family with an income of 400% or greater of the federal poverty level. These results show that poorer families are at more risk to have a child with limited ability.

In Georgia, conditioning on other factors in the model, the odds of a child having limited ability for a household education level that is less than high school is 5.209 (1.581, 16.442) times higher than the household with an education level with more than high school. However, in the rest of the combined states it has no effect. This result shows that educated families are at more risk for children with limited ability in Georgia. This may be because less educated families are unaware about the conditions related to a child with limited ability and thus, report of such conditions may be lacking.

In Georgia, conditioning on other factors in the model, the odds of a child having limited ability when he/she has asthma is 3.192 (1.638, 6.204) times higher than those without asthma. However, in the rest of the combined states, conditioning on other factors in the model, the odds of a child having limited ability when the child has asthma is 2.202 (1.780, 2.723) times higher than those without asthma. The odds of asthma for a child having limited ability in Georgia are higher as compared to the rest of the combined states.

In Georgia, conditioning on other factors in the model, the odds of a child having limited ability when he/she has bone, joint or muscle problems is 4.716 (1.953, 11.283) times higher than those without bone, joint or muscle problems. However, in the rest of the combined states these conditions have no effect. In Georgia, conditioning on other factors in the model, the odds of a child having limited ability when he/she has developmental delay or physical impairment is 24.920 (9.698, 67.678) times higher than those without developmental delay or physical impairment. However, in the rest of the combined states these conditions have no effect. It seems that development delay or physical impairment is prominent in children with limited ability in Georgia as compared to all other states combined.

Table 10. Child with limited ability

Factors		Georgia Odds ratio (95% CI)	Rest of Combined States Odds ratio (95% CI)
Gender	Male	2.38 (1.23, 4.79)	1.35 (1.25, 1.46)
Age	0-5 yrs old vs 12-17 yrs old	0.54 (0.21, 1.34)	0.63 (0.57, 0.69)
	6-11 yrs old vs 12-17 yrs old	1.84 (0.93, 3.77)	0.83 (0.78, 0.89)
Race	Black vs White	1.26 (0.593, 2.67)	1.24(1.12, 1.37)
	Hispanic vs white	0.32 (0.06, 1.26)	0.71 (0.64, 0.79)
	Multi racial vs white	2.28 (0.261, 11.41)	1.26 (1.08, 1.46)
	Other vs white	2.35 (0.27, 12.88)	1.15 (0.98, 1.34)
Poverty level (Income)	0-99% FPL vs 400% FPL or greater	10.93 (3.39, 38.22)	3.00 (2.71, 3.33)
	100-199% FPL vs 400% FPL or greater	2.11 (0.69, 6.73)	1.96 (1.79, 2.15)
	200-399% FPL vs 400% FPL or greater	3.170 (1.236 , 8.986)	1.22 (1.12, 1.33)
Education	< High school vs > High School	5.21 (1.58, 16.44)	
	High school vs > High school	2.01 (0.93, 4.34)	
Asthma		3.19 (1.64, 6.20)	2.20 (1.78, 2.72)
ADD/ADHD		0.90 (0.38, 2.08)	
Depression or anxiety problems		1.45 (0.50, 4.04)	
Bone, joint or muscle problems		4.72 (1.95, 11.28)	
Diabetes		9.08 (0.95, 65.86)	4.30 (3.19, 5.72)
Autism		24.92 (9.70, 67.68)	37.89 (18.43, 77.23)
Developmental delay or Physical impairment		11.12 (5.47, 23.12)	
Child with special care needs			

In Georgia, conditioning on other factors in the model, the odds of a child having limited ability when he/she has special care needs is 11.117 (5.471, 23.118) times higher than those without special care needs. However, in the rest of the combined states, special care needs status has no significant impact in the model.

This section discussed the disparities in Georgia of children with limited ability. In Georgia, boys, children with asthma, children living in poverty (and lower familial incomes below 400% federal poverty level), higher levels of household education above high school, bone, joint and muscle problems, and children with special care needs are more susceptible to have limited ability.

From Table 4.2 in the combined states with Georgia removed, conditioning on other factors in the model, the odds of a child having limited ability for the Black racial category is 1.239 (1.123, 1.365) times higher than that of the White racial category, and the odds for those categorized as Multiracial is 1.256 (1.079, 1.455) times higher than those in the White racial category. These results show that children in the racial categories of Black and Multiracial are at higher risk for limited ability in the combined states with Georgia removed.

In the combined states with Georgia removed, conditioning on other factors in the model, the odds of a child having limited ability when he/she has diabetes is 4.299 (3.188, 5.724) times higher than those without diabetes. This shows that children with diabetes are at higher risk to have limited ability.

In the combined states with Georgia removed, conditioning on other factors in the model, the odds of a child having limited ability when he/she has autism is 37.885 (18.430, 77.232) times higher than those without autism. This result shows that children with autism are at higher risk to have limited ability.

In comparing Georgia with the rest of the combined states for children with special care needs and limited ability, this study revealed the similarities and differences of factors that contribute to susceptibility for inclusion in these special populations. The factors as provided in the tables demonstrate the comparisons.

Children with asthma, ADD/ADHD, depression or anxiety problems, behavioral and conduct problems, bone, joint and muscle problems, developmental delay or physical impairment and children living in poverty are significantly more susceptible for requiring special care needs in Georgia. While, also in Georgia, boys, children with asthma, children living in poverty (and lower familial incomes below 400% federal poverty level), higher levels of household education above high school, bone, joint and muscle problems, and children with special care needs are more susceptible to have limited ability.

ACKNOWLEDGMENTS

We are grateful to the Center for Child and Adolescent Health for providing us with the 2003 National Survey of Children's Health. Also, we would like to thank the referees and the associate editor for their valuable comments which improved the manuscript.

REFERENCES

[1]   Children with Special Health Care Needs (CSHCN) 2006 North Carolina Statewide CHAMP Survey Results.North Caroline State Center for Health Statistics. Accessed 2009 July 9. URL:http://www.schs.state.nc.us/SCHS/champ/2006/k14q01.html

[2]   Children with Special Health Care Needs (CSHCN) 2007. North Carolina Statewide CHAMP Survey Results.North Caroline State Center for Health Statistics. Accessed 2009 July 9. URL: http://www.schs.state.nc.us/SCHS/champ/2007/k13q07.html

[3]   Child and Adolescent Health Measurement Initiative 2003. National survey of children with special health care needs: Indicator dataset 6. Data Resource Center for Child and Adoles-cent Health website. Accessed 2009 July 9. URL: www.childhealthdata.org.

[4]   HRSA:2009. Maternal and Child Health Bureau – Accessed 2009 July 9. URL:

[5]   http://mchb.hrsa.gov/programs/

[6]   Mental Health in the United States: Health Care and Well Being of Children with Chronic Emotional, Behavioral, or Developmental Problems --- United States, 2001. MMWR weekly October 7, 2005 / 54(39);985-989. Accessed 2009 July 9. URL: http://www.cdc.gov/mmwr/preview/mmwrhtml /mm5439a3.htm

[7]   Oftedahl E, Benedict R, Katcher ML. National Survey of Children with Special Health Care Needs: Wisconsin-Specific Area. Wisconsin Med J 2006;105(3):88-90.

[8]   Fox HB, McManus MA, Zarit M, Fairbrother G, Cassedy AE, Bethell CD, et al. Racial and ethnic disparities in adolescent health and access to care. Incenter Strateties: The National Allliance to Advance Adolescent Health January 2007, Fact Sheet No. 1.

[9]   Fox HB, McManus MA, Zarit M, Fairbrother G, Cassedy AE, Bethell CD, et al. Racial and ethnic disparities in health and access to care among older adolescents. Incenter Strateties: The National Allliance to Advance Adolescent Health January 2007, Fact Sheet No. 2.

[10]   Lo K, Fulda KG. Impact of predisposing, enabling, and need factors in accessing preventive medical care among U.S. children: results of the national survey of children's health. Osteopath Med Prim Care 2008;2:12.

[11]   The national survey of children with special care needs: Chart book 2005-2006. Accessed 2009 July 9. URL: http://mchb.hrsa.gov/cshcn05/

[12]   Porterfield S, McBride TD. The effect of poverty and caregiver education on perceived need and access to health services among children with special health care needs. Am J Public Health 2007;97(2):323-9.

[13]   U.S. Department of Commerce (2000). United States Census: 2000 Census of Population and Housing. Washington, DC: U.S. Department of Commerce. Accessed 2009 July 9. URL: http://www.census.gov/prod/cen2000/index.html

[14]   SAS Institute, Inc. SAS/STAT Version 9.1. Cary, NC: SAS Institute, Inc.:2010.

[15]   Agresti A. Categorical data analysis. New York, NY: John Wiley, 1990.

[16]   Hosmer DW, Lemeshow S. Applied logistic regression. New York: John Wiley, 1989.

Submitted: June 07, 2011. *Revised:* August 10, 2011. *Accepted:*August 26, 2011.

SECTION TWO - TROPICAL PEDIATRICS

In: Public Health Yearbook 2012
Editor: Joav Merrick

ISBN: 978-1-62808-078-0
© 2013 Nova Science Publishers, Inc.

Chapter 7

RECOGNIZING COMMUNITY PRIORITIES, NEEDS AND WATER SAFETY

Linda S Vail, BS, MPA and Douglas N Homnick, MD, MPH*

Kalamazoo County Health and Community Services, Nazareth, Michigan,
Division of Pediatric Pulmonology, Pediatrics and Human Development,
Michigan State University College of Human Medicine,
Michigan State University/Kalamazoo Center for Medical Studies,
Kalamazoo, Michigan, United States of America

ABSTRACT

Waterborne disease remains a significant worldwide cause of human morbidity and mortality. This occurs commonly in developing countries where sanitation of common and individual household drinking water supplies is lacking or with transmigration of displaced persons into camps due to political turmoil and war. In addition, a number of natural disasters including earthquakes, tsunamis, and hurricanes have proven the vulnerability of centralized source water treatment facilities. Bioterrorism also remains a threat to centralized systems with potential for widespread dissemination of toxic and infectious agents. In developing countries or with the need for rehabilitation or reconstruction of existing infrastructure, a consideration of point-of-use or individual household water sanitation systems versus central source systems is logical. This will depend on a social and economic examination of societal needs but point-of-use systems, particularly with widespread rural populations, may offer considerable improvement over current household water management. In addition, they may be more resistant to natural and manmade disruptions to the safe drinking water supply. This article reviews issues related to community needs, community priorities, and water safety.

Keywords: Community, waterborne disease, drinking water, environment, public health

---

* Correspondence: Linda S. Vail, BS, MPA, Director, Health Officer, Kalamazoo County Health and Community Services, 3299 Gull Road, P. O. Box 42, Nazareth, Michigan 49074-0042, United States. E-mail: lsvail@kalcounty.com

INTRODUCTION

An estimated 1.1 billion people worldwide lack clean drinking water and 2.4 billion lack access to basic sanitation. Targets adopted by the United Nations in September, 2000 aim to halve these figures by 2015; but projections suggest those goals, which would require more than 100,000 people every day to be connected to clean water supplies, will not be met

Patricia Brett. Water supply bogs down in complexity. Int Herald Tribune 2005 Aug 20.

Water is basic to life and civilizations have always congregated and established themselves around water supplies. For over 4,000 years there have been references to water quality with both Sanskrit and Greek writings discussing water treatment methods including filtering, boiling, straining, and exposure to sunlight (1). Knowledge of disease associated with impure water began to emerge in the 19th Century, most notably with the demonstration by British epidemiologist John Snow (1813-1858) of cholera as a waterborne disease linked to an outbreak from a public well contaminated by human waste. This was followed later in this century by the isolation of the causal agent of cholera (*V. cholera*) by the German physician Heinrich Hermann Robert Koch (1843-1910) and by the demonstration of the French chemist and microbiologist Louis Pasteur (1822-1895) of the "germ theory" whereby microbes could transmit disease through water.

At this time in the United States, it was recognized that cloudiness or turbidity associated with water sources could not only be a source of unpleasant particulates but could contain disease-causing sewage particles. With the isolation of the etiologic agent of typhoid fever (*S. typhi*) in 1884, it was also recognized that this was a significant contributor to water-borne disease. An experimental sand filtration system in Lawerence, Massachusetts, USA was established and proved to be effective in dramatically decreasing the death rate from typhoid fever in that community by 79% resulting in a proliferation of communities using both mechanical and sand filters occurred over the next few years (2).

Chlorination of municipal water supplies began in Jersey City, New Jersey, USA in 1908 to combat occasional sewage contamination. Over the next 10 years, both filtration and chlorination became accepted water purification techniques thus establishing the first effective means to effectively reduce and prevent water borne disease outbreaks in the United States. The introduction of disinfectants such as chlorine is considered to have played the most important role in reducing this disease burden.

Regulation of federal drinking water standards began in 1893 with the Interstate Quarantine Act. This act authorized the US Surgeon General to make and enforce regulations controlling the introduction and transmission of communicable diseases. A national law to address the spread of major epidemic diseases in the United States was passed by the US Congress in 1878. The Marine Hospital Service, fore runner to the United States Public Health Service, and initially serving as a relief organization for ill seamen, was assigned the task of inspection, investigation, and prevention of transmissible disease in order to reduce epidemics such as yellow fever.

The initial standards for bacteriological quality began in 1914 and only applied to water systems of interstate carriers and only to prevention of disease caused by infectious agents. These standards were expanded and between 1942 and 1946 with regulations requiring bacteriological sampling of all water supplies in the US and up until the early 1970's, subsequent legislation to prescribe and enforce drinking water standards by municipalities was directed at prevention of communicable diseases. Passage of the Safe Drinking Act of 1974 (PL 93-523) recognized the potential harm to the public health of not only communicable diseases but of the growing body of evidence supporting the importance of other contaminants, such as chemical carcinogens.

It mandated that the US Environmental Protection Agency (EPA) set national standards to protect the public from all varieties of water contaminants. The Act has been subsequently reauthorized and listings and standards for contaminant levels expanded as scientific knowledge of actual and potential health effects of these has also expanded. The evolution of water quality standards from communicable diseases to a long list of other environmental contaminants, sometimes with long time intervals from exposure to manifestation of disease, parallels the story of a developing nation (United States) from one that was primarily rural and agrarian to one that is urban and industrialized. The public demand for centralized services including clean water also parallels this development as traditional point-of-use supplies in densely populated urban settings, such as individual wells, are clearly impractical and impossible to achieve.

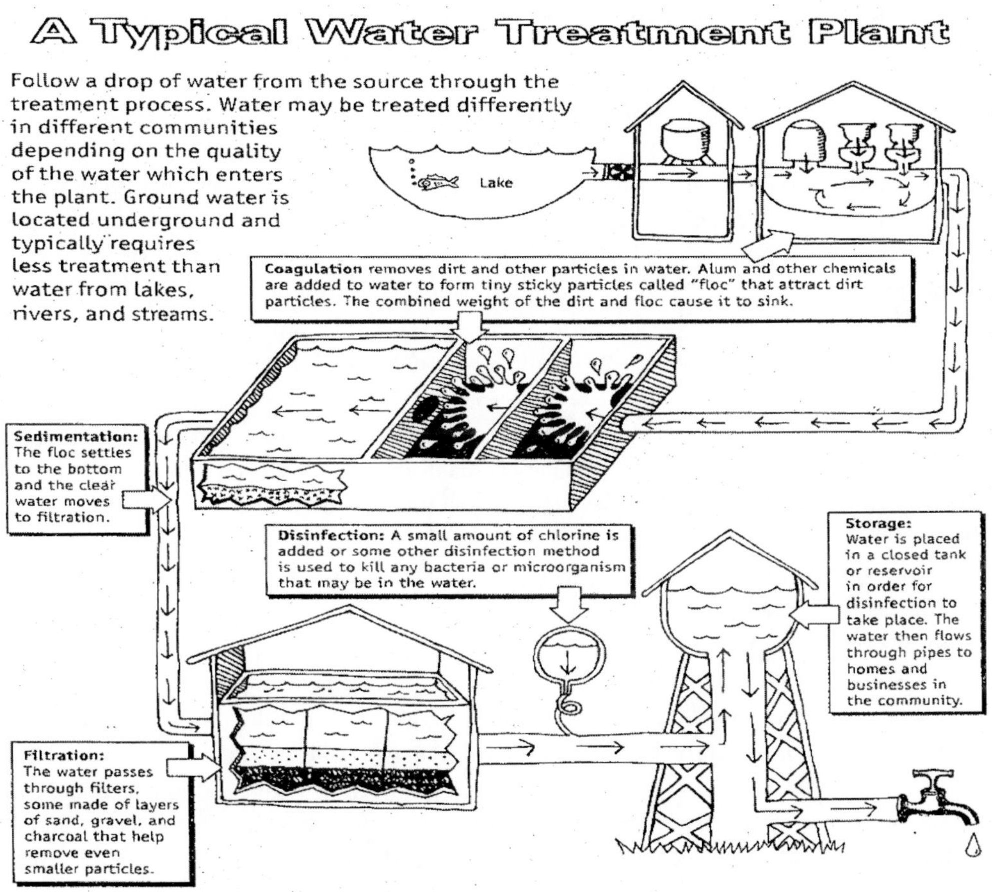

Figure 1. A typical water treatment plant. Adapted from reference 1.

The components of the central source water system have changeed little over the last century. A typical system consists of a primary water source (reservoir, lake, river, stream, well, etc.), a treatment plant (to clear the turbidity by removing dirt and other particulates), a filtration unit (to remove bacteria and other smaller particles), a disinfection unit (to kill remaining bacteria or other microorganisms), a storage unit (for the decontaminated effluent), and a distribution system (to piping to take the water to individuals and businesses) (see figure 1). With a multi-layered system, there is room for breakdown either from natural disaster, mechanical breakdown, or human error. Although this system is efficient in delivering clean water to large populations, a breakdown in the system would likewise put a larger population at risk. This is in contrast to a breakdown in an individual household's point-of-use system whereby only the individual family members are at primary risk. Breakdown in a central source system can occur at each point in the treatment cascade leading to insufficient decontamination and the subsequent potential for widespread disease. In addition, central source water systems are potential targets for bioterrorism. EPA regulation and prudent management with backup safety systems minimize this risk. The next section discusses examples of how public water systems have failed and provides lessons on the breakdown of water systems due to design and natural disasters. In addition, the relative benefit of modern point-of-use water systems versus central source water systems as a choice for developing countries will be considered.

WHEN THINGS GO WRONG

A sophisticated multi-layered, modern water system is seen as a hallmark of well-developed countries and has virtually eliminated widespread waterborne illnesses formerly commonplace in the pre-industrial age. In less developed parts of the world, these well planned, consistent mechanisms for maintaining clean water supplies are not readily available and as a result devastating waterborne illnesses are still problematic. This has been particularly true in Africa and Asia. However, one can see that the advancements in well-developed parts of the world with regard to clean water supply do not come without numerous risks. J Edgar Hoover (1895-1972), director of the US Federal Bureau of Investigation (FBI), made note of water supply facilities as particularly vulnerable to attack by foreign agents as the modern water supply system is strategically positioned to keep the "wheels of industry turning" and "preserving the health and morale" of the nation (3).

Hoover alluded to the vast interdependency of water and wastewater systems within the critical infrastructure of this nation. In identifying the water supply system as both a part of the critical infrastructure and having infrastructure interdependency, it is recognized that the system has impact well beyond the water supply itself and outages in the system will quickly escalate and ultimately have significant cascading effects on many other critical infrastructure components. As seen in figure 2, the impact of disruption to the water supply system is far reaching (4). Natural disasters (e.g., floods, hurricanes, tsunamis, and earthquakes) and man-made disasters (e.g. accidents, system failure including power outages, and terrorist attacks) both reveal these interdependencies and the potential devastation caused by failure of the water supply system.

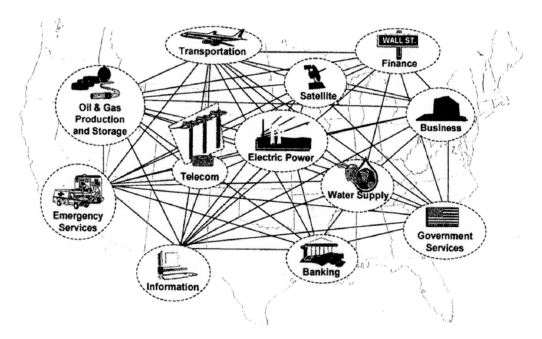

Figure 2. The interdependence of critical infrastructure. Adapted from reference 4.

MAN MADE DISASTERS

To date, the modern water supply system has not knowingly been compromised in a bioterrorist attack, though a credible threat was received by the FBI in January 2001. A terrorist group indicated their intent to disrupt the water supply system (whether or not this was to be biologic in nature is unknown) in 28 cities within the United States (3). A threat such as this exposes the potential devastation of such a disruption. With regard to a bioterrorist attack by dispersal in the water supply system, experts believe the risk is minimal. It is, however, possible and protection against such an attack is part of the preparedness efforts across the nation. According to Nelson Moyer of the University of Iowa Hygienic Laboratory, "the ideal waterborne agent of bioterrorism has a low infectious dose, produces severe gastrointestinal disease in a population with little or no immunity, and results in a higher percentage of systemic complications leading to death" (3).

Although not the result of a bioterrorist attack, contamination of the Milwaukee water supply system in 1993 provides ample evidence that, in fact, a biological agent introduced into the water supply system can have devastating effects (5). The Cryptosporidium outbreak in Milwaukee, Wisconsin in 1993 is the largest waterborne disease outbreak ever documented in the history of the United States. The root cause of the outbreak was not initially identified; however, it was determined that Cryptosoridium oocysts passed through the filtration system of one of the city's water treatment plants.

Recent evidence supports a theory regarding the source of contamination. The Cryptosporidium source was identified as human, and modeling theories proposed that the three rivers that flow into Milwaukee forming the bay were contaminated by sewage overflow after heavy rains in March 1993 (6). It was estimated that 403,000 residents became ill during the outbreak. A total of 880,000 of Milwaukee's 1.61 million residents were served by the identified malfunctioning treatment plant. The experience in Milwaukee demonstrates the potential risk of a waterborne agent being introduced into a central water supply system and such an agent evading the layers of protection afforded by a modern water treatment plant.

The massive power outage causing a blackout that swept the entire east coast of the United States in August of 2003 brings to bear the potential risk to critical infrastructure when systems are no longer functioning to deliver clean water to a large portion of the population, as well as the interdependence and vulnerability of an aging water supply system (7). In Cleveland, Ohio the city's four water pumping stations shut down leaving all residents without a water supply. Despite backup systems in the Detroit area, there was not sufficient backup power for the entire metropolitan area. In Macomb County, Michigan, 4.3 million residents were temporarily without a safe water supply source. In New York City, backup generators serving several wastewater treatment plants failed and approximately 500 million gallons of untreated sewage overflowed past the treatment facilities and into the waterways surrounding the city. Although a breach into the public drinking water supply system from the overflow of untreated sewage was not reported as an issue, the experience with the Milwaukee outbreak demonstrates the potential impact that failure of wastewater treatment facilities can have on public drinking water supply systems.

NATURAL DISASTERS

Information can be drawn from a number of recent natural disasters both in the United States and other countries as to how drinking water supply systems can be at risk from the forces of nature. Focusing on the effects of hurricanes Katrina and Rita, the Indonesian tsunami of 2004, and the earthquake in Haiti in 2010 provides a good sampling for examination of the impact of these types disasters to the water supply in areas where the critical infrastructure was devastated.

The surge of ocean water into the coastal areas affected by the December 2004 Indonesian tsunami submerged the sources of safe drinking water placing them at immediate risk of microbial contamination (8). Survivors were immediately at increased risk of waterborne diseases such as cholera, hepatitis A, shigellosis, and typhoid fever. Tamilnadu was among the worst affected areas in India. Analysis of water samples from multiple types of drinking water sources demonstrates the disruption of various systems for supplying clean drinking water. Bacteriological analysis revealed that 76.5% of public wells, 60.9% of bore wells, 39.5% of overhead tanks, 31% of plastic storage tanks, and 11% of public fountains were contaminated with coliform bacteria (8). Subsequent attempts to treat water making it suitable for consumption showed that point-of-use chlorination was effective in reducing risk of coliforms in the water, and, on the contrary, boiling water at point-of-use was not shown to significantly improve water quality (9). Safe drinking water was available from government supplies, from numerous natural springs in the mountains nearby, and from the use of membrane technology in temporary camp areas that were established as shelters for affected residents. In the aftermath of the tsunami disaster, the Thai government has promoted increased use of natural resources, such as artesian wells, for ongoing supply of safe drinking water (10).

Hurricanes Katrina and Rita devastated the coast of the U.S. southern states, particularly Alabama, Louisiana, and Mississippi, during the hurricane season of 2005. As with the tsunami, the storm surge was significant and impacted coastal areas particularly in Mississippi and Alabama. Complicating the actual storm surge were breeches in the levee system in New Orleans causing substantial flooding of approximately 80% of the city. Water treatment and wastewater treatment facilities were impaired. In Mississippi, 28 wastewater facilities were damaged. In New Orleans, every major water and wastewater treatment facility was affected (10). For numerous reasons, including the breakdown of wastewater treatment facilities and human and animal bodies that could not be retrieved for long periods of time, the media reported the flood waters to be a "toxic soup." In the end, however, toxic effects of contaminated water were not a significant issue in these storm surges. Similar to the Indonesian tsunami, efforts to mitigate the effects of contaminated water were significantly effective in averting the potential public health impacts of a contaminated water supply. Essentially, the water, contaminated with raw sewage, was not a significant danger unless it was consumed or came into contact with untreated wounds. Efforts such as importing water, super-chlorination, and boil water alerts were effective in preventing a major waterborne disease outbreak.

Rehabilitation of storm surge areas where water and wastewater facilities are significantly impacted present the next challenge in reestablishing the critical infrastructure of severely affected areas as the repair and restoration process can be problematic and lengthy (11). A centralized water system that is multilayered not only has multiple points where breakdown can occur, but also requires multiple steps to restore the system and ensure that the water supply is safe again. These steps, including immediate disinfection, replacement and repair of system components, and reintegration of the system, also require government funding in the aftermath of a declared disaster (11). The technology of our modern multilayered water supply system drives an expensive, lengthy, and multistep recovery process due to the nature of how our water supply systems developed over time.

A final example of the disruption of a safe drinking water supply is illustrated in the aftermath of the devastating earthquake in Haiti on January 12, 2010. The day after the earthquake, an article in Time magazine questioned whether disease outbreaks would be able to be prevented given the vulnerability of the country pre-earthquake. Stating that "vulnerability will be felt first in the water", the article continues to relay the good news that major infectious disease outbreaks are rarely seen after these types of natural disasters (12). While that was the case in the tsumai and hurricanes noted above, ultimately, an infectious disease outbreak did follow the earthquake in Haiti. By October 2010, an epidemiologic investigation confirmed that a large number of illnesses, hospitalizations, and deaths were caused by *V. cholera*. While cholera outbreaks are common in Asia and Africa, one had not been reported in the Caribbean since the 1990s. A cholera outbreak had not been reported in Haiti for more than a century, despite the fact that no city in Haiti currently has a sewer system or waste treatment facility. Months after devastation and deaths caused by the earthquake in January 2010, Haiti faced more devastation including 992 cholera deaths and 16,111 cholera hospitalizations (13). Distribution of the illnesses was widespread, affecting seven of Haiti's 10 departments.

CENTRAL SOURCE VERSUS POINT-OF-USE WATER TREATMENT

There are considerations of complexity, cost, and vulnerability in the development of central source water systems versus individual household or point-of-use systems for effective drinking water treatment. We have seen how complex these systems are (figures 1 and 2) and the effort (and associated expense) in recovering these systems after natural or manmade disruption. In a developing country without an established water treatment system or with a an inadequate or deteriorating central source water distribution infrastructure, development of point-of-use water purification systems are akin to adoption of wireless cellular phone systems versus the expensive and intrusive, centralized, as well as vulnerable, hard-wired systems.

Point-of use systems have been shown to be effective in providing adequate quantities of drinking water to individual households and reduce the primary risk to human health from contaminating fecal organisms. Candidate systems include boiling, solar disinfection by the combined action of heat and ultra violet (UV) radiation, solar disinfection by heat alone, UV disinfection with lamps, chlorination plus storage in an appropriate vessel, and combined systems of chemical coagulation-filtration and chlorine disinfection (14). The last may be especially important where turbid source water is present as decrease in microbial load is impaired by the presence of suspended matter (14). Methods to pre-treat water to remove suspended material includes settling (sedimentation), fiber, cloth or membrane filters, granular media filters, and slow sand filtration (14). Of the above systems, chlorination and storage in a safe container and solar disinfection plus heat have been systematically studied and shown to reduce risk from waterborne disease.

Shannon and Burnham showed significant reductions of diarrheal diseases in a controlled study of flocculation plus chlorine disinfection versus improved water storage only in 400 households located in a Liberian displaced persons camp (15). In this study diarrheal illness incidence was reduced by 90% and prevalence by 83%.

In another controlled study of point-of use water treatment, Quick et al. (16) evaluated bacteriologic contamination and diarrheal illness in two Zambian communities by comparing 166 households implementing chlorine disinfection plus safe storage to 94 control households using usual storage methods for their drinking water. Both communities used a shallow well as their local source. Coliform contamination of stored water was significantly less in the intervention group than in control households and diarrheal disease risk 48% lower than controls over the 13 week study.

The effectiveness of point-of-use water treatment on the reduction of life threatening diarrheal illness has been well documented in other controlled trials (17-19). Establishing a safe water system as a community priority must take into consideration not only the economic impact but also the educational, behavioral, and related socio-cultural aspects.

Table 1. Relative cost of point-of-use drinking water treatment systems. Adapted from 14

	Imported Items	Initial cost of hardware (per capita; per household)	Annual operating cost per capita and household
Boiling	None	None (assumes use of a cook pot)	Varies with fuel price; expensive
Ceramic filter	Filter candles	$5; $25	$1, $5 for annual replacement
SODIS and SOLAIR (solar disinfection by UV radiation and heat)	None (assumes spent bottles available)	Cost of black paint for bottles or alternative dark surface (roofing)	None
Solar heating (solar disinfection by heat only)	Solar cooker or other solar reflector	Initial cost of solar cooker or reflector & water exposure and storage vessels	Replacement costs of solar reflectors and water exposure and storage vessels
UV Lamp Systems	UV lamps and housings	Initial cost of UV system: US$100-300), $20-60	Power (energy); lamp replacement ($10-100) every 1-3 years
On-site generated or other chlorine and narrow-mouth storage vessel ("USA CDC Safewater" system)	Hypochlorite generator and associated hardware for production and bulk storage	$1.60; $8.00	$0.60/$3.00 (estimated by USA CDC); costs may be higher for different sources of chlorine and for different water storage vessels
Combined coagulation-filtration and chlorination systems	Chemical coagulant and chlorine mixture, as powder or tablet	Use existing storage vessel or buy a special treatment and storage vessels (US$5-10 each)	Chemical costs at about $US7-11 per capita per year ($35-55 per household per year, assuming about 2 liters per capita (10 liters per household)/day

The World Health Organization (WHO) emphasizes that "the introduction of water treatment technology without consideration of the socio-cultural aspects of the community and without behavioral motivational, educational, and participatory activities within the community is unlikely to be successful or sustainable" (14). An example of a program that that has been successful in promoting community "buy in" to water sanitation improvement is the WHO Participatory Hygiene and Sanitation Transformation (PHAST) program (15). This program engages the community in education and training, and promotes community changes in hygiene and sanitation behaviors in order to effect disease risk reduction.

Are point-of-use water treatment systems cost effective? Costs and costs savings must be calculated not only in terms of equipment and labor required to implement and sustain these systems but also in the savings impact on the community due to disease reduction, including reduced medical costs and lost time from work, disability, or even deaths of providers of household income. Initial and operating costs of various point-of-use water treatment and storage systems in US dollars are found in table 1.

Initial capital expenditure to install systems may come from philanthropic non-governmental organizations or government, but in all cases some cost recovery will be necessary for sustainability of the program just as a stable tax revenue base is necessary to maintain and sustain a centralized source system (14). In some developing countries, this cost recovery may necessarily be delayed or subsidized until economic improvements in individual household can be realized and some costs transferred to the consumer or reductions in health care costs due to disease reduction can be transferred as revenue to support disease prevention programs such as clean water. The long term costs of point-of-use systems compared to the construction and maintenance of central source systems is unknown in similar societies.

SUMMARY

Clean drinking water is an essential component of a established, growing, economically stable, and one could argue, politically stable society. With recent and historical breakdown in central source water treatment systems, the threat of bioterrorism, and large displacements of populations due to political unrest and war, the development of practical and relatively inexpensive point-of-use household water treatment and safe storage systems and their implementation becomes more practical. This is particularly true for developing countries, who still face significant morbidity and mortality from water borne illness and who have yet to develop the infrastructure to provide adequately treated water for their populations.

REFERENCES

[1]   United States Environmental Protection. The history of drinking water treatment. Washington, DC: EPA-816-F-00-006, 2000.

[2]   Raucher RS. Public health and regulatory considerations of the safe drinking water act. Annu Rev Public Health 1996;17:179-202.

[3]   DeNileon GP. Critical infrastructure protection: The who, what, why, and how of counterterrorism issues, 2001. Accessed 2011 Jul 01. URL: www.mrws.org/terror /counterterrorism.htm.

[4]   Gillette J, Fisher R, Peerenboom J, Whitfield R. Analyzing water/wastewater infrastructure interdependencies, 2002. Accessed 2011 Jul 01. URL: www.dis.anl.gov/pubs/42598.pdf.

[5]   Mac Kenzie WR, Hoxie NJ, Proctor ME, et.al. A massive outbreak in Milwaukee of Cryptosporidium infection transmitted through the public water supply. New Engl J Med1994;331:161-7.

[6]   Cryptosporidium in Milwaukee's water supply caused widespread illness, 2007. Accessed 2011 Jul 01. URL: www.infectiousdiseasenews.com.

[7]   Beatty ME, Phelps S, Rohner C, Weisfuse I. Blackout of 2003: Public health effects and emergency response. Public Health Rep 2006;121:36-44.

[8]   Rajendran P, Murugan S, Raju S, et al. Bacteriological analysis of water samples from Tsunami hit costal areas of Kanyakumari District, Tamil Nadu. Indian J Med Microbiol 2006;24:114-6.

[9]   Gupta SK, Suantio A, Gray A, et al. Factors associated with E. coli contamination of household drinking water among tsunami and earthquake survivors, Indonesia. Am J Trop Med Hyg 2007;76(6):1158-62.

[10]   Englande Jr AJ. Katrina and the Thai tsunami—water quality and public health aspects mitigation and research needs. Int J Environ Res Public Health 2008;5(5):384-93.

[11]   Muthuramalingam R. The effects of hurricanes Katrina and Rita on the water and wastewater infrastructure, 2005. Accessed 2011 Jul 01. URL: http://www.frost.com /prod/servlet/market-insight-top.pag?docid=50091110.

[12]   Walsh B. After the quake comes the disease. Can Haiti cope? Accessed 2011 Jul 01. URL: http://www.time.com/time/specials/packages/article/0,28804,1953379_ 19534 94_1953675,00.html.

[13]   Centers for Disease Control and Prevention. Update: Cholera outbreak. Haiti, 2010. MMWR 2010;59 (45):1473-9.

[14]   WHO. Managing water in the home: Accelerated health gains from improved water supply. Water Sanitation and Health (WSH). Accessed 2011 Jul 01. URL: www.who.int/water_sanitation_ health/dwq/wsh0207/en/index7.html.

[15]   Doocy S, Burnham G. Point-of-use water treatment and diarrhea reduction in the emergency context: an effectiveness trail in Liberia. Trop Med Int Med 2006;2(10):1542-52.

[16]   Quick RE, Kimura A, Thevos A, et al. Diarrhea prevention through household-level water disinfection and safe storage in Zambia. Am J Trop Med Hyg 2002;66(5):584-9.

[17]   Reller ME, Mendoza CE, Lopez MB, et al. A randomized controlled trial of household-based flocculant-disinfectant drinking water treatment for diarrhea prevention in rural Guatemala. Am J Trop med Hyg 2003;69(4):411-9.

[18]   Rangel J, Lopez B, Mejia MA, Mendoza C, Luby S. a novel technology to improve drinking water quality: a microbiological evaluation of in-home flocculation and chlorination in rural Guatemala. J Water Health 2003;1:15-22.

[19]   Sobsey PF, Hanzel T, Venczel. Chlorination and safe storage of household drinking water in developing countries to reduce waterborne disease. Water Sci Technol 2003;47:221-8.

[20]   WHO. Participatory hygiene and sanitation transformation: A new approach to working with communities, 1996. Accessed 2011 Jul 01. URL: http://www.who.int/water_sanitation_health /hygiene/envsan/phast/en/

Submitted: August 01, 2011. Revised: September 02, 2011. Accepted: October 03, 2011.

In: Public Health Yearbook 2012
Editor: Joav Merrick

ISBN: 978-1-62808-078-0
© 2013 Nova Science Publishers, Inc.

Chapter 8

PERSPECTIVES ON IMMUNIZATIONS

Donald E Greydanus, MD, Dr HC (ATHENS), Daiva Olipra, MD, Jocelyn De Leon, MD and Anjana Neupaney, MD*

Western Michigan University School of Medicine
The Departments of Pediatric & Adolescent Medicine and Internal Medicine

ABSTRACT

Immunizations for all citizens of the world should be an important goal of all clinicians including those dealing with children and adolescents in developing and developed countries. Vaccine preventable diseases continue to take a devastating toll on these vulnerable human beings. This article summarizes concepts of immunizations with the caveat that widespread travel brings many diseases around the globe whether one lives in a tropical or subtropical area or anywhere in the world. The current anti-vaccine hysteria now prevalent in developed countries threatens to explode into epidemics of diseases now controlled by vaccinology with significant increase in morbidity and mortality.

Keywords: Pediatrics, immunization, prevention, public health

INTRODUCTION

Proper immunizations of all children, adolescents, and adults should be a mission of all clinicians (1,2). Global travel allows easy dispersal of dangerous organisms that can infect and injury the person who has not been exposed to these microbes and thus, has no immunity against them. Fortunately, some of these disorders are preventable because there are vaccines that have been developed to allow the vaccinated person to avoid the growing list of these vaccine preventable diseases (VPDs).

---

* Correspondence: Professor Donald E Greydanus, MD, Western Michigan University School of Medicine; The Departments of Pediatric & Adolescent Medicine; and Internal Medicine, United States. E-mail: Donald.Greydanus@med.wmich.edu.

After millions of years without protection against these microbes, much progress has been made after the historic work of Dr. Edward Jenner (1749-1823) in 1796 against the smallpox virus, one of the deadliest epidemics haunting humans, killing over one-third of those infected for thousands of years. One hundred and eighty one years after Jenner inoculated 8 year old James Phipps with cowpow vaccine in 1796 using what was then called the "Turkish" method, smallpox was eliminated from the world except for stockpiles of this virus in some countries (3). This monumental achievement in medicine was started in the 800s in India with oral snake venom, continued in China in the 1100s, stimulated by Jenner in 1796, sparked by the Spanish government for the world's first immunization campaign from 1803 to 1813 (4), and improved greatly with scientific progress in immunology and microbiology in the 20th and now 21st centuries.

As a result of such progress, many diseases have been reduced or even eliminated in some parts of the world. For example, infectious poliomyelitis has been eliminated from the Western Hemisphere and in the United States, diphtheria and congenital rubella syndrome are rarely seen. In the United States inactivated polio vaccine (IPV) is given at 2,4,6-18 months, and 4-6 years; it is not routinely given at or after age 18 years in the U.S. Oral polio vaccine (OPV) is used in some developing countries.

Unfortunately, controversy arose against vaccines as soon as vaccinology began, with a number of people in the 19th century mounting an antivaccine campaign, as is noted today even in the 21st century (4,5). Such controversy has reduced the number of people in the globe who have received immunization against vaccine preventable diseases (VPDs).

Other issues with regard to providing comprehensive coverage of VPDs to the public have continued. Some people do not have access to immunizations because of poverty, have limited access to clinicians, or have clinicians who do not emphasize vaccinations in health care. Despite World Health Organization's (WHO, Geneva, Switzerland) and the Centers for Disease Control and Prevention's (CDC, Atlanta, Georgia, US) guidelines, immunizations schedule and recommendations can be vary from country to country. Some people do not receive comprehensive health care, were vaccinated at the wrong time or given a wrong schedule because of clinician error.

Estimates in the United States note that over 35 million American adolescents are missing one or more recommended vaccinations (6,7) Some may have been vaccinated at the wrong time or with a wrong schedule because of error by the busy health care system (8). Sometimes an opportunity to vaccine an individual is missed because the health care system uses incorrect contraindications for vaccinations. Some vaccines (such as for hepatitis B and varicella) were not part of the recommended vaccine schedule when some youth or college students were children.

Some of the VPDs considered in this discussion are listed in Table 1. More vaccines are being developed and their safety is important to provide to a sometimes skeptical public that may receive the wrong information from the media (5,9) (www.cdc.gov/od/science.iso/). In this discussion, the immunization schedule used in the United States is considered (10,11). The exact recommendations and schedule will vary from country to country depending on the issues within that country and the precise recommendations of the experts in that particular country—as for example, in Argentina (12).

Clinicians should pay close attention to the contraindications or precautions to use of vaccines (13). Sometimes precautions are noted for vaccines in which the person has a condition in which the vaccine might increase the chance of or the severity of an adverse reaction or compromise the ability of the vaccine to produce immunity. Absolute or permanent contraindications are rare and include anaphylactic reaction to a vaccine or a component of the vaccine. Temporary contraindications include moderate or severe illness; additional contraindications for live, attenuated vaccine include pregnancy and immunosuppressive disorders. Clinicians should note that contraindications do not include low grade fever, upper respiratory infections, ear infections, or mild gastroenteritis.

Consultation with experts may be necessary for immunosuppressive conditions. In general, these vaccines are acceptable for those with HIV/AIDS patients with an adequate CD4 count (at or over 25%), those with leukemia or other cancers if healthy and 3 to 6 months post-chemotherapy, those on less than 2 mg/kg/day of corticosteroids, and on a dose of steroids of 2 or more mg/kg/day if less than 2 weeks. If two or more live viral vaccines are given they should be given at the same time; if one vaccine is missed in this fashion, separate them by 28 days to avoid possible interference from circulating antibodies to the first vaccine.

Children and adults are at risk for morbidity and mortality from vaccine preventative diseases. Many adults are at considerable risk because of low vaccination rates.

Table 1. Vaccine Preventable Diseases (Partial List)

1. Tetanus, Diphtheria, Pertussis (Td/Tdap)
2. Measles, Mumps, Rubella (MMR)
3. Meningococcal
4. Human Papillomavirus (HPV)
5. Hepatitis A vaccine
6. Hepatitis B vaccine
7. Varicella vaccine
8. Influenza vaccine
9. Pneumococcal (polysaccharide): PPV23 Rotavirus
10. Cholera vaccine
11. Rabies vaccine
12. Japanese encephalitis vaccine
13. Typhoid vaccine
14. Yellow fever vaccine
15. Lyme disease vaccine
16. Others

For example, the combination of influenza and pneumococcal disease represent the 5th leading cause of death in adults in the US over 65 years of age. Annual mortality in US adults include as many as 48,000 deaths (average over 23,000) annually from influenza, 6,000 from hepatitis B, and over 5,000 from invasive pneumococcal disease (7,11). If clinicians caring for adults to not provide these vaccines, death rates to vulnerable adults will continue.

New developments in vaccinology include the production of new vaccines and combination vaccines. New vaccines in preparation include vaccines for cytomegalovirus, herpes simplex virus, Mycoplasma pneumoniae, Neisseria gonorrhoeae, Chlamydia trachomatis, and others. New vaccine delivery systems are under development including patch vaccines, nasal vaccines, microencapsulation, and use of bioengineered plants.

TETANUS/DIPHTHERIA/PERTUSSIS (TdaP/Td) VACCINES

Children are usually protected against tetanus, diphtheria, and pertussis by receiving a combination vaccine which covers all three and which occurs in a series of immunizations in early childhood (DTaP at 2, 4, 6, and 15 to 18 months). A DTaP booster is given at 4 to 6 years of age, and then one between 11 and 12 years, usually 5 years after the primary childhood series. The early adolescent booster was a Td immunization but now a combination of all three is recommended in the United States (Tdap) because of recent rise in pertussis. After that, a booster for tetanus and diphtheria is recommended every 10 years. If one is over 7 years of age and did not receive the recommended primary childhood series, the primary series is started as soon as possible with a second dose 4 weeks after the first, a third primary dose 5 to 12 months later, and then a booster every 10 years.

Children between 7 and 10 years of age who did not complete a DTaP series can receive the Tdap. Those 11-12 years who have received a full DTaP series can receive a Tdap vaccine and those who are 13-18 years of age can receive a Tdap if not given at 11-12 years. Older persons who are due for a tetanus-diphtheria booster can be given a Tdap booster. Only one immunization for all three diseases (Tdap) is recommended after the primary series at this time (14).

TETANUS

Tetanus (Greek word for taut or stretch) is caused by the Clostridium tetani exotoxin and there are about 40 to 50 cases of tetanus in the United States each year, ranging from a low of 34 in 2004 to a high of 601 in 1948. It is usually found in the elderly adult whose immunization never occurred or was many years earlier. Clostridium tetani is a Gram-positive, rod-shaped, obligate, anaerobic bacterium that lives in the soil as well as the intestinal tract. It causes the classic tetanus disorder with skeletal muscle spasms and lockjaw in generalized tetanus; other forms include neonatal, local, and cephalic tetanus (15).

The WHO estimates 59,000 newborns died from neonatal tetanus around the world in 2008 (15). Neonatal tetanus can develop if the mother does not have antibodies to this organism. The mortality rate of tetanus varies from 48% to 75%. The tetanus vaccine was first introduced in the US in 1927 and this tetanus toxoid vaccine develops serum IgG antibodies to prevent tetanus. Protection against this organism is noted with a serum tetanus antitoxin level of 0.1 IU/ml or more as measured by ELISA technology. Coverage for tetanus in pregnant women can dramatically reduce the incidence of neonatal tetanus in tropical regions (16).

DIPHTHERIA

Diphtheria is caused by the Corynebacterium diphtheriae toxin produced by this Gram positive, pleomorphic, facultative, anaerobic bacterium also known as the Klebs-Loffler bacillus. It gains entry into the person via the respiratory tract and induces a severe infection with local inflammatory membrane involvement (pseudomembrane), myocarditis, and distal neuritis. The mortality rate is 10%-20% and though no cases have been reported in the United

States recently, there was a high of 206,939 cases in 1921. The diphtheria toxoid vaccine was introduced in the United States in 1923 and develops both serum IgG and mucosal IgG antibodies to prevent diphtheria. Diphtheria is common in various parts of the world including Latin America and the Caribbean countries. Cases increased dramatically in the USSR after its breakup in 1989; by 1998, there were 200,000 cases with 5,000 deaths (17).

PERTUSSIS

Pertussis is due to Bordetella pertussis, a Gram-negative, aerobic, coccobaccilus in which humans are the only hosts (18). It was isolated by the Belgian microbiologist, Jules Bordet (1870-1961), in 1906. It causes a highly contagious infection of the respiratory tract with a classic cough lasting over 2 weeks and up to 180 days; the classic cough is characterized by coughing paroxysms, post-tussive emesis, and/or a respiratory whoop (19,20). Pertussis diagnosis is with a nasopharyngeal swab or polymerase chain reaction (PCR) technology. There are over 300,000 pediatric deaths in the world each year due to pertussis (19).

The highest number of pertussis cases in the United States was 256,269 in 1934, though the first pertussis vaccine (whole cell vaccine) was developed in the early part of the 20th century. Dr. Louis Sauer (1885-1980) developed an inactivated whole cell vaccine in the 1920s in Evanston, Illinois and the Danish scientist, Dr. Thorvald Madsen (1870-1957), accomplished the first large scale test of the pertussis vaccine in the Faroe Islands of the North Sea in 1925 (17). In 1942 Pearl Kendrick (1890-1980) produced the first combined DTP vaccine with toxoid tetanus as well as diphtheria vaccine and an inactivated whole cell pertussis compenent. Before the pertussis vaccine was developed, 10,000 persons were dying each year in the United States from this infection.

Though cases of pertussis and numbers of infant deaths dropped dramatically after widespread use of the DPT vaccine in the United States, anti-vaccine forces launched an assault on this vaccine with a charge that the whole cell pertussis vaccine produced encephalopathy in infants. The power of the media was witnessed by a one-hour television documentary that aired on April 19, 1982 in the Washington, DC area called "DTP: Vaccine Roulette"; it alleged that pertussis vaccine induced severe neurological damage in infants (21) Though these charges were later noted to be spurious, the damage was done and many parents withheld this vaccine from their children leading to increase in pertussis infections and increase in infant deaths (22).

Though pertussis infections reached a nadir in 1976 with 1,020 cases in the United States, importation of unvaccinated persons to the U.S. along with a decrease in DTP vaccinations lead to a rise of pertussis case after that with over 25,000 cases in 2004. Cases are often to adolescents and adults who have lost their immunity to this infection. Experts suggest there are over 600,000 cases each year in the US and perhaps over three million (17, 23). Unfortunately adolescents and adults without full immunity to pertussis can transmit this infection to infants with severe consequences. Approximately half of infants under one year of age who develop pertussis are hospitalized, one in twenty develops pneumonia, one in 100 develops seizures, and death can occur. Pertussis has a waning immunity in which the immunity from the vaccine or natural infection can begin to lower as early as 7 years after the infection or vaccine. This drop in protection from the natural disease or vaccine may also be due to genetic changes in Bordetella pertussis representing an ability that other organisms possess in the evolutionary dance for survival. An inactivated acellular pertussis vaccine was developed by Dr. Yuji Sato in 1981 and an acellular vaccine received FDA approval in 2005. This has resulted in the Tdap vaccine that is recommended as a one-time dose for adolescents (as noted earlier) and adults who need a booster (18,24-28). It is important to protect ("cocoon") these infants by vaccinating those around the infant until these infants can complete their own primary pertussis series. This includes those living with an infant less than 12 months of age and health care personnel.

MEASLES, MUMPS, RUBELLA VACCINE (MMR)

Measles, mumps, and rubella are well-known contagious viral infections that are spread via the respiratory tract with episodic outbreaks. Measles (rubeola or morbilli) is caused by a paramyxovirus of the genus Morbillivirus. Unfortunately 900,000 persons die from measles annual around the world. Two doses of this live viral vaccine (MMR—Edmonston-Enders strain) are given to children with recommendations in the US since 1989; the first one is given at or after 12 months of age (12-15 months) and the second one at 4 to 6 years of age. Fortunately, measles, and rubella are rare in the United States due to the high coverage of children with vaccination. In 2004, there were 37 cases of reported measles cases in the U.S. in contrast to over 600 cases in 1996 (one-third of which were in adolescents) and a high of 894,000 in 1941.

Failure to vaccinate individuals leads to increases in measles. In 2005, a 17 year old unvaccinated female returned to the US from a visit to Romania; during that time she attended a family gathering of 500 people. After her return from visiting relatives, 34 cases of measles were confirmed that were traced to her (29). Such examples are increasing because of failure for immunizations among all ages with an increase in the number and percentage of measles cases in those over age 20. In 1973 measles was noted in 3% of cases in those over 19 years of age and this increased to 34% in 2000.

College students who leave their countries to study in the US are advised to be fully vaccinated against measles to protect them from a potential outbreak at their university and also prevent them from staring the epidemic (30). Adults born in the United States in 1957 or later can receive one MMR dose while adults who need 2 doses are those at high risk for disease and include health care workers, international travelers, and college students. Though measles has been targeted by the Centers for Disease Control and Prevention (CDC) for eradication from the United States and beyond, the recent surge has set this goal on hold for now (31,32).

RUBELLA

Rubella was reported at its highest level in the US at 57,000 in 1969 and vaccination with the MMR vaccine has practically removed it from the U.S. with very few if any cases reported each year; the few cases noted are mostly in adults with no immunity. Unfortunately rubella cases are noted around the world where vaccination rates are low. Congenital rubella syndrome (CRS) is a serious condition in which rubella infection during pregnancy results in an infant with many congenital defects including mental retardation, deafness, cardiac defects, cataracts, encephalitis, and others. The US had a high of 20,000 cases in the 1964 to 1965 period and now has none thanks to the official rubella vaccination program that began in the US in 1969. It is a tragic result when an infant is born with CRS in the world when it is a preventable condition. Waiver of the rubella vaccine may be acceptable in a female who may become pregnant and who either has a positive serological test for rubella or has documentation of acceptable vaccination. Ironically, though the MMR vaccine has been falsely linked with an increase in autism, its use has been shown to reduce autism in addition to measles, mump, rubella, and CRS (5,33).

MUMPS

Mumps is due to a paramyxovirus that can lead to classic parotitis but also orchitis, epididymitis, spontaneous miscarriage, meningitis (usually mild), oophoritis, pancreatitis, and even rare encephalitis. It reached its highest 20th century level in the US at over 152,000 cases in 1968 and vaccination reduced its prevalence to less than 1 case per 1 million population in the early 2000s. The mumps vaccine was introduced in the US in 1976 with one dose and then 2 doses (MMR) as of 1989.

A resurgence of mumps is noted in the US since the early 2000s with over 250 cases per year since then and a number of outbreaks in many states (34). In 2006 there were 6,300 mumps cases in the middle of the US with the state of Iowa as the epicenter, but eventually involved 45 states and the District of Columbia (2). During this epidemic mumps occurred in over 2 per 100,000 in 8 midwestern states with over 6 per 100,000 in those 18 to 24 years of age. In this epidemic, complications included orchitis (9.6%), meningitis (0.5%), encephalitis (0.4%), and deafness (0.4%); 2.1% of these students were hospitalized. Failure for some to have 2 MMR vaccinations was the cause for some students, but decreasing immunity to the mumps vaccine may have been the main factor in this epidemic. The vaccine seems to be 80 to 85% effective and thus, vaccine failure, played (2) a part in this outbreak.

ANTIVACCINE CONCERNS

Perhaps a much greater problem than limited vaccine failure is the growing movement in the United States and Europe against vaccinations including the MMR vaccine. The movement against vaccines began as soon as vaccinology began with the work of Edward Jenner on smallpox (5). Concerns with vaccines over the past two centuries have focused on a myriad of issues such as claims of greater efficacy with natural infection versus vaccination, anger at compulsory vaccine programs, concerns with mercury in vaccines, worries about side effects from vaccines, worries about the low efficacy of vaccines, and others.

The MMR vaccine has been the epicenter of current antivaccine angst due to false clams linking it with causing autism (5).The first salvo in this current movement was fired by the 1982 television documentary falsely alleging brain damage from the pertussis vaccine (5). Then Bernhard Rimland PhD (1928-2006), a highly respected psychologist in the field of developmental-behavioral disorders (i.e., autism, ADHD, learning disorders, and learning disorders) asserted that thiomersal was linked to what he saw was an epidemic rise in autism.

He was the Autism Society of America founder in 1965 and also founder (1967) as well as the Autism Research Institute director in San Diego, California, USA).

Adding to this belief was the work of Andrew Wakefield who is a medical researcher and surgeon from England. In 1998 he published a highly-publizied study in the well-known medical journal, Lancet, in 1998 claiming a link between the MMR vaccine and what he called "autistic enterocolitis" (35). Though this research was later discredited and his article recalled by the Journal that published it, the pebble-in-the-pond effect continued, as increasing numbers of alarmed mothers stopped and/or delayed allowing their children to receive the MMR vaccination resulting in increased numbers of infections such as measles (5,36-40). The public remains concerned even though science has clearly shown there is no link of autism with vaccines or with mercury (41-45). Even so, the lawsuits continue in the United States, the media continues to pursue such stories, and some chose to ignore science as in the past (46-50). Globally there were an estimated 873,000 deaths from measles in 1999 and 345,000 deaths in 2005; mortality in some countries is about 1 in 1,000 with about 450 deaths in children each day in sub-Saharan Africa (51). Mumps is increasing and children remain at risk to be born with the preventable congenital rubella syndrome.

Alice in Alice in Wonderland, 1865:

> If I had a world of my own, everything would be nonsense.
> Nothing would be what it is because everything would be what it isn't.
> And contrary-wise; what it is it wouldn't be, and what it wouldn't be, it would. You see?

(Lewis Carroll [Charles Lutwidge Dodgson])

MENINGOCOCCAL VACCINES

There are approximately 3,000 meningitis cases of meningitis each year due to Neisseria meningitidis in the United States and it has a mortality rate of 14% in addition to a high risk for complications in the survivors that include deafness, mental retardation, and loss of limbs (52-54). N meningitidis is a leading cause of meningitis and bacterial sepsis in the US and the world, especially among adolescents and young adults.

Infectious rates can range from 0.5 to 1.3 per 100,000 and 1.4 in selected young adults in a college or university setting (55). Those immunized at 11-12 years of age may have decreased protective immunity when 16 to 21 years of age and thus, a booster immunization is recommended. If a dose is given at 16 years of age or older, a booster is not needed later unless the person remains at high risk for this infection (Table 2) (56). MCV4 contains 48 micrograms of diphtheria toxoid but does not provide any protection against diphtheria.

In the US, most cases (98%) are sporadic and 62% involve those over 11 years of age. Thus, a university with 40,000 students in the US can expect one case of invasive meningococcal disease every 1 to 2 years unless these students are protected by a meningococcal vaccine (57). Table 2 notes those at high risk for N meningitidis meningitis, including university students in crowded dormitory situations with increased smoking and nasopharyngeal carriage of this microbe (58-61). Those in college who are 21 years of age and young should have received an MCV4 dose within the past 5 years; if not, they can be given this vaccine. Those who are 22 or older do not need a routine MCV4 vaccination.

Table 2. Persons at Increased N. Meningitidis risk

First year university students living in crowded places (as dormitories)
Military recruits
Persons exposed during an acute epidemic or outbreak
Those traveling to West Africa or other areas with a high rate of infection
Individuals with some conditions that lower immunity
-HIV infection,
-Functional or anatomical asplenia
-Terminal complement component
Persons working in labs with *N. meningitidis*

Though a polysaccharide meningococcal vaccine is available, the meningococcal conjugate vaccine is preferred for those 2 to 55 years of age. The polysaccharide vaccine produces (MPSV4) is a less effective T-cell independent immune response but can be used if the conjugate vaccine is not available. Conjugate vaccine technology was developed in the 1980s and utilizes chemical conjugation to carrier proteins that leads to an induced T-cell dependent response for improved protection against this organism. This vaccine (MVC4) was first licensed by the FDA in 2006. Both the polysaccharide and conjugate meningitis vaccine protect against 4 subtypes: A, C, Y, and W-135. MCV4 is given intramuscularly and MPSV4 is given subcutaneously. Protection from the B subtype does not occur and B can cause 20% of invasive meningococcemia in the U.S.

HUMAN PAPILLOMAVIRUS (HPV) VACCINE

The human papillomavirus (HPV) is the most common sexually transmitted disease microbe that infects over 20 million individuals in the United States with over 6 million new cases each year (53). Over half of sexually active persons are infected including over 80% before 50 years of age. Over 100 HPV serotypes are classified including 40 that affect the genitals and 15 that are listed as oncogenc—particularly types 16,18,31,33, and 45. HPV is a global infection and found throughout the world (62). Chronic HPV infection can lead to cervical cancer with over 10,000 cases diagnosed in adult females each year in the U.S. and over 4000 deaths annually. Globally there are over 250,000 deaths annually from cervical cancer.

The first infection usually occurs soon after sexual behavior initiates (sexarche) and infection with more than one HPV type often occurs. Use of condoms is not fully protective and rare genital infection may develop from non-penetrative sexual contact as well as underclothes transmission and even surgical gloves as agents of transmission. Though HPV infection is typically cleared from the female within 2 years after initial infection, it can become a persistent infection in about 10% of females leading to an increased risk for cervical and other anogenital cancers.

Recombinant DNA technology led to the development of the HPV vaccine (HPV4) that includes VLPs (viral-like particles) of the oncogenic types 16 and 18 and in one vaccine, the addition of two types causing over 90% of anogenital warts—6 and 11. Serotypes 16 and 18 result in over 70% of cervical cancer and cross-over immunogenicity may lead to proposed protection from 80% of cervical cancer (63).The HPV vaccine contains the L1 protein that self-assemble into VLPs that are immunogenic but non-infectious by mimicking the HPV viron.

It is given in three intramuscular injections at 0, 2, and 6 months apart with minimal intervals between dose 1 and 4 at 4 weeks and 12 weeks between dose 2 and 3. HPV-4 (contains serotypes 6,11,16, and 18) is US. It is FDA-approved for females and males between 9 and 26 years of age; it is recommended to give this vaccine before sexual behavior starts. Even if one is infected with one HPV, the vaccine is recommended since it is unlikely one has each cancer type. Providing the HPV vaccine does not replace the recommendation for cervical cancer screening for females (64). Though there is no evidence of teratogenicity, it is not given to pregnant females since data on this is still limited. Contraindications to the HPV vaccine include history of allergic reaction to a previous HPV vaccine injection, Baker's yeast, or other vaccine components. Other anti-STD vaccines under research include vaccines against Neisseria gonorrhoeae, herpes simplex virus, Chlamydia trachomatis, and the HIV virus (65).

HEPATITIS A IMMUNIZATION

In 2006 the CDC recommended that all children 12 to 23 months of age receive two doses of the Hepatitis A vaccine since data revealed it was widespread in the United States and was capable of causing significant morbidity with increased health care cost and loss of days from work or school; rates of hospitalization vary from 11 to 22% and adults loose an average of 27 days from work. Those older than 23 months who are were not vaccinated can be covered as well. High-risk conditions for this virus include traveling to countries with a high Hepatitis A prevalence, those using illegal drugs, those with chronic liver disease, and men having sex with men (66). Pre-vaccination serologic testing may be useful for some adults, such as those over 40 years of age, those born or living for a prolonged time in places with high hepatitis A infection, and certain populations in the US (such as Hispanics, native Americans, or Alaskan natives).

HEPATITIS B IMMUNIZATION

There are approximately annual 140,000 cases of Hepatitis B infections with 70% noted in adolescents and young adults in the U.S.; overall there are 1.2 million persons infected in the U.S. and the incidence is about 2.8 per 100,000 population (67). Hepatitis B infection leads to hepatitis of various types: acute, chronic, and fulminant. Table 3 lists known risk factors for infection from this DNA virus, though these are not found in 25% of infected persons. Most adults with diabetes mellitus will develop high risk conditions for hepatitis B infection due to the development of chronic liver disease and end stage renal disease; thus, those with diabetes are at risk for increased morbidity and mortality from hepatitis B. This vaccine is given intramuscularly in a three dose schedule or a two dose vaccine that is only available for adolescents between 11 and 15 years of age. There is no proven link between Hepatitis B vaccination and the development of multiple sclerosis (68).

Hepatitis B vaccine is a recombination of antigenic groups (hepatitis B incorporated into plasmids) and has been available in the U.S. since the mid-1980s. Coverage should insure protection of newborns by beginning the hepatitis B series within 12 hours of birth.

Table 3. Risk Factors for Hepatitis B Infection

Multiple sex partners (including more than one partner in last 6 months)
History of sexually transmitted diseases
Male-male sexual behavior
Intravenous drug use
Use of contaminated needle (body piercing, tattooing)
Requiring hemodialysis or clotting factor
Person from a country where hepatitis B infection is common
Caring for or living with a person with hepatitis B infection
Health care workers

If a mother is positive for HBsAg and HBeAg, 70%-90% of the infants become infected without postexposure prophylaxis; the risk of perinatal transmission is 10% if the mother is positive only for HBsAg. An infant is born to an HBsAg+ mother should receive the hepatitis B vaccine and also HBIG within 12 hours of birth. Up to 90% of infected infants develop a chronic infection with HBV.

VARICELLA IMMUNIZATION

Varicella (chickenpox) is the most common vaccine preventable disease in the United States and immunization begins with the 12 to 15 month old and the routine second dose is recommended for all children 4 to 6 years of age. The vaccine (Oka-Merck strain) is also suggested for all adolescents and adults who have not been infected with the varicella virus in a schedule of 2 doses with a minimal interval of 3 months if under age 13 years and 4 weeks if over 13 years of age (69). Antibodies develop after the first dose in 78% and 99% after the second dose. Infection can develop after immunization, though it is much milder with less than 50 lesions that are mainly macular-papular and not vesicular. Efficacy of the vaccine is up to 95% against moderate to severe disease and over 90% retain antibody levels for at least 6 years. Criteria for evidence of immunity to varicella are noted in Table 4 (70).

Prior to the introduction of this varicella vaccine in the United States in 1995, 11,000 persons were hospitalized each year from varicella infection (2-3 per 1,000 healthy children and 8 per 1,000 adults) with one child and one adult dying each week from this infection, 80% in previous "healthy" individuals (69).

The fatality rate of varicella infection is 1 per 100,000 for those 1 to 14 years of age, 2.7 per 100,000 if 15 to 19 years of age, 8 per 100,00 for those 20 to 29 years of age, and 25.2 if 30 to 49 years of age (69).

Persons over 19 years of age account for 5% of varicella cases in the United States but also 35% of the deaths. The implementation of the varicella vaccine program in the United

States resulted in a 97% decrease in deaths from this virus in persons under age 20 years and 96% decrease in those under age 50 years (71).

Table 4. Criteria for Evidence of Varicella Immunity

1. Born in the US before 1980
2. Documentation of appropriate vaccination
3. Laboratory documentation of immunity
4. Clinician report of herpex zoster history
5. Others

PNEUMOCOCCUS IMMUNIZATIONS

Streptococcus pneumoniae is a bacteria that can causes serious infection in individuals of all ages, especially in those with chronic illness (72,73) (Table 5). Children should receive the pneumococcal conjugate vaccine (PCV) at 2,4,6, and 12-15 months of age; PCV-13 has replaced the PCV-7 in which 13 serotypes are covered versus 7. The pneumococcal polysaccharide vaccine (PPV23) is recommended for persons (2 years of age and older) at high risk of S. pneumonia infections, as noted in Table 5. It reduces the rate of drug-resistant Streptococcus pneumoniae (especially type 19A) and provides coverage for 23 of the 90 pneumococcal serotypes (73).

Those at high risk for pneumococcal infection can receive the PPV-23 vaccine including those 19 to 64 years of age who have asthma or smoke cigarettes and all those 65 years of age and older.

One dose is given and a second dose can be given 5 years or more after the first dose; no more than 2 lifetime doses are recommended for those at high risk for complications from infection with Streptococcus pneumonia (72). Efficacy of PPV23 is about 60% to 70% in preventing invasive pneumococcal disease.

Table 5. Conditions with Increased Streptococcus pnemoniae risk

1. Age (at or over 65 years)
2. Alcoholism
3. Asplenia (anatomical or functional)
4. Cancer
5. Chronic cardiovascular disorders
6. Chronic pulmonary disorders
7. Chronic renal failure
8. Diabetes mellitus
9. HIV infection
10. Nephrotic syndrome
11. Sickle cell disease
12. Others.

INFLUENZA VACCINES

Influenza is due to a RNA orthomyxovirus that annually leads to millions of symptomatic infections globally and four pandemics in the world over the past century that includes the infamous Spanish influenza pandemic of 1918-1920 (Table 6) (74). During each influenza season in the United States, 200,000 are hospitalized with over 35,000 deaths, mostly in the elderly and those under 5 years of age. Mortality rates are 2.7% higher when H3N2 is predominant.

Table 6. Influenza Type A Pandemics

Year Subtype Severity of Pandemic:
1889 H3N2 Moderate
1918 H1N1 Severe
1957 H2N2 Severe
1968 H3N2 Moderate
1977 H1N1 Mild

VIRAL CHANGES FROM GENETIC REASSORTMENT (ANTIGENIC DRIFT OR SHIFT)

Alters one's immunity to influenza each year, particularly the ability to deal with the changing hemagglutinin antigen. The vaccine induced immunity does not last from year to year and thus, a new vaccine is introduced each year in attempts to deal with these viral changes. Unfortunately, millions of humans avoid this vaccine each year with potentially devastating results. Starting with the 2011 to 2012 influenza season, allergy to eggs is a precaution and not a contraindication to the influenza vaccine.

Table 7 lists conditions that place individuals at high risk for morbidity and mortality from influenza infection, though anyone can become very ill from this infection with death a potential risk (75-77). Current CDC recommendations include universal influenza vaccination each year for all those over 6 months, since all are at potential risk from this infection. This is in addition to recommendations to cover those at high risk that have been in place since the early 1960s in the United States. Pregnant females, even without other high risk conditions, are at 3 to 4 times increased risk for hospitalization and even death from influenza infection because of the pregnancy. This high risk situation is substantially lowered with receiving the intramuscular influenza vaccination. Though fears have increased for an Avian influenza (H5N1) epidemic or pandemic in the United States and the world, there is no evidence that such an event is imminent—though certainly possible (78).

Two basic types of influenza vaccines are produced, the LAIV and the TIV. The LAIV is the live, attenuated influenza vaccine that is given intranasally for healthy persons between 2 and 49 years of age. It is not given to pregnant females since there is not enough data to assess its safety in pregnancy, though there is no data to indicate toxicity or teratogenicity in this situation.

Table 7. High risk groups for Influenza Complications

1. Diabetes mellitus and other metabolic disorders
2. Cardiovascular disorders (not hypertension)
3. Asthma and other chronic pulmonary disorders
4. Nephrotic syndrome and renal failure
5. HIV infection and other immunosuppressive disorders
6. Those with spinal cord injuries that increase aspiration risks
7. Sickle cell disease; other hemoglobinopathies
8. Pregnancy
9. Children and adolescents (to 18 years of age) on long term aspirin management

The trivalent (inactivated) influenza vaccine (TIV) is an intramuscular immunization given to anyone 6 months of age and older during the influenza season, which is October to May in the United States. The influenza vaccine for the 2011 to 2012 season in the U.S. was the same for the previous year: A/California/7/2009 (H1N1)-like virus, an A/Perth/16/2009 (H3N2)-like virus, and a B/Brisbane/60/2008-like virus. Immunity wanes after 8 to 10 months. It is up to 80% effective in healthy individuals under 65 years of age. Among sickly elderly individuals, the influenza vaccine is less effective: 80% effective in prevention of death, up to 60% effective in prevention of hospitalization, and up to 40% overall efficacy (76).

ROTAVIRUS VACCINES

Rotavirus is a viral infection that results in up to 70,000 hospitalizations in infants and young children in the U.S. with 20 to 60 deaths annually (79). It leads to over 500,000 deaths in children under age 5 years each year in developing countries (80). Rotavirus infection leads to viral gastroenteritis with severe emesis, diarrhea, and dehydration. It is the most common case of diarrheal diseases in young children in the world. Prior to the current rotavirus immunization program that was begun the U.S. in 2006, 95% of children had this infection by age 5 (79).

Two live oral rotavirus vaccines are now available in the U.S. and many other countries (79-81). One is derived from an attenuated human strain (89-12) rotavirus and the other contains five bovine-human reassortant strains (80). Both vaccines have high efficacy rates and are not associated with increased rates of intussusceptions that were noted in 1999 with the previous vaccine.

Table 8. Contraindications to the Rotavirus Vaccines

> Demonstrated history of hypersensitivity to the vaccine or any of its components
> History of intussusception
> History of uncorrected congenital gastrointestinal tract malformation that may lead to intussusception
> History of SCID
> (severe combine immunodeficiency)

Contraindications to these vaccines are noted in Table 8, which includes intussusceptions due to the previous risk as noted. The vaccines are given to young infants, one at 2 and 4 months of age versus the other one that is given in three doses: 2,4, and 6 months.

IMMUNIZATIONS FOR PREGNANT FEMALES

Pregnant females should be fully protected from vaccine preventable disorders both for the health of the mother and her offspring. Very low risk is conferred to the pregnancy female or offspring by use of killed vaccines. Though there is no evidence of teratogenicity using US FDA approved, attenuated, live viral vaccines (i.e., MMR, Varivax, LAIV), they should be avoided on theoretical basis one month prior to and during pregnancy. Women should be advised to avoid contraception for one month after receiving live vaccines. Neither killed nor live vaccines are contraindicated for breast-feeding females. Varicella and MMR vaccines should be given to susceptible females immediately postpartum.

The pregnant female should be protected from influenza, hepatitis B disease, tetanus, and diphtheria. Immunologic protection in the pregnant mother can confer protection for her newborn with various diseases, including influenza, tetanus, pertussis, diphtheria, respiratory syncytial virus, Group B streptococcus, and Haemophilus influenzae type b (82). Vaccination of the pregnancy female to protect both mother and fetus has been strongly emphasized by leading health care organizations in the U.S. since 1957. Tdap is approved for women after 20 weeks of gestation and is typically given, if needed, during the third or late 2nd trimester. If Tdap is not given during the pregnancy, it can be given immediately postpartum. It is not clear whether or not Tdap given during pregnancy leads to protection of the infant against pertussis via transplancetal antibodies.

COMMENTARY ON IMMUNIZATIONS IN VARIOUS COUNTRIES

As noted previously, immunization schedules and issues vary from country to country based on various factors in each place. This section provides an overview of immunization concepts in three representative countries: Lithuania, the Philippines, and Nepal.

IMMUNIZATION IN LITHUANIA

Lithuania was under the health insurance system of the Soviet Union from 1940-1990. The health insurance plan was an integral part of what was called social insurance or universal care. The advantage of this system is that medical service is accessible to all residents. In 1990 Lithuania restored its independence so health care moved out of the centralized Soviet Union model. The authorities decided to reform the health care system with a decentralized management system. In 1991 Lithuania joined the World Health Organization.

While there has been some attempt to privatize the system, Lithuania's National Immunization program is overwhelmingly regulated by the Ministry of Health. Vaccinations are performed mostly by the state but also some private health centers. According to Lithuanian law only medical doctors (pediatricians or general practitioners) can administer vaccinations.

Health institutions report the number of vaccinations and the number of children that were vaccinated in each age group to public health centers. The public health centers then report to the national level Centre for Communicable Diseases, Prevention and Control. Sufficient high coverage of vaccination is maintained in Lithuania (94-99 percent for DTP3, HepB3, Hib, MMR1 in age groups under 2 years old). The Republic of Lithuania preventive vaccination calendar includes children vaccinated against tuberculosis, hepatitis B, pertussis, diphtheria, tetanus, polio, measles, mumps, rubella, and Haemophilus influenzae type B infection (83-86). All of these vaccines are 100 percent covered by the Lithuanian health system.

Under the current immunization schedule, public funds now cover acellular pertussis-diphtheria-tetanus vaccine for all infants at 2 months of age. Another innovation is inactivated polio vaccine (IPV) used instead of live polio vaccine (OPV). Not all vaccines in Lithuania are covered by the Lithuanian Health System. Additionally offered are: tick-born encephalitis, Influenza, rabies, varicella, hepatitis A, and human papillomavirus (87,88). Since 2007 Rota virus vaccine is also registered in Lithuania. Since 2010 conjugated Pneumococcal vaccine (7 components) is available and recommended. All of these vaccines are at the parent's expense. Plans are under discussion for the Lithuanian immunization program to include the pneumococcal conjugated vaccine.

IMMUNIZATION IN THE PHILIPPINES

The government of the Philippines has an Expanded Program on Immunizations (EPI) which is made available to infants at no cost throughout the whole country. This includes BCG, OPV #s 1-3, DPT #s 1-3, Hep B #1-3 and measles vaccine (89,90). It does not include some vaccines, such as Hib, MMR, varicella, influenza, pneumococcal, rotavirus, meningococcal, boosters of said vaccines, and others (91-96). The government provides the EPI vaccines in health centers and government municipalities on a monthly basis. Recently, because of an increase in cases of measles in 2010, the government had a door-to-door administration of measles vaccine. Most the third world countries, such as the Philippines, do not have national insurance and if they do, vaccines are typically not covered. Those with private insurance are less likely to have such difficulties in vaccine procurement.

A large percentage of the Philippine population is below the poverty line especially in rural areas. Vaccines other than the ones provided by the government are relatively expensive and are not afforded by those in poverty. This is the primary reason why those families are not able to get these vaccines for their children even if they want it. Consequently, it is not surprising that diseases prevented by these vaccines still occur in this country.

Lack of education and lack of dissemination of correct information to parents is another major factor in limited vaccine implementation. Indirectly, this is associated with poverty. Mothers from these families are not aware of all the vaccines nor their schedules, diseases that it may lead to when not given, their sequelae, and their complications.

These mothers feel that their infants are completely immunized' after receiving the vaccines provided by the government.

Primary care physicians in the Philippines still follow the American Academy of Pediatrics' guidelines with regard to the schedule and types of vaccines.

These patients are lost to follow up after 9 months when the measles vaccine, which is the last vaccine in the EPI, is administered. Primary care physicians should be aware that if mothers tell them that their children have completed 'their vaccines', that just means to say that these only refer to the EPI vaccines.

There are still a number of children who get H. influenza meningitis, measles, rubella/congenital rubella syndrome, mumps and chicken pox. Unfortunately, there continues to be considerable morbidity and mortality as a result.

These illnesses and their severe complications might have been prevented only if these vaccines had been given. Herd immunity is not even applicable to a country where the majority of people are not given vaccines. It is been a struggle for the government, physicians and patients to do what should and could be done in this regard. These groups should work closely to improve this situation in the Philippines.

IMMUNIZATION IN NEPAL

Nepal is a land-locked country with an area of approximately 147,181 square kilometers. The country is divided into three geographic regions: the mountain zone (16 districts) makes up the northern part of the country; the hill zone (39 districts) parallels the mountain zone through the central part of the country from east to west; and the Terai zone (20 districts) which is in the lower elevation of the country and borders India.

These three zones cover 35%, 42% and 23% of the total land area but around 7%, 44% and 49% of the population, respectively.

Health care in Nepal is under the Government of Nepal Ministry of health. Health system in Nepal and includes district hospitals, zonal hospitals, referral hospitals, nursing homes, private hospitals, primary health care centers, health posts and sub-health posts.

Nepal started the Expanded Program on Immunization (EPI) in 1979 in three districts and extended it throughout the country by 1988. EPI is one of the priority programs of Government of Nepal. It is considered to be one of the most cost-effective health interventions.

Vaccine preventable diseases (VPDs) are routinely reported through the Health Management Information System (HMIS) complemented by appropriate surveillance.

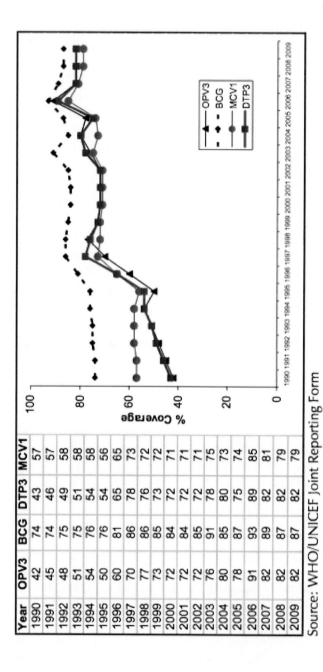

Year	OPV3	BCG	DTP3	MCV1
1990	42	74	43	57
1991	45	74	46	57
1992	48	75	49	58
1993	51	75	51	58
1994	54	76	54	58
1995	50	76	54	56
1996	60	81	65	65
1997	70	86	78	73
1998	77	86	76	72
1999	73	85	73	72
2000	72	84	72	71
2001	72	84	72	71
2002	72	85	72	71
2003	76	91	78	75
2004	80	85	80	73
2005	78	87	75	74
2006	91	93	89	85
2007	82	89	82	81
2008	82	87	82	79
2009	82	87	82	79

Source: WHO/UNICEF Joint Reporting Form

Figure 1. Estimated routine immunization coverage, Nepal 1990-2009.

Antigen	2005		2006		2007		2008		2009	
	Country Official	WHO UNICEF (estimate)	Country Official	WHO UNICEF (estimate)	Country Official	WHO UNICEF (estimate)	Country Official	WHO UNICEF (estimate)	Country Official	WHO UNICEF (estimate)
BCG	87	87	93	93	89	89	87	87	94	87
MCV1	74	74	85	85	81	81	79	79	90	79
DTP3	75	75	89	89	82	82	82	82	89	82
OPV3	78	78	91	91	82	82	82	82	93	82

Source: WHO/UNICEF Estimates and Country Official Estimates (WHO/UNICEF JRF)

Figure 2. Routine immunization coverage, Nepal, 2005-2009.

A World Health Organization (WHO) review team recently observed that overall, through both public and private sector involvement, it appears that the immunization system is able to provide coverage greater than 80% for all antigens. Currently the national immunization program provides a birth dose of BCG; DPT-hepatitis B- Hib combination vaccine with oral polio vaccine at 6, 10 and 14 weeks (97); also, the measles vaccine is provided at nine months (98). Japanese encephalitis vaccine is being phased in high-risk district of the country for children 12-23 months of age. Pentavalent vaccine containing DPT, hepatitis B and Haemophilus influenzae type B antigens was introduced in 2009. Additional vaccinations include tetanus toxoid for pregnant women.

Figure one shows routine immunization coverage estimates from 1990 to 2009 while Figure two shows estimate of WHO and country official's coverage of routine immunization in the last 5 years. In conclusion, the EPI program has had significant effect in decreasing child mortality in Nepal. The coverage is good and is increasing.

There are many remote and inaccessible mountainous areas where coverage is poor and maintenance of a cold chain is difficult. There are also surveillance programs in place involving WHO and other private sectors.

Additional progress would be made if other vaccines are made available to the general public, such as Hepatitis A and B virus vaccines since Hepatitis A and B are endemic in Nepal. Many people are not aware of these disorders More awareness is also needed for rotavirus and HPV vaccinations (99).

SUMMARY

Immunizations for all citizens of the world should be an important goal of all clinicians including those dealing with children and adolescents in developing and developed countries. Vaccine preventable diseases (VPDs) continue to take a devastating toll on these vulnerable human beings. Failure to provide available vaccines is a common problem in the world for various reasons, including poverty, limited health care systems, ignorance on the part of individuals or governments, difficulty in keeping up with ever more complex and changing immunization schedules, and the growing influence of anti-vaccine movements fueled by false information the media. Despite these issues, vaccinology has been one of the greatest advances in modern medicine in the 21st century that can potentially benefit billions of human beings on earth (100-106).

REFERENCES

[1]   Kaul P, Kaplan DW. Caring for adolescents in the office. In: Greydanus DE, Patel DR, Pratt HD, eds. Essential adolescent medicine. New York: McGraw-Hill Medical Publishers, 2006:17-27.

[2]   Greydanus DE, Patel DR. Vaccines for adolescents leaving for higher studies in the USA. In: Bhave S, Parthasarathy A, Yadav S, eds. A ready manual for vaccinations: Adult, adolescents, and pediatric. New Delhi, India: Jaypee Brothers Medical Publishers, 2010:154-72.

[3]   Huygelen C. Jenner's cowpox vaccine in light of current vaccinology. Verh K Acad Geneedskd Belg 1996;58:479-536. [Dutch].

[4]   Mark C, Rigau-Pérez JG. The world's first immunization campaign: The Spanish smallpox vaccine expedition, 1803-1813. Bull Hist Med 2009; 83:63-94.

[5]   Greydanus DE, Toledo L. Historical perspectives on autism: Its past record of discovery and its present state of solipsism, skepticism, and sorrowful suspicion. Pediatr Clin North Am 2012;59(1):5-12.

[6]   Recommended immunization schedules for persons aged 0-18 years—United States, 2007. MMWR 2007;55(51):Q1-Q4.

[7]   Infectious Diseases Society of America. Actions to strengthen adult and adolescent immunization coverage in the United States: policy principles of the Infectious Diseases Society of America. Clin Infect Dis 2007;44(e):104-11.

[8]   Kimmel SR, Burns IT, Wolff RM, Zimmerman RK. Addressing immunization barriers, benefits, and risks. J Fam Pract 2007;56: S61-9.

[9]   Ellenberg SS, Foulkes, MA, Midthun K, et al. Evaluating the safety of new vaccines: summary of a workshop. Am J Publ Health 2005;95:800-7.

[10]   Recommended immunization schedules for persons aged 0-18 years—United States, 2011. MMWR 2011;55(51).

[11]   Recommended immunization schedules for persons aged 19+ years—United States, 2011. MMWR 2011;55(51).

[12]   Calendario National de vacunaci?n de la rep?blica Argentina, 2011. Congresso del Centenario de la Sociedad Argentina de Pediatría. September, 2011.

[13]   Cohen NJ, Laudendale DS, et al. Physician knowledge of catch-up regimens and contraindications for childhood vaccinations. Pediatrics 2003;111:925-32.

[14]   Updated recommendations for use of Tetanus toxoid, reduced diphtheria toxoid and pertussis (Tdap) Vaccine from the Advisory Committee on Immunization Practices, 2010. January 4, 2011.

[15]   Tetanus. Accessed 2011 Oct 01. URL: Http://en.wikipedia.org/wiki/tetanus.

[16]   Personal Communication, Richard Roach MD, Reduction of neonatal tetanus in Madagascar, 2011.

[17]   Diphtheria. Accessed 2011 Oct 01. URL: Http://en.wikipedia.org/wiki/diphtheria.

[18]   Atkinson W, Wolfe S, Hamborsky J, eds. Epidemiology and prevention of vaccine-preventable diseases, 12th Ed. Centers for Disease Control and Prevention. Washington, DC: Public Health Foundation, 2011:215-32.

[19]   Crowcroft NS, Pebody RG. Recent developments in pertussis. Lancet 2006;367:1926-36.

[20]   Purdy KW. Pertussis in the United States. Clin Infect Dis 2004;39:20-8.

[21]   Adashi EY, Offit PA. Paul Offit on the dangers of the anti-vaccine movement. Accessed 2011 Oct 01. URL: http://www.medscape.com/viewarticle/741343?src=mpandsponCommittee on Cherry J. 'Pertussis vaccine encephalopathy': It is time to recognize it as the myth that it is. JAMA 1990;263:1679-80.

[22]   Cherry JD. Ghe epidemiology of pertussis: a comparison of the epidemiology of the disease pertussis with the epidemiology of Bordetella pertussis infection. Pediatrics 2005;115:1422-7.

[23]   Infectious Diseases: Prevention of pertussis among adolescents: Recommendations for use of tetanus toxoid, reduced diphtheria toxoid, and acellular pertussis (Tdap) vaccine. Pediatrics 2006;117(3):965-78.

[24]   Preventing tetanus, diphtheria among adolescents; Use of tetanus toxoid, reduced diphtheria toxoid, and acellular pertussis vaccines. MMWR 2006;55:1-34.

[25]   Pichichero ME, Rennels MB, Edwards KM, et al. Combined tetanus, diphtheria, and 5-component pertussis vaccine for use in adolescents and adults. JAMA 2005;293:3003-11.

[26]   Marshall GS, Happe LE, Lunacsek OE, et al. Use of combination vaccines is associated with improved coverage rates. Pediatr Infect Dis J 2007;26:496-500.

[27]   MMWR, Dec 15, 2006: Preventing Tetanus, Diphtheria, and Pertussis Among Adults: Use of Tetanus Toxoid, Reduced Diphtheria Toxoid, and Acellular Pertussis Vaccine.Recommendations of the ACIP, supported by the Healthcare Infection Control Practices Advisory Committee (HICPAC) for use of Tdap among health-care personnel. MMWR 2006;55(RR17):1-43.

[28]   Parker AA, Staggs W, Dayan GH, et al. Implications of a 2005 Measles outbreak in Indiana for sustained elimination of measles in the United States. N Engl J Med 2006;355:447-55.

[29]   Baughman AL, Williams WW, Atkinson WL, et al. The impact of college prematriculation immunization requirements on risk for measles outbreaks. JAMA 1994;272:1127-32.

[30]   Meissner HC, Reef SE, Chochi S. Elimination of rubella from the United States: A milestone on the road to global elimination. Pediatrics 2006;117:933-35.

[31]   Progress in global measles control and mortality reduction, 2000-2006. MMWR 2007;56(47):1237-41.

[32]   Berger BE, Navar-Boggan Am, Omer SB. Congenital rubella syndrome and autism spectrum disorder prevented by rubella vaccination—United States, 2001-2010. BMC Public Health 2011;11:340.

[33]   Parker AA, Staggs W, Dayan GH, et al. Implications of a 2005 Measles outbreak in Indiana for sustained elimination of measles in the United States. N Engl J Med 2006;355:447-55.

[34]   Wakefield AJ, Murch SH, Anthony A, et al. Ileal-lymphoid-nodular hyperplasia, non-specific colitis, and pervasive developmental disorder in children. Lancet 1998;351:637-41.

[35]   Eggertson L. Lancet retracts 12-year-old article linking autism to MMR vaccines. CMAJ 2010;182:E199-200.

[36]   Godlee F, Smith J, Marcovitch H. Wakefield's article linking MMR vaccine and autism was fraudulent. BMJ 2011;342:c7452.

[37]   Rapin I. High hopes, shoddy research, and elusive therapies for autism examined and exposed. Neurol Today 2009; 9:23.

[38]   Offit PA. Autism's false prophets. Bad science, risky medicine, and the search for a cure. New York: Columbia University Press, 2008.

[39]   Freed GL, Clark SJ, Butchart AT, et al. Parental vaccine safety concerns in 2009. Pediatrics 2010;125:654-9.

[40]   Mrozek-Budzyn D, Kieltyka A, Majewska R. Lack of association between measles-mumps-rubella vaccination and autism in children: a case-control study. Pediatr Infect Dis J 2010;29:397-400.

[41]   Thompson WW, Price C, Goodson B et al. Early thimersol exposure and neuropsychological outcomes at 7 to 10 years. N Engl J Med 2007; 357:1281-92.

[42]   DeStefano F, Chen RT. Autism and measles, mumps, and rubella vaccine: No epidemiological evidence for a causal association. J Pediatr 2000;136:125-6.

[43]   Institute of Medicine Immunizaition Safety Review Committee. Immunization safety review: Vaccines and autism. Washington, DC: National Academies Press, 2004.

[44]   Institute of Medicine. Adverse effects of vaccines: Evidence and causality, 2011. Accessed 2011 Oct 01. URL: http://www.iom.edu/vaccineadverseeffects.

[45]   Sugarman SD. Cases in vaccine court—legal battles over vaccines and autism. N Engl J Med 2007; 357:1275-1279.

[46]   Goodman NW. MMR scare stories: some things are just too attractive to the media. BMJ 2007;335:222.

[47]   Chatterjee A, O'Keefe C. Current controversies in the USA regarding vaccine safety. Expert Rev Vaccines 2010;9:497-502.

[48]   Gerber JS, Offit PA. Vaccines and autism: A tale of shifting hypotheses. Clin Infect Dis (CID) 2009;48:456-61.

[49]   Tafuri S, Martinelli D, Prato R, Germinario C. From the struggle for freedom to the denial of scientific evidence: history of antivaccinationists in Europe. Ann Ig 2011;23:93-9. [Italian]

[50]   Measles. Accessed 2011 Oct 01. URL: http://enwikipedia.org/wiki/measles#epidemiology.

[51]   Gardner P. Prevention of meningococcal disease. N Engl J Med 2006; 355(14):1466-72.

[52]   Middleman AB. Immunization update: Pertussis, meningococcus, and human papillomavirus. Adolesc Med 2006;17:233-140.

[53]   Ellenberg SS, Foulkes, MA, Midthun K, et al. Evaluating the safety of new vaccines: Summary of a workshop. Am J Publ Health 2005; 95:800-7.

[54]   Harrison CH, Dwyer DM, Maples CT et al. Risk of meningococcal infection in college students. JAMA 1999;281:1906-10.

[55]   CDC. Updated recommendations for meningococcal conjugate vaccines. ACIP. MMWR 2011;60:72-6.

[56]   Kumar A, Murray DL, Havlicheck DH. Immunizations for the college student: A campus perspective of an outbreak and national and international considerations. Pediatr Clin 2005;52:229-41.

[57]   Bruce MG, Rosenstein NE, Capparella JM, et al. Risk factors for meningococcal disease in college students. JAMA 2001;286:688-93.

[58] Meningococcal disease and college students. Recommendations of Advisory Committee on Immunizations Practices (ACIP). MMWR 2000;49(RR07):1-20.

[59] Prevention and control of meningococcal disease. recommendations of the Advisory Committee on Immunization Practices (ACIP). MMWR Recomm Rep 2005;54 (RR-7):1-21.

[60] Offit PA, Peter G. The meningococcal vaccine—public policy and individual choices. N Engl J Med 2003;349:2353-6.

[61] Galano A. Vacuna contra el virus del Papiloma Humano (VPH). Argentina. Buenos Aires,Argentian: Ministerio de Salud Presidencia de la Nacion, 2011. Accessed 2011 Oct 01. URL: www.msal.gov.ar.

[62] Bryan JT. Developing an HPV vaccine to prevent cervical cancer and genital warts.Vaccine 2007;25:3001-6.

[63] Franco EL, Mayrand M-H, Ratnam S. HPV DNA versus Papanicolaou screening tests for cervical cancer. N Engl J Med 2008;358:643-4.

[64] Johnston MI, Fauci AS. An HIV vaccine---evolving concepts. N Engl J Med 2007;356:2073-81.

[65] CDC Pink Book: Epidemiology and prevention of vaccine preventable diseases, 9th ed. Atlanta, GA: Centers Disease Control Prevention, 2006:182-3,194,263-4.

[66] Incidence of acute hepatitis B—United States, 1990-2002. MMWR 2004;52(51):1252-4.

[67] Asherio A, Zhang SM. Hepatitis B vaccination and the risk of multiple sclerosis. N Engl J Med 2001;344:327-32.

[68] Meyer P, Seward JF, Jumaan AO, et al. Varicella mortality: trends before vaccine licensure in the United States, 1970-1994. J Infect Dis 2000;182:383-90.

[69] CDC Pink Book: Epidemiology and prevention of vaccine preventable diseases, 11th ed. Atlanta, GA: Centers Disease Control Prevention, 2011:292.

[70] Marin M, Zhang JX, Seward JF. Near elimination of varicella deaths in the US after implementation of the vaccination program. Pediatrics 2011;128:214-20.

[71] Huang SS, Johnson KM, Ray GT, et al. Healthcare utilization and cost of pneumococcal disease in the United States. Vaccine 2011;29:3398-3412.

[72] Kyaw MH, Lynfield R, Schaffner W, et al. Effect of introduction of the pneumococcal conjugate vaccine on drug-resistant Streptococcus pneumoniae. N Engl J Med 2006;354:1455-63.

[73] Centers for Disease Control and Prevention. Prevention and control of influenza: Recommendations of the Advisory Committee on Immunization Practices (ACIP). MMWR Recomm Rep 2007;56 (RR-6):1-60.

[74] Centers for Disease Control and Prevention. Prevention and control of influenza with vaccines. Recommendations of the Advisory Committee on Immunization Practices (ACIP). MMWR 2010;59(RR-8):1-62.

[75] Atkinson W, Wolfe S, Hamborsky J, eds. Epidemiology and prevention of vaccine-preventable diseases, 11th ed. Washington, DC: Public Health Foundation, 2011:142-3.

[76] Zerr DM, Englund JA, Robertson AS, et al. Hospital-based influenza vaccination of children: An opportunity to prevent subsequent hospitalization. Pediatrics 2008;121:345-8.

[77] Writing Committee of the Second WHO consultation on Clinical Aspects of human infection with Avian influenza (H5N1) virus. Update on Avian Influenza (H5N1) virus infection in humans. N Engl J Med 2008;358:261-73.

[78] Atkinson W, Wolfe S, Hamborsky J, eds. Epidemiology and prevention of vaccine-preventable diseases, 11th ed. Washington, DC: Public Health Foundation, 2011:263-74.

[79] Glass RI, Parashar UD, Bresee JS, et al. Rotavirus vaccines: current prospects and future challenges. Lancet 2006;368:323-32.

[80] Centers for Disease Control and Prevention. Prevention of rotavirus gastroenteritis among infants and children. MMWR 2009;58(RR-2):1-25.

[81] Glezen WP, Alpers M. Maternal immunizations. Clin Infect Dis 1999; 28:219-24.

[82] Lutsar I, Anca I, Bakir M, et al. Epidemiologic characteristics of pertussis in Estonia, Lithuania, Romania, the Czech Republic, Poland, and Turdy—1945-2005. Eur J Pediatr 2009;168:407-15.

[83] Usonis V, Bakasenas V, Morkunas B, et al. Diphtheria in Lithuania, 1986-1996. J Infect Dis 2000;181(Suppl 1):S55-9.

[84]   Rix BA, Zhobakas A, Wachmann CH, et al. Immunity from diphtheria, tetanus, poliomyelitis, measles, mumps, and rubella among adults in Lithuania. Scand J Infect Dis 1994;26:459-67.

[85]   Usonis V, Bakasenas V, Taylor D, Vandepapeliere P. Immunogenicity and reactogenicity of a combined DTPw-hepatitis B vaccine in Lithuanian infants. Eur J Pediatr 1996;155:189-93.

[86]   Laiskonis A, Bareisiene MV, Velyvyte D, et al. Surveillance of animal and human rabies in Lithuania from 1991 to 2001. Med Mai Infect 2006; 36:4-8.

[87]   Vanagas G, Padaiga Z, Kurtinaitis J, Logminiene Z. Cost-effectiveness of 12- and 15-year-old girls' human papillomavirus 16/18 population-based vaccination programmes in Lithuania. Scand J Public Health 2010;38:639-47.

[88]   Sobel H, Docusin J, De Quiroz M et al. The Philippines 2004 measles campaign: a success story towards elimination. Trop Doct 2009;39:36-8.

[89]   Sobel HL, Mantaring JB 3rd, Cuevas F, et al. Implementing a national policy for hepatitis B birth dose vaccination in Philippines; lessons for improved delivery. Vaccine 2011;29:941-5.

[90]   Young AM, Crosby RA, Jagger KS, et al. HPV vaccine acceptability among women in the Philippines. Asian Pac J Cancer Prev 2010; 11:1781-7.

[91]   Lucero MG, Nohynek H, Williams G, et al. Efficacy of an 11-valent pneumococcal conjugate vaccine against radiologically confirmed pneumonia among children less than 2 yars of age in the Philippines: a randomized, double-blind, placebo-controlled trial. Pediatr Infect Dis 2009;28:455-62.

[92]   Carlos CC, Inobaya MT, Bresee JS et al. The burden of hospitalizations and clinic visits for rotavirus disease in children aged <5 years in the Philippines. J Infect Dis 2009;200(Suppl 1):S174-81.

[93]   Anh DD, Carlos CC, Thiem DV, et al. Immunogenicity, reactogenicity, and safety of the human rotavirus RIX4414 (RotarixTM) oral suspension (liquid formulation) when co-administered with expanded program on immunization (EPI) vaccines in Vietnam and the Philippines in 2006-2007. Vaccine 2011;29:2029-36.

[94]   Capeding RZ, Lunai IA, Bomasang E, et al. Live-attenuated, tetravalent dengue vaccine in children, adolescents, and adults in a dengue endemic country: randomized controlled phase I trial in the Philippines. Vaccine 2011; 29:3863-72.

[95]   Teyssou R. Dengue fever: from disease to vaccination. Med Trop (Mars) 2009; 69:333-4.

[96]   Jha N, Kumar S. Are we progressing towards the elimination of diphtheria, pertussis, tetanus from Nepal? Kathmandu Univ Med J 2008; 6:520-5.

[97]   Upreti SR, Thapa K, Pradhan YV. et al. Developing rubella vaccination policy in Nepal—results from rubella surveillance and seroprevalence and congenital rubella syndrome studies. J Infect Dis 2011;204(Suppl 1):S433-8.

[98]   Singh Y, Shah A, Singh M et al. Human papilloma virus vaccination in Nepal: An initial experience in Nepal. Asian Pac J Cancer Prev 2010; 11:615-7.

[99]   Plotkin SA, Robinson JM. How and why vaccines are made. In: Kaufmann HE, Lambert PH, eds: The great challenge for the future. Basel, Switzerland: Birkhäuser Basel, 2005:23-36.

[100]   Orenstein WA, Douglas RG, Rodewald LE, Hinman AR. Immunization in the United States: Ssuccess, structure, and stress. Health Aff (Millwood). 2005;24:599-610.

[101]   Hinman AR. Control of communicable diseases. In: Wallace HM, Patrick K, Parcel GS, Igoe JB, eds. Principles and practices of student health. Oakland, CA: Third Party Publishing Company, 1992:53-62.

[102]   Centers for Disease Control and Prevention (CDC). Ten great public achievements-United States. 1900-1999. MMWR 1999;48:241-3.

[103]   Centers for Disease Control and Prevention (CDC). Vaccine preventable diseases. Improving vaccination coverage in children, adolescents and adults. A report on recommendations from the Task Force on Community Preventable services. MMWR 1999;48(RR-8):1-5.

[104]   Centers for Disease Control and Prevention (CDC). Ten great public health achievements—United States, 2001-2010. MMWR 2011; 60:619-23.

[105]   Centers for Disease Control and Prevention (CDC). Ten great public health achievements—worldwide, 2001-2010. MMWR 2011; 60:814-8.

Submitted: September 01, 2011. *Revised:* October 20, 2011. *Accepted:* November 01, 2011.

In: Public Health Yearbook 2012
Editor: Joav Merrick

Chapter 9

MALNUTRITION

*Dilip R Patel, MD**

Department of Pediatrics and Human Development,
Michigan State University College of Human Medicine,
Kalamazoo Center for Medical Studies, Kalamazoo, Michigan, United States of America

ABSTRACT

Food insecurity and malnutrition remain significant public health problems in the developing countries. Malnutrition affects an estimated 900 million peoples worldwide with long term adverse health and economic consequences both at individual and societal levels. Although progress has been made with effective treatment and preventive interventions, the overall burden of malnutrition remains significant. This article reviews key aspects of prevalence, clinical features, and intervention strategies for malnutrition.

Keywords: Malnutrition, public health

INTRODUCTION

Food insecurity and malnutrition are significant concerns worldwide. Food security is defined as "access by all people at all time to sufficient food in terms of quality, quantity and diversity for an active and healthy life without risk of loss of such access" (1-5). Food security thus comprises 3 dimensions, namely availability, access, and utilization (see table 1) (1-3).

The spectrum of malnutrition ranges from undernutrition (see table 2) at one end to obesity at the other end (3-9). The Food and Agriculture Organization measure of malnourishment refers to "number of persons who are assumed to be unable to meet daily calorie requirements necessary for light activities (1).

An estimated 900 million people worldwide are reported to be undernourished, of whom 97% live in developing countries (2-5). About 16% of infants in developing countries are

---

* Correspondence: Professor Dilip R Patel, MD, Department of Pediatrics and Human Development, Michigan State University College of Human Medicine, Kalamazoo Center for Medical Studies, 1000 Oakland Drive, Kalamazoo, MI 49008 USA. E-mail: patel@kcms.msu.edu

born low birth weight. Forty two percent of pregnant women and 47% of children younger than 5 years of age have been reported to have anemia; 1 billion people worldwide have iron deficiency anemia; 2 billion have zinc deficiency and 100-400 million have vitamin A deficiency (10-12).

Malnutrition can have wide ranging adverse impact for the individual and society. Major consequences of chronic undernutrition are listed in table 3 (13).

Table 1. Three dimensions of food security

Dimension	Comments
Availability	Refers to market level supply of food and is generally a reflection of economic conditions of production and trade
Access	Refers to household level ability to purchase food as well as equity of food distribution within household
Utilization	Refers to appropriate use of food in the presence of availability and access

Table 2. Spectrum of undernutrition

Category	Definition or comments
Underweight	Weight that is ≤ 2 SD for age
Stunting	Height that is ≤ 2 SD for age Reflects chronic undernutrition
Wasting	Weight that is ≤ 2 SD for height for age Reflects acute malnutrition
Micronutrient deficiencies	Major deficiencies are for vitamin A, iron, zinc, iodine, and folic acid

Table 3. Major consequences of chronic undernutrition

Consequence	Comments
Premature death	35% of child mortality result from undernutrition Vitamin A deficiency account for 0.6 million deaths per year Zinc deficiency account for 0.4 million deaths per year
Overutilization of health care resources	Low birth weight infant need increased use of neonatal servies Malnourished infants and children more prone to illnesses need more medical care Long term effects in development of diabetes mellitus and cardiovascular diseases
Loss of productivity during adult life	Reduced cognitive abilities and educational achievement result in reduced economic and work productivity in adult years
Effects of future generations	Deficit maternal nutrition result in adverse consequences on future generations

CLINICAL FEATURES OF MALNUTRITION

The clinical features of nonedamatous malnutrition or marasmus include failure to gain weight, weight loss leasing to emaciation (2-3,12). The infant or child is irritable. Child with edematous malnutrition presents with lethargy, apathy and edema. Infants and children with malnutrition show a number of signs affecting many systems. In kwashiorkar the face is described as moon face whereas in marasmus simian facies is noted. The skin may be shiny, edematous and dry. Follicular hyperkeratosis, hyper or hypopigmentation are common. Nail plates are thin and soft with fissuring or ridges.

Oral mucosa shows angular stomatitis, cheilitis and glossitis. Children have dull, sparse and brittle hair with patchy bands of light and normal color. Abdomen is distended and hepatomegaly or ascites can be present. Cardiovascular manifestations include hypotension, reduced cardiac output and small vessel vasculopathy. Neurologic manifestations include developmental delay, impaired cognition and depressed deep tendon reflexes.

Causes, manifestations and management of major micronutrient deficiencies are summarized in table 4 (2,4,11).

Table 4. Causes, manifestations, management and prevention of the major micronutrient deficiencies

Nutrient	Essential for the production or function of	Causes of deficiency	Manifestations of isolated deficiency	Management and prevention
Iron	Hemoglobin Various enzymes Myoglobin	Poor diet Elevated needs (e.g., while pregnant, in early childhood) Chronic loss from parasite infections (e.g., hookworms, schistosomiasis, whipworm)	Anemia and fatigue Impaired cognitive development Reduced growth and physical strength	Foods richer in iron and with fewer absorption inhibitors Iron-fortified weaning foods Low-dose supplements in childhood and pregnancy Cooking in iron pots
Iodine	Thyroid hormone	Except where seafood or salt fortified with iodine is readily available, most diets, worldwide, are deficient	Goiter, hypothyroidism, constipation Growth retardation Endemic cretinism	Iodine supplement Fortified salt Seafood
Vitamin A	Eyes Immune system	Diets poor in vegetables and animal products	Night blindness, xerophthalmia Immune deficiency Increased childhood illness, early death Contributes to development of anemia	More dark green leafy vegetables, animal products Fortification of oils and fats Regular supplementation
Zinc	Many enzymes Immune system	Diets poor in animal products Diets based on refined cereals (e.g., white bread, pasta, polished rice)	Immune deficiency Acrodermatitis Increased childhood illness, early death Complications in pregnancy, childbirth	Zinc treatment for diarrhea and severe malnutrition Improved diet

Reproduced from "Malnutrition and health in developing countries". CMAJ. 2005 Aug 2; 173(3):279-86.

TREATMENT

Treatment of infants and children with malnutrition generally progresses through gradually progressive phases (14-18). The initial treatment usually lasts for the first week followed by rehabilitation of 2-6 weeks and additional 4-6 weeks of final follow-up phase.

During the initial stabilization phase, dehydration is corrected and appropriate antibiotic treatment is started if indicated. Oral feeding is started with WHO F75 diet (75 kcal/100 ml) followed gradually by WHO F100 diet (100 kcal/100 ml). Twelve smaller feedings are gradually transitioned to about 8 feedings/24 hours. Ready to use therapeutic foods (RUTFs) can also be used. RUTF is an oil-based paste which is a mixture of powdered milk, peanuts, sugar, vitamins and minerals.

As the feedings are tolerated, they can be switched to ad lib and during later phase of rehabilitation, environmental stimulation is integrated in the treatment regimen. Infants and children with severe acute malnutrition without complications are treated in the community setting and those with complications need treatment in the healthcare facility.

Refeeding syndrome is a potential complication during initial phase of nutritional rehabilitation in malnourished infants and children. Refeednig syndrome is characterized by development of severe hypophosphatemia and its consequences (see table 5) (19-21). Infants and children at risk for refeeding syndrome require careful management and general principles of management are as follows as described by Mehanna and colleagues (20):

- Identify patients at risk for refeeding syndrome
- Check potassium, calcium, phosphate and magnesium
- Administer thiamine 200-300 mg daily orally, vitamin B high potency 1-2 tablets 3 times daily, multivitamin or trace supplements once daily
- Start feeding 0.0418 MJ/kg/day (If the patient is severely malnourished or if intake is negligible for = 2 weeks, start feeding at a maximum of 0.0209 MJ/kg/day)
- Slowly increase feeding over next 7 days
- Rehydrate carefully and supplement and/or correct levels of potassium, phosphate, calcium and magnesium
- Monitor potassium, phosphate, calcium and magnesium for first 2 weeks and amend treatment as appropriate.

Table 5. Consequences of hypophosphatemia

Weakness
Rhabdomyolysis
Hypotension
Cardiorespiratory failure
Cardiac arrhythmias
Seizures
Coma
Hemolysis
Thrombocytosis
Death
Leukocyte dysfunction

Patients with severe acute malnutrition with complications need treatment in a healthcare facility. These include patients with bilateral pitting sever edema, significant loss weight, anorexia, associated infections, severe anemia or severe dehydration.

PREVENTION

Public health and population based interventions can effective in prevention and treatment of malnutrition (21-24). Some of such key interventions for undernutrition include:

- Promotion of breast feeding for all infants. For mothers with HIV/AIDS breast feeding is recommended for first 6 months in developing countries with rapid weaning at 6 months.
- Adequate and timely complementary feeding, starting at 6 months of age
- Promotion of personal hygiene and sanitation practices
- Giving micronutrient supplements to pregnant women, infants, and children
- Deworming of mothers and infected children
- Fortifying commonly consumed food with micronutrients and minerals
- Presumptive treatment of malaria for pregnant women in endemic regions

Prevention efforts should focus on interventions during pregnancy and first two years of life. The adverse effects of malnutrition on brain development to fetus and during first two years are potentially irreversible. Large scale public health efforts can be effective.

Supplement of folic acid in pregnancy has been successful in preventing neural tube defects. Two thirds of people in developing world now have access to iodized salt that has improved care significantly for iodine deficiency and anemia that affect 3.5 billion people. About 450 million children a year receive Vitamin A capsules, reducing blindness and childhood mortality.

CONCLUSION

Food insecurity and malnutrition are persistent problems in developing world affecting millions of people. The long term consequences of malnutrition are significant both at individual and societal levels. Although effective treatment and prevention interventions have made significant impact in reducing the burden of malnutrition, enormous challenges still remain to meet the needs of populations worldwide.

REFERENCES

[1]   Food and Agriculture Organization of the United Nations. Undernourishment around the world. In: The state of food insecurity in the world 2004. Rome: Food Agriculture Organization United Nations, 2004.

[2]   Brabin BJ, Coulter JBS. Nutrition-associated disease. In: Cook GC, Zumla AI, eds. Manson's tropical diseases. London: Saunders, 2003:561-80.

[3]   Pinstrup-Andersen P, Burger S, Habicht JP, Peterson K. Protein-energy malnutrition. In: Jamison DT, Mosley WH, Measham AR, Bobadilla JL, eds. Disease control priorities in developing countries, 2nd ed. Oxford: Oxford University Press, 1993:391-420.

[4]   Levin HM, Pollitt E, Galloway R, McGuire J. Micronutrient deficiency disorders. In: Jamison DT, Mosley WH, Measham AR, Bobadilla JL, eds. Disease control priorities in developing countries, 2nd ed. Oxford: Oxford University Press, 1993:421-51.

[5]   World Health Organization. World health report. Geneva: WHO, 2004.

[6]   World Health Organization and the United Nations Children's Fund: WHO child growth standards and the identification of severe acute malnutrition in infants and children. Accessed 2011 Sep 01. URL: www.who.int/nutrition/publications/severemalnutrition/9789241598163/en/index.html 2009.

[7]   Word Health Organization. Informal consultation to review current literature on severe malnutrition. Gevena: WHO, 2005.

[8]   Behrman JHR, Alderman H, Hoddinott J. Hunger and malnutrition. In: Lomborg B, ed. Global crises, global solutions, Cambridge: Cambridge University Press, 2004.

[9]   Black RE, Allen LH, Bhutta ZA, et al. Maternal and child undernutrition: global and regional exposures and health consequences. Lancet 2008;371:243-60.

[10]   Rice AL, Sacco L, Hyder A, Black RE. Malnutrition as an underlying cause of childhood deaths associated with infectious diseases in developing countries. Bull World Health Organ 2000;78:1207-21.

[11]   Black R. Micronutrient deficiency – an underlying cause for morbidity and mortality. Bull World Health Organ 2003;81:79.

[12]   Grover Z, Ee LC. Protein energy malnutrition. Pediatr Clin N Am 2009;56:1055-1068.

[13]   Collins S, Dent N, Binns P, et al. Management of severe acute malnutrition in children. Lancet 2006;368:1992-2000.

[14]   Collins S. Treating severe acute malnutrition seriously. Arch Dis Child 2007;92:453-461.

[15]   World Health Organization, United Nations Children's Fund. Joint statement on the management of acute diarrhea. Geneva: The Organization, 2004.

[16]   World Health Organization. Management of the child with a serious infection or severe malnutrition. Guidelines for care at the first-referral level in developing countries. Geneva: The Organization, 2000.

[17]   World Health Organization. Management of severe malnutrition: a manual for physicians and other senior health workers. Geneva: The Organization, 1999.

[18]   Bhan MK, Bhandari N, Bahl R. Management of the severely malnourished child: perspective from developing countries. BMJ 2003;326:146-51.

[19]   Fuentebella J, Kerner JA. Refeeding syndrome. Pediatr Clin N Am 2009;56:1201-10.

[20]   Mehanna HM, Moledina J, Travis J: Refeeding syndrome: what it is and how to prevent and treat it. BMJ 2008;336:1495-8.

[21]   Manary MJ, Sandige HL: Management of acute moderate and severe childhood malnutrition. BMJ 2008;337:1227-30.

[22]   Nemer L, Gelban H, Jha P; Commission on Macroeconomics and Health. The evidence base for interventions to reduce malnutrition in children under five and school-age children in low- and middle-income countries. CMH working paper no WG5:11. Geneva: World Health Organization, 2001.

[23]   Collins S, Sadler K, Dent N, et al: Key issues in the success of community-based management of severe malnutrition. Food Nutr Bull 2006;27(suppl 3):S49-S82.

[24]   World Bank: Repositioning nutrition as central to development: a strategy for large-scale action. Washington, DC, World Bank, 2006.

Submitted: September 01, 2011. *Revised:* November 02, 2011. *Accepted:* November 16, 2011.

In: Public Health Yearbook 2012
Editor: Joav Merrick

ISBN: 978-1-62808-078-0
© 2013 Nova Science Publishers, Inc.

Chapter 10

THE HUMAN IMMUNODEFICIENCY VIRUS IN PEDIATRICS

Amanda Gittus, MD[*]

Internal Medicine/Pediatrics, Michigan State University, MSU/Kalamazoo Center for
Medical Studies, Kalamazoo, Michigan, United States of America

ABSTRACT

As we enter the 4th decade of a world-wide epidemic, it is clear that few diseases
have so widely shaped our world's health, economy, and society in the modern age as the
acquired immunodeficiency syndrome (AIDS).This article will review the history,
pathophysiology, and diagnosis of infection with HIV. It will also discuss the basics of
prevention as well as treatment and provide the primary care doctor with a reference to
care for HIV infected children, including immunization recommendations, and expectant
management of comorbidities. Finally, this article contains a review of the most recent
literature relating to pathogenesis, treatment options, medication side-effects, and
progress toward halting disease progression and ultimately finding a cure.

Keywords: Human immunodeficiency virus, acquired immunodeficiency syndrome,
HIV, AIDS, children

INTRODUCTION

As we enter the 4th decade of a world-wide epidemic, it is clear that few diseases have so
widely shaped our world's health, economy, and society in the modern age as the Acquired
Immunodeficiency Syndrome (AIDS). As of 2009 the World Health Organization (WHO)
estimated that nearly 2.5 million children under 15 years of age are living with HIV, with
1,000 new infections appearing in this age group every day(1). Seven hundred children die

---
[*] Correspondence: Amanda Gittus MD, Assistant Professor, Internal Medicine/Pediatrics, Michigan State
University, MSU/Kalamazoo Center for Medical Studies, 1000 Oakland Drive, Kalamazoo, MI, 49008-1284,
United States. E-mail: Gittus@kcms.msu.edu

from AIDS related diseases in the world every 24 hours and in 2009 alone a quarter of a million children under the age of 15 years, died of the disease (1-3). In areas of high prevalence of Human Immunodeficiency Virus (HIV) infection, AIDS has single-handedly reversed the progress that was made in reducing childhood mortality throughout the 20th century. In rural South Africa, for example, AIDS is currently the single largest cause of death in children less than15 years of age (4).

THE HISTORY OF HIV

It is now widely accepted that HIV became a human pathogen following exposure to Simian Immunodeficiency Virus (SIV) in the blood of primates in West and Central Africa at some point in the middle of the 20th century (5) (see figure 1). What is not clear is how and why this virus mutated to not only infect humans, but to become capable of human to human transmission. The SIV virus has likely been present in these primates for more than 1,000 years and humans have hunted and been exposed to their blood for centuries without the emergence of HIV (5). How and why not just one, but two versions of the HIV virus suddenly appeared at a single point in history, after years of exposure, is still the topic of much debate. The conversion of SIV into the human pathogen HIV is believed to have happened at some point in the 1950's. The first documented serologic response to HIV was found in a blood sample collected in Zaire in 1959 (6). The years of 1950 to 1970 is considered the "critical period" during which all epidemic strains of HIV emerged in Africa.

There are several theories about why the Simian viruses waited until the 20th century to mutate into HIV. Many of these theories involve the introduction of the hypodermic needle and the practice of mass, unsterile, injection practices. It is possible that HIV had occasionally emerged at several points throughout history, but was contained in small villages or rural areas and therefore, never progressed to epidemic proportions. The use of unsterile, mass, injections for immunization and antibiotic delivery may have provided the environmental pressure for an epidemic to emerge.

Additionally, there is some thought that repeated contamination of one person's blood to another, during stages of active viremia with SIV, allowed the evolutionary pressure that ultimately resulted in mutation to the human form of the virus (5). Certain 20th century changes, such as war, mass migrations, and changes in sexual practices, likely also contributed to the fast spread of this disease.

By the late 1970's doctors in Zaire and Burundi began noticing an increase in opportunistic diseases, wasting, and diarrhea among their patients (7). In 1981, doctors in California and New York had recognized an immunodeficiency syndrome in numerous patients for which they coined the term GRID (gay related immunodeficiency virus), as most of their patients, at that time, were men who have sex with men.

As time went on, the disease was recognized first in intravenous drug abusers in Haiti and then in women and children. By 1983, 3,000 infected US women and children had been identified, of which 1,000 were already dead (7). Concurrently, doctors in Uganda were battling a new and fatal disease that involved chronic diarrhea, wasting, and death that they were calling "Slim".

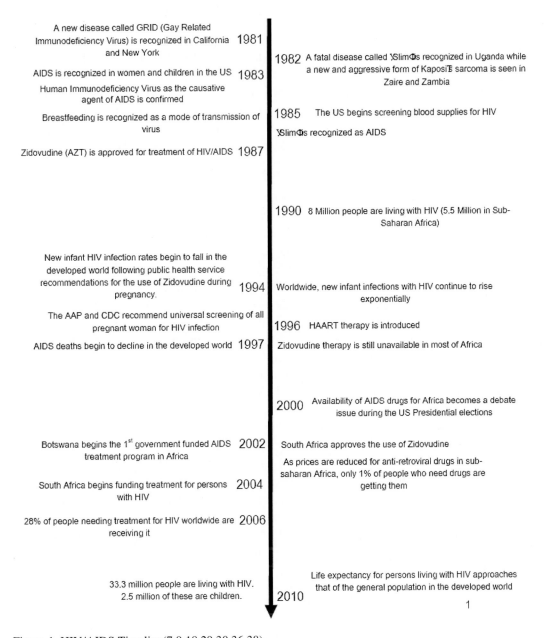

Figure 1. HIV/AIDS Timeline(7,9,18,29,30,36,38).

By the mid-1980's HIV was identified as the causative infective organism behind this fatal immunodeficiency syndrome, and doctors internationally had recognized that the new and deadly disease causing "Slim" in so many people in Sub-Saharan Africa was the same disease that Westerners were now calling AIDS. Over the course of the next 30 years, AIDS has become one of the most deadly pandemics in human history (5).

PATHOGENESIS

HIV is a retrovirus of the genus Lentivirus and the family Retroviridae. Two HIV viruses are known to cause human disease, HIV-1 and HIV-2. HIV-1 is the most prevalent virus infecting North Americans. HIV-2 virus has traditionally been associated with disease in West Africa, but infection in pockets outside of this region has been on the rise. When a patient infected with the HIV virus develops severe immunodeficiency, as evidenced either by the presence of opportunistic infections or by falling levels of the body's immune cells, they are considered to have the disease AIDS.

As a retrovirus, HIV is an RNA virus that uses the enzyme reverse transcriptase to replicate, using the host cell's molecular machinery. After entering the host, glycoprotein 120 on the surface of the HIV molecule attaches itself to CD4 receptors on the host cell surface (8). It therefore tends to infect lymphocytes and macrophages which express the CD4 surface molecule. Viral replication within the human host impairs cellular and subsequently, humoral immunity. This immune impairment not only allows for viral replication to continue unchecked, but as the immune system is further hijacked, the host becomes unable to protect itself from common and opportunistic pathogens.

Reverse transcriptase is an error-prone enzyme that does not contain the capacity for proof reading (8,9). HIV virus is therefore prone to frequent and numerous mutations in the individual host. These mutations have provided a significant challenge to treatment, prevention, and the hope for vaccination from this virus.

The virus is able to enter the cell through the use of chemokine coreceptors, which help with cell-cell surface fusion and entry of virus particles (9). The two most commonly used chemokines of this type have been identified as CCR5 and CXR4 (9-11). These chemokines have become important players in the further understanding of HIV disease and future hope for therapy and cure.

As early as the 1990's, persons had been identified that appeared to be "resistant" to infection with HIV in spite of repeated and adequate exposure (12). These people were found to be homozygous for a base pair deletion in the gene that encodes for the CCR5 co-receptor (10-12). This mutation is referred to as CCR5 ?32/?32 mutation and is present in 1% of the Caucasian population around the world (10,11). Individuals with this mutation are considered to be "highly protected" from infection with HIV-1 and as discussed in this article, this mutation has already proven to be a promising target for future cure of this disease (8).

PRESENTATION

HIV infection often presents with non-specific symptoms which are summarized in Table 1. Within 3-6 weeks following acute infection, 50-70% of people will develop these symptoms (8). Following this initial flu-like phase, the infected individual may not have any further symptoms until signs of immunodeficiency begin to appear, often several years following primary infection. This is the disease pattern most commonly seen in adolescents and adults. Infection in infants often presents with a much more rapid progression of disease than that seen in older children and adults (8). The neonatal period is characterized by a rapid proliferation of lymphocytes. When initial viral infection occurs within this period, an aggressive expansion of virus infected cells throughout the entire body can result (8). As these cells migrate to host tissues, the remainder of the infant's immature immune system is not equipped to suppress further viral expansion.

Table 1. Presenting Symptoms of Pediatric HIV infection (8,13)

- Generalized lymphadenopathy
- Hepatomegaly
- Splenomegaly
- Failure to thrive
- Oral candidiasis
- Recurrent diarrhea
- Parotitis
- Cardiomyopathy
- Hepatitis
- Nephropathy
- CNS disease (including microcephaly, hyperreflexia, clonus, and developmental delay)
- Lymphoid interstitial pneumonia
- Recurrent invasive bacterial infections
- Opportunistic infections
- Malignant neoplasms

The lymphocytosis observed in infancy persists, though to a lesser extent, throughout childhood. Therefore, school aged children who have been newly infected with HIV have presentations that are something of a cross between that seen in infants and that seen in adolescents. Without antiretroviral treatment, three distinct patterns of presentation have been observed in children. Fifteen to twenty-five percent of children have a rapid and fatal disease course that results in death within 6-9 months of primary infection. The majority (60-80%) experience a slower progression with a median survival of 6 years from the time of initial infection. The minority of patients (<5%) are classified as "long-term survivors." These children can have normal CD4 lymphocyte counts and very low viral loads for 8 years or more (8).

The Centers for Disease Control and Prevention (CDC, Atlanta, Georga, USA) has created a classification system for children less than 13 years of age who have known infection with HIV. This classification helps with disease staging, prognosis, and in determining treatment strategies. The full classification system is presented in Table 2.

DIAGNOSIS

HIV disease can be detected both by direct nucleic acid detection or by antibody based assays. In adolescents and adults, ELISA antibody testing is the preferred initial screening tool. If an ELISA is positive, a second, confirmatory ELISA test is performed. If the test remains positive, the more specific, Western blot, antibody test is performed. A positive result by Western Blot using this algorithm is highly sensitive and specific for HIV infection and a confirmatory diagnosis has been made.

In infants, antibody tests are far less reliable due to trans-placental transfer of maternal antibodies.

Table 2. Clinical Categories of HIV for Children less than 13 years of Age(13)

Category N: Not Symptomatic	• Lymphoid interestistial pneumonia or pulmonary lymphoid hyperplasia complex.
Category A: Mildly Symptomatic.	• Nephropathy
2 or more of the following:	• Nocardiosis
• Lymphadenopathy	• Persistent fever > 1 mo in duration
• Hepatomegaly	• Toxoplasmosis prior to 1 mo of age
• Splenomegaly	• Disseminated varicella
• Dermatitis	*Category C: Severely Symptomatic.*
• Parotitis	• Multiple or recurrent serious bacterial infections.
• Recurrent or persistent upper respiratory infections, sinusitis, or otitis media.	• Esophageal or pulmonary candidiasis
Category B: Moderately Symptomatic	• Disseminated Coccidioidomycosis
• Any of the following attributed to HIV infection:	• Extrapulmonary Cryptococcosis
• Anemia	• Cryptosporidiosis or isosporiasis with diarrhea for >1 month
• Single episode of bacterial meningitis, pneumonia, or sepsis.	• CMV with onset after 1 mo of age
• Candidiasis or thrush persisting for >2 months in children over 6 months of age.	• Lymphoma –Burkitt's, Large cell of B-lymphocyte or unknown immunologic phenotype
• Cardiomyopathy	• Disseminated or extrapulmonary *Mycobacterium tuberculosis*
• CMV onset prior to 1 mo of age	• Other disseminated *Mycobacterial* infections
• Recurrent or chronic diarrhea	• *Pneumocystis jiroveci* pneumonia
• Hepatitis	• Progressive multifocal leukoencephalopathy.
• Recurrent HSV stomatitis.	• Recurrent *Salmonella* septicemia
• HSV bronchitis, pneumonitis, or esophatitis with onset before 1 mo of age	• Toxoplasmosis of the brain with onset >1 mo of age
• Herpes zoster in 2 distinct episodes or in two dermatomes.	• Wasting syndrome in the absence of concurrent illness.
• Leiomyosarcoma	

Therefore, prior to 18 months of age, when maternal antibodies have totally cleared the infant's circulation, nucleic acid detection by PCR is the preferred test and antibody tests are considered unreliable (14). Waiting until a child is more than 18 months in order to complete antibody testing is inappropriate, as half of children infected in utero will die before their HIV status is even known (2). Disease can also be suggested, though not confirmed, by measurement of CD4 count and percentage. In an infant, infected in utero, there is a 30% chance that they will have a positive HIV DNA PCR within the first 48 hours of life (13). By 2 weeks, 93% of HIV infected infants will have a positive HIV DNA PCR and by 1 month, this number increases to nearly 100% (13). The HIV DNA PCR test is 95% sensitive and 97% specific for HIV infection in this age group (13).

Children born to mothers with known HIV infection should therefore be screened with HIV DNA PCR within 14-21 days of life (14). This screening should be repeated at 1-2 months of age and again at 4-6 months of age. If the infant is at high risk for HIV infection in utero, HIV PCR testing can be considered within the 1st 48 hours after birth (13,14). Any non-breastfed child who has at least two negative HIV PCR tests, one at >1 month of age and one at >4 months of age is considered negative for HIV infection. Some recommend additional antibody testing at 12-18 months of age to further confirm lack of seroconversion, but this is not considered necessary to exclude the diagnosis (13,14). If a child presents at greater than 18 months of age, antibody testing alone can be done to confirm or exclude this diagnosis (14). If at any point, PCR testing comes back positive, a new blood sample should be drawn and HIV PCR assay should be repeated. Two positive results are considered confirmation of disease (13).

There are now several commercially available rapid antibody-based HIV tests that can be done to facilitate fast access to HIV status in emergency departments and clinics. These tests can often be performed on either blood or an oral swab. Physicians should be aware, that most of these rapid tests only screen for HIV-1 disease. In the United States, a positive result on a rapid test should be followed by either further antibody testing or HIV PCR testing. In the developed world, however, two positive rapid results performed with two different brands of rapid HIV tests is considered confirmation of disease (13).

Following sexual exposure, it may take several months for either seroconversion or detectable viral load to occur. Therefore, antibody testing should be done at 4-6 weeks, 12 weeks, and at 6 months following contact with an infected person or with someone in whom HIV status is unknown (13). If antibody testing remains negative after 6 months, a person is considered HIV negative.

Assessing immune status in infants and young children is especially difficult because maternal antibodies may influence test results and a relative lymphocytosis makes absolute numbers unreliable. For example, a child with an absolute CD4 count of <1500 cells/mm3 is comparable to an adult with an absolute number <200 cells/mm3. Percentage of CD4 cells as a fraction of total lymphocytes is therefore, much more predictive of disease in younger children. A CD4% of less than 25% of the total is considered evidence of CD4 lymphocytopenia and T-cell immunodeficiency(15).

TRANSMISSION

The Human Immunodeficiency Virus is acquired through three main modes of transmission: vertical, sexual, and from exposure to contaminated blood products. Individual risk varies throughout the pediatric age groups. Because all of these modes of transmission are preventable, including the use of universal precautions when exposed to blood products, there is no obligation to report disease status to schools, care-givers or coaches. Though parents certainly have the right to share their child's HIV status with anyone they like, reporting is not mandatory.

Ninety percent of new HIV infections in children occur from maternal to child transmission (16). Infants most commonly acquire HIV during the peripartum period as they are directly exposed to maternal blood (13). This risk is increased in low birth weight and premature infants. It is hypothesized that these infants are at increased risk because of decreased skin barrier protection and greater immaturity of the immune system (9). Infants can also acquire HIV in utero or through breast milk. The risk of acquiring the infection through breast milk is higher if the woman acquires the virus as a primary infection during the breastfeeding period (8). This is particularly concerning because there are no current protocols for the continued screening of women who are breastfeeding their infants if they have already had a negative test result during pregnancy.

School aged children are at greatest risk of exposure to HIV through blood transfusions and sexual abuse by infected adults. This risk is, of course, greatest in the developing world, where the blood supplies are not always screened for HIV and in areas where the prevalence of HIV is very high among the adult population.

The primary mode of transmission in the adolescent age group is through unprotected sexual intercourse and through intravenous drug abuse. Adolescent males and females are both at risk, even though exposure is often though different modes of transmission. Girls are more likely to be infected at a younger age and through sexual contact with men. Boys are more likely to be infected at a more advanced age and are more likely to acquire the virus through sexual contact with other adolescent males or through drug abuse.

TREATMENT

In 1987, 6 years after the appearance of AIDS in North America, zidovudine, a drug initially developed for the treatment of cancer, was approved for the treatment of HIV. Major advances in the medical management of HIV have been made since that time. Sadly, access to care, costs and even political influence have at times presented significant road blocks in providing care to those who are most in need. These challenges are particularly pronounced in the pediatric age group. Even with good access to care and availability of anti-retroviral therapies, many drugs have either not been tested, have not been approved for use in children, or are not available in a pediatric friendly form (e.g., liquids, powders, or dispersible capsules) (17). Unfortunately, the near elimination of HIV disease in children in the developed world has resulted in even less incentive for pharmaceutical companies to research and produce antiretroviral drugs for children (2).

There are currently, 6 classes of drugs used in the treatment of HIV. Within these classes18 of the 20 drugs have been approved for the use in children less than 16 year of age and 12 exist in child-friendly forms (17). A summary of these drugs is listed in Table 3.

In 1996, the concept of highly active antiretroviral therapy (HAART) was introduced. This consists of the use of 3 different drugs from at least 2 different pharmaceutical families (18). This typically involves 2 nucleoside analogue reverse transcriptase inhibitors plus either a protease inhibitor or a non-nucleoside reverse transcriptase inhibitor (13). The use of HAART has been shown to suppress viral replication and allow immune reconstitution within the 1st few months of initiating therapy (19).

When to initiate antiretroviral therapy for infants with known HIV exposure has long been a debate among health care providers. This decision is further complicated in resource poor areas, where antibody testing is the only means of detecting infection and therefore, a reliable diagnosis cannot be confirmed until 18 months of age. Since many HIV infected children will already be dead by this age without treatment, there is a push to begin treatment at earlier stages, even in the absence of confirmed disease (16).

Current guidelines recommend initiating zidovudine therapy in all HIV exposed infants until HIV infection is either definitively positive or definitively negative. If the patient is negative for HIV and is not breastfeeding from an HIV positive mother, zidovudine therapy may be discontinued at this point. If the patient is found to have HIV infection, zidovudine should be stopped and referral should be made to an infectious disease specialist if available to evaluate and make treatment decisions about combination therapy (14).

Another concern about the initiation of early treatment of HIV is that the safety profiles of most antiretroviral medications are based solely upon adult studies. The long term effects of these medications are not well known. Resistance and compliance issues worsen the longer that a person is on treatment, which for children could be more than 40 years. For all of these reasons, consultation with a specialist in infectious diseases is needed to help with treatment and timing of treatment decisions.

The traditional treatment plan for infants with known HIV disease was to wait to initiate therapy until the CD4 count had fallen to <20%, there was evidence of HIV progression, or there was a high viral load. Recent studies, however, suggest that early treatment of HIV disease in known HIV positive children can reduce early infant mortality by 76% and HIV progression by 75% (15). Cessation of therapy can be considered after initial immune reconstitution and suppression of viremia is achieved. Even though this method involves earlier treatment than traditional therapy, it has been shown to ultimately delay the time to initiation of continuous antiretroviral therapy (15).

In pregnant woman already receiving HAART therapy, treatment should be continued throughout the pregnancy. If a pregnant woman is HIV positive, but does not require anti-retroviral therapy for her own health, it is recommended that zidovudine therapy be initiated at 14 to 34 weeks of gestation and continued into the post-partum period. Children exposed to HIV in utero should also be treated with zidovudine for the first 6 weeks of life. This strategy has been shown to decrease the risk of maternal to child transmission of virus by up to two-thirds (13).

Table 3. Approved Antiretroviral Agents in the United States (17)

Nucleoside Reverse Transcriptase Inhibitors
• Zidovudine(a,b)
• Stavudine(a,b)
• Lamivudine(a,b)
• Abacavir(a,b)
• Didanosine(a,b)
• Emtricitabine(a,b)
Non-Nucleoside Reverse Transcriptase Inhibitors
• Delaviridine
• Nevaripine(a,b)
• Efavirenz(a,b)
• Etravirine
Nucleotide Reverse Transcriptase Inhibitors
• Tenofovir

Table 3. (Continued)

Protease Inhibitors
• Indinavir(b)
• Ritonavir(a,b)
• Saquinavir(b)
• Nelfinavir(a,b)
• Lopirnavir(a,b)
• Atazanavir(b)
• Fosamprenavir(a,b)
• Tipranavir(b)
• Darunavir(b)
Integrase Inhibitor
• Raltegravir
CCR5 Receptor Inhibitor
• Maraviroc
Fusion Inhibitor
• Enfuvirtide(b)
a – Child-friendly formulation available
b – US FDA-approved for patients <16 years of age

In the developed world, women are strongly discouraged from breastfeeding if they are known to be HIV positive; however, in many of the areas where HIV has the highest prevalence, bottle feeding poses a greater risk than breast feeding, even when the mother is HIV infected. Bottle fed infants may be subject to malnutrion and chronic diarrheal illnesses from contaminated water. Therefore, the World Health Organization (WHO—Geneva, Switzerland) recommends that in areas where supplemental feeding is either not available or is unsafe, HIV positive women should continue to breastfeed their infants for up to 6 months, followed by rapid weaning (8). During this period, both the mother and the infant should be treated with antiretroviral therapy.

MEDICATION SIDE-EFFECTS

The use of antiretroviral medication has changed the course of the HIV epidemic; however, like all medications, these come with their own inherent risks and side-effect profiles. While the full list of interactions and side-effects to anti-retroviral medications is beyond the scope of this article, there are certain concerns of which all physicians who care for children affected by HIV should be aware.

As the use of antiretroviral medications for the prevention of maternal to child transmission of HIV increases, there is a growing population of non-HIV infected children who have been exposed to these medications in utero and through breast milk. Little is known about the risks of these exposures or their implications in future health (20).

There is growing evidence that the use of protease inhibitors during pregnancy can increase the incidence of low birth weight and prematurity compared to those on a non-protease inhibitor containing HAART regimens (17,20,21). Prolonged in utero exposure to zidovudine alone has also been associated with low birth weight in infants(17). Exposure to tenofovir in utero may cause renal phosphate wasting and a Fanconi's syndrome like picture in the neonate (17). Finally, anemia may be seen in infants who have been exposed to combination antiretrovirals in utero, but these changes typically resolve in the first few months of life (20). No formal guidelines exist for screening these infants; however, physicians caring for an infant who has been exposed to antiretroviral medications should be aware of, and prepared to deal with all of these complications.

Likewise, recent studies have shown that exposure to antiretrovirals in utero is associated with changes in cardiac development and function (22). Whether or not these changes are permanent or in any way affect mature cardiac function is unknown. In animal models, in utero exposure to antiretroviral medications has been associated with long term cardiotoxicity, but this has not yet been shown in humans (22).

MEDICATION COMPLIANCE

Because HIV-1 reverse transcriptase is both error prone and lacks error correcting mechanisms, a wide variety of HIV mutations can be seen, even within the same patient (8). For this reason, HIV infected patients on antiretroviral medications may develop resistance to their medications over time. These mutations occur with greater frequency when there are interruptions in treatment.

Access to care and compliance with medications present unique challenges in the care of children with HIV. Even small deviations from a prescribed antiretroviral regimen can have a pronounced effect on drug efficacy. Less than 95% adherence to prescribed doses of antiretroviral medications at any level can result in accumulations of mutated, drug resistant strains of HIV (17). Strict compliance with a treatment program is therefore necessary to maintain low or undetectable viral loads.

In patients with compliance issues, treatment options become fewer as more and more mutations occur. For children, this is especially serious as they are likely to need treatment for a longer period of time than adults and early resistance to medications can seriously compromise long term survival. These concerns only increase as children reach adolescents. Furthermore, social and governmental programs in place to ensure that care and treatment are available to all children affected with HIV disease may disappear as the child reaches their 18th or 21st birthdays, so transition of care in the adolescent age group should be paid extra attention.

IMMUNIZATIONS

Because children with HIV infection are immunocompromised, immunizations must be tailored to their current state of immunodeficiency. Not only are symptomatic HIV infected children at greater risk from live vaccines, they are also likely to have a poor immunologic response to vaccines. Measles infections, for example, can be particularly severe and life-threatening in HIV-infected patients (23). MMR vaccine should therefore be given to all HIV-infected children according to routine CDC/American Academy of Pediatrics (AAP)-approved immunization schedules at 12 months of age unless they are severely immunocompromised (19). The second dose should not be delayed until school entry, but should be given at 4 weeks after the 1st dose (13,23).

Likewise, children with Class N or A (see Table 2 for disease classification) disease should receive varicella vaccine at 12 months with the second dose repeated at 3 months of age (13,23). Household contacts of patients with HIV may receive live vaccines, even if the HIV-infected child is severely immunosuppressed (23).

There is no data supporting the use of rotavirus vaccination in those who are immunocompromised, including children infected with HIV (19). It is therefore recommended that decisions regarding this vaccine should be made in conjunction with a local infectious disease specialist and careful consideration of the patient's current immune status should be considered.

Because of the high likelihood of an inadequate immune response to vaccination, HIV-infected children should receive special care when exposed to vaccine preventable disease. In the setting of an outbreak, the MMR vaccine can be given as early as 6 to 9 months of age (13,23). If a child is severely immunosuppressed, treatment with immunoglogulin therapy should be considered in patients and their families, when indicated (13).

As many as 20% of the diseases that cause serious illness in children with AIDS are caused by encapsulated organisms including Pneumococcus and Meningococcus (8). HIV infected children should therefore receive the full series of conjugated Pneumococcal vaccine, followed by the 23-valent polysaccharide vaccination at 2 years of age and meningococcal vaccination at 2 years of age according to current AAP/CDC guidelines (24).

CHALLENGES TO CARE

For the pediatrician, there are numerous unique challenges to caring for children with HIV disease. HIV infected children are at greater risk for developing certain malignancies, growth parameters may be different than in their non-infected peers, immune reconstitution may result in worsening of opportunistic disease, and as children are living into adulthood, long term health effects from both the disease and its treatment are becoming more apparent.

Though they are not common, certain malignancies are significantly more common in children infected with HIV when compared with their peers. The majority of these malignancies are leiomyosarcomas and lymphomas. In particular, the types of lymphomas that pose the greatest risk to HIV positive children are CNS lymphoma and Burkitt's lymphoma. Kaposi's sarcoma, which is much more commonly seen in adults with HIV, can occur frequently in children living in areas of high endemic prevalence of the virus, but has not been reported among children in the United States (13).

One of the hallmark features of untreated HIV disease in children is progressive failure to thrive and severe wasting disease. These changes show dramatic improvement in children treated with HAART therapy; however, early changes in growth parameters might be the first clues of treatment failure or non-compliance. Height velocity, more so than weight velocity has been shown to be the best predictor of progression of HIV disease. Increases in height velocity correlate with decrease in clinical progression of disease and with increase in immune reconstitution (25).

Children with HIV infection and who are taking antiretroviral therapy are also at risk for developing fat redistribution changes compared to age matched controls. This is characterized by lipoatrophy, with a wasted appearance in the face and periphery, and an increase in fat accumulation centrally (17). Therefore, weight and height measurements should be taken at every visit for children with HIV disease and physical exam should pay particular attention to fat distribution. Because protease inhibitors have been particularly linked to thinness and lipoatrophy, the appearance of these features should prompt evaluation of current therapy and risks versus benefits of a change.

Metabolic derangements can also be seen in HIV infected children undergoing treatment. Up to 62% of children with HIV will eventually develop lipid abnormalities (17). Hypercholesterolemia has been found to be common among children who were perinatally infected with HIV (26). These changes can be exacerbated by the changes in fat distribution commonly seen in these children. Insulin resistance and diabetes mellitus are also seen in association with lipoatrophy. It is therefore recommended that blood lipid profiles be checked every 3-6 months once treatment of HIV infection has begun in children (17).

Finally, use of tenofovir in children has been associated with osteopenia and osteoporosis. In children taking tenofovir, yearly DEXA scans should be performed to assess bone mineral density and adequate Vitamin D and calcium should be encouraged in the diet (17).

As the first generation of persons initially infected with HIV in childhood has now entered early adulthood, there is rapidly evolving information about the long term health consequences of this disease and its treatments. In particular, it is now clear that HIV infection confers an increased risk of cardiovascular disease (27). The continued use of anti-retroviral therapies decreases, but does not eliminate this risk. Therefore, in spite of the lipid abnormalities associated with some anti-retroviral medications, treatment is better than no treatment in the progression of cardiovascular effects.

While there are clear guidelines for how often lipids should be screened in HIV infected children, there is no consensus about when treatment should be initiated (26-28). There are recommendations by the American Academy of Pediatrics (AAP) for the treatment of hyperlipidemia in otherwise healthy children; however, there has neither been enough time nor enough patients to develop treatment strategies and risk profiles for children infected with HIV. The AAP does have separate guidelines for the treatment of hypercholesterolemia in children who are considered "high-risk" secondary to inflammatory conditions and these guidelines could be used to help in guiding therapy (27).

Opportunistic infections are one of the greatest threats to HIV infected children. While most opportunistic infections in adults are the result of reactivation, the majority of these infections in children are primary infections, which can often be much more severe (19). Pneumocytis jerovecii pneumonia can present a life-threatening complication of perinatally acquired HIV infection. Therefore, all children exposed to HIV in utero should receive PCP prophylaxis beginning at 4-6 months of age and continuing until the 1st year of life or until infection has been ruled out (13). Furthermore, HIV infected infants who are living with an HIV infected parent should be followed closely for opportunistic infections as the immunocompromised parent is often much more contagious than a non-infected caregiver who carries one of these pathogens (19).

Mycobacterium avium complex infection can present a serious risk to HIV-infected individuals who are immunocompromised. It is currently recommended that all patients with severe immunosuppresion (CD4 cell count less than 50 cells/mm3 in persons over 6 years of age, less than 500 cells/mm3 in children aged 1-2 years, or less than 750 cells/mm3 in children less than 1 year) should be treated with prophylactic doses of azithromycin (14).

After initiation of antiretroviral therapy, as immune reconstitution occurs, a profound, systemic inflammatory response may arise. This syndrome, referred to as IRIS (Immune Reconstitution Inflammatory Syndrome), has primarily been described in adults, but also has been reported in pediatrics (19). This inflammation can result in apparent worsening of symptoms soon after the initiation of therapy and can be a major cause of non-compliance with treatment. It is believed that this reaction is secondary to the newly re-established immune systems response to both infectious and non-infectious antigens within the host. If symptoms are severe, treatment with steroids may be initiated and interruption of HAART therapy should be avoided.

PREVENTION

Great strides have occurred in the prevention of maternal to child transmission of HIV in utero, at birth and through breast feeding. Through appropriate treatment with antiretroviral therapy, the risk of vertical transmission of HIV can be reduced to less than 2% (29). These prevention strategies have decreased the transmission of HIV from mother to child by almost 95% and have virtually eliminated mother to child transmission in the developed world (30).

In spite of this progress, the risk of maternal to child transmission remains high among women who are either unaware of their HIV status or do not have access to care. There is a greater risk of transmitting infection during the intrapartum period than in utero, especially if the maternal viral load is high (13). Therefore, in patients with no treatment or undertreatment of disease, the USPHSTF (United States Preventative Health Service Task Force) recommends that scheduled cesarean delivery be considered if viral levels exceed 1,000 copies near the time of delivery (13,30). Delivery prior to rupture of membranes is a clear goal as the risk of transmission is directly proportional to the number of hours that membranes are ruptured prior to cesarean delivery (13).

One third to one half of all cases of maternal to child transmission of HIV worldwide are caused by breastfeeding (33). The use of HAART throughout pregnancy and for an additional 6 months post-partum, with rapid weaning thereafter, can reduce the risk of HIV transmission through breast milk to less than 1%, compared to 35% without antiretrovirals (21,31). The reduction of transmission through breast feeding is therefore one of the most important and effective means of preventing pediatric HIV infections.

Beyond the neonatal time period, the next age group that can be most affected by prevention strategies are adolescents. In the United States, almost 50% of new cases of HIV occur in people between the ages of 13 and 24 (13). Among younger adolescents, girls are at higher risk and in older adolescents, boys are at higher risk (13). Prevention strategies such as safe needle programs, encouraging condom use, and offering HIV testing should all be encouraged in this age group. Additionally, in areas of high prevalence of HIV, three independent studies have shown a proven benefit to male circumcision in preventing men from acquiring HIV through sexual contact (32).

PROGRESS

The number of people living with HIV worldwide continues to grow. This trend is not a result of growing spread of disease, but rather from the improvement in the care of HIV infected individuals. The number of newly infected persons per year peaked on an International level in 1996 and has been steadily declining ever since (3). This improvement can be attributed mostly to education, screening of blood supplies, and prevention strategies. The next significant leap in worldwide progress occurred after 2004 when antiretroviral medications were finally available to enough persons that AIDS deaths peaked and have since been declining (3).

Young people are leading the way in halting the progression of HIV transmission on a worldwide scale. Young men and women have participated in increased antenatal care, more routine screening, safer sex practices, and improved education in both the developed and developing worlds. These efforts have resulted in a 25% decrease in the number of children contracting HIV during delivery or breastfeeding from 2001 to 2004, a 19% decrease in AIDS related deaths among children, and a steady decline in the number of persons newly contracting HIV between 2001 and 2009 (32).

Not only have numerous children been infected with the HIV virus, but many more have suffered the consequences of losing one or both parents to the disease. In spite of declining numbers of new infections, the number of children orphaned by AIDS continues to rise, with 90% of them living in sub-Saharan Africa (32). The protection of and provision for children who have been orphaned by AIDS has become a major goal in our global efforts to address the disaster that lies in the wake of this disease. Though orphan rates are rising, there has been progress in the protection of these children. Recent reports show that children who have been orphaned by AIDS are now almost as likely to attend school as their peers (32).

FUTURE

Goals for the prevention, treatment, and elimination of HIV have been proposed by several international organizations, most notably the World Health Organization, through its Millennium Development Goals and the Joint United Nations program's UNAIDS.

Millennium Development Goals 4 and 5 address broad social changes that will ultimately result in improved care for woman and children and Millennium Goal number 6 specifically addresses international targets for halting the progression of HIV/AIDS. Millennium Development Goals 4 through 6 are outlined in Table 4. The deadline for Target 6b, has already passed and while much progress was made between 2000 and 2010 toward meeting this goal, it is still far from complete.

Table 4. Millennium Development Goals Relating to HIV/AIDS(3)

MDG 4: Reduce Child Mortality MDG 5: Improve Maternal Health MDG 6: Combat HIV/AIDS, malaria and other diseases

Table 4. (Continued)

• Target a: Halt, by 2015 and begin to reverse the spread of HIV/AIDS • Target b: By 2010, provide universal access to treatment for HIV/AIDS for all who need it

The spread of HIV was halted on an international level around 2009; however, target 6a is far from being met in many parts of the world (3,32). In addition to these goals, UNAIDS has also called for the elimination of mother to child transmission by 2015.

The future of HIV care will likely involve not only progression of antiretroviral medications, but also more advanced prevention and prophylaxis strategies, including vaccination. In an effort to further halt the transmission of HIV to women, a tenofovir-based vaginal gel is currently under evaluation for prevention of sexual transmission of disease (32).

Vaccination against the HIV virus has long eluded scientists, largely due to the high degree of heterogeneity of gp120, the cell surface receptor found on the HIV virus. and the most logical target for research (8). Recently HIV immunoglobulin therapy for the prevention of maternal to child transmission of the virus reached phase three clinical trials in the United States. Unfortunately, while this therapy was found to be safe, it was no more efficacious than antiretroviral therapy in preventing transmission of disease (33).

Great promise for the future of HIV prevention and treatment lies in the use of the natural resistance to HIV-1 seen in homozygotes for the ?32/?32 base pair deletion mutation that codes for the cell surface co-receptor CCR5. In 2007, German scientists performed a bone marrow transplant for an HIV infected man who had acute myelogenous leukemia. They selectively chose a bone marrow donor possessing the ?32/?32 mutation in the hope that the donor resistance would be passed on to the recipient. At the time of transplantation, all antiretroviral medications were stopped. In March of 2011, the same scientists issued a report, that at three and a half years post-transplantation, their patient was still not taking antiretrovirals, has no signs of HIV infection and no detectable viral particles (even in dormant macrophages and lymphocytes) and has experienced full immune reconstitution (10,11).

CONCLUSION

Real progress in our fight against the HIV/AIDS epidemic will not occur until universal access is achieved for prevention, treatment, care, and support for all those infected with the virus. In spite of significant advancement in the treatment and prevention of HIV in much of the developed world, certain populations are still facing serious risk and many lack access to care. Though antiretroviral treatment is now available in Sub-Saharan Africa at prices that are significantly reduced, the number of new infections still outweighs those who are getting care. In Southern Africa, for every two patients who are starting treatment, five are becoming newly infected (34). In many areas of high HIV prevalence, HIV/AIDS is the single leading cause of death in children under the age of 5 (4,32).

A progress report by WHO in 2010 showed that worldwide, only one-quarter of pregnant women had received an HIV test and of those who were found to be HIV positive, only one-half had received any form of antiretroviral therapy (2). AIDS is the single leading cause of maternal mortality in South Africa and child mortality has continued to increase since the 1990's (32).

Thanks to worldwide efforts in education and prevention, the number of people newly infected with HIV has steadily been declining since 2009 (32) In spite of this overall progress, several regions of the world have remained isolated from these prevention strategies. These areas include the Middle East and North Africa, many parts of Asia, Oceana, Central and South America, and multiple areas within Europe, in which AIDS related deaths and newly acquired infections with HIV have been on the rise (32).

Lack of access to care and costs are not the only barriers to prevention of HIV. Even within the developed world, certain populations are at increased risk for exposure and infection with HIV. In the United States, African American women are 19 times more likely to contract HIV than their Caucasian counterparts and rates of HIV infection in African American infants have been slowly rising while rates among all other races have remained stable (32,35,36). Men who have sex with men, commercial sex workers, and intravenous drug users are all likewise, disproportionately affected by the disease in the developed world and should be counseled about prevention strategies at every opportunity. Failure to address the human rights issues that affect those who have been marginalized by society has only facilitated the further growth of the epidemic (32). In spite of significant public education and prevention strategies, male to male sexual contact remains the primary mode of transmission in adolescents and young adults with rates that continue to climb (35).

Progress in the prevention and treatment of HIV in the pediatric population has fallen behind that seen in adults. Only 28% of the children who are in need of treatment for HIV/AIDS worldwide, are receiving it (32). In most areas where there is access to antiretroviral medications, children are significantly less likely to receive care than adults.

In 2010 it was reported that for adults living with HIV, who have sustained CD4 cell counts of more than 500 and who have been on antiretroviral therapy for more than 5 years, the life expectancy of these individuals approaches that of the general population (37). Unfortunately, these positive results only apply to those with full access to medications and appropriate treatment. Worldwide, the life expectancy for HIV infected persons remains at only 45 years of age (7).

As we enter the 4th decade of HIV disease in the world, there has been much progress in our treatment options, prevention strategies, and understanding of the virus. In spite of all of this, continued international efforts must continue to keep the disease from spreading further and ultimately put a stop to the epidemic.

REFERENCES

[1]   World Health Organization. Global summary of the AIDS epidemic: 2009. Accessed 2011 Sep 01. URL: http://www.who.int/hiv/data/2009_global_summary.png.

[2]   Lallemant M, et al. Pediatric HIV –a neglected disease? N Engl J Med 2011;365(7):581-3

[3]   World Health Organization. Millennium Development Goals. Accessed 2011 Sep 01. URL: http://www.who.int/topics/millennium_development_goals/en/.

[4]   Garrib A, Jaffar S, Knight S, Bradshaw D, Bennish ML. Rates and causes of child mortality in an area of high HIV prevalence in rural South Africa. Trop Med Int Health 2006;11(12):1841-8.

[5]   Marx PA, Apetrei C, Drucker E. AIDS as a zoonosis? Confusion over the origin of the virus and the origin of epidemics. J Med Primatol 2004;33(5-6):220-6.

[6]   Quinn TC, Mann J, Curran J, Piot P. AIDS in Africa: An epidemiologic paradigm. Science 1986;234(4779):955-63.

[7]   Greene MF. There is no me without you. New York: Bloomsbury, 2006.

[8]   Yogev R, Chadwick EG. Acquired immunodeficiency syndrome (human immunodeficiency virus). In: Kliegman R, Behrman R, Jenson H, Stanton B, eds. Nelson textbook of pediatrics, 18th ed. Philadelphia, PA: WB Saunders, 2010:1427-42.

[9]   Rivera DM, et al. Pediatric HIV. Medscape. Accessed 2011 Sep 01. URL: http://emedicine.medscape.com/article/965086-overview.

[10]   Hütter G, et al. Long-term control of HIV by CCR5 Delta32/Delta32 stem cell transplant. N Engl J Medicine 2009;360(7):692-8.

[11]   Allers K, Hütter G, et al. Evidence for the cure of HIV infection by CCR5 Delta32/Delta32 stem cell transplant. Blood 2011;117(10):2791-9.

[12]   Carrington DM, Winker C, et al. Genetic restriction of HIV-1 infection and Progression to AIDS by a deletion allele of the CKR5 Structural Gene. Hemophilia growth and Development Study, Multicenter AIDS Cohort Study, Multicenter Hemophilia Cohort Study, San Fransisco City Cohort Study, ALIVE Study. Science 1996;273(5283):1856-62.

[13]   Red Book. 2006 Report of the Committee on Infectious Diseases, 27th edition. Elk Grove Village, IL: American Academy of Pediatrics, 2006:378-401.

[14]   AIDS information. Accessed 2011 Sep 01. URL: http://aidsinfo.nih.gov/contentfiles /Recommendations_Only_Ped_2011.pdf.

[15]   Violari A, Cotton MF, Gibb DM, Babiker AG, Steyn J, Madhi SA, et al. Early antiretroviral therapy and mortality among HIV-infected infants. N Engl J Med 2008;359(21):2233-44.

[16]   World Health Organization. Strategic Vision. World Health Organization. Accessed 2011 Sep 01. URL: http://www.who.int/hiv/pub/mtct/strategic_vision.pdf.

[17]   Kim RJ, Rutstein RM. Impact of antiretroviral therapy on growth, body composition and metabolism in pediatric HIV patients. Paediatric Drugs 2010;12(3):187-99.

[18]   Editorial. 30 years of pediatric HIV/AIDS treatment: A time of breakthroughs, innovation. Pediatric Ann 2011;40(7):340-1.

[19]   Mofenson LM, et al. Guidelines for the prevention and treatment of opportunistic infections among HIV-exposed and HIV-infected children: Recommendations from CDC, the National Institutes of Health, the HIV Medicine Association of the Infectious Diseases Society of America, the Pediatric Infectious Diseases Society, and the American Academy of Pediatrics. MMWR Recomm Rep 2009;58(RR-11)1-166.

[20]   Heidari S, Mofenson L, Cotton MF, Marlink R, Cahn P, Katabira E. Antiretroviral drugs for preventing mother-to-child transmission of HIV: A review of potential effects on HIV-exposed but uninfected children. J Acquir Immune Defic Syndr 2011;57(4):290-6.

[21]   Shapiro RL, Hughes MD, Ogwu A, Kitch D, Lockman S, Moffat C, et al. Antiretroviral regimens in pregnancy and breast-feeding in Botswana. N Engl J Med 2010;362(24):2282-94.

[22]   Lipshultz SE, Shearer WT, Thompson B, et al. Cardiac effects of antiretroviral therapy in HIV-negative infants born to HIV-positive mothers:NHLBI CHAART-1 (National Heart, Lung, and Blood Institute Cardiovascular Status of HAART Therapy in HIV-Exposed Infants and Children cohort study). J Am Coll Cardiol 2011;57(1):76-85.

[23]   Epidemiology and Prevention of Vaccine Preventable Diseases. The Pink Book 12th edition April 2011. Accessed 2011 Sep 01. URL: http://www.cdc.gov/vaccines/pubs/pinkbook/.

[24]   Vaccines. Accessed 2011 Sep 01. URL: http://www.cdc.gov/vaccines/recs/schedules/downloads /child/0-6yrs-schedule-pr.pdf.

[25]   Benjamin DKJr, Miller WC, Benjamin DK, Ryder RW, Weber DJ, Walter E, et al. A comparison of height and weight velocity as a part of the composite endpoint in pediatric HIV. AIDS 2003;17(16):2331-6.

[26] Jacobson DL, et al. Clinical management and follow-up of hypercholesterolemia among perinatally HIV-infected children enrolled in the PACTG 219C study. J Acquir Immune Defic Syndr 2011;57(5):413-20.

[27] Ross AC, McComsey GA. Cardiovascular disease risk in pediatric HIV: The need for population-specific guidelines. J Acquir Immune Defic Syndr 2011;57(5):351-4.

[28] Rhoads MP, et al. Effect of specific ART drugs on lipid changes and the need for lipid management in children with HIV. J Acquir Immune Defic Syndr 2011;57(5):404-12.

[29] World Health Organization. Paediatric HIV and treatment of children living with HIV. Accessed 2011 Sep 01. URL: http://www.who.int/hiv/paediatric/ed/index.html.

[30] Centers for Disease Control and Prevention. Achievements in public health. Reduction in perinatal transmission of HIV infection –United States, 1985-2005. MMWR 2006;55(21):592-7.

[31] WHO. Antiretroviral drugs for treating pregnant women and preventing HIV infections in infants, 2010 version. Accessed 2011 Sep 01. URL: http://whqlibdoc.who.int/publications/2010 /9789241599818_eng.pdf.

[32] UNAIDS Report on the Global AIDS Epidemic 2010. Accessed 2011 Sep 01. URL: http://www.unaids.org/global report/Global_report.htm.

[33] Onyango-Makumbi C, Omer SB, Mubiru M, Moulton LH, Nakabiito C, Musoke P, et al. Safety and efficacy of HIV hyperimmune globulin (HIVIGLOB) for prevention of mother-to-child HIV transmission in HIV-1 infected pregnant women and their infants in Kampala, Uganda (HIVIGLOB/NVP STUDY). J Acquir Immune Defic Syndr 2011;58(4):399-407.

[34] Katsidzira L, Hakim JG. HIV prevention in southern Africa: why we must reassess our strategies? Trop Med Int Health 2011;16(9):1120-30.

[35] HIV Surveillance in Adolescents and Young Adults. Accessed 2011 Sep 01. URL: http://www.cdc.gov/hiv/topics/serveillance/resources/slides/adolescents/index.htm

[36] Pediatric HIV Surveilance (through 2009) Accessed 2011 Sep 01. URL: http://www.cdc.gov/hiv/topics/surveillance/resources/slides/pediatric/index.htm.

[37] Hill A, Pozniak A. A normal life expectancy, despite HIV infection? AIDS 2010;24(10):1583-4

[38] Centers for Disease Control and Prevention. HIV Surveillance , United States, 1981-2008. MMWR 2011;60(21):689-93.

Submitted: September 03, 2011. *Revised:* November 03, 2011. *Accepted:* November 10, 2011.

In: Public Health Yearbook 2012
Editor: Joav Merrick

ISBN: 978-1-62808-078-0
© 2013 Nova Science Publishers, Inc.

Chapter 11

TROPICAL NEPHROLOGY

*Valerie Duhn, MD**

Department of Internal Medicine, Nephrology, Michigan State University/Kalamazoo
Center for Medical Studies, Kalamazoo, Michigan, USA

ABSTRACT

Tropical nephrology includes a broad spectrum of pathologic changes of the kidney in response to infectious organisms, natural toxins, or environmental toxins specific to that region of the world between the tropic of cancer and the tropic of capricorn. It must also include diseases of the kidney that are encountered in both the tropical region and the western world. Clinical syndromes observed in tropical nephrology include asymptomatic urine abnormalities, macroscopic hematuria, acute kidney injury, and glomerular disease. Glomerular disease may be primary or secondary to a variety of infectious organisms. Clinical syndromes are reviewed along with proposed causative organisms. Special attention is given to malaria and schistosomiasis as major contributors to renal disease in this region of the world. Of note, recent evidence has questioned the existence of a distinct "topical nephrotic syndrome" previously ascribed to quartan malaria. Whether this reflects a changing spectrum of disease in the region or a history of inaccurate assignment of a single cause and effect relationship to the malarial pathogen and the nephrotic syndrome remains to be determined. Finally, treatment options are discussed including a suggested approach to persistent proteinuria of unknown cause.

Keywords: Nephrology, tropics, public health

INTRODUCTION

Tropical nephrology encompasses a broad spectrum of pathologic changes of the kidney in response to infectious organisms, natural toxins, or environmental toxins specific to that

* Correspondence: Valerie Duhn, MD, Assistant Professor, Department of Internal Medicine, Nephrology, Michigan State University/Kalamazoo Center for Medical Studies, 1000 Oakland Drive, Kalamazoo, Michigan 49008, E-mail: vsduhn@kcms.msu.edu or Duhn@kcms.msu.edu

region of the world between the tropic of cancer and the tropic of capricorn. In addition, tropical nephrology must also account for the spectrum of primary glomerular diseases that are also observed in western countries. In fact, primary glomerular diseases including IgA nephropathy, IgM nephropathy, membranous nephropathy, and lupus nephritis, have been reported to have a prevalence in the tropics of 2.5 times that of the western world (1).

Clinical syndromes can range from asymptomatic hematuria or proteinuria, to self-limited episodes of acute kidney injury, or to progressive chronic glomerulonephritis that persists despite eradication of the offending organism. The host's immune response and subsequent inflammatory process play a critical role in the renal lesions observed. Treatment is often directed at the offending pathogen, with little benefit observed from immunosuppression directed at the resultant inflammatory process in most cases.

CLINICAL SYNDROMES

Clinical syndromes observed include asymptomatic urine abnormalities, macroscopic hematuria, acute kidney injury, and glomerular disease. Glomerular disease may be primary or secondary to a variety of infectious organisms.

Nonspecific urinary sediment changes are often observed in the setting of febrile infectious diseases. These include microscopic hematuria, proteinuria, pyuria, or the presence of granular casts. Usually these changes resolve as the disease improves. Proteinuria can range from mild and transient to severe and persistent despite treatment of the offending pathogen.

Transient proteinuria often less than 1gram per 24 hours can be seen in any acute febrile illness as well as in the setting of dehydration, intense exercise, or severe emotional stress. Orthostatic proteinuria, which can be diagnosed with a split urine collection, should also be considered in the adolescent population with less than 1 gram per 24 hours, although its occurrence in the tropical region is unclear. Proteinuria of over 1 gram and especially over 2 grams per 24 hours that persists beyond 4 weeks suggests a glomerular cause.

Macroscopic hematuria is often suspected in setting of red to brown urine. It should be noted that hemoglobinuria and myoglobinuria can also present similarly. When possible a centrifugation of a fresh urine sample should be performed. If the red/brown color is limited to the sediment with a clear supernatant, then hematuria is responsible. However, if the supernatant is a red/brown color, it should be tested and if heme positive, then either hemoglobinuria or myoglobinuria should be suspected. It is important to study a fresh sample of urine, as red blood cells may lyse with prolonged standing and result in a false positive heme test of the supernatant (2).

The differential diagnosis of macroscopic hematuria observed in the tropics should include schistosomiasis as well as bacterial infection, but should also take into consideration IgA nephropathy, post-streptococcal glomerulonephritis, trauma, nephrolithiasis, sickle cell disease, and malignancy. Schistosomiasis affecting the lower urinary tract typically presents with painful terminal gross hematuria and will be discussed in detail below. Gross hematuria that occurs within one to three days of an upper respiratory infection ("synpharyngitic hematuria") suggests the diagnosis of IgA nephropathy. Gross hematuria that occurs 10-21 days after an episode of pharyngitis or cellulitis suggests the diagnosis of post-streptococcal glomerulonephritis.

Hemoglobinuria is a common finding in tropical diseases and often a result of intravascular hemolysis. Significant intravascular hemolysis has been documented after viper bites as well as after wasp or hornet stings (3-7). In addition, glucose 6 phosphate dehydrogenase deficiency is common in tropical countries and may account for episodes of intravascular hemolysis after infection or exposure to certain medications (1). Myoglobinuria may be seen in the setting of rhabdomyolysis that results from infections including leptospirosis, trichinosis, malaria, typhoid fever, and viral infection (1). Often the renal injury in the setting of significant intravascular hemolysis or rhabdomyolysis progresses to acute tubular necrosis requiring renal replacement therapy.

Acute kidney injury in the tropics includes acute tubular necrosis (ATN), acute tubulointerstitial nephritis (ATIN), and thrombotic microangiopathy (TMA) (8). ATN in the setting of malaria results from *Plasmodium falciparum* infection associated with heavy parasitemia and intravascular hemolysis. The hemolysis can result from the infection itself or secondary to the use of anti-malarial drugs in patients with underlying glucose-6-phosphate dehydrogenase deficiency. Mortality in this setting has been reported to range between 15% and 50% (9-11). ATN is also observed as a result of rhabdomyolysis with infections such as leptospirosis, trichinosis, malaria, typhoid fever, and viral infection.

Plasmodium falciparum can also produce acute kidney injury via severe inflammation of the renal interstitium, also known as acute tubulointerstitial nephritis either alone or in combination with ATN. ATIN is also observed in the setting of severe infection with leptospirosis (8). Acute kidney injury in the tropics is also seen as a result of thrombotic microangiopathy. Hemolytic uremic syndrome can be observed in adults and children infected with Shigella dysenteriae type I as well as Escherichia Coli O157:H7.

Glomerular disease in the tropics includes both primary diseases of the glomerulus as well as secondary causes. Primary causes include minimal change disease, focal segmental glomerulosclerosis, and IgA nephropathy among others. In Thailand, immunoglobulin M nephropathy, a variant of minimal change disease, accounts for 50% of primary glomerular diseases (1). It should be noted that the incidence of diabetic nephropathy in tropical regions is expected to have a sharp increase in the years ahead. It is expected that by 2030, 81% of those with diabetes will live in the developing world with a 88% increase in the number of people with diabetes in Latin America, 98% increase in Africa, and 91% increase in Asia in the next 25 years (12).

Secondary glomerular disease in the tropics can result from a variety of infectious agents with a corresponding spectrum of pathologic lesions in the kidney. These include but are not limited to viral hepatitis B (13,14), hepatitis ((15,16), schistosomiasis (17), leprosy (18,19), filariasis (20,21), and malaria (11,22-24). *Plasmodium malariae* has been considered an important cause of chronic malarial nephropathy or "quartan malarial nephropathy" with a proposed immune complex pathology (11,22,24,25).

Recently, the link between nephrotic syndrome and quartan malaria presenting in children from tropical regions has been questioned with the proposition that the link is only circumstantial rather than causative. It should also be noted that the term "tropical nephrotic syndrome" has also been used widely in the literature. The term was first credited to Liliane Morel-Maroger et al. in a 1975 publication describing a unique observed pathology in 16 patients from Senegal with nephrotic syndrome that was in some ways similar to "quartan malarial nephropathy", but lacked immune complex deposits (26).

More recently, a review of 32 children with nephrotic syndrome in Ghana between the years of 2000 and 2003 found no evidence of a dominant role of steroid-resistant "tropical glomerulopathy" that had previously been ascribed to quartan malaria. The review identified minimal change disease and focal segmental glomerulosclerosis as the most frequent findings on histology in African children from Ghana and South Africa (27). Another review pointed out that the association of nephrotic syndrome and quartan malaria was mostly described prior to 1975 and may have been coincidental (28). It can be argued that the term "topical nephrotic syndrome" should be eliminated as evidence suggests that there is not a distinct glomerular pathology specific to this region of the world, but rather a myriad of glomerular patterns of injury in response to various pathogens often in combination (29). Furthermore, while antigens specific to various infectious organisms have been identified in glomerular lesions, one most proceed with caution in concluding that this is substantial proof that the organism in question is solely responsible for the observed glomerular pathology. Certainly, the observed progression of some glomerular diseases in the tropics despite eradication of the proposed offending organism supports the unlikely nature of this single cause and effect scenario.

MALARIA AND KIDNEY DISEASE

Infection with malaria can result in acute kidney injury as well as chronic glomerular disease and is becoming a recognized complication of renal transplantations. With the rising trend of medical tourism, malaria has been increasingly reported as either a new infection or as reactivation disease in the immunocompromised recipient (11,30). Of the four species of Plasmodium that are pathogenic in humans, *Plasmodium falciparum* and *Plasmodium malariae* are generally considered to be the major contributors to renal disease in the tropical region. Renal disease attributed to the other types of malaria, *Plasmodium vivax* and *Plasmodium ovale*, is characterized by nonspecific and benign renal lesions. There have been occasional reports of acute kidney injury and nephritic syndrome associated with *P. ovale* (24).

It is important to note that *Plasmodium malariae* infects only older red blood cells whereas *Plasmodium falciparum* disregards the ages of erythrocytes. This corresponds to the intensity of infection observed and has implications for the resultant kidney disease. In general *P. falciparum* can produce fluid and electrolyte abnormalities, acute kidney injury that ranges from transient to severe and life-threatening, and also glomerulopathy that tends to reverse within 2 to 6 weeks after eradication of the infection (11,31). *Plasmodium malariae* on the other hand has been long associated with a progressive glomerulonephritis termed "quartan malarial nephropathy." As described above, this association has been questioned in the more recent literature.

Plasmodium falciparum

Infection with *Plasmodium falciparum* has been associated with three different renal complications. These are acute kidney injury due to acute tubular necrosis (ATN) with concomitant electrolyte abnormalities, acute tubulointerstitial nephritis, and acute proliferative glomerulonephritis. The first complication, ATN often proves to be the most frequent as well as the most grave.

Acute tubular necrosis can occur in 1-4% of all cases of *P. falciparum*, but up to 60% in cases defined as "malignant malaria (11)." The World Health Organization (WHO) defines malarial acute kidney injury as a serum creatinine concentration of more than 3 mg/dl (265 μmol/L) with urine output of less than 400 ml over 24 hours despite rehydration in patients with documented asexual forms of *P. falciparum* in their peripheral blood smear (9). It is predominantly seen in adults and older children. One study from Orissa, India reported 1,857 patients admitted with falciparum malaria in whom 61 adults and only one child (age 11) developed acute kidney injury (32). In adults, severe disease usually appears after 3-7 days of nonspecific fevers. The condition seems to be more common in males and this may be due to the higher incidence of falciparum malaria in men in areas of low or unstable transmission (24).

Acute kidney injury due to falciparum malaria tends to be oliguric and hypercatabolic. *P. falciparum* activates both the alternative pathway of complement and the intrinsic coagulation cascade which may explain the pathogenesis of thrombotic complications (11). Acute kidney injury can occur either as an isolated complication or as part of the spectrum of multi-organ failure (10). The latter cases are associated with a profound micro-circulatory disorder characterized by peripheral vasodilatation, with or without hemolysis, rhabdomyolysis, and disseminated intravascular coagulation (11). Jaundice is the most common association with malarial acute kidney injury, occurring in approximately 75% of cases (33). Hyperkalemia due to the combination of hemolysis, rhabdomyolysis, acidosis, and impaired renal function can be severe and often fatal. Prognosis depends on the severity of infection, extra-renal manifestations, response to anti-malarial medications, and the availability of renal replacement therapy. Mortality ranges from 15-45% (23).

TREATMENT OF FALCIPARUM INDUCED ACUTE KIDNEY INJURY

Treatment is directed at early implementation of appropriate anti-malarial drugs, maintenance of fluid and electrolyte levels, renal replacement therapy, and treatment of associated complications.

Chloroquine has long been the gold standard for treatment of malaria but its use must be avoided in areas of widespread resistance. It should be noted that these areas of chloroquine-resistance tend to be the same regions where acute kidney injury from *P. falciparum* is the most common. Preferred anti-malarial drugs in these regions include artesunate or quinine given parenterally (10). Treatment with quinine may produce prolonged QT interval, premature atrial or ventricular beats, as well as hypotension. Some authors advise initiating a maintenance dose of quinine at 10 mg/kg/body weight given every 8 hours for the first 48 hours regardless of acute kidney injury (10).

Ideally quinine levels should be monitored closely in the setting of oliguric acute kidney injury; however, testing is not readily available at many centers. Presumably under-dosing of quinine early in the disease course may have a profound effect on renal outcome and mortality. Caution is advised, however, with the use of intravenous quinine in patients with underlying glucose-6-phosphate dehydrogenase deficiency as massive intravascular hemolysis may ensue. This clinical scenario has become known as fatal "black water fever."

The introduction of artemisinin derivatives has improved outcomes in those with severe malaria (34,35). They have been shown to clear parasitemia quickly and effectively with limited side effects. Intravenous artesunate is given at a dose 2 mg/kg/body weight at 0, 12, and 24 hours, and then once daily for a total of 7 days (10).

Fluid resuscitation should be aggressive but with careful monitoring to avoid fluid overload. Diuretics have been used in the setting of continued oliguria despite fluid resuscitation; however, they are often ineffective in increasing urine output and there is no evidence that their use improves outcome.

When renal replacement therapy becomes necessary, intermittent hemodialysis or continuous renal replacement therapy in the form of continuous veno-venous hemofiltration or continuous arterio-venous hemofiltration is preferred. While peritoneal dialysis may be less effective due to circulatory disturbances, unfortunately it is often the only modality available. Indications for dialysis include uremic symptoms, intractable volume overload, pericardial rub, severe metabolic acidosis, or severe hyperkalemia. Exchange transfusion should be considered in patients with heavy parasitemia and severe jaundice. Corticosteroids have no role in the treatment of falciparum-induced acute kidney injury and have been reported to be detrimental in the outcomes in cerebral malaria (23).

Plasmodium malariae

Plasmodium malariae (quartan malaria) has a reported association with a chronic, progressive, immune-complex mediated glomerulopathy dating back to the 1960s and 1970s (22,25,26,36). More recent reviews have pointed out the lack of data on this association since that time (27-29). Whether the conflicting data on the existence of quartan malarial nephropathy is due to a changing pattern of underlying nephrotic syndrome in the region over the past 30 years or due to incorrect prior assumptions regarding cause and effect remains to be determined. The most significant epidemiologic observation in support of the existence of a "tropical nephrotic syndrome" is the change in incidence of renal disease following eradication of malaria in British Guiana (29,37). This observation is limited by the paucity of pathology to support the firm conclusion that malaria was in fact the causative agent of glomerular disease pre-eradication.

The quartan malarial nephrotic syndrome has been described to affect mostly children with a mean age of 5 years (11). Proteinuria is the presenting feature in most cases with occasional episodes of microscopic hematuria that more often occur in adults. A proportion of patients will go on to develop nephrotic syndrome with hypertension as a late manifestation. Hyperlipidemia is usually absent presumably due to concomitant malnutrition. Based on animal models, the pathology of malaria induced glomerulonephritis has been believed to be an immune complex mediated process either from circulating immune complexes formed by malarial antigens or immune complexes formed *in situ* in the renal glomeruli (1).

The clinical course usually includes persistent proteinuria with slow deterioration in renal function. The mechanisms underlying the progression of renal disease to advanced chronic stages are not well understood. While anti-malarial therapy can eliminate the organisms, it does not always prevent the progression of glomerular disease suggesting additional contributions to the pathology other than malarial immune complexes (8). There is no evidence to support treatment of quartan malarial nephropathy with corticosteroids or alternate immunosuppressants as they do not alter the course of nephropathy and may worsen the course of the underlying infection.

SCHISTOSOMIASIS

Schistosomiasis is a disease caused by parasitic trematode worms called schistosomes. It was known in ancient Egypt as "the bloody urine disease" and has also been known as "bilharziasis" in honor of Theodore Bilharz (1825-1862), the German physician practicing in Egypt who discovered schistosomiasis in the 1850s (38). Often the parasite is acquired during the teenage years and leads to complications that can extend into the fourth or fifth decades of life. Three species of schistosomes are responsible for the majority of morbidity in humans. These are *Schistosoma haematobium*, *Schistosoma mansoni*, and *Schistosoma japonicum*. Each has a varying geographic distribution: *S. haematobium* is present throughout Africa and adjacent regions; *S. mansoni* is present in Africa, South America, and the Carribean islands; *S. japonicum* is present in the Far East. According to the World Health Organization (WHO), a total of 700 million people in 74 endemic countries worldwide are at risk for infection given contact with contaminated water sources. Of the estimated 207 million people living with schistosomiasis worldwide, 85% live in Africa (39).

Human infections follow direct contact with fresh water that contains the free-swimming larval form of the parasite known as cercaria. The cercaria penetrate the skin of the human host and then shed their bifid tails. The worms then enter capillaries and lymphatic vessels and eventually make their way to the lungs, and finally to the portal venous system, where they mature into sexually differentiated adult worms and live in almost continuous copulation. The females leave the males only to lay eggs usually in the bladder or rectal mucosa. The eggs are driven out of the human host during defecation or urination and eventually hatch to release miracidia which then infect specific snails. Within this intermediate host, the miracidia mature asexually into cercaria, thus completing the life cycle (17,40).

Schistosomes can cause disease of the kidney and lower urinary tract via two major mechanisms. The first is through local reactions around the ova deposited in tissue. The second is through systemic effects of the host's immune reaction to circulating antigens released from the worm or the ova. The host immune response to schistosomiasis can be notably altered by concomitant infections with Salmonella or Hepatitis C amongst others.

Past history of infection with schistosomiasis is an independent risk factor for end- stage renal disease (41). The first mechanism of injury, chronic granulomatous inflammation leading to obstructive uropathy, is responsible for end-stage renal disease in approximately 7% of the Egyptian dialysis population (42). A prospective study from Yemen identified schistosomiasis with resultant obstructive uropathy as the cause of end stage renal disease in 4.75% (43). In many Arab countries obstructive uropathy, from either renal calculi or schistosomiasis, accounts for the cause of ESRD in an estimated 40% of cases. The second immune-mediated mechanism of renal injury progresses to end stage renal disease in approximately 15% of patients, and accounts for the etiology of renal failure in 2% of the Egyptian dialysis population (42).

Lower urinary tract schistosomiasis: *Schistosoma haematobium*

The lower urinary tract tends to be the site of local granulomatous response to schistosomes and typically *S. haematobium* is the pathogen. The local reaction is the cell mediated immune response to soluble egg antigens that eventually leads to granuloma formation. With time fibrotic granulomas in the bladder, lower ureters, and seminal vessels can become calcified (38).

Multiple granulomas can eventually form small "pseudotubercles" in the bladder mucosa. These are distinct from true tubercles associated with genitourinary tuberculosis due to their surrounding vascular congestion (17). These pseudotubercles can then coalesce to form a sessile mass or even ulcerate resulting in painful terminal hematuria. This is the typical presenting feature of lower urinary tract schistosomiasis in up to 90% of cases. Examination of the urine at this stage is essentially diagnostic with visualization of live schistosomal ova with characteristic terminal spikes in conjunction with red and white blood cells in the urine sediment.

Eventually these granulomas may become fibrotic and calcify. Calcified granulomas beneath atrophic mucosa give the characteristic cystoscopic appearance of sandy patches as well as the radiologic appearance of linear bladder calcifications (38). Comparative studies have validated ultrasonography as a highly sensitive modality and is comparable to cystoscopy and intravenous pyelography for detecting bladder pathology in infected individuals (44,45).

With time, scarring and contracture of these lesions can lead to many complications including ureteral strictures, outflow obstruction, reduction of bladder volume, detrusor muscle contraction abnormalities, ureteral obstruction, or vesicoureteral reflux (17). In addition, the bladder lesions can predispose to bacterial infection with Pseudomonas or Proteus infection especially following instrumentation. Proteus infection can then predispose to stone formation making the picture even more complicated.

In most instances, the upper ureter musculature is able to hypertrophy and overcome lower urinary tract partial obstruction by urinary schistosomiasis. However, complications of schistosomiasis in the lower urinary tract can eventually lead to upper urinary tract pathology. Hydronephrosis and progressive renal failure can occur, as well as chronic tubulointerstitial nephritis.

Bladder cancer is a dreaded complication of chronic schistosomal cystitis. Clinically, bilharzial bladder cancer presents with an escalation in symptoms of chronic cystitis, necroturia, resistance to antibacterial therapy, and recurrence of hematuria (17). Chronic bladder involvement, also known as chronic bilharzial cystitis, is essentially a precancerous state. A case series of 1,026 cases of bladder cancer that underwent surgical cystectomy in Egypt detected schistosomal ova in more than 85% of subjects (46). While typically associated with squamous cell carcinoma, this study revealed approximately 60% squamous cell, 20% transitional cell carcinoma, 10% adenocarcinoma, and the rest were of mixed pathology (46). Due to the fibrosis of the surrounding lymphatics in the setting of chronic schistosomal cystitis, the tumor, especially when squamous cell in origin, tends to be localized for an extended period of time prior to metastasis (17).

GLOMERULAR DISEASE AND SCHISTOSOMIASIS

Glomerular disease due to schistosomiasis is believed to result from a systemic, humoral immune response to schistosomal antigens circulating in the host rather than a local reaction in the tissue. Glomerular disease with schistosomiasis is typically associated with *S. mansoni* although it is also reported with *S. haematobium* and *S. japonicum*. The responsible circulating antigens originate mostly from the worm's gut antigens (47,48). Studies have demonstrated that the host kidneys play an important role in clearance of these antigens from the peripheral blood. Deposition of schistosomal antigens in the mesangial cell is critical to the pathology. The mesangial cell is believed to be the site of the initial processing of schistosomal antigens. Hamsters inoculated with schistosomal antigens demonstrate a mesangioproliferative glomerulonephritis with associated deposition of IgG, IgM, and C3 together with schistosomal antigens (49).

Additional impairment of the hepatic mononuclear phagocyte system in the setting of hepatosplenic schistosomiasis further increases the severity of the glomerulopathy (50). Immune complexes containing these gut antigens have been identified in mesangial, subendothelial, and intramembranous locations in both experimental and human infection (17,38). A correlation between the kidney disease and the duration and load of *S. mansoni* infection has been documented in animal models (51,52).

Proteinuria is the most frequent clinical manifestation of glomerular disease associated with schistosomiasis. Affected patients tend to be males between the ages of 20 and 40 years-old usually with hepatosplenic schistosomiasis. Renal disease can be asymptomatic in up to 40% of these patients, usually detected as various grades of proteinuria or microscopic hematuria on surveillance urine dipstick. Another 15% however, present with overt disease manifested by the nephrotic syndrome, hypertension, or impaired renal function.

There are six classes of schistosoma-associated glomerular lesions (16,17,38). Three of these classes (I – mesangioproliferative glomerulonephritis, III – membranoproliferative glomerulonephritis, and IV – focal segmental glomerulosclerosis) represent different stages in the evolution of pure schistosomal hepatosplenic disease. Class II, diffuse proliferative exudative glomerulonephritis, is associated with co-infection with salmonella strains. Amyloid A deposits can be detected in up to 15% of biopsy samples from patients with class III or IV disease.

In class V disease, however, amyloidosis is the predominant lesion. Recently a class VI lesion, cryoglobulinemic glomerulonephritis, has been described especially in Egyptian patients co-infected with hepatitis C (16). It is noted that in class II (co-infection with schistosomiasis and salmonella) and class VI (co-infection with schistosomiasis and hepatitis C virus), the pathology in the glomerulus does not fit with either infection alone. The concomitant helminthic and viral or bacterial infection is believed to provoke a unique immune response in the glomerulus (16).

Class I is mesangioproliferative glomerulonephritis due to *S. haematobium, mansoni, or japonicum*. Clinically these patients tend to present with microscopic hematuria and various grade of proteinuria. On biopsy, immunofluorescence reveals the presence of IgM, C3, and schistosomal gut antigens in the mesangium. Treatment of the parasite in this stage can be curative, but up to 60% may be asymptomatic at this stage.

Class II is diffuse proliferative exudative glomerulonephritis due to co-infection of *S. haematobium or mansoni* with *Salmonella paratyphi A* in Africa or *Salmonella typhimurium* in Brazil. The glomerular lesion seen with co-infection of schistosomiasis and salmonella is unique from that observed from either infection alone. Studies have demonstrated that the salmonella endotoxin provokes the release of macrophage inhibitory factor by interaction with the pituitary gland in the brain (16,53). This eventually leads to upregulation of a macrophage receptor known as toll-like receptor-4 (54). Increased activation of the antigen presenting cells eventually leads to a florid inflammatory response that results in the diffuse proliferative exudative glomerulonephritis seen in class II schistosomal glomerulopathy.

This is distinct from the glomerular lesions seen in typhoid fever in an otherwise healthy individual which is much less severe and often subclinical. In this class, the glomeruli is essentially "primed" by the immune response to schistosomiasis (16). Clinically, these patients present with the picture of acute nephritic syndrome associated with salmonella-related toxemia which can include fever, exanthema, and severe anemia. Serum C3 is often low. Biopsy reveals the presence of C3 and salmonella antigens by immunofluorescence in the glomerular capillary walls and mesangium. Eradication of schistosoma in conjunction with antibiotics targeted at salmonella can be curative.

Class III is membranoproliferative glomerulonephritis (usually MPGN Type I or Type III without cryoglobulinemia) due mostly to *S. mansoni* with some question of contribution by *S. haematobium*. In this stage, 80% present with overt renal disease including nephrotic syndrome, hypertension, and decline in glomerular filtration rate; hepatosplenomegaly is also seen. Biopsy reveals the presence of IgG, IgA, C3, and schistosomal antigens by immunofluorescence. Immune complex deposition is located in the mesangium, subendothelial, as well as subepithelial location. Glomerular IgA deposits have been shown to be markers of significant renal involvement with hepatosplenic schistosomiasis (55). Eradication of the parasite at this stage, unfortunately, does not seem to abate the progression of glomerulopathy (56).

Class IV is focal segmental glomerulosclerosis due almost exclusively to *S. mansoni*. Its clinical presentation is similar to Class III with nephrotic syndrome, hypertension, renal failure, and hepatosplenomegaly. Biopsy reveals IgM, IgG, and occasionally IgA usually with noted absence of schistosomal antigens. As documented in class III, the IgA deposits tend to parallel the severity of proteinuria and mesangial proliferation. The presence of impaired hepatic clearance and increased mucosal synthesis of IgA has been documented in these patients (55).

Hypoalbuminemia can be severe and reflects not only urinary losses, but also associated hepatic dysfunction and nutritional deficiency. Interestingly hypolipidemia is usually encountered for these reasons, rather than the hyperlipidemia usually associated with nephrotic syndrome (17). The lesions of class III and IV disease do not respond to corticosteroids or immunosuppression (57). It is a progressive glomerular disease regardless of presence or absence of the organism at this stage.

Class V schistosomal glomerulopathy is amyloidosis due to either *S. mansoni* or *S. haematobium*. While up to 15% of biopsy samples in class III and IV can have amyloid A protein detected by special stains or electron microscopy, in class V the predominant lesion is amyloidosis. This occurs in less than 5% of patients and is associated with a heavy burden of infection. Typical of amyloidosis, these patients present with heavy proteinuria, nephrotic syndrome, and the clinical picture is progressive to end stage renal disease regardless of attempted treatment with anti-schistosomal drugs, corticosteroids, or colchicines (56).

Class VI is cryoglobulinemic glomerulonephritis that was recently described in patients co-infected with *S. mansoni* and hepatitis C mostly in Egypt (16). In addition to hepatosplenomegaly, these patients present with nephrotic syndrome, purpura, vasculitis, arthritis, hypertension, as well as renal failure. Biopsy reveals a mixture of mesangial proliferation, amyloid deposition, fibrinoid necrosis, and cyroglobulinemic thrombi in glomerular capillaries with tubular casts (40).

SCHISTOSOMIASIS AND THE KIDNEY: TREATMENT

Praziquantal remains the agent of choice in treatment of schistosomes of all species. Of note it is active only against mature worms. Artemisinin derivatives have demonstrated activity against cercariae, maturing schistosomulae, as well as mature worms, although their use is still being studied.

Complications of chronic fibrotic lesions in the lower urinary tract may require surgical intervention to relieve obstruction. Unfortunately, surgical intervention can then induce vesicoureteral reflux, further complicating the situation. Plastic surgery to correct bladder, ureteral, and urethral distortion can also be performed.

Treatment of class I schistosomal mesangioproliferative glomerulonephritis is aimed at eradication of the organism. The same is true for class II schistosomal diffuse proliferative exudative glomerulonephritis but in conjunction with treatment for salmonella. Unfortunately classes III – VI schistosomal glomerular disease tends to progress regardless of anti-schistosomal treatment, glucocorticoids, or immunosuppression.

Patients who go on to develop end stage renal disease can be considered for renal transplantation when available. The impact of schistosomiasis on patient and graft outcome over 10 years of follow-up has been studied (58). While there is a higher incidence of schistosoma-related complications after renal transplantation, including higher incidence of urinary tract infection and urological complications, schistosomal infection is not a major risk factor for transplantation. Infected patients can be considered suitable donors or recipients after proper treatment 1 month prior to transplantation with aim to eradicate the organism.

EMPIRIC TREATMENT OF PROTEINURIA WITH UNCERTAIN DIAGNOSIS

Treatments for falciparum acute kidney injury, quartan malarial nephropathy, and the various renal manifestation of schistosomiasis are described above. Unfortunately for the practicing physician in many tropical regions, resources may limit the evaluation of a patient who presents with proteinuria of unknown etiology.

For proteinuria in the pediatric population that is persistent and above 40 mg/h/m^2, the treatment of nephrotic syndrome should mirror the treatment plan in the western world where the presumed diagnosis is minimal change disease. Renal biopsy is deemed unnecessary unless the patient does not respond to corticosteroids. A diligent search for active infectious disease should be performed prior to the initiation of corticosteroids. Empiric corticosteroids should be initiated at a dose of 60 mg/m^2/day with a maximum of 80 mg/day. Weight should be based on estimated dry weight.

Intravenous corticosteroids should be considered in those with severe edema or diarrhea since edema of the gut wall may limit absorption. Of those children that respond to corticosteroids 75% will respond within 2 weeks, 80-85% within 4 weeks, and over 90% within 8 weeks (59). When remission is achieved, defined by proteinuria of less than 4 mg/h/m^2, then full dose prednisone should be continued for an additional 4 weeks and then switched to alternate-day dosing for an additional 4-8 weeks. Subsequent tapering should be slow with reduction in dose by 15 mg/m2 on alternate days every 2 weeks until withdrawn (60).

For proteinuria that is persistent and above 2 grams daily in the adult population, renal biopsy should be pursued when available. If biopsy is not available, investigation should be aimed at excluding active infectious diseases such as hepatitis B, hepatitis C, HIV, syphilis, malaria, and schistosomiasis as resources permit. If clinical suspicion is high for any of these diseases, then it is quite possible that the nephrotic syndrome observed is secondary in nature and treatment should be aimed at the primary infectious disease. Even if specific syndromes such as "quartan malarial nephropathy" do in fact exist, then treatment should be directed at malaria rather than focus on corticosteroids which have shown to be of little benefit and may have adverse effects.

If a diligent search does not identify an active infectious disease and biopsy is unavailable, then it is reasonable to consider an empiric course of corticosteroids at 1 mg/kg/day or 2 mg/kg every other day for 6-8 weeks with subsequent slow taper of dose and continued therapy until remission or up to 6 months (61).

Steroids should ideally be combined with angiotensin converting enzyme inhibitors or angiotensin receptor blockers. It is worth noting that corticosteroids in the setting of IgA nephropathy have proven to be most useful in the clinical setting of acute onset nephrotic syndrome or rapidly progressive glomerulonephritis. They are of limited utility in the setting of IgA nephropathy characterized by isolated hematuria, where prognosis is excellent.

Steroid resistance should be suspected when no reduction in proteinuria is achieved despite maximum dose steroids of up to 16 weeks. Ideally if no response is observed within 6-8 weeks, renal biopsy should be performed in the pediatric population. Given that this is unlikely to be available, it is reasonable to continue steroids for the full 16 weeks or even up to 6 months in children, thus treating empirically for focal segmental glomerulosclerosis. The prognosis for non-responders in this region of the world, without access to renal biopsy, alternate immunosuppressive agents, or renal replacement therapy, is poor.

These recommendations are based on newer data from the tropical region that suggests the most common glomerular pathology may in fact be focal segmental glomerulosclerosis and minimal change disease rather than a distinct "topical nephrotic syndrome (27,61)."

Regarding therapy of nephrotic syndrome under tropical conditions it should be emphasized that over half of the patients especially in the pediatric population may benefit from corticosteroids (27).

SUMMARY

Tropical nephrology includes a broad spectrum of pathologic changes of the kidney in response to infectious organisms, natural toxins, or environmental toxins specific to that region of the world between the tropic of cancer and the tropic of capricorn. It also includes renal disorders that are encountered in both the tropical region and the western world. This article considers clinical syndromes that are observed in tropical nephrology such as asymptomatic urine abnormalities, macroscopic hematuria, acute kidney injury, and glomerular disease. Glomerular disease may be primary or secondary to a variety of infectious organisms. Clinical syndromes are reviewed along with proposed causative organisms. Special attention is given to malaria and schistosomiasis as major contributors to renal disease in this region of the world. Of note, recent evidence has questioned the existence of a distinct "topical nephrotic syndrome" previously ascribed to quartan malaria. Whether this reflects a changing spectrum of disease in the region or a history of inaccurate assignment of a single cause and effect relationship to the malarial pathogen and the nephrotic syndrome remains to be determined. Finally, treatment options are discussed including a suggested approach to persistent proteinuria of unknown cause. Concepts of evaluation and management are also considered when resources are limited.

REFERENCES

[1]   Sitprija V. Overview of tropical nephrology. Semin Nephrol 2003;23(1):3-11.

[2]   Rose BD. Pathophysiology of renal disease, 2nd. New York : McGraw-Hill, 1987:11-6.

[3]   Chugh KS. Snake-bite-induced acute renal failure in India. Kidney Int 1989;35:891-907.

[4]   Chugh KS, Aikat BK, Sharma BK, et al. Acute renal failure following snakebite. Am J Trop Med Hyg 1975;24(4):692-7.

[5]   Hoh TK, Soong CL. Fatal haemolysis from wasp and hornet sting. Singapore Med J 1966;7(2):122-6.

[6]   Thiruventhiran T, Goh BL, Leong CL, et. al. Acute renal failure following multiple wasp stings. Nephrol Dial Transplant 1999;14:214-7.

[7]   Bhalla VS, Pereira BJG, Kapoor MM, et al. Acute renal failure following multiple hornet stings. Nephron 1988;49:319-21.

[8]   Boonpucknavig V, Soontorniyomkij V. Pathology of renal diseases in the tropics. Semin Nephrol 2003;23(1):88-106.

[9]   World Health Organization. Severe falciparum malaria. Trans R Soc Trop Med Hyg 2000;94(Suppl 1):S1-S90.

[10]   Mishra SK, Das BS. Malaria and acute kidney injury. Semin Nephrol 2008;28(4):395-408.

[11]   Barsoum R. Malarial nephropathies. Nephrol Dial Transplant 1998;13:1588-97.

[12]   Atkins R. The changing patterns of chronic kidney disease: The need to develop strategies for prevention relevant to different regions and countries. Kidney Int Suppl 2005;98:S83-S85.

[13]   Lai KN, Lai FM. Clinical features and the natural course of hepatitis B virus-related glomerulpathy in adults. Kidney Int Suppl 1991;35:S40-S45.

[14]   Johnson RJ, Couser WG. Hepatitis B infection and renal disease: Clinical, immunopathogenetic, and therapeutic considerations. Kidney Int 1990;37:663-76.

[15]   Burnstein DM, Rodby RA. Membranoproliferative glomerulonephritis associated with hepatitis C virus infection. J Am Soc Nephrol 1993;4:1288-93.

[16]   Barsoum RS. The changing face of schistosomal glomerulopathy. Kidney Int 2004;66:2472-84.

[17]   Barsoum RS. Schistosomiasis and the kidney. Semin Nephrol 2003;23:34-41.

[18]   Nakayama EE, Ura A, Fleury RN, et al. Renal lesions in leprosy: a retrospective study of 199 autopsies. Am J Kidney Dis 2001;38(1):26-30.

[19] Da Silva Jr GB, De Francesco DE. Renal involvement in leprosy: Retrospective anaylsis of 461 cases in Brazil. Brazilian J Infect Dis 2006;10(2):107-12.

[20] Ngu JL, Chatelanat F, Leke R, et al. Nephropathy in Cameroon: Evidence for filarial derived immune-complex pathogenesis in some cases. Clin Nephrol 1985;24(3):128-34.

[21] Langhammer J, Birk WH, Zahner H. Renal disease in lymphatic filariasis: evidence for tubular and glomerular disorders at various stages of the infection. Trop Med Int Health 1997;2(9):875-84.

[22] Hendrickse RG, Adeniyi A. Quartan malarial nephrotic syndrome in children. Kidney Int 1979;16:64-74.

[23] Barsoum, Rashad. Malarial acute renal failure. J Am Soc Nephrol 2000;11:2147-54.

[24] Eiam-Ong S. Malarial nephropathy. Semin Nephrol 2003;23(1):21-33.

[25] Gilles HM, Hendrickse RG. Nephrosis in Nigerian children: Role of plasmodium malariae and effect of antimalarial treatment. BMJ 1963;2(5348):27-31.

[26] More-Maroger L, Saimot AG, Sloper JC, et al. Tropical nephropathy and tropical extramembranous glomerulonephritis of unknown etiology in Senegal. BMJ 1975;1:541-6.

[27] Doe JY, Funk M, Mengel M, et al. Nephrotic syndrome in African children: lack of evidence for "tropical nephrotic syndrome"? Nephrol Dial Transplant 2006;21:672-6.

[28] Ehrick JHH, Eke FU. Malaria-induced renal damage: facts and myths. Pediatr Nephrol 2007;22:626-37.

[29] Davies DR, Wing AJ. Malaria, microscopy, and marmosets: the saga of the tropical nephrotic syndrome. Quart J Med 1990;75(278):533-5.

[30] Sajjad I, Baines LS, Patel P, et al. Commercialization of kidney transplants: a systemic review of outcomes in recipients and donors. Am J Nephrol 2008;28(5):744-54.

[31] Sitprija V. Nephropathy in falciparum malaria. Kidney Int 1988;34:867-77.

[32] Mohanty S, Mishra SK, Pati SS, et al. Complications and mortality patterns due to Plasmodium falciparum malaria in hospitalized adults and children, Rourkela, Orissa, India. Trans R Soc Trop Med 2003;97:69-70.

[33] Wilairatana P, Looareesuwan S, Charoenlarp P. Liver profile changes and complications in jaundiced patients with falciparum malria. Trop Med Parisitol 1994;45:298-302.

[34] Mohanty S, Mishra SK, Satpathy SK, et al. Alpha, beta-Arteether for the treatment of complicated falciparum malaria. Trans R Soc Trop Med Hyg 1997;91:328-30.

[35] Dondorp A, Nosten F, Stepniewska K, et al. South East Asian Quinine Artesunate Malaria Trial (SEAQUAMAT) group. Artesunate versus quinine for treatment of severe falciparum malaria; a randomised trial. Lancet 2005;366:717-25.

[36] Wing AJ, Hutt MSR, Kibukamusoke JW. Progression and remission in the nephrotic syndrome associated with quartan malaria in Uganda. Quart J Med 1972;163:273-89.

[37] Giglioli G. Malaria and renal disease with special reference to British Guiana. II. The effect of malaria eradication on the incidence of renal disease in British Guiana. Anna Trop Med Parasitol 1962;56:224-41.

[38] Barsoum R. The kidney in schistosomiasis. In: Floege J, Johnson RJ, Feehally J, eds. Comprehensive clinical nephrology, 3rd. Philadelphia, PA: Mosby, 2007:631-9.

[39] World Health Organization. Schistosomiasis: Fact Sheet. Accessed 2011 Sep 01. URL: http://www.who.int/ mediacentre/factsheets/fs115/en/.

[40] Ross AG, Bartley PB, Sleigh AC, et al. Schistosomiasis. N Engl J Med 2002;346(16):1212-20.

[41] El-Gaafary M, Abou El-Fetouh A, Zaki M, et al. Some epidemiological aspects of patients with end-stage renal diseases. J Egypt Public Health Assoc 2000;75(1-2):107-29.

[42] Barsoum RS. End-stage renal disease in North Africa. Kidney Int Suppl 2003;83:S111-4.

[43] Al-Rohani M. Renal failure in Yemen. Transplant Proceed 2004;36:1777-9.

[44] Degremont A, Burki A, Brunier E, et al. Value of ultrasonography in investing morbidity due to Schistosoma haematobium infection. Lancet 1985;325(8530):662-5.

[45] Abdel-Wabab MR, Ramzy I, Esmat G, et al. Ultrasound for detecting Schistosoma haematobium urinary tract complications: comparison with radiographic procedures. J Urology 1992;148:346-50.

[46] Ghoneim Ma, El-Mekresh MM, El-Baz MA, et al. Radical cystectomy for carcinoma of the bladder: critical evaluation of the results in 1,026 cases. J Urology 1997;158:393-9.

[47] deWater R, Van Marck EA, Fransen JAM, et al. Schistosoma mansoni: Ultrastructural localization of the circulating anodic antigen and the circulating cathodic antigen in the mouse kidney glomerulus. Am J Trop Med Hyg 1988;38:118-24.

[48] Quian Z, Lu P, Wang Z, et al. Isolation and specific detection of two major schistosoma gut-associated circulating antigens. Chinese Med J (English) 2001;114(6):614-17.

[49] De Brito T, Carneiro CR, Nakhle MC, et al. Localization by immunoelectron microscopy of Schistosoma mansoni antigens in the glomerulus of the hamster kidney. Exp Nephrol 1998;6:368-76.

[50] Barsoum RS, Sersawy G, Haddad S, et al. Hepatic macrophage function in schistosomal glomerulopathy. Nephrol Dial Transplant 1988;3:612-6.

[51] Vaclav H. Experimental renal disease due to schistosomiasis. Kidney Int 1979;16: 30-43.

[52] Sobh M, Moustafa F, Ramzy R, et al. Schistosoma mansoni nephropathy in Syrian golden hamsters: effect of dose and duration of infection. Nephron 1991;59:121-30.

[53] Koebernick H, Grode L, David JR, et al. Macrophage migration inhibitory factor (MIF) plays a pivotal role in immunity against Salmonella typhimurium. Proceed Natl Acad Sci 2002;99:13681-6.

[54] Li Q, Cherayil BJ. Roll of toll-like receptor 4 in macrophage activation and tolerance during Salmonella enterica serovar typhimurium infection. Infect Immun 2003;71:4873-82.

[55] Barsoum RS, Nabil M, Saady G. Immunoglobulin-A and the pathogenesis of schistosomal glomerulopathy. Kidney Int 1996;50:920-8.

[56] Martinelli R, Noblat AC, Brito E, et al. Schistosoma mansoni-induced mesangiocapillary glomerulonephritis: Influence of therapy. Kidney Int 1989;35:1227-33.

[57] Martinelli R, Pereira LJ, Rocha H. The influence of anti-parasitic therapy on the course of the glomerulopathy associated with schistosomiasis mansoni. Clin Nephrol 1987;27(5):229-32.

[58] Mahmoud KM, Sobh MA, El-Agroudy AE, et al. Impact of schistosomiasis on patient and graft outcome after renal transplantation: 10 years follow-up. Nephrol Dial Transplant 2001;16:2214-21.

[59] Barnett Hl, Edelman CM, Greifer I, et al. The primary nephrotic syndrome in children: Identification of patients with minimal change nephrotic syndrome from initial response to prednisone: A report of the International Study of Kidney Disease in Children. J Pediatrics 1981;98:561-4.

[60] Mason, Philip D. Minimal change disease. In: Floege J, Johnson RJ, Feehally J, eds. Comprehensive clinical nephrology, 3rd. Philadelphia, PA: Mosby, 2007:209-16.

[61] Appel GB, Pollack MR, D'Agati V. Focal segmental glomerulosclerosis. In: Floege J, Johnson RJ, Feehally J, eds. Comprehensive clinical nephrology, 3rd. Philadelphia, PA: Mosby, 2007:217-30.

Submitted: September 01, 2011. *Revised:* November 02, 2011. *Accepted:* November 10, 2011.

In: Public Health Yearbook 2012
Editor: Joav Merrick

ISBN: 978-1-62808-078-0
© 2013 Nova Science Publishers, Inc.

Chapter 12

MALARIA

*Richard R Roach, MD, FACP**

Internal Medicine Department, Michigan State University/Kalamazoo Center for Medical Studies, Kalamazoo, Michigan, United States of America

ABSTRACT

Malaria remains a major cause of death among children in the world. Recent research has led to dramatic insights as to the cause of pathology and a better understanding of treatment. *Plasmodium falciparim* is well known to cause cerebral malaria and most of the mortality, but P. vivax is now recognized for causing pulmonary vascular damage and significant mortality as well. Artemesin products have given new life to treatment but resistant parasites threaten the future. Research into vaccines is plodding along demonstrating that a number of single antigens may not be effective but a vaccine of the future may require a combination of antigens. This review examines the recent research of malaria.

Keywords: Malaria, plasmodium falciparim, public health

INTRODUCTION

Malaria continues to cause profound morbidity and mortality with estimated annual death tolls ranging between 0.7 to 2.7 million worldwide. Mortality of children represents greater than half of the total each year. *Plasmodium falciparum* causes 90% of the mortality primarily through central nervous system vascular damage and secondarily through renal and red cell damage (1.) New research recognizes *Plasmodium vivax* as causing mortality mainly through pulmonary vascular damage, comprising 0-20% of cases depending on the local prevalence of *P. vivax* (2).

* Correspondence: Richard R. Roach, MD, FACP, Assistant Professor, Internal Medicine Department, Michigan State University/ Kalamazoo Center for Medical Studies, 1000 Oakland Drive, Kalamazoo, Michigan 49008, United States. E-mail: roach@ kcms.msu.edu

Due to increased international travel, countries where malaria is not endemic are experiencing increasing numbers of imported cases. The Swedish Institute for Infectious Disease Control reported a risk that varied from 1 per 100,000 travelers from Central America to 357 per 100,000 travelers to Central Africa (3). The Sentinel Surveillance Report, data collected by TropNetEurop which monitors 16 European countries, reported an average incidence of eight hundred cases a year since 2000 (4). Consistent with European data, the Epidemic Intelligence Service which conducts malaria surveillance in the United States, reported 1278 cases of malaria in 2003 and 1324 cases in 2004. The following species were implicated: *P. falciparum* 53.3 (49.6) %, *vivax* 22.9 (23.8) %, *malariae* 3.6(3.6) %, and *ovale* 2.6(2.0) % (5).

VECTOR

Malaria is characteristically spread by the bite of the parasitically infected female *Anopheles* mosquito. Of the 400 species of mosquitoes, at least 80 are capable of transmitting the parasite. Recent research has identified *A. quadrimaculatus* and *A. punctipennis* as competent vectors. Although each vector has its own feeding behavior, the majority of competent vectors feed between sunset and early morning. Some have a seasonal maturation so that in parts of the Gambia, for instance, malaria only occurs during the rainy season. Recent studies of global warming in the tropics have demonstrated more rapid maturation of vectors which may increase the incidence of human disease.

PARASITE

Human disease is caused by 1 of 4 major and a few minor species of the genus *Plasmodium* (6), protozoan parasites of red blood cells [RBC's]. *Plasmodium* species infect many non-human hosts including cattle, birds, reptiles and other mammals such as macaque monkeys. A unique *Plasmodium* species discovered by the Pasteur Institute infects lemurs of Madagascar. The *Plasmodium* that infects humans is phylogenetically most similar to the species that infects birds.

Genomes for *P. falciparim* and *P. vivax* have been sequenced. *P. falciparim* remains fairly constant genetically. Forms found in Egyptian mummies have almost identical genetic sequences to modern forms. In contrast, *P. vivax* demonstrates such dramatic genetic shifts that it is impossible to distinguish re-infection from persistent infection by genome studies.

P. vivax and *P. ovale* have hypnozoite stages that reside in the liver. This means that they can cause clinical relapses since hypnozoites are immune to the drugs used to treat acute disease. Hypnozoites require specific treatment. The other *Plasmodium* species do not have such liver forms and therefore do not cause clinical relapses.

P. falciparim prefers young RBC's but is capable of invading all ages of RBC's, while *P. vivax* and *P. ovale* prefer reticulocytes. Mixed infections of *P. falciparim* and *P. vivax* can be difficult to diagnose because *P. vivax* decreases the number of cells *P. falciparim* can invade which can cause microscopic false negative results on microscopic examination. *P. malariae* which prefers older RBC's, is uncommon even in Africa where it is endemic. *P. ovale* is common only in West Africa, but is found in Madagascar. *P. knowlesi* is becoming more recognized as a lethal form of malaria in Borneo and Southeast Asia where it also infects macaque monkeys, the only known animal reservoir for *Plasmodium* species.

CLINICAL MANIFESTATIONS

The clinical manifestations of malaria are variable and nonspecific. Table 1 lists factors of severity which include fever, chills, myalgias as well as the laboratory abnormalities of anemia, thrombocytopenia, and renal dysfunction. These clinical findings are too non-specific to raise the suspicion of malaria in areas where the disease is not endemic. Therefore, a clinical diagnosis of malaria can be missed for extended periods of time in locations where the disease is uncommon.

In endemic areas the opposite is true. Patients are treated for malaria before other causes of their symptoms are investigated. Therefore, a careful history of exposure, laboratory expertise, and clinical suspicion must be combined to form a correct diagnosis and provide timely treatment. Delay in diagnosis and treatment leads to significant morbidity and mortality as evidenced by 4 fatal cases reported by the Centers for Disease Control in 2004.

Lack of familiarity with chemoprophylaxis for people traveling to endemic areas has been an important cause of preventable morbidity and mortality due to malaria.

Table 1. Features of Severe Malaria

- Acidosis pH<7.3
- Hypoglycemia
- Hemaglobin < 8g/dl
- Shock BP< 90/60
- Disseminated intravascular coagulation
- Renal failure
- Hemaglobinuria
- Pulmonary edema
- Cerebral infarction and edema

Equally important but less recognized has been the risk incurred by foreign nationals returning to endemic areas without prophylaxis because they did not take prophylaxis while residing there previously. Furthermore, malaria is frequently not considered when the patient reports compliance with appropriate prophylaxis, despite the fact that prophylaxis is incomplete. *P. vivax* has shown as great as 50% resistance to CDC recommended prophylactic regimens (7).

The diagnosis of malaria is particularly challenging when a patient presents a year after parasitic exposure. This prolonged period between exposure and presentation results in a number of alternative diagnoses taking priority, specifically idiopathic thrombocytopenic purpura (ITP) because of the reduced platelet count and the course of the illness. Such delays cause severe morbidity such as renal failure requiring dialysis and even mortality to a disease that is potentially curable.

P. vivax and *P. ovale* develop dormant hypnozoites that may persist in the liver for months to years. The latency period exceeds 3 months in 40% of patients, and relapses occur in 18% of patients after an acute infection (8). Treatment of hypnozoite forms is essential since as many as 29-40% of patients relapse without primaquine therapy. Even the difference between the 2 species producing hypnozoites is important clinically as *P. vivax* infections often require a higher dose primaquine therapy, whereas only 2 cases of *P. ovale* treatment failure have been reported in the world literature (9,10). Primaquine is the only available hypnozoicide and a concerted effort to find alternative drugs is ongoing.

Acute renal failure is second only to cerebral malaria as the most important cause of malarial mortality. *P. falciparum* has the ability to sequester within the microvasculature, to conglomerate infected erythrocytes, to elaborate tumor necrosis factor, and to produce microparticles from endothelial cell membranes. These microparticles alone in serum depleted of parasites, have been shown to cause vascular damage to the renal and cerebral vasculature in mice. *P. falciparum* causes infected erythrocytes to form "knobs" that adhere to vascular endothelium, other erythrocytes, and platelets, ultimately leading to sequestration in the venules and capillaries (11). Timely treatment dramatically improves the clinical course of these complications. Dialysis may be necessary but return of adequate renal function is the rule. Therefore, even in the face of minimal resources, peritoneal dialysis should be considered, anticipating restored renal function.

Pulmonary involvement has been reported with *P. falciparum* and *P. vivax*. In some regions, serious, life-threatening malaria has always been considered to be a *P. falciparum* infection, but recent reports have made physicians aware of the pulmonary manifestations of *P. vivax*. In addition, the pathology of the parasites is different at autopsy. In severe *P. falciparum* malaria, parasitized RBC's, leucocytes and platelets are found in the microvasculature of the lung, similar to cerebral pathology (12). In contrast, with *P. vivax* infection the microcirculation is congested with monocytes and parasitized red blood cells are rarely found. This difference suggests different pathophysiology (13,14).

Anstey et al. (2) reported respiratory symptoms in 53% of patients with uncomplicated *P. vivax* malaria, although 1 of their patients was found to have *P. ovale* infection. Since *P vivax* only infects reticulocytes, it is often sparsely present in erythrocyte smears during the initial onset of clinical disease and may even be absent at the onset of pulmonary symptoms. Physicians are becoming increasingly aware that pulmonary malaria is more likely to be caused by *P. vivax* than *P. falciparum*.

Mixed infections with predominance of one species are not uncommon especially with *P. vivax*. Since it parasitizes only reticulocytes, infection reduces the peripheral population of *P. falciparum*. Appropriate treatment is required for both parasites, including hypnozoite treatment.

Even though polymerase chain reaction [PCR] testing for malaria is available, the thick smear with Geimsa stain remains the main diagnostic tool in most hospital laboratories. Recently developed rapid test strips can be helpful in facilitating early treatment, but numerous false negative results require further investigation when malaria is the clinical diagnosis. The morphological appearance, discerning the different forms, is dependent on technical experience, a frequent problem according to the professional literature. A large study in the United Kingdom of technicians trained and familiar with malarial parasites, concluded that the diagnosis was missed when there were mixed infections or low parasite numbers (15).

PREVENTION

Bed nets are important and even popular in developing countries for the prevention of malaria. In areas of consistent use and high malaria prevalence bed nets are the most significant factor decreasing child mortality from malaria. Insect-repellant bed nets have proven even more effective. However, there have been concerns regarding their use. For example, initial cost has often been mediated by philanthropic donors or subsidized by governments. Will this continue? Will bed nets be affordable in the future?

If the bed net develops a hole, will this admit mosquitoes? Studies of bed net holes demonstrate that small holes less than 3cm actually cause laminar flow of carbon dioxide, improving the ability of the mosquito to find a host. Larger holes, measuring more than 3 cm, although allowing insect access, diffuse carbon dioxide flow, and challenge the mosquito to find the host source.

Insecticide permeated bed nets have been shown to kill more than 50% of mosquitoes lured to the net, but initial studies demonstrated that washing decreases the effectiveness. More recent long-lasting insecticide-treated nets have more stability and effectiveness after multiple washings (16-18). Several different insecticides have been used including detamethrin and deltamethrin-piperonyl butoxide combination which is effective against pyrethroid-resistant *anopheles*.

Some research has studied bed net use comparing use in valleys to mountain regions of central Africa and found bed nets to be effective in the valleys where there was high malaria transmission but not in mountain regions where the percentage of infected mosquitoes was low. There is no statistical difference in the incidence of malaria cases for mountain dwellers whether they used bed nets or not. Therefore, there is a threshold of malaria prevalence before bed nets become clinically relevant in prevention.

Several investigators in Africa have reported higher mortality from malaria in teenagers when bed nets are used extensively for young children. The hypothesis is that teenagers who used bed nets as young children do not have endemic immunity and when their nocturnal behavior changes during the dating years, they are more susceptible to serious infection.

Prophylaxis has focused on prevention of *P. falciparum* mortality. Studies in endemic areas have shown that other forms of malaria have relatively high resistance to recommended prophylactic drugs; however, since *P. ovale* and *P. malariae* cause minimal mortality, this is not considered sufficient reason to change the current recommendations. Excluding chloroquine use in areas of parasite resistance, proper prophylaxis still does not exclude *P. falciparum* from the differential diagnosis, and *in vitro* testing has shown significant resistance by *Plasmodium* species to recommended drugs (19).

Loss of endemic tolerance has been a significant problem in many countries where people migrate to urban areas and where students seeking advanced education migrate to areas where they are not exposed to malaria-carrying mosquitoes. Even physicians who come from countries where malaria is endemic do not recognize the need for prophylaxis when they return to their country of origin.

Living in a region of frequent exposure has been shown to result in tolerance to parasitemia (20). How persistent this tolerance is when a person is exposed again to malaria is not well understood. Relative protection to infection has been reported to be lost within two years of leaving an endemic zone (21). Yet compared with naïve individuals, people raised in malaria areas exposed to the parasite experience decreased severity of illness and accelerated parasite clearing for years after leaving an endemic area. Bouchaud studied individuals raised in an endemic area, who then resided 10 or more years in an area without malaria exposure. He demonstrated that when they returned to an area of malaria exposure, that they had a decreased risk of cerebral malaria (22).

A Unites States study in 2003 demonstrated that only 17.3% of civilians who acquired malaria while traveling abroad reported taking prophylaxis. Prophylaxis is effective. Many immigrants, even physicians from malaria-endemic areas are not aware that acquired partial immunity is lost after residing outside an endemic area for only a few months. Thus, immigrants constitute a significant percentage of people who do not take prophylaxis and return from visiting their homeland with clinical malaria.

Apparently contradictory results from these cited studies stem from the complex immune response to malaria, the lack of understanding of the cause of clinical malaria, and the acquired tolerance to the parasite that occurs without clinical disease. In their review article, Struik and Riley explain the complexities of the immune response and current understanding of parasite tolerance (23,24). Without constant exposure to *Plasmoduim* parasites, certain antibodies are undetectable within weeks, but this fact still does not explain the tolerant state (25). Immune response to antitoxic components is currently under investigation as a means of explaining clinical disease as well as the variability of host response to the parasite to produce endothelial microparticles. In any case, without frequent exposure, expatriates should consider prophylaxis when returning to endemic countries, especially if they intend to return to a non-endemic area.

HOST FACTORS

Danquah et al. (26) have recently defined the occurrence of parasitemia in children with hemaglobinopathies. They examined blood samples taken between January and April of 2002 from children in Ghana who lived in an area where malaria was hyper-endemic. HgAA children had 55.9% positive results where as the children with hemaglobinopathies had the following results: HgAC 59.3%, HgAS 47.8%, HgSC 29.4%, HgCC 43.8% and HgSS 28.6%. This study provides the objective evidence of a discernable benefit of hemaglobinopathies as protection from clinical malaria. In population studies, evaluating hospital admissions for clinical malaria HgSS children seem to be at lower risk (27). However, when HgSS children develop clinical malaria they have a higher mortality with equivalent treatment (28).

TREATMENT

The World Health Organization [WHO] reports 'Artemisinin-based combination therapy [ACTs] has transformed the treatment of malaria, but if not used properly the medicine could become ineffective'. Most developing countries with endemic malaria are requiring Artemisinin-based combination therapy as a government regulation. Combination pills and blister packs have provided easily administered proper treatment even in physician deprived areas. In order to avoid resistance to Artemisinin, WHO has convinced the majority of pharmaceutical companies who manufacture therapy for malaria treatment to stop producing monotherapy medications. Artemisinin resistance is already a problem where quality/quantity control, previous use of monotherapy or fake medications have been distributed. When Artemisinin fails there is no novel treatment on the horizon.

Initial therapy (Tables 2 and 3) of children who require hospitalization and/or have cerebral malaria should be intravenous.

Table 2. Intravenous therapy doses

Quinine: loading dose of 20 mg/kg quinine dihydrochloride in 5% dextrose or dextrose saline over 4 h. Followed by 10 mg/kg every 8 h for first 48 h or until patient can swallow. [Maximum quinine concentration in infusion fluid should be 2 mg/ml]

Artesunate 2·4 mg/kg bodyweight loading dose, then at 12 h, 24 h, then once daily until patient can swallow. [Anhydrous artesunic acid 60 mg vial dissolved in 1 mL 5% sodium bicarbonate is mixed with 5 mL of 5% dextrose before injecting as a bolus into indwelling IV.]

Table 3. Treatment Table

Oral quinine 10 mg/kg (of quinine salt) 8 hourly for 7 days
And Clindamycin 7e13 mg/kg/dose 8 hourly for 7 days
Or Doxycycline (children >12 years old) 200 mg once daily for 7 days
Or Fansidar_ up to 4 years (>5 kg) ½ tablet as a single dose

- 5e6 years 1 tablet as a single dose
- 7e9 years 1 ½ tablets as a single dose
- 10e14 years 2 tablets as a single dose
- 14e18 years 3 tablets as a single dose

Atovaquoneeproguanil Over 40 kg: 4 'standard' tablets daily for 3 days (Malarone_)

- 31e40 kg 3 'standard' tablets daily for 3 days
- 21e30 kg 2 'standard' tablets daily for 3 days
- 11e20 kg 1 'standard' tablet daily for 3 days
- 9e10 kg 3 'paediatric' tablets daily for 3 days
- 5e8 kg 2 ' paediatric' tablets daily for 3 days

Co-artem (Riamet_)
children > 12 years or over 35 kg)

- >35 kg, 4 tablets then 4 tablets at 8, 24, 36, 48 and 60 h
- 25e35 kg 3 tablets then 3 tablets at 8, 24, 36, 48 and 60 h
- 15e24 kg 2 tablets then 2 tablets at 8, 24, 36, 48 and 60 h
- 5e14 kg 1 tablet then 1 tablet at 8, 24, 36, 48 and 60 h

Intravenous quinine therapy should also be used if the patient is unable swallow, is vomiting or has decreased level of consciousness.

The South East Asian Quinine Artesunate Malaria Trial (SEAQUAMAT) showed a 33% reduction in mortality of treatment with IV artesunate as opposed to quinine (29). Thirteen percent of their patients who received artesunate were under 15 years of age and 17% were pregnant suggesting that this treatment is safe for children and pregnant women. However, this study was done in an area of high chloroquine resistance. Pregnant women and patients with high parasite loads [greater than 2% of RBC's parasitized] should receive initial IV therapy.

Malaria in pregnancy poses a difficult treatment challenge. Not only is malaria more severe in the pregnant woman but it is associated with premature labor and stillbirth. The parasites are sequestered in the placenta and make the peripheral smear a less reliable diagnostic tool. Treatment protocols still use quinine. Clindamycin is safe as an adjunct, while tetracyclines are not. Chloroquine prophylaxis is recommended until delivery even in chloroquine resistant areas. Primaquine is contraindicated in pregnancy but should be used for eradication of hypnozoites of *P. vivax* and *P. ovale* after delivery.

CONCLUSION

P. falciparum is recognized as having the greatest risk of morbidity and mortality due to cerebral malaria, pulmonary edema, hypoglycemia, lactic acidosis, and renal failure, and therefore warrants the prophylactic emphasis recommended by the CDC. However, this regimen does not completely exclude *P. falciparum* infection and is even less effective for non- *falciparum* malaria. A 25% failure rate among "adherent" patients is noted. In addition, recommended prophylaxis has no ability to eradicate hypnozoites of *P. vivax* or *P. ovale* and is ineffective at preventing recrudescence of latent erythrocytic stages of *P malariae* (8).

P. vivax in particular, is associated with persistent hypnozoites that reappear months or years after the initial infection may become resistant to low dose primaquine. Malaria needs to be considered in the differential diagnosis if the clinical illness is consistent with clinical disease as long as a year after exposure.

P. vivax is demonstrating significant morbidity and mortality that has previously not been recognized. Reports from India, the Middle East, and the Far East have associated *P. Vivax* with acute renal failure, acute respiratory distress syndrome, shock, and splenic rupture (30).

REFERENCES

[1]   Wilson JF. Advancing the war on malaria. Ann Intern Med 2003;138(8): 693-6.
[2]   Anstey N, Jacups S, Cain T, Pearson T, Ziesing P, Fisher D. Pulmonary manifestations of uncomplicated falciparum and vivax malaria: cough, small airways obstruction, impaired gas transfer and increased pulmonary phagocytic activity. JID 2002;185:1326-34.
[3]   Askling HH, Milsson J, Tegnell A, Janzon R, Ekdahl K. Malaria Risk in Travelers. Emerg Infect Dis 2005;11(3):436-41.
[4]   Bottieau E, Clerinx J, Van Den Enden E, Van Esbroeck M, Colebunders R, Van Bompel A, et al. Imported non-plasmodium falciparum malaria: A five-year prospective study in a European referral center. Am J Trop Med Hyg 2006;75(1): 138-9.

[5]   Chotivanich K, Udomsangpetch R, Chierakul W, Newton P, Ruangveerayuth R, Pukrittayakamee S et al. In vitro efficacy of antimalarial drugs against plasmodium vivax on the western border of Thailand. Am J Trop Med Hyg 2004;70(4):395-7.

[6]   Clark IA, Cowden WB. Why is the pathology of falciparum worse than that of vivax malaria? Parasitol Today 1999;15(11):458-61.

[7]   Combes V, Coltel N, Faille D, Wassmer SC, Grau GE. Cerebral malaria: role of microparticles and platelets in alterations of the blood-brain barrier. Int J Parasitol 2006;36(5):541-6.

[8]   Dondorp AM, Pongponratn E, White NJ. Reduced microcirculatory flow in sever falciparum malaria: pathophysiology and electron-microscopic pathology. Acta Tropica 2004;89(3):309-17.

[9]   Eliades MJ, Snehal S, Nguyen-Dinh P, et al. Malaria surveillance—United States, 2003. MMWR 2005;54:25-39.

[10]   Gatton ML, Cheng Q. Modeling the development of acquired clinical immunity to Plasmodium falciparum malaria. Infect Immun 2004;72(11):6538-45.

[11]   Gentilini M, Duflo B. Médecine Tropicale: Paludisme, 5th ed. Paris: Flammarion: 1986:90.

[12]   Kirchgatter K, Del Portillo H. Clinical and molecular aspects of severe malaria. An Acad Bras Cienc 2005;77:455-75.

[13]   Koh KH, Chew PH, Kiya A. A retrospective study of malaria infections in an intensive care unit of a general hospital in Malaysia. Singapore Med J 2004; 45(1):28-36.

[14]   Lomar AV, Vidal JE, Lomar FP, Barbas CV, Janot de Matos G, Boulos J. Acute respiratory distress syndrome due to vivax malaria: case report and literature review. Braz J Infect Dis 2005;9(5):425-30.

[15]   Maguire G, Handojo T, Pain M, Kenangalem E, Price R, Tjitra E, et al. Lung injury in uncomplicated and severe falciprum malaria: a longitudinal study in Papua, Indonesia. JID 2005;192:1966-74.

[16]   Mandell G, Bennett JE, Dolin R, eds. Principles and practice of infectious diseases, 6th ed. Philadelphia, PA: Churchill Livingstone, 2005.

[17]   Manson-Cook GC, Zumla AI, eds. Manson's tropical diseases, 21st ed. Philadelphia, PA: Saunders, 2002.

[18]   McQueen PG, McKenzie FE, Competition for red blood cells can enhance Plasmodium vivax parasitemia in mixed-species malaria infections. Am J Trop Med Hyg 2006;75(1):112-25.

[19]   Milne LM, Kyi MS, Chiodini PL, Warhurst DC. Accuracy of routine laboratory diagnosis of malaria in the United Kingdom. J Clin Pathol 1994;47:740-2.

[20]   Sunstrum J, Lawrenchuk D, Tait K, Hall W, Johnson D, Wilcox K, et al. Mosquito-transmitted malaria. Michigan, 1995. MMWRep 199;45(19):398-400.

[21]   CDC. Local transmission of plasmodium vivax malaria.Virginia, 2002. MMWR 2002;51(41):921-3.

[22]   CDC. Local transmission of plasmodium vivax malaria. Palm Beach County, Florida, 2003. MMWR 2003;52(38):908-11.

[23]   CDC. Local transmission of plasmodium vivax malaria. Houston, Texas, 1994. MMWR 1995;44(15):295;301-3.

[24]   Nathwani D, Currie PF, Smith CC, Khaund R. Recurrent plasmodium ovale infection from Papua New Guinea--chloroquine resistance or inadequate primaquine therapy? J Infect 1991;23(3):343-4.

[25]   Ozsoy MF, Oncul O, Pekkafali Z, Pahsa A, Yenen OS. Splenic complications in malaria: report of two cases from Turkey. J Med Microbiol 2004;53(Pt 12):1255-8.

[26]   Prakash J, Singh AK, Kumar NS, Saxena RK. Acute renal failure in Plasmodium vivax malaria. J Assoc Physicians India 2003;51:265-7.

[27]   Singh KS, Wester WC, Trenholme GM. Problems in the therapy for imported malaria in the United States. Arch Intern Med 2003;163:2027-30.

[28]   Siske S, Riley E. Does malaria suffer from lack of memory? Immun Rev 2004; 201:268-90.

[29]   Strickland GT. ed. Hunter's yropical medicine and emerging infectious disease, 8th ed. Philadelphia, PA: WB Saunders, 2000.

[30]   Tanios MA, Kogelman L, McGovern B, Hassoun P. Acute respiratory distress syndrome complicating Plasmodium vivax malaria. Crit Care Med 2001;29:665-7.

Submitted: September 04, 2011. *Revised:* November 02, 2011. *Accepted:* November 11, 2011.

In: Public Health Yearbook 2012
Editor: Joav Merrick

ISBN: 978-1-62808-078-0
© 2013 Nova Science Publishers, Inc.

Chapter 13

DENGUE VIRUS INFECTION

Richard R Roach, MD, FACP and Sapna Sadarangani, MD*

Internal Medicine Department, Michigan State University/Kalamazoo Center for Medical
Studies, Kalamazoo, Michigan, United States of America

ABSTRACT

Dengue infection is rapidly becoming a world-wide disease and the mortality is
casting a profound pall on children. Understanding the vector, the different types of the
virus, and the stages of infection can dramatically impact the mortality of this burgeoning
disease. Though no anti-viral agent exists at present, careful attention to the stages of the
disease and management of the fluid, electrolyte, red cell, and platelet abnormalities can
result in successful intervention.

Keywords: Public health, tropical medicine, Dengue virus infection

INTRODUCTION

Dengue virus infection is a common tropical infection, and the most rapidly spreading
mosquito born disease in the world (1). In the last two years the incidence world-wide has
quadrupled. It inflicts a significant health, social, and economic burden on affected
populations.

Areas with the highest incidence are South East Asia, South Asia (India), non-tropical
Asia (China), Caribbean, Africa, Europe, Australia, and America (Central and South). Most
dengue cases in the U.S. occur in Puerto Rico, the U.S. Virgin Islands, Samoa and Guam,
which are endemic for the virus. Temperate area reports are imported cases. Hawaii had a
small outbreak in 2001, several cases were reported following Katrina, and locally acquired
dengue was documented in Florida in 2009 (2, 3).

---

* Correspondence: Richard R Roach, MD, FACP, Internal Medicine Department, 1000 Oakland Drive, Kalamazoo,
Michigan 49008 United States. E-mail: roach@ kcms.msu.edu

The emergence and re-emergence of dengue virus infection is a global threat with 2.5 billion (40% of global population) people at risk of infection (4). A range of 50-100 million cases are diagnosed annually, of which 500, 000 are dengue hemorrhagic fever with 25, 000 annual deaths attributed to dengue fever. Figure 1 shows the countries at risk for dengue and figure 2 illustrates the exponential rise in the global burden of disease. The case fatality ratio of dengue infection is 1-5%, and may increase to 20% in certain epidemic situations. The more severe forms of the illness are dengue hemorrhagic fever (DHF) and dengue shock syndrome (DSS).

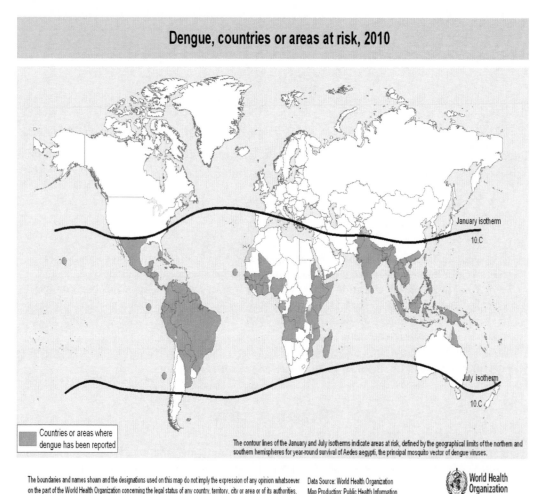

Figure 1.

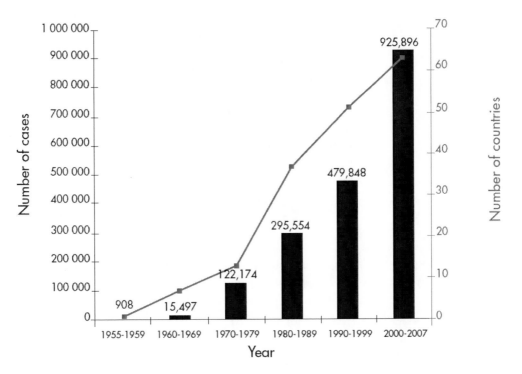

Figure 2.

DENGUE: THE VIRUS

Dengue is a single stranded RNA flavivirus, 40-50 nm in diameter. The vector, an infected mosquito is usually *Aedes aegypti*; occasionally *Aedes albopictus* can also transmit the infection (4). Humans are the natural hosts, and the incubation period ranges from 2-7 days. Four serotyes are known to cause disease--DEN1-4 and these are antigenically related different species. The "Asian" genotypes of DEN-2 and DEN-3 have been associated with the most severe infections. The envelope of dengue virus consists of an E and M protein. The E protein, responsible for attachment to cellular receptors and fusion with cell membranes, contains the main epitopes recognized by neutralizing antibodies, which provide protective immunity against that particular serotype (5). This protein is dengue virus specific but cross reactive with other flaviviruses.

THE VECTOR

The *Aedes aegypti* mosquito, the main vector (see figure 3), is a tropical and subtropical species widely distributed around the world, mostly between latitudes 35 0N and 35 0S. This region corresponds to a winter isotherm of greater than 10 0C. The *Aedes aegypti* mosquitoes have be found as far north as 45 0N, but this occurs during warmer months and the mosquitoes do not survive the winters.

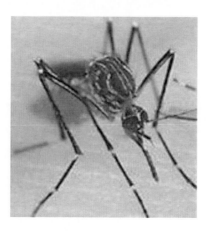

Figure 3.

Due to lower temperatures at higher elevations, Ae. *aegypti* is relatively uncommon above 1,000 meters, although they have been reported to survive altitudes above 2,000 m. Other vectors that may transmit dengue virus are *Aedes albopictus*, *Aedes polynesiensis* and several species of the *Aedes scutellaris* complex, but they have the same habitat requirements (2).

The *Aedes* mosquitoe feeds during the day, in contrast to *Anopheles*, the malaria vector, which feeds during the evening and early night. Immature stages (larvae) prefer water-filled habitats, often artificial containers associated with human dwellings typically found indoors. Studies suggest that most female *Ae. aegypti* spend their lifetime in or around the houses where they emerged as adults. In contrast, *Anopheles* mosquitoes have been documented to fly several miles from their source of pupation. Therefore, people, rather than mosquitoes, rapidly spread the virus within communities and are the main amplifying host of the virus.

In order for transmission to occur the mosquito must feed on a patient during a 5- day period the patient is viremic, which begins before the onset of symptoms. Some individuals never manifest symptoms and yet are viremic and able to infect mosquitoes. After entering the mosquito in a blood meal, the virus requires an additional 8-12 days incubation before it can be transmitted to another human. The mosquito remains infected for the remainder of its life (days- few weeks).

The challenges of vector control and prevention are that the *Aedes aegypti* eggs have an ability to withstand desiccation and to survive without water for several months on the inner walls of containers while bed nets do not prevent human infection from a mosquito that feeds during the day.

CLINICAL FEATURES: THE SPECTRUM OF THE DISEASE

The incubation period is typically 2-7 days and then a wide spectrum of clinical manifestations. A significant proportion of patients remain asymptomatic during infection. When symptoms occur, they manifest both severe and non-severe clinical forms. The World Health Organization (WHO) case definition of dengue fever (DF) and the lab criteria for diagnosis are illustrated in Table 1 (2).

Table 1. WHO definition of dengue fever (9)

Probable:
• An acute febrile illness with 2 or more the following manifestations
• Headache
• Retro-orbital pain
• Myalgia
• Arthralgia
• Rash (a generalized blanchable morbilliform maculopapular rash appears 1-2 days after defervescence)
• Hemorrhagic manifestations
• Leucopenia and
• Various degrees of thrombocytopenia
• Supportive serology (Ab titer by HI> 1280, + IgM Ab on a late acute or convalescent serum specimen)
• Occurrence at same time and location as other confirmed dengue cases
Confirmed by lab criteria:
• Isolation of dengue virus from serum samples (or autopsy)
• Atleast a 4 fold rise in reciprocal IgG or IgM Ab titers to 1 or more dengue virus Ag in paired serum samples (6-30 days of illness onset)
• Dengue virus Ag in autopsy tissue, serum or CSF by immunohistochemistry, immunofluorescence, or ELISA
• Dengue virus RNA PCR detection in serum/ autopsy tissue/ CSF samples

Table 2. Dengue Hemorrhagic fever WHO criteria (9)

The following must all be present:
1. Fever or hx of fever lasting 2-7 days, occasionally biphasic
2. Hemorrhagic tendencies, evidenced by atleast 1 of the following:
• A positive tourniquet test
• Petechiae, ecchymoses or purpura
• Bleeding from mucosa, GIT, injection sites or other locations
3. Hematemesis or malena Thrombocytopenia (100,000/mm3 or less)
4. Evidence of plasma leakage due to increased vascular permeability:
• Rise in Hct > 20% above average for age, sex, and population;
• Drop in Hct following volume replacement Rx > 20% of baseline;
• Signs of plasma leakage such as pleural effusion, ascites, and hypoproteinemia

In addition, dengue fever may present with ocular manifestations such as macular or retinal hemorrhages, maculopathy, optic neuritis, and retinal vessel occlusion.

It is beneficial to prospectively consider a patient's clinical course (see figure 4).

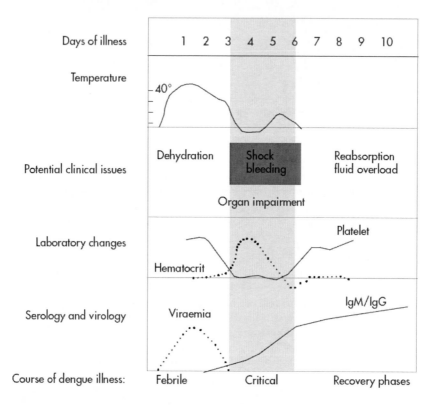

Figure 4. WHO (9).

The following illustrates the different potential phases of the illness (1,2,5):

a) *Febrile phase:* the acute phase of the patient's presentation is a sudden onset of high grade fever, skin erythema, body aches, arthralgia, and headache. Some report sore throat and conjunctival injection. Due to this non-specific clinical picture, multiple viral febrile syndromes may be confused with dengue. This phase includes hemorrhagic manifestations such as petechiae and mucous membrane bleeding. A positive tourniquet test (a test for capillary fragility) increases the probability of dengue in contrast to other viral syndromes. The tourniquet test requires inflating the blood pressure cuff on a patient's arm to a value between the diastolic and systolic pressure, and then keeping it inflated for 5 minutes. A positive test is more than 10 petechiae noted per square inch of skin; a definite positive is more than 20 petechiae noted per square inch. This test, although useful in endemic areas, is not highly specific. Leukopenia is another important manifestation. When the patient is viremic, dengue serology may be falsely negative. Perinatal transmission is possible during this viremic phase, giving rise to neonatal disease. Monitoring for warning signs of progression to the critical phase is important in this phase.

b) *Critical phase.* The hallmark of this phase is increased capillary permeability and plasma leakage. It occurs at the time of defervescence, days 3-7 into the illness. Progressive leucopenia, rapid fall in platelet count precedes capillary leakage. Patients with clinical dengue fever, will not develop this marked increased capillary permeability, and their platelet counts and clinical course will improve. A generalized maculopapular rash develops, described as "erythematous rash with islands of sparing" (See Figure 5). The rash usually spares the hands and the soles. Infants and children may have an undifferentiated febrile illness associated with the maculopapular rash.

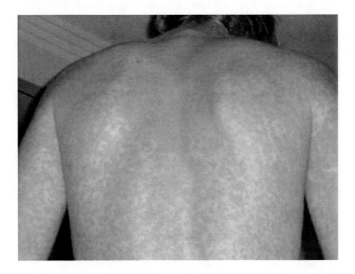

Figure 5. http/denguefever.co.in accessed 11 October 2011.

Those who develop capillary leakage manifest a rise in hematocrit as well asBUN and a fall in serum protein. This is known as Dengue hemorrhagic fever (DHF) and it may progress to dengue shock syndrome if not recognized. Capillary plasma leakage manifests as pleural effusions and ascites. Monitoring for a narrow pulse pressure, tachycardia, urine output (at least 0.5 ml/kg/hr in an adult and older child; 1 ml/kg/hr in an infant) and hypotension are critical signs require vigilance.

Children should be monitored for mental status changes and signs of shock with close attention to capillary refill, urine output, skin turgor, and fontanelle depression (if open). Hematocrit and hemodynamic status should be monitored and these patients require hospitalization. Young children may not compensate for these fluid shifts and are at increased risk for dengue shock. Some patients present already in the "critical" phase. A drop in the hematocrit after intravenous hydration indicates that the patient is hemo-concentrated and hence has DHF. In this phase certain "warning signs" may be present:

a) abdominal pain or tenderness,
b) persistent vomiting,
c) mucosal bleeding,
d) severe plasma leakage,
e) severe hemorrhage,

f)   severe organ impairment, (severe hepatitis, encephalitis, myocarditis)
g)   liver enlargement > 2 cm
h)   Lab: increase in hematocrit with concurrent rapid decrease in platelet count

Once the patient is in decompensated shock syndrome (DSS), manifested by hypotension and a narrow pulse pressure, a critical loss of plasma leakage occurs. Consider DHF a continuum of DHF grades 3 and 4 or severe DHF DSS. In fact, capillary leakage occurs as a continuum (see Figure 6). Refer to Table 2 for the WHO case definition for diagnosis of DHF, and to Table 3 for DSS.

Dengue serology is helpful if obtained at the time the patient has defervesced. A positive IgM and IgG point towards a secondary dengue infection. This is because antibody dependent enhancement, as in the setting of a secondary dengue infection, is discussed as one of the proposed theories for the pathogenesis of DHF.

Table 3. Dengue Shock syndrome (DHF grade 3,4) WHO criteria (9)

All of the criteria for DHF must be present plus evidence of circulatory failure manifested by:
1.   Rapid and weak pulse, and
2.   Narrow pulse pressure (< 20 mmHg) or manifested by:
3.   Hypotension for age, and
4.   Cold, clammy skin and restlessness

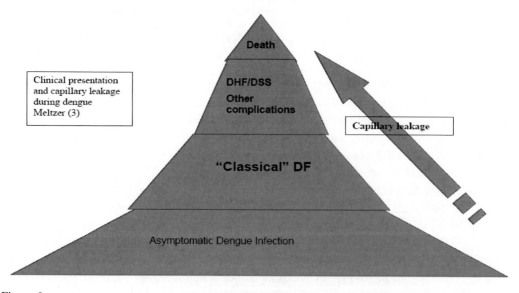

Figure 6.

RECOVERY PHASE

If the patient survives the critical phase, recovery ensues with decreased plasma leakage and reabsorbtion of extracellular fluid over the next 2-3 days. Platelet recovery takes longer than white cell and red cell recovery. Extreme vigilance is needed to the patient's fluid status as increased reabsorption of fluid may lead to fluid overload, especially if aggressive intravenous fluids are not adjusted. Clinical criteria such as urine output, heart rate, pulse pressure, blood pressure, and improving hematocrit and BUN are key to decision making.

PATHOGENESIS: DENGUE HEMORRHAGIC FEVER

The underlying pathogenesis of dengue hemorrhagic fever is not completely understood. Hypotheses suggest a complex, synergistic pathologic process. There is overwhelming evidence that of DHF is mediated by host immune responses. Non-neutralizing cross-reactive antibodies play a critical role in DHF. A majority of DHF cases occur in the setting of secondary dengue infection. During secondary infection, the dengue virus and non-neutralizing antibodies against a previous exposed and recognized dengue serotype, form complexes that bind to Fc receptors on target cells.

Subsequently infection augments the immune response resulting in antibody dependent enhancement (ADE). The increased numbers of infected cells means a greater viral burden. The host immune response cascade, including increased activation of inflammatory cytokines, TNF-α, complement, and endothelial tissue activation contribute to increased capillary permeability and plasma leakage. Hemorrhagic manifestations are partly due to vascular endothelial cell dysfunction.

An additional hypothesis is that the virulence of the infecting dengue virus is important. This stems from the observation that DHF occurs in some primary infections (1). Since antibody dependent enhancement is not a possible in primary infection, it is possible that some virulent strains cause DHF. Several virulence factors show evidence of the role of cytokine stimulation.

DENGUE DIAGNOSTICS

In endemic areas, diagnostic tests may not be available or are cost prohibitive.

Laboratory methods for confirming dengue infection may involve detection of the virus, viral nucleic acid, antigens or antibodies, or a combination of the above. During the early stage of the disease, when the patient is still febrile and viremic, tests such as virus isolation, nucleic acid or antigen detection can be diagnostic. Serology is often falsely negative at this stage. Antibody response to an infection depends on the host response.

Immunological based tests for dengue include hemagglutination inhibition, neutralization, and IgM and IgG ELISA assays. Dengue IgM is the first antibody to appear. There is varied response and false negatives are possible. Fifty percent of patients have detectable IgM by day 3-5 of illness, rising to 80% by day 5; also, by day 6-10, 93-99% have detectable IgM (2, 4).

This IgM may persist over 90 days after the primary infection; hence, it is not predictive of when the infection occurred. If the test is ordered during a febrile illness it may not be indicative of dengue, even if positive because dengue IgM cross reacts with other flaviviruses, such as Japanese Encephalitis, St. Louis Encephalitis, and yellow fever. The distribution of these diseases often coincides with dengue endemic areas.

Dengue IgG on the other hand, appears at low titers at the end of the first week of the primary infection and then increases gradually. In a secondary dengue infection, the IgG titers rise rapidly over the course of 2 weeks (6).

After primary infection, the antibodies confer lifelong protective immunity against the infecting serotype. They provide cross protective immunity to other serotypes for about 2-3 months but not long term. Therefore, if dengue serology obtained at day 5 of a febrile illness reveals positive IgM and IgG, then this is most likely a secondary dengue infection. If dengue IgM is positive and dengue IgG is negative then this is a primary infection. IgM/IgG ratios may be used to differentiate primary and secondary infection (2).

DIRECT VIRUS DETECTION

Available tests include virus isolation in cell culture, detection of viral RNA by nucleic acid amplification (NAAT), and detection of viral antigens by ELISA or rapid tests. Isolation by cell culture takes several days and therefore, does not influence clinical decision making. Nucleic acid detection assays detect dengue viral RNA within 24-48 hours; they have good sensitivity and specificity but are expensive (4, 7). Rapid diagnostic tests, yielding results in an hour are available.

DIFFERENTIAL DIAGNOSIS

The differential diagnosis changes according to febrile illnesses endemic in the area, but there are several treatable diseases that can mimic dengue. Malaria has almost identical geographic endemnicity and should be considered in the differential diagnosis. Co-infections have been documented. Malaria has different fever patterns, tertian or quartian as opposed to high, unremitting fevers for 3-4 days with defervescence and then development of rash or hemorrhagic manifestations of DHF. The transmitting mosquito is different, Anopheles being a night-feeding mosquito, whereas dengue is transmitted by a daytime-feeding mosquito. Also, dengue is more of an urban disease whereas malaria is more prevalent in rural areas. But these distinctions are difficult to discern when a febrile child presents for care (6).

HIV acute seroconversion is also a possible differential for dengue fever, given appropriate risk factors and clinical suspicion. Chikungunya virus is an arbovirus of the Togaviridae family and is also transmitted by Aedes aegytpi and Aedes albopictus mosquitoes. Clinical features include fever, arthralgia, myalgia, headache, and eye pain. The joint symptoms in chikungunya are more prominent, specifically arthritis, compared to dengue and may take months to resolve. Although dengue is known as "break-bone fever", it does not typically cause joint inflammation or serositis. The outcome of chikungunya is also not as fatal compared to DHF/DSS. Leptospirosis, rubella infection, yellow fever, Japanese encephalitis, St Louis encephalitis, rickettsial infections, and influenza all present with a febrile child and need to be considered in the differential diagnosis.

MANAGEMENT

The clinical manifestations and the pathophysiology of dengue may be complex but the management is relatively simple and inexpensive; however, it requires the health care provider to have a keen understanding of the phases of the disease. Management is generally supportive, including symptom relief. Vigilance for complications to limit morbidity and mortality is crucial. Prompt fluid resuscitation under close observation is essential to the management of DHF/ DSS. Antipyretics may be used such as acetaminophen; however, NSAIDs and aspirin should be avoided due to the increased bleeding risk. In addition, it should be noted that aspirin may give rise to Reye syndrome.

Intravenous fluids should be given as a bolus of 20 ml/kg/h x 2 h and then 10 ml/kg/hr x 6 h; it is then adjusted based on clinical response and monitoring (2). The pulse pressure and blood pressure are critical to warn the clinician of possible DHF/ DSS. A narrow pulse pressure is an impending sign as well. One should monitor the hematocrit over time, as increasing hematocrit suggests hemo-concentration and plasma leakage. Blood urea nitrogen and protein level are important parameters. The BUN will rise with increased capillary leakage and the protein level will fall. Thrombocytopenia is worrisome, but the cause of bleeding in dengue and the hemorrhagic manifestations are multi-factorial and not due to thrombocytopenia alone. Platelet dysfunction, vascular endothelial dysfunction, and sometimes disseminated intravascular coagulation (DIC) are all contributing factors.

Lye et al. (8) studied the role of prophylactic transfusion with platelets and fresh frozen plasma in patients who were not actively bleeding but had severe thrombocytopenia (platelet count < 20,000) and demonstrated no benefit when there was no clinical bleeding (8). Similarly, in pediatric studies, clinical bleeding was independent of platelet count. Prophylactic transfusion may cause fluid overload leading to prolong hospitalization and does not expedite platelet recovery. Therefore, it is not recommended to transfuse platelets and blood products without clinical bleeding.

If frank bleeding is present, then platelet and blood transfusions are indicated. The level of the hematocrit may be falsely elevated despite significant bleeding in an unstable patient because of concurrent hemo-concentration. The decision to transfuse should be clinical, and not based on the hematocrit. IVIG has been used in DHF due to the immune pathogenesis postulated, but has not hastened recovery. Experimental use of corticosteroids has not shown benefit.

It is clear that patients with DHF and DSS are important to identify early in order to limit morbidity and mortality. While some clinical signs or 'warning signs' may help define this, a clinical predictor model based on certain lab criteria has prevented unnecessary hospitalization and use of critical resources without missing potential high risk cases of DHF/ DSS. Lee et al. found certain factors were independent and significant indicators of high risk (7):

1. Bleeding from any site (OR= 237)
2. Serum total protein (unit decrease in g/L, OR= 1.28)
3. Serum urea (unit increase in mmmol/L OR= 1.31)
4. Lymphocyte proportion (unit decrease in proportion %, OR= 1.08).

Other known DHF risk factors in the literature are infection with dengue-serotype 2, Asian genotype or prior dengue infections in children.

FUTURE TREATMENT

An antiviral drug is being studied, but is not yet available (9). A dengue vaccine is also not yet available. An effective vaccine must be a tetravalent vaccine, which will induce protective immunity against all homologous serotypes or it could theoretically cause DHF/ DSS. Neutralizing antibodies against homologous serotypes is the most important immunity. Protection against heterologous serotypes might be short lived or have different immune responses (4). Based on the antibody dependent enhancement theory this could prove harmful or even fatal.

SUMMARY: PUBLIC HEALTH CONSIDERATIONS

Dengue fever is a global emerging disease with significant morbidity and mortality (DHF/ DSS). Clinical research to detect early clinical diagnosis is important. From the public health stand point, expansive population growth and unplanned urbanization lead to substandard housing and inadequate water, sewage and waste management systems including proliferation of man-made containers that serve as mosquito-breeding habitats (2). These all contribute to the current global dengue epidemic. Increased international travel has also been important in spreading the disease to non-endemic areas as well as contributing to morbidity and mortality in temperate climates where dengue is less likely to be recognized. Adequate vector control is imperative. Improved infrastructure and management of waste and proper disposal of containers and abandoned tires the mosquito uses for breeding will limit the disease. Regular and thorough vector surveillance and clinical surveillance are pillars of management from the public health stand-point. Strong political initiative is important for communities to address these needs.

REFERENCES

[1]   Meltzer E, Schwartz E. A travel medicine view of dengue and dengue hemorrhagic fever. Travel Med Infect Dis 2009;7:278-83.
[2]   WHO- Dengue-guidelines for diagnosis, treatment, prevention and control. Accessed 2011 Sep 01. URL: http://whqlibdoc.who.int/publications/2009/9789241547871_eng.pdf
[3]   CDC. Dengue virus infection. Accessed 2011 Sep 01. URL: http://www.cdc.gov/Dengue/
[4]   Guzman MG, Kouri G. Dengue diagnosis, advances and challenges. Intern J Infect Dis 2004;8:69-80.
[5]   Kurane I. Dengue hemorrhagic fever with special emphasis on immunopathogenesis. Comparative immunology, Microbiol Infect Dis 2007;30:329-40.
[6]   Gregory CJ, Santiago LM, Arguello DF, et al. Clinical and laboratory features that differentiate dengue from other febrile illnesses in an endemic area--Puerto Rico, 2007-2008. Am J Trop Med Hyg 2010;82(5):922-9.
[7]   Lee V, Lye D. Predictive value of simple clinical and laboratory variables for dengue hemorrhagic fever in adults. J Clin Virology 2008;42:34-9.

[8]   Lye D, Lee V. Lack of efficacy of Prophylactic platelet transfusion for severe thrombocytopenia in Adults with Acute uncomplicated dengue infection. CID 2009:48: 1262-5.

[9]   Wiwanitkit V. Dengue fever: diagnosis and treatment. Expert Rev Anti Infect Ther 2010; 8(7):841-5.

Submitted: September 03, 2011. *Revised:* November 05, 2011. *Accepted:* November 10, 2011.

In: Public Health Yearbook 2012
Editor: Joav Merrick

ISBN: 978-1-62808-078-0
© 2013 Nova Science Publishers, Inc.

Chapter 14

SCHISTOSOMIASIS

*Richard R Roach, MD, FACP**

Internal Medicine Department, Michigan State University/Kalamazoo Center for Medical
Studies, Kalamazoo, Michigan, United States of America

ABSTRACT

Schistosomiasis is a mammalian blood fluke that causes profound pathology through
specific snails in freshwater environments. Though sixteen species are capable of
infecting humans only five produce the majority of mortality and morbidity.
Schistosomiasis has a long history of human pathology. *S. hematobium* has been
demonstrated in Egyptian mummies and continues to cause bladder and renal disease in
Egypt. *S. mansoni* was described in 1902 by Manson in a West Indian patient in London
and still is a major cause of hepatic failure worldwide. *S. japonicum* was described in the
Katayama Memoir in 1847 and since has continued to be a major cause of seizures in
Southeast Asia; *S. intercalatum*, not described until 1934, causes bloody diarrhea. Other
human schistosomes such as avium flukes, *Trichobilharzia*, *Ornithobilharszia* and
Gigantobilharzia are ubiquitous even in temperate climates but only cause transient
irritation to swimmers. This article reviews schistosomiasis in humans.

Keywords: Public health, tropical medicine, schistosomiasis

INTRODUCTION

In the Malagasy language of Madagascar schistosomiasis is called *sakoratzy*, the 'bad worm'.
This is appropriate since Madagascar has both *S. hematobium* and *S. mansoni* and the
Malagasy people recognize that this worm causes more morbidity and mortality than any of
the other numerous parasitic 'worms' on this island. Young children often contract the disease
during play in contaminated water, while older children contract the parasite as they learn

---

* Correspondence: Richard R Roach, MD, FACP, Internal Medicine Department, 1000 Oakland Drive, Kalamazoo,
Michigan 49008 United States. E-mail: roach@ kcms.msu.edu

adult work activities, preparing aquatic fields, and planting as well as harvesting rice. As a World Health Organization (WHO) targeted schistosomiasis as a *neglected tropical disease*, recent research has brought new hope to managing this problematic parasite of antiguity.

EPIDEMIOLOGY

Schistosomiasis is endemic in almost eighty countries of the world 55 of which have *S. mansoni* and 53 have *S. hematobium*. *S. intercalatum* is limited to Sub-Saharan Africa while *S. japonicum* and *S. mekongi* are in Southeast Asia.

LIFE CYCLE

The miracidia hatch from eggs in fresh water and infect their molluscan intermediate host. Lytic enzymes secreted from the gut allow penetration of the snail. Most are usually destroyed by snail phagocytosis, but some persist and mature to sporocysts which eventually develop into larval cercariae. Cercariae swim in fresh water and penetrate human skin in minutes. *S. hematobium* can penetrate the skin and reach the lymphatics in six minutes (1). Avium species penetrate the skin even faster but are destroyed and cause the inflammatory reaction of 'swimmer's itch'.

Unfortunately, the more pathologic species evade the skin's immune system, migrate to the lungs as well as the hepatic portal system and mature in the hepatic portal venous system pairing as male and female worms that produce eggs daily throughout their lives. The eggs migrate to the genitourinary tract (*S. hematobium*) to be excreted in the urine or they migrate to the bowel (*S. mansoni, japonicum, mekoni* and *inercalatum*) to be excreted in stool.

The snails for each form are unique and the *Institute Pasteur de Madagascar* has demonstrated that the snails compete for the same ecologic environment. Therefore, the two parasites, *S. mansoni* and *S. hematobium* never occur in the same body of water. Their research has also demonstrated that cercariae release is temperature dependant and survival is ρH dependant. These requirements may provide future preventative management.

PATHOLOGY

Although most of the morbidity and mortality occur in adults, the infection usually occurs or initiates in childhood. The clinical syndromes relate primarily to the patient's inflammatory response to egg deposition. Each egg type has specific migratory properties; thus, the chronic diseases result from granulomatous responses to egg deposition in tissue. Unfortunately, colon cancer is related to *S. mansoni* while bladder cancer, squamous (not transitional) cell, and cervical cancer are related to *S. hematobium* (2). Even this predilection to cancer is probably caused by the immunologic response of the host to the eggs as apposed to some tumor-inducing protein secreted by the eggs.

Katayama syndrome is an acute toxic, febrile response to parasite invasion. In contrast, the relative resistance to penetration of the cercariea among people living in endemic areas is host-immune mediated protective response. The relatively benign nature of avium species invasion is because the immune system destroys the parasite in the skin.

S. hematobium

S. hematobium implants eggs primarily in the bladder wall. Young teens often report hematuria and in some cultures this is considered a 'male menarche'. Bladder deposition causes a granulomatous reaction that calcifies which can be seen on ultrasound. Most patients maintain bladder wall elasticity but some patients, after extensive chronic bladder wall calcification, develop renal failure attributed to a non-distensible bladder as evidenced by bladder drainage returning renal function to normal.

Eggs are common in both male and female genitalia. Male infertility caused by *S. hematobium* is debated but eggs can be found in the seminal vesicles. The female genitalia demonstrate egg deposition in the vulva, vagina and cervix. Extensive investigation in Tanzania demonstrated that granulomas around eggs in the fallopian tubes was associated with infertility compared to patients that had schistosome eggs in the female genital tract but not in the fallopian tubes (3). A case report of a tourist without HPV and cervical cancer, demonstrated *S. hematobium* in the pathology specimen; she had contracted the parasite in a single fresh-water exposure (2). This is the strongest evidence for a causal role of *S. hematobium* causing cervical cancer. For years there have been epidemiologic reports that demonstrated a higher incidence of cervical cancer where *S. hematobium* was endemic. However the argument with these studies has been that there may be a disparity of HPV infection among the populations studied. Multiple studies show that genital ulcers from *S. hematobium* increase the transmission of HIV. In addition, *S. hematobium* is not only found in the semen of infected men but decreases the sperm count and induces sperm apoptosis (4).

S. hematobium eggs are found in the gastrointestinal tract with a particular propensity for the appendix. Ulcerated inflammatory polyps have demonstrated *S. hematobium* within the polyps but eggs seen on rectal biopsy are usually dead. In contrast, *S. mansoni* causes much more extensive gastrointestinal pathology [see below]. Skin lesions with *S. hematobium* eggs are well known but cause minimal pathology. Egg deposits have occurred in the liver, spinal cord, pericardium and even the brain; however, these tissues are much more likely to be infested with *S. mansoni*.

S. mansoni

S. mansoni is well known to cause periportal hepatic fibrosis due to deposition of eggs in the liver. Since the hepatic parenchyma is normal, this is not cirrhosis by definition, although the clinical effects of ascites, esophageal varices, and redirection of portal blood flow are similar. Chaotic inflammation leads to fibrosis and pyelophlebitis because of the eosinophilic infiltrates surrounding the eggs. Portal blockage leads to hepatic artery enlargement and neovascular capillaries. The resulting presinusoidal portal hypertension produces compensatory intrahepatic blood flow, maintaining hepatic function such as coagulation factors and protein production. Thus, the natural history is a slow progression, with hepatic decompensation a late phenomenon. But in areas of endemic viral hepatitis, co-infection with resulting hepatic pathology from viral hepatitis, may appear to the clinician as accelerated decompensation presumed to be related to *S. mansoni*.

The inflammatory response does seem to be related to gender, and genetic factors. Men tend to have a more dramatic fibrotic response than women (5). Genetic factors may also have a role as studies in diverse populations show a differing response to the same degree of infestation (6). Other factors such as alcohol ingestion, diet, and the age at which an individual becomes infected may be important to the overall prognosis and fibrotic response (7).

Splenomegaly from portal venous hypertension causes reticuloendothelial hyperplasia. The spleen then becomes a sequestering organ causing pancytopenia and thrombocytopenia; focal infarct and intra-splenic hemorrhages result while he fibrotic response aggravates the problem. Egg deposition in the spleen does occur but it is uncertain if this inflammatory response influences the degree of splenic pathology. An increase in splenic follicular lymphomas have been reported (8,9) and this may indeed be related to egg deposition in the spleen and not to splenic congestion.

Esophageal varices are an important cause of morbidity and mortality. The patient with bleeding from esophageal varices may present with hematemesis or in severe cases, shock requiring massive volume expansion. This can be aggravated by the increased blood volume, so it is not uncommon for the first episode of frank hematemesis to be related to pregnancy. Chronic variceal bleeding can also present with profound anemia. Propranalol is documented to decrease bleeding from esophageal varices caused by alcoholic cirrhosis. It is presumed to be beneficial with schistosomiasis-induced esophageal varices. A higher dose may be required in shistosomiasis patients compared to cirrhotic patients because the catabolism of β-blockers remains normal in schistosomiasis.

Renal involvement is multi-factorial and is discussed in the renal article (chapter 6). A variety of glomerular and tubular syndromes are described related to immunologic response, but egg deposition is rare and not thought to be related to any pathology. Amyloidosis has been noted on renal biopsy consistent with the chronicity of the renal response.

Neurologic manifestations of *S. mansoni* are fortunately rare, but they can be devastating. *S. japonicum* was the first to be associated with granulomas in the central nervous system (9). Subsequent reports described space occupying lesions diagnosed by brain biopsy as *S. mansoni*. The patients present with seizures (10) or ventricular dilation from obstruction (11). Treatment with praziquantel and steroids has been successful (12). Often neuroleptic drugs can be discontinued one year after praziquantel without recurrent seizures.

Spinal cord involvement, even more rare than central nervous system involvement, is also devastating. Two forms are described: when eggs migrate to the vaso-nevorum at T12 causing vascular compromise to the spinal cord and when granulomas form in proximity to the spinal cord leading to compression. Often children who are schistosomal naïve present with transverse myelopathy when they first start helping their parents in the rice fields. Without any immune response inhibiting skin migration, they have a massive infestation. Subsequent massive egg migration results in vaso-nevorum obstruction, T12 being the most vulnerable site. Some case reports suggest that immediate steroid therapy may decrease the morbidity but often patients present to clinical attention days after lower extremity weakness presents (13). Unfortunately there is little clinical response to steroids.

In contrast, neurologic deficits from granuloma formations, due to egg deposits that enlarge and compress neurologic structures, do respond to removal. These deposits can occur from the foramen magnum to the cauda equina. Case reports of dramatic improvement with surgical intervention are described (14). In areas where MRI or CT scans are available, a distinction between vascular obstruction and granulomas compression directs therapy.

S. japonicum and S. mekongi

The intestinal and hepatic pathology of *S. japonicum* is similar to *S. mansoni*. Both produce a T cell-mediated inflammatory reaction but *S. japonicum* seems to have a B cell response that is more prominent to the pathogenesis. Gastric lesions are more prominent but conflicting studies have not verified an association with gastric cancer. Association of *S. japonicum* with colonic and rectal cancer is more complex. Rectal cancer has strong associative evidence whereas there are mixed results to colonic cancer. Confusion about a relationship to hepatic cancer is confounded by the high incidence of hepatitis B in the areas of greatest infestation. Thus, carcinogenicity of *S. japonicum* is speculative at present.

Of greatest concern is the intracranial egg deposition and embolization of *S. japonicum*. The predilection to vascular embolization is thought to be related to the size and shape of the eggs. Meningoencephalitis is a well-recognized phenomenon with signs of increased intracranial pressure, headache, vomiting, blurred vision, and cognitive dysfunction,. Egg deposition results in seizures, usually focal, Jacksonian type, stroke syndrome or as a space-occupying lesion.

Studies of *S. mekongi* suggest a similar relationship to intestinal and hepatic pathology (15). In animal models, subtle differences in granulomas formation are reported (16); however, there is little clinical difference in disease in humans. Co-infection with *Opisthorcis viverrini* does confound the specificity of pathology in areas where both parasites are endemic. Objective descriptions of human pathogenesis have been suspended because of mass treatment in endemic areas has reduced transmission and political interruption has impaired research. Historical observation described severe intestinal and hepatic disease (17). This series of three patients illustrates the spectrum of pathology from hepatic involvement to asymptomatic (18):

> "One patient had severe portal hypertension with bleeding esophageal varices requiring a splenorenal shunt; studies of her liver biopsy showed S. mekongi eggs and periportal fibrosis. A second patient had abnormal liver function tests, and a third patient was asymptomatic. (18)"

Despite the miniature size of this study it does demonstrate the diverse clinical spectrum. Future studies need to be initiated when the political situation in endemic areas resolves.

DIAGNOSIS

For decades, rectal biopsy was the diagnostic technique most utilized for intestinal infections of *S. mansoni*. Even central nervous system (CNS) lesions were determined to be related to schistosomal infestation by rectal biopsy. Stool specimens are less diagnostic for intestinal schistosomes as the parasitic eggs are not reliably evacuated in the stool. For *S. hematobium*, first morning urine was the favored diagnostic technique. Bladder, cervix, and vaginal biopsies have also proven to be diagnostic. However, recently a number of diagnostic chemical reagent strips have become available for both parasites. Immunodiagnostic techniques have been simplified and developed to be cost-effective even in areas with poor technologic support. These techniques have been supported by WHO and other health care non-government organizations (NGO's). Even some governments in developing countries have supported the availability of these diagnostic tests.

Ultrasound techniques are non-invasive, portable, and in the last decade have become affordable in countries with inadequate technology. The specificity and sensitivity are adequate for making clinical decisions. Research in Madagascar has demonstrated that liver fibrosis from *S. mansoni* can be graded, can correlate with parasite load, and predict clinical outcome (19). In addition, spleen size can be evaluated for portal diversion (20). In skilled hands fibrosis related to *S. mansoni* can be distinguished from cirrhosis of other causes. For *S. hematobium* field techniques utilized in Egypt can distinguish bladder wall lesions and renal obstruction. Studies in Madagascar have even demonstrated ultrasound correlations with *S. hematobium* egg counts (21).

TREATMENT

Curing the individual patient by eradicating the infection not only benefits that patient but has therapeutic and prognostic implications for community health as well. In contrast, molluscacide interventions have been fraught with failure (22). There is initial benefit, but when fresh water becomes repopulated with snails, mortality and morbidity are worse. Trying to prevent repopulation with snails is futile since the snails are repopulated by waterfowl.

Praziquantel is still the drug of first choice. Even when egg excretion continues, the patient has lower morbidity and mortality. It is still effective despite decades of use for schistosomiasis and decades of use for other parasites. A single oral dose of 40mg/kg is effective for *S. hematobium, S. mansoni*, and *S. intercalatum*. For *S. japonicum* a higher dose was recommended but studies have shown that the same dose is adequate. With *S. mekongi* a repeat dose may be needed. It is well tolerated with confirmed absence of hepatic, renal or hemapoetic toxicity and it can be given with albendazole and ivermectin with no increase risk of toxicity (23). Caution is necessary if there is co-infection with central nervous system cystocercosis which requires pre-treatment with corticosteroids. Failures have been reported related to intense infestation with maturing worms (24). Some patients persist in egg excretion which may relate to their immune tolerance as opposed to praziquantel being ineffective.

Tetrahydroquinolone compounds are effective but only against *S. mansoni*. In animal studies, male worms were more susceptible than female worms. Oxamniquine is available in South America and also in Africa in 250mg capsules or syrup (50mg/cc). Adults can be cured with a single dose of 15mg/kg and children 20mg/kg given in two divided doses.

SUMMARY AND FUTURE DEVELOPMENTS

Schistosomiasis is a mammalian blood fluke that causes profound pathology through specific snails in freshwater environments. Principles of epidemiology, diagnosis, and current management are reviewed. *Institut Pasteur de Madagascar* has demonstrated that periportal hepatic fibrosis and the associated morbidity and mortality from *S. mansoni* can be dramatically ameliorated with once-a-year praziquantil treatment, even when it does not eradicate the parasite (25). Since praziquantel is relatively inexpensive, developing country governments can afford community therapy in endemic areas. It may even decrease the extent of infection if maintained for several decades. Unfortunately, treatment of *S. hematobium*, with annual therapy has not shown any beneficial effects. Treating *S. japonicum* on an annual basis in the Dongting Lake region of China has not yet demonstrated benefit but has shown a 20% annual re-infection rate (26).

Schistosomiasis produces polo-like kinases that regulate cell mitosis and parasite replication. These kinases may be useful in directing the development of new cancer chemotherapy. They may also be useful in therapeutic drug development for parasite eradication since cancer chemotherapy drugs, that are known to be polo-like kinases type 1 inhibitors, induce profound alterations in Schistosome gonads (27).

REFERENCES

[1] Bayssade-Dufour C, Vuong PN, Farhati K, et al. Speed of skin penetration and initial migration route of infective larvae of Schistosoma haematobium in Meriones unguiculatus. Comptes Rendus de l'Academie des Sciences 1994;317(6):529-33.

[2] Dzeing-Ella A, Mechai F, Consigny PH, et al. Cervical schistosomiasis as a risk factor of cervical uterine dysplasia in a traveler. Am J Trop Med Hyg 2009;81(4):549-50.

[3] Swai B, Poggensee G, Mtweve S, Krantz I. Female genital schistosomiasis as an evidence of a neglected cause for reproductive ill-health: a retrospective histopathological study from Tanzania. BMC Infect Dis 2006;6:134.

[4] Leutscher PD, Host E, Reimert CM. Semen quality in Schistosoma haematobium infected men in Madagascar. Acta Tropica 2009;109(1):41-4.

[5] Malenganisho WL, Magnussen P, Friis H, et al. Schistosoma mansoni morbidity among adults in two villages along Lake Victoria shores in Mwanza District, Tanzania. Trans Rl Soc Trop Med Hyg 2008;102(6):532-41.

[6] Rahoud SA, Mergani A, Khamis AH, et al. Factors controlling the effect of praziquantel on liver fibrosis in Schistosoma mansoni-infected patients. FEMS Immun Med Microbiol 2010;58(1):106-12.

[7] Conceicao MJ, Lenzi HL, Coura JR. Human study and experimental behavior of Schistosoma mansoni isolates from patients with different clinical forms of schistosomiasis. Acta Tropica 2008;108(2-3):98-103.

[8] Andrade ZA, Abreu WN. Follicular lymphoma of the spleen in patients with hepatosplenic Schistosomiasis mansoni. Am J Trop Med Hyg 1971;20(2):237-43.

[9] Kirchhoff LV, Nash TE. A case of schistosomiasis japonica: resolution of CAT-scan detected cerebral abnormalities without specific therapy. Am J Trop Med Hyg 1984; 33(6):1155-8.

[10] Carod-Artal FJ. Tropical causes of epilepsy. Revista Neurologia. 2009;49(9):475-82.

[11] Pittella JE. Neuroschistosomiasis. Brain Pathol (Zurich) 1997;7(1):649-62.

[12] Ross AG, Bartley PB, Sleigh AC, et al. Schistosomiasis. *N Engl J Med* 2002;346(16): 1212–20.

[13] Ahmed AF, Idris AS, Kareem AM, Dawoud TA. Acute toxemic schistosomiasis complicated by acute flaccid paraplegia due to schistosomal myeloradiculopathy in Sudan. Saudi Med J 2008;29(5):770-3.

[14] Dar J, Zimmerman RR. Schistosomiasis of the spinal cord. Surg Neurol 1977;8(6):416-8.

[15]   Keang H, Odermatt P, Odermatt-Biays S, et al. Liver morbidity due to Schistosoma mekongi in Cambodia after seven rounds of mass drug administration. Trans R Soc Trop Med Hyg 2007;101(8):759-65.

[16]   Shimada M, Kirinoki M, Shimizu K, et al. Characteristics of granuloma formation and liver fibrosis in murine schistosomiasis mekongi: a morphological comparison between Schistosoma mekongi and S. japonicum infection. Parasitology 2010;137(12):1781-9.

[17]   Muth S, Sayasone S, Odermatt-Biays S, et al. Schistosoma mekongi in Cambodia and Lao People's Democratic Republic. Adv Parasitology 2005;72:179-203.

[18]   Wittes R, MacLean JD, Law C, Lough JO. Three cases of schistosomiasis mekongi from northern Laos. Am J Trop Med Hyg 1984;33(6):1159-65.

[19]   Raobelison A, Rabarijaona L, Ramarokoto CE, et al. [Ultrasonographic evaluation of Schistosoma mansoni morbidity: comparison of Cairo/WHO and Managil-Hannover classifications]. Arch l'Institut Pasteur de Madagascar 1996;63(1-2):43-5. [French]

[20]   Hoffmann H, Esterre P, Ravaoalimalala VA, et al. Morbidity of schistosomiasis mansoni in the highlands of Madagascar and comparison of current sonographical classification systems. Trans R Soc Trop Med Hygiene 2001;95(6):623-9.

[21]   Leutscher PD, Reimert CM, Vennervald BJ, et al. Morbidity assessment in urinary schistosomiasis infection through ultrasonography and measurement of eosinophil cationic protein (ECP) in urine. Trop Med Int Health 2000;5(2):88-93.

[22]   Erko B, Abebe F, Berhe N, et al. Control of Schistosoma mansoni by the soapberry Endod (Phytolacca dodecandra) in Wollo, northeastern Ethiopia: post-intervention prevalence. East African Med J 2002;79(4):198-201.

[23]   Namwanje H, Kabatereine N, Olsen A. A randomised controlled clinical trial on the safety of co-administration of albendazole, ivermectin and praziquantel in infected schoolchildren in Uganda. Trans R Soc Trop Med Hyg 2011;105(4):181-8.

[24]   Gryseels B, Stelma FF, Talla I, et al. Epidemiology, immunology and chemotherapy of Schistosoma mansoni infections in a recently exposed community in Senegal. Trop Geographical Med 1994;46(4):209-19.

[25]   Boisier P, Ramarokoto CE, Ravaoalimalala VE, et al. Reversibility of Schistosoma mansoni-associated morbidity after yearly mass praziquantel therapy: ultrasonographic assessment. Trans R Soc Trop Med Hyg 1998;92(4):451-3.

[26]   Li YS, Sleigh AC, Ross AG, et al. Williams GM, Tanner M, McManus DP. Epidemiology of Schistosoma japonicum in China: morbidity and strategies for control in the Dongting Lake region. Internat J Parasitol 2000;30(3):273-81.

[27]   Dissous C, Grevelding CG, Long T. Schistosoma mansoni polo-like kinases and their function in control of mitosis and parasite reproduction. Anais da Academia Brasileira de Ciencias 2011;83(2):627-35.

Submitted: September 03, 2011. *Revised:* November 05, 2011. *Accepted:* November 10, 2011.

In: Public Health Yearbook 2012
Editor: Joav Merrick

ISBN: 978-1-62808-078-0
© 2013 Nova Science Publishers, Inc.

Chapter 15

SOIL-TRANSMITTED HELMINTHS

Richard R Roach, MD, FACP and Jashan Octain, MD*

Internal Medicine Department, Michigan State University/Kalamazoo Center for Medical
Studies, Kalamazoo, Michigan, United States of America

ABSTRACT

Helminths currently infect over two billion people worldwide. A quarter of world's
population has been infected at some time in their lives. Sobering statistics from a World
Health Organization [WHO] March 2008 report that 80% of the "Bottom Billion"
impoverished population of the world have *Ascaris*, 60% have *Trichuris* and 57% have
hookworm. This would only be a matter of pharmacologic distribution were it not for
additional disturbing reports that standard therapy has a 50% failure to clear *Trichuris*
and 90% failure to clear hookworm. These reports challenge tropical physicians who
have had years of confidence in mebendazole and albendazole to adequately treat
children. This is even more of a challenge to physicians in temperate climates who may
be less familiar with standard treatment. This article presents the recent data, the
approach to treatment failure, and concepts of new therapeutic approaches.

Keywords: Public health, tropical medicine, helminths

INTRODUCTION

Intestinal parasites cause substantial morbidity and mortality, particularly in children in whom
they have detrimental effects on growth and cognitive performance (1-4).

Parasitic infestation leads to deformities, long-term disabilities, and often stigmatizes the
child. Parasitized pregnant women are anemic, have increased fetal wastage, and have low
birth weight newborns (4).

Though tropical diseases affect a large portion of the world's population, less than one
percent of new drug development over the past 30 years has been aimed at tropical disease

---

* Correspondence: Richard R Roach, MD, FACP, Internal Medicine Department, 1000 Oakland Drive, Kalamazoo,
Michigan 49008 United States. E-mail: roach@ kcms.msu.edu

(4). In recent years, philanthropic interest has resulted in research, long tardy, for this group of children.

EPIDEMIOLOGY

The three soil-transmitted helminth infections: *Ascaris*, hookworm and *Trichuris* are often called the "Unholy Trinity" by WHO. They are ubiquitous to tropical climates and even temperate rural areas in poverty that are stricken communities with poor sanitation (5,6) (see Table 1). *Ascaris* and *Trichuris* increase in prevalence from infancy to puberty, and then decreases in adulthood. In contrast hookworm, the leading cause of anemia throughout the world, increases throughout life, not reaching a plateau until age forty (7). Significantly, this affects women of childbearing age and is associated with small-for-gestation newborns as well as increasing fetal loss.

SYMPTOMATOLOGY

WHO has classified parasitic infestation by egg intensity to clarify symptomatic and asymptomatic infestations (see table 2). Children with light worm loads are often asymptomatic, but children form the greatest proportion of the heavy intensity group. Even children who are clinically asymptomatic may have subtle differences in learning and intellectual achievement.

Clinical presentation is often related to parasite migration in the skin, viscera, and gastrointestinal tract. *Trichuris* and *Ascaris* are a result of fecal-oral ingestion. Features such as wheezing, dyspnea, non-productive cough, fever, bloody sputum, chest x-ray infiltrates, and systemic eosinophilia are associated with pulmonary vascular migration. Once swallowed, the larvae mature and their migration in the gastrointestinal tract causes abdominal pain, distention, and malabsorption.

If adult *Ascaris* worms migrate into the biliary tree, then pancreatitis, cholangitis or cholecystitis can result. Even hepatic abscesses and appendicitis have been attributed to *Ascaris* worm migration. In younger children, heavy loads of worms can cause partial or complete bowel obstruction in the ileum. Swelling of Peyer's patches can lead to intussusception or cause volvulus. On occasion, unrecognized obstruction leads to bowel infarction and perforation with peritonitis.

Trichuris infects the colon, preferring the cecum. Eggs release the larvae in the small intestine and the worms mature in the colon where they tunnel into the mucosa causing inflammation. Heavy infestation causes a dysentery syndrome severe enough to cause rectal prolapse. Impaired growth and anemia are the result of the chronic disease state.

Hookworm infects through skin penetration. An itching, erythematous rash from multiple skin penetrations causes severe pruritus of the feet or hands. The larvae use the pulmonary vasculature to access the bronchial secretions and then when swallowed, mature in to adults in the gastrointestinal tract. The bronchial migration can present as a clinical pneumonitis, or can be mistaken for asthma, but seldom are the pulmonary symptoms or clinical response as serious as *Ascaris* worm migration. The significant sequelae of infection are related to intestinal blood loss. An infestation of as few as 40 worms can reduce hemoglobin to below 11g/dl. Heavy infestations can lead to hypoproteinemia and even anasarca.

Table 1. Impact of Soil-Transmitted Helminths WHO 2008

Disease	Global Prevalence (millions)[25]	Population at Risk (billions)	Estimated global disease burden (disability adjusted life years in millions)	Vulnerable Population
Ascariasis	807	4.2	1.8 – 10.5	School-age children
Trichuriasis	604	3.2	1.8 – 6.4	School-age children
Hookworm	576	3.2	1.5 – 22.1	School-age children, women of reproductive age

Table 2. Soil-Transmitted Helminth Infection Intensity (WHO)

Intensity	Ascaris	Hookworms	Trichuris
Light	1 – 4,999 epg	1 – 1,999 epg	1 – 999 epg
Moderate	5,000 – 49,999 epg	2,000 – 3,999 epg	1,000 – 9,999 epg
Heavy	≥ 50,000 epg	≥ 4,000 epg	≥ 10,000 epg

epg: eggs per gram of feces.

Helminths cause anemia and malnutrition, growth stunting and cognitive deficits associated with poor school attendance and performance (8). Since helminth infestation occurs in impoverished areas of poor nutrition, intestinal worms cause even more severe malnutrition to the children's limited diet. If this occurs in an area where malaria is prevalent, the anemia of the helminths compounds the anemia caused by malaria (9). Infected women have a 3 fold increase in anemia (10) and are 2.6 times more likely to have preterm deliveries and 3.5 times more likely to have small-for-gestational-age infants (11).

PHARMACOLOGIC TREATMENT

There are four medications currently available to treat soil-transmitted helminth infections (12) (see Table 3). The benzimidazoles impede the microtubular system, in particular β-tubulin, in the worm. As a result these drugs are well tolerated, even though some patients report nausea, vomiting, headache, and rare allergic reactions with fever; however, heavy worm loads increase the risk of abdominal pain, bloating, and diarrhea (13). Levamisole and pyrantel pamoate are nicotinic acetylcholine receptor agonists which paralyze the worms and precipitate their expulsion. Mild gastrointestinal symptoms, headache, dizziness, fever, and rash are usually mild and self-limited.

Since the drugs are well tolerated, the remaining consideration of treatment is efficacy. Cure rates and egg reduction rates are high for all four drugs when treating *Ascaris* (12,14) [see table 4].

Table 3. Treatment of Soil-Transmitted Helminth Infections

Infection	Drug	Dose
Ascariasis	Albendazole*	400 mg once
	Mebendazole	100 mg twice daily x 3 days or 500 mg once
	Pyrantel pamoate	11 mg/kg (max 1 g) x 3 days
	Levamisole	2.5 mg/kg once
Hookworm	Albendazole*	400 mg once
	Mebendazole	100 mg twice daily x 3 days
	Pyrantel pamoate	11 mg/kg (max 1 g) x 3 days
	Levamiosle	2.5 mg/kg once, repeat after 7 days for heavy infection
Trichuris	Mebendazole	100 mg twice daily x 3 days or 500 mg once
	Albendazole*	400 mg x 3 days
	(* in children 1-2 years old, use 200 mg)	

Table 4. Efficacy of single and multiple dose anthelminthic drugs against common soil transmittedhelminth infections [26]

Parasite	Drug	Dose	Cure rate (%)	Egg reduction rate (%)
A. lumbricoides	Albendazole	400 mg once	88[a,b]	87–100[a]
	Mebendazole	500 mg once	95[a,b]	96–100[a]
		100 mg twice a day for 3 days	92[c]	91–100[c]
	Pyrantel pamoate	10 mg/kg once	88[a,b]	88[a]
		10 mg/kg for 3 days	92[d]	99[d]
	Levamisole	2.5 mg/kg once	92[a]	92–100[a]
Hookworm	Albendazole	400 mg once	72[a,b]	64–100[a]
	Mebendazole	500 mg once	15[a,b]	0–98[a]
		100 mg twice a day for 3 days	80[c]	41–100[c]
	Pyrantel pamoate	10 mg/kg once	31[a,b]	56–75[a]
		10 mg/kg for 3 days	68[d]	77–99[d]
	Levamisole	2.5 mg/kg once	38[a]	68–100[a]
T. trichiura	Albendazole	400 mg once	28[a,b]	0–90[a]
	Albendazole	400 mg for 3 days	53[f]	81–100[f]
	Mebendazole	500 mg once	36[a,b]	81–93[a]
		100 mg twice a day for 3 days	63[g] / 80[h]	38–99[g]
	Pyrantel pamoate	10 mg/kg once	31[a]	52[a]
		10 mg/kg for 3 days	27[d]	77[d]
	Levamisole	2.5 mg/kg once	10[a]	42[a]
S. stercoralis	Ivermectin	200 µg/kg once	88[i]	N/A
	Ivermectin	200 µg/kg for 2 days	96[j]	N/A
	Albendazole	400 mg once	69[k]	N/A
	Albendazole	400 mg twice daily for 3 days	62[k]	N/A

N/A, not applicable.
[a] Data derived from recent systematic review and meta-analysis (Keiser and Utzinger, 2008).
[b] Data from randomised controlled trials.
[c] Overall cure rate and egg reduction rates based on 29 trials.
[d] Overall cure rate and egg reduction rates based on three trials (Botero and Castano, 1973; Kale et al., 1982; Seah, 1973).
[e] Overall cure rate and egg reduction rates based on 27 trials.
[f] Overall cure rate and egg reduction rates based on five trials (Adams et al., 2004; Marti et al., 1996; Okelo, 1984; Sirivichayakul et al., 2001; Zhang et al., 1990).
[g] Overall cure rate and egg reduction rates based on 33 trials.
[h] Combined pooled relative risk of four randomised controlled trials (Davison, 1979; Sargent et al., 1975; Vandepitte et al., 1973; Wesche and Barnish, 1994).
[i] Overall cure rate based on six trials (Datry et al., 1994; Gann et al., 1994; Igual-Adell et al., 2004; Marti et al., 1996; Shikiya et al., 1991b, 1992).
[j] Overall cure rate based on three trials (Gann et al., 1994; Igual-Adell et al., 2004; Ordonez and Angulo, 2004).
[k] Based on literature review by Horton (2000).

Recent studies, however, have documented ineffective and inconsistent treatment of *Trichuris* and hookworm. The concern is that the lack of efficacy is due to drug resistance, but lack of previous investigations means that these drugs were only presumed to be effective in the past. Until recently, the efficacy was determined based on mass drug administration to animals in endemic areas by veterinarians. Subsequent studies of adults suggested adequate efficacy, but these studies excluded children and pregnant women, who are the most vulnerable population.

Currently, benzimidazoles are established as safe for children greater than one year of age. Teratogenic potential was seen in animal studies, so benefit/risk must be carefully evaluated in pregnant women; however, WHO recommends treatment of hookworm in pregnancy because of the devastating effect of anemia. Limited studies demonstrated no congenital anomalies or perinatal mortality with the use of albendazole, mebendazole or ivermectin, although use in first trimester is still discouraged. There are no adequate studies in pregnancy of levamisole and pyrantel.

PUBLIC HEALTH CONCEPTS

Considering the large burden of disease, prevention needs to be at the forefront in improving community health. Sanitation, access to clean sources of water, and careful food preparation limit fecal-oral contamination. Careful disposal of feces and protective footwear limits hookworm exposure. Hand washing prior to meals and secure storage of food and water also reduce exposure to parasites.

Periodic treatments decrease morbidity in endemic communities (15). The school system has been the logical institution to study the impact of periodic treatment (16). The most profound impact occurs when de-worming school children on an annual basis or when the focus is on women of reproductive age. These approaches reach a minimum of 75% of the at-risk population. GlaxoSmithKline has made the medication affordable at $0.02 USD per treatment, per patient. One study done in Zanzibar examined the co-administration of ivermectin, albendazole and praziquantedl in 5,055 children and adults (17,18). The integration of mass drug administration with efficacy studies resulted in important data regarding parasite eradication and produced great the community benefit.

SUMMARY: FUTURE RESEARCH AND MANAGEMENT CONCEPTS

As noted, helminths currently infect over two billion people worldwide resulting in devastating morbidity and mortality (1-4). Considering the prevalence of soil-transmitted helminths and the established resistance, other treatment options are needed. This has provoked enthusiasm for vaccines and novel drugs, but unfortunately there has been little financial incentive to develop human vaccines or new drugs for poverty stricken areas. Veterinary medicine provides the necessary financial incentive of animal herd management, so most of the novel treatments have come from veterinary research (19).

Nicotinic acetylcholine receptor seems to be unique to helminthes and nematodes, although possibly are present in malaria parasites as well. This receptor does not exist in humans, so medications blocking this receptor, or a vaccines against this receptor, have logical potential to be realistic and safe options (20). Tribendimidine was thought to be a L-type nicotinic acetyl-choline receptor agonist and is very effective in animals. Clinical trials in humans resulted in approval in China in 2004 (21). Despite the difference in chemical structure and the hypothesized receptor agonist effect, it unfortunately proved to have the same mechanism of action as benzimidazoles and showed no clinical advantage.

Monepantel was developed as a nicotinic acetyl-choline receptor agonist. It is highly effective in animals and is licensed for sheep (22), and thus, studies in humans have been initiated (12). It appears to have a unique mechanism of action and has been effective in treating multi-drug resistant nematode infections in animals.

Developing a vaccine requires an antigen, and developers have struggled with which antigen to use that would provoke a sufficient and effective antigenic response in order to prevent helminthic infection (23). Vaccines for soil-transmitted helminths have been developed that are effective in animals. A vaccine to the hookworm antigen, Na-ASP-2, was shown to be effective for dogs (24). Vaccinated when puppies, the adult dogs were resistant to hookworm infection. This success led to a limited phase 1 trial in Brazil. Unfortunately, 30% of the patients developed urticaria and one patient developed anaphylaxis, causing the trial to be stopped. Speculation as to the cause of this intense reaction led to the hypothesis that the patients were already exposed to the antigen in this endemic area. Thus, further research in the effective management of soil-transmitted helminthes is urgently needed in the early part of the 21st century (25,26).

REFERENCES

[1]   Moon TD, Oberhelman RA. Antiparasitic therapy in children. Pediatr Clin North Am 2005;52(3):917-48.

[2]   Bethony J, Brooker S, Albonico M, et al. Soil-transmitted helminth infections: Ascariasis, trichuriasis, and hookworm. Lancet 2006;367:1521-32.

[3]   Uneke CJ. Soil transmitted helminth infections and schistosomiasis in school age children in sub-Saharan Africa: efficacy of chemotherapeutic intervention since World Health Assembly Resolution. Tanzania J Health Res 2001;12:86-99.

[4]   Reddy M, Gill SS, Kalkar SR, et al. Oral drug therapy for multiple neglected tropical diseases: a systematic review. JAMA 2007;298:1911-24.

[5]   Hotez P. Hookworm and poverty. Ann NY Acad Sci 2008;1136:38-44.

[6]   Hotez PJ, Fenwick A, Savioli L, Molyneux DH. Rescuing the bottom billion through control of neglected tropical diseases. Lancet 2009;373:1570-5.

[7]   Harhay MO, Horton J, Olliaro PL. Epidemiology and control of human gastrointestinal parasites in children. Exp Rev Anti-infective Ther 2010; 8:219-34.

[8]   Taylor-Robinson DC, Jones AP, Garner P. Deworming drugs for treating soil- transmitted intestinal worms in children: effects on growth and school performance. Cochrane Database Syst Rev 2007;4:CD000371.

[9]   Kung'u JK, Goodman D, Haji HJ, et al. Early helminth infections are inversely related to anemia, malnutrition, and malaria and are not associated with inflammation in 6- to 23-month-old Zanzibari children. Am J Trop Med Hyg 2009;81:1062-70.

[10]   Sousa-Figueiredo JC, Basanez MG, Mgeni AF, et al. A parasitological survey, in rural Zanzibar, of pre-school children and their mothers for urinary schistosomiasis, soil-transmitted helminthiases and malaria, with observations on the prevalence of anaemia. Ann Trop Med Parasitology 2008:102:679-92.

[11]   Yatich NJ, Jolly PE, Funkhouser E, et al. The effect of malaria and intestinal helminth coinfection on birth outcomes in Kumasi, Ghana. Am J Trop Med Hyg 2010;82:28-34.

[12] Keiser J, Utzinger J. The drugs we have and the drugs we need against major helminth infections. Adv Parasitology 2006;73:197-230.

[13] Van den Enden E. Pharmacotherapy of helminth infection. Expert Opinion Pharmacother 2009;10:435-51.

[14] Keiser J, Utzinger J. Efficacy of current drugs against soil-transmitted helminth infections: systematic review and meta-analysis. JAMA 2008;299:1937-48.

[15] Zhang Y, Koukounari A, Kabatereine N, et al. Parasitological impact of 2-year preventive chemotherapy on schistosomiasis and soil-transmitted helminthiasis in Uganda. BMC Med 2007;5:27-30.

[16] Vercruysse J, Behnke JM, Albonico M, et al. Assessment of the anthelmintic efficacy of albendazole in school children in seven countries where soil- transmitted helminths are endemic. PLoS Neglect Trop Dis 2011; 5(3):e948.

[17] Montresor A, Ramsan M, Chwaya HM, et al. School enrollment in Zanzibar linked to children's age and helminth infections. Trop Med Int Health. 2001; 6(3):227-31.

[18] Mohammed KA, Haji HJ, Gabrielli AF, et al. Triple co-administration of ivermectin, albendazole and praziquantel in zanzibar: a safety study. PLoS Neglect Trop Dis 2008;2:e171.

[19] Geary TG, Woo K, McCarthy JS, et al. Unresolved issues in anthelmintic pharmacology for helminthiases of humans. Int J Parasitology 2010;40:1-13.

[20] Kaminsky R, Ducray P, Jung M, et al. A new class of anthelmintics effective against drug-resistant nematodes. Nature 2008;452:176-80.

[21] Steinmann P, Zhou XN, Du ZW, et al. Tribendimidine and albendazole for treating soil-transmitted helminths, Strongyloides stercoralis and Taenia spp.: open-label randomized trial. PLoS Neglect Trop Dis 2008;2(10):e322.

[22] Hosking BC, Griffiths TM, Woodgate RG, et al. Clinical field study to evaluate the efficacy and safety of the amino-acetonitrile derivative, monepantel, compared with registered anthelmintics against gastrointestinal nematodes of sheep in Australia. Aust Veterinary J 2009;87(11):455-62.

[23] Hotez PJ, Bethony JM, Diemert DJ, et al. Developing vaccines to combat hookworm infection and intestinal schistosomiasis. Nature Rev 2008;8(11):814-26.

[24] Bethony J, Loukas A, Smout M, et. al. Antibodies against a secreted protein from hookworm larvae reduce the intensity of hookworm infection in humans and vaccinated laboratory animals. Faseb J 2005;19(12):1743-5.

[25] Hotez PJ, Molyneux DH, Fenwick A, et al. Control of neglected tropical Diseases. N Engl J Med 2007;357(10):1018-27.

[26] Keiser J, Utzinger J. The drugs we have and the drugs we need against major helminth infections. In: Xiao-Nong Zhou RBRO, Jürg U, eds. Advances in parasitology: Philadelphia, PA: Elsevier/Academic Press 2010:197-230.

Submitted: September 03, 2011. *Revised:* November 05, 2011. *Accepted:* November 10, 2011.

In: Public Health Yearbook 2012
Editor: Joav Merrick

ISBN: 978-1-62808-078-0
© 2013 Nova Science Publishers, Inc.

Chapter 16

INTESTINAL, LUNG AND LIVER FLUKES

Richard R Roach, MD, FACP and Elizabeth Friedman, MD*

Internal Medicine Department, Michigan State University/Kalamazoo Center for Medical Studies, Kalamazoo, Michigan, United States of America

ABSTRACT

Current estimates indicate that 50 million people are infected with food-borne trematodes. This is a significant public health problem but still a neglected tropical disease because the burden of disease is in rural areas where health care is limited. Traditional ingestion of raw or poorly cooked food contaminated by unrestrained defecation maintains the cycle of disease, and school-age children bear the predominant burden.

Clinical patterns of infection as well as current means of diagnosis, treatment, and treatment failure are reviewed in sections on intestinal flukes, liver flukes and lung flukes. New therapeutic approaches are emphasized in this discussion.

Keywords: Trematodes, food-born disease, public health

INTRODUCTION

Of the 50 million people infected with trematodes, most are in China, Japan, Korea, and parts of Southeast Asia including Indonesia, Vietnam, Thailand, Laos and Myanmar (1).

Paramphistomatidae occurs in Africa, Echinostomatidae is endemic in Inda, and Hereophyidae has been reported in Brazil. International travel has also made this a world-wide problem.

People contract this infection by eating raw or undercooked fresh-water fish or water plants such as watercress with encysted metacercaria. Infestation of human trematodes is related to their migration. Intestinal, pulmonary, and liver flukes present distinct clinical and

---

* Correspondence: Richard R. Roach, MD, FACP, Assistant Professor, Internal Medicine Department, Michigan State University/ Kalamazoo Center for Medical Studies, 1000 Oakland Drive, Kalamazoo, Michigan 49008, United States. E-mail: roach@ kcms.msu.edu

diagnostic problems to physicians and health care workers who care for patients with neglected tropical diseases.

INTESTINAL FLUKES

More than 70 species of intestinal flukes have been reported in humans (2). The most common are *Fasciolopsis, Echinostoma, Gymnophallidae*, and *Heterophye* species. The cysts of *Fasciolopsis* are ingested when eating aquatic plants such as water hyacinth, water chestnuts, water bamboo, and water lotuses, many of which are preferred raw. *Echinostoma* is encysted in fish, mollusks and amphibians which are eaten raw or incompletely cooked. Freshwater fish, carp, and mullet, contain *Heterophye* cysts. *Gymnophallidae* contaminate both mollusks and vegetation. The ingested cysts, released in the duodenum, attach to the mucosa and mature into adult worms over a period of 3 months.

Epidemiology

Fasciolopsiasis is endemic to Southeast Asia and the Orient. The disease has the highest prevalence in school-age children (3). Reported prevalence is 57% in mainland China, 25% in Taiwan, 50% in Bangladesh, 60% in India, and 10% in Thailand. Control programs with effective medications have not achieved success due to continued traditions of eating raw aquatic plants and contact with domestic pigs. Change in traditional practices is slow. Athough simply drying plant products kills the parasite, this practice is not acceptable in many local customs, and cooking is thought to destroy the flavor.

Recognition of the disease in Africa and reports of the disease in Brazil, Russia, Spain, Turkey, and the Philippines have raised awareness of this neglected disease. The economic impact of the disease is difficult to assess but clearly affects rural communities depending on subsistence agriculture.

Clinical features

Food-borne trematodes predominantly infect children in endemic areas. Many are asymptomatic but heavy infections produce severe diarrhea, abdominal pain, low-grade fever, and fatigue. High inoculums cause malabsorption due to villous edema and atrophy. When cysts attach to the mucosa in duodenum and jejunum they cause inflammation, ulceration, and micro-abscesses. Eosinophilia occurs as an immunologic response to trematode protein and toxins and is directly related to worm load (4). Children tend to become re-infected after treatment, amplifying the clinical problems and confusing the understanding of which treatments are effective, and when and if eradication occurs with treatment. Flukes mature in 3 months and have an average life span of 1 year in humans (2).

Although a few flukes are asymptomatic, heavy worm burdens, identified as > 500 worms, cause intermittent diarrhea, constipation, anorexia, nausea, and vomiting (5). Diagnosis depends on the detection of *Fasciolopsis* eggs in stool samples. Morbidity in endemic areas is related to anemia from chronic blood loss, malnutrition due to malabsorption from villous damage, and toxic worm metabolites which are thought to cause a variety of symptoms and immunologic reactions that result in facial as well as generalized edema (6). Mortality is related to malnutrition, intestinal obstruction, and electrolyte abnormalities.

The *Heterophyids* infect humans eating fish or shrimp infected with viable metacercariae. Infected fish-eating mammals and birds contain the egg-producing *heterophyids*. Feces from these creatures contaminate the water and release eggs. Ingested by snails cercariae are released from the snails and then penetrate fish and shrimp in which they encyst. An Egyptian study showed fish to have the greatest intensity of infestation during the summer months (7).

Human prevalence studies in Korea showed the highest prevalence in young and middle aged adults (4). A national survey to determine the prevalence among primary school children in Laos was unable to differentiate *Opisthorchis viverrini* (a liver fluke) from intestinal flukes (1); thus, most studies just report stool collection samples as '*Opisthorchis*-like' eggs. Verification of disease burden by purging and stool analysis is therefore complicated by infection with multiple species that cannot be differentiated. A study of cysts in fish dishes in Vietnam restaurants showed a greater prevalence in freshwater than in brackish water fish [8]. Prevalence in Vietnam is as high as 70% depending on the region [7]. *H. tauchi* infection, though rare, is different from other flukes because it enters the mesenteric lymphatics and migrates to the heart causing myocarditis, chronic congestive heart failure, and death.

Gymnophallidae

Gymnophalloides seoi contaminates raw oysters. Infestation tends to be restricted to focal geographic areas. One village in Korea had a 70% infestation rate (9), dramatically higher than the neighboring populations. The usual symptoms are indigestion, constipation, and diarrhea. Microscopic examination of gastric mucosa in animal models demonstrates stimulated goblet cell production. In humans, infestation has been associated with diabetes mellitus because it causes acute pancreatitis. One study noted subsequent insulin deficiency in 46% of 37 infected patients (1,10). A case study described patients with polyuria and polydipsia but without increased blood glucose or glucosuria (10); however, the cause was not elucidated. Infections with *Gymnophalloides seoi* are associated with polyuria and polydipsia and are probably toxin related (11).

Diagnostics

There are three approaches to diagnosing fishborne zoonotic trematodes: detection of parasite eggs in stool, immunodiagnostics (indirect diagnosis), and molecular biologic testing. Detection of eggs is the most common approach, especially in epidemiological surveys. Methods include fecal flotation in salt and sugar solutions, the Kato-Katz technique, and the formalin-ethyl-acetate technique (1). Trematode species identification based on egg morphology is challenging because *F. buski*, *F. hepatica* and echinostomes all appear similar. *Heterophyids* egg-laying capacity is low, 2-28 eggs per worm (*Ascaris* by contrast produce hundreds of thousands of eggs per day) and the eggs resemble *Clonorchis* spp. A definite diagnosis can be obtained by examination of adult worms after chemotherapy expulsion.

Several tests to detect specific antibodies are available but many have low specificity and cross-reactivity. Enzyme-linked immune-absorbent assays have been developed, but consensus on their use has not been established. Recently, polymerase chain reaction (PCR) methods have been developed to identify trematode eggs (12). They will likely prove to be an effective research tools, but use in endemic areas are likely to be impractical in the near future. While metabolic profiling is a new approach to research, its application with intestinal trematodes is presently limited.

Treatment

A single 15mg/kg dose of praziquantel is generally adequate for children, but adults should receive 25mg/kg (3). Various authors have reported that a single dose ranging from10–40 mg/kg is curative and safe (1). Praziquantel is not approved for children under the age of four, but its use may be therapeutically necessary. Ivermectin is an alternative choice for children under 4 who weigh greater than 15 kg. Pregnant women should not take praziquantel. Treatment should be delayed until after delivery unless life-saving treatment is required. Breast-feeding should be avoided for 72 hours after praziquantel treatment.

Prevention

The key to prevention is education and avoidance of raw, water-derived food (for preventing *F. Buski*), raw fish (for preventing intestinal trematodes) and raw oysters from endemic contaminated locations. This has been difficult because of culinary traditions in endemic areas. Other prevention methods include treatment of infected people as well as livestock and increased sanitation methods to prevent infected humans and pigs from defecating near water sources. Ironically, industrialization has polluted streams and rivers, destroying the environment for aquatic animals and breaking the ecosystem life cycle which had reduced the incidence and prevalence of disease in previously endemic areas (13).

Public programs address the role of animal carriers including dogs, cats, pigs, and wildlife. In Vietnam, studies of fish-borne trematodes showed prevalence in cats, dogs, and pigs of 48.6%, 70.2%, 35-56.9% and 7.7-14.4% respectively (14). While pigs are generally confined and their prevalence rates are lower, their total fecal contribution is huge which makes pigs significant contributors to endemic regions. Education is important to avoid feeding domestic animals contaminated feed such as raw fish and oysters. However this is impractical for free-roaming animal reservoirs such as cats and dogs. In the commercial fish farms, practices that prevent introduction of infection and quality control are of the utmost importance.

LIVER FLUKES

Opisthorciasis and clonorchiasis are primarily diseases of Southeast Asia, ranging from China to Indonesia and from Thailand to the Philippines. Clonorchins sinensis eggs have been found in a corpse buried in the 4th century BCE (15). These trematodes, of which 18 varieties are known, penetrate the skin and encyst fresh water fish. Consumption of raw or undercooked fish release the harbored metacercariae to migrate in the human host.

Clinical

Liver flukes migrate through the ampulla of Vater into the common bile duct and from there infest the intrahepatic bile ducts where they cause hepatomegaly, cholangitis and periportal fibrosis. This infestation precipitates gallstones and causes cholecystitis. Ultrasonography often demonstrates gallbladder sludge and poor contractile function. In one study, intrahepatic duct dilation was noted in 68% of egg positive patients with sludge reported in 20.8% (1,16). Higher grade dilation was found to correlate with higher egg counts. Periductal fibrosis was also a common finding (16). Treatment with praziquantel improves biliary function and decreases intrahepatic duct dilation.

More important than the acute manifestations is the predisposition these parasites cause for bile duct cancer and cholangiocarcinoma. Thailand has the highest incidence of liver cancer in the world. Recent research has noted an exacerbation of hepatic carcinoma by N-nitrosamine. Noteworthy is the fact that N-nitrosamine levels are highest in tobacco, but it is also found in beer, fish, and pickles. Tobacco product marketing in Southeast Asia historically correlates with a dramatic increase in hepatic carcinoma. Although this may be due to better case identification, cigarette smoking may be exacerbating the parasitic predisposition to hepatic cancer.

Treatment

A single 40mg/kg oral dose of praziquantel is effective, but some authors note three divided doses of 25mg/kg as a more effective dose for treating clonorchiasis (1,16,17). This higher dose is associated with dizziness, vomiting, and abdominal pain; however, these side-effects tend to be transient. Other treatment options have been investigated and tribendimidine seems to be as effective as praziquantel for *Opisthorchis* (17).

Prevention

If culture continues to mandate eating raw fish, then improved sanitation is the only prevention and control measure available. Molluscicides are not proven effective, are expensive, and are associated with an increase incidence in community disease when the snails inevitably return. Prevention should be focused on community education, especially school-aged children, for long-term control.

LUNG FLUKES

Paragonimus species, lung flukes, are contracted from eating raw freshwater crabs and other crustaceans (15). Although known to be a problem in Southeast Asia, recent literature has demonstrated significant prevalence in South America (18,19) and Africa (20). There are about 15 species known to infect humans world-wide.

Clinical features

Infection occurs when the parasite migrates into the human body and releases toxins as well as other proteins during migration. Pulmonary infection with cough is often non-productive, but when it is productive, gelatinous, brown sputum from pulmonary hemorrhage is characteristic. Hemorrhage is associated with leukocyte infiltrate and necrosis of the lung parenchyma. The tissue reaction leads to fibrotic encapsulation, but opening in the capsule releases fluke eggs. Hemoptosis with exertion is often reported. The prominent bronchospasm is often misinterpreted as asthma. Prominent eosinophilia (20-25%) is common. Persistent pleural effusions, unresponsive to parasitic treatment, are related to chronic granuloma reaction. It is not uncommon that lung fluke infestation is diagnosed as tuberculosis, especially in communities where both diseases are endemic. Pneumothorax related to the inflammatory reaction and secondary bacterial infection in the infracted lung has been reported. The immune response eventually modulates and calcification surrounds the cysts.

Extra-pulmonary syndromes

Cerebral migration causes eosinophilic meningitis with headache and seizures. This extra-pulmonary syndrome seems to have a predilection for male children who are under ten years of age. Spinal cord migration causes spastic paraplegia and the neurologic manifestations are usually accompanied by pulmonary symptoms. Neurologic complications such as mass effect and intracranial hemorrhage have required surgical intervention (21).

Diagnosis

The differential diagnosis of lung flukes includes tuberculosis as well as common causes of pneumonia. Clinicians need to be aware of the diagnosis in endemic areas, especially when there is eosinophilia. A careful history of exposure in travelers or patients who have migrated from endemic areas is essential since the parasite can persist for decades. Smear examination of expectorated sputum, gastric washings, pleural fluid, feces reveal eggs in infected individuals; however, tissue biopsy is sometimes required.

Immunodiagnostic tests are highly sensitive (22). Complement fixation and enzyme-linked immunosorbent assay (ELISA) tests are able to diagnose chronic infection and can monitor treatment since they decline with cure.

Treatment

Praziquantel appears to be the treatment of choice, but treatment with bithionol is still reported to be effective (23). Treatment causes an inflammatory response and thus, skin lesions can flair, cerebral edema can result from neurologic infestation, and pulmonary symptoms may worsen.

Prevention

Discouraging consumption of raw crustaceans is still the best prevention, but dietary custom and culture often mitigate this solution. Local customs of soaking raw crustaceans in brine or alcohol (24) to kill parasites does not appear to be effective. Community awareness and environmental sanitation can be successful. Cobalt-60 irradiation of crustaceans can prevent parasite infectivity but this requires significant economic and public health commitment.

SUMMARY

Current studies estimate there are 50 million humans infected with food-borne trematodes involving intestinal, lung, and liver flukes. The ensuing morbidity and mortality is enormous and more research is urgently needed in the management of this potentially devastating infestation.

Consumption of raw foods is a major problem and complicates preventative health attempts. Clinical patterns of infection as well as current means of diagnosis, treatment, and treatment failure are reviewed in sections on intestinal flukes, liver flukes and lung flukes. New therapeutic approaches are emphasized in this discussion.

REFERENCES

[1] Keiser J, Utzinger J. Food-borne trematodiases. Clin Microbiol Rev 2009;22(3):466-83.

[2] Liu LX, Harinasuta KT. Liver and intestinal flukes. Gastroenterol Clin North Am 1996; 25(3):627-36.

[3] Graczyk TK, Gilman RH, Fried B. Fasciolopsiasis: is it a controllable food-borne disease? Parasitology Res 2001;87(1):80-3.

[4] Chai JY, Shin EH, Lee SH, Rim HJ. Foodborne intestinal flukes in Southeast Asia. Korean J Parasitol 2009;47(Suppl):S69-102.

[5] Most H. Drug therapy. Treatment of common parasitic infections of man encountered in the United States. N Engl J Med 1972;287(14):698-702.

[6] Mas-Coma S, Bargues MD, Valero MA. Fascioliasis and other plant-borne trematode zoonoses. Int J Parasitol 2005;35(11-12):1255-78.

[7] Trung Dung D, Van De N, Waikagul J, et al. Fishborne zoonotic intestinal trematodes, Vietnam. Emerg Infect Dis 2007;13(12):1828-33.

[8] Tran TK, Murrell KD, Madsen H, et al. Fishborne zoonotic trematodes in raw fish dishes served in restaurants in Nam Dinh Province and Hanoi, Vietnam. J Food Protection 2009;72(11):2394-9.

[9] Lee SH, Chai JY, Lee HJ, et al. High prevalence of Gymnophalloides seoi infection in a village on a southwestern island of the Republic of Korea. Am J Trop Med Hyg 1994; 51(3):281-5.

[10] Chai JY, Choi MH, Yu JR, Lee SH. Gymnophalloides seoi: a new human intestinal trematode. Trends Parasitol 2003;19(3):109-12.

[11] Park JH, Guk SM, Shin EH, et al. A new endemic focus of Gymnophalloides seoi infection on Aphae Island, Shinan-gun, Jeollanam-do. Korean J Parasitol 2007;45(1):39-44.

[12] Prasad PK, Goswami LM, Tandon V, Chatterjee A. PCR-based molecular characterization and insilico analysis of food-borne trematode parasites Paragonimus westermani, Fasciolopsis buski and Fasciola gigantica from Northeast India using ITS2 rDNA. Bioinformation 2006;6(2):64-8.

[13] Lu SC. Echinostomiasis in Taiwan. Int J Zoonoses 1982;9(1):33-8.

[14] Lan-Anh NT, Phuong NT, Murrell KD, et al. Animal reservoir hosts and fish-borne zoonotic trematode infections on fish farms, Vietnam. Emerg Infect Dis 2009;15(4):540-6.

[15]   Sripa B, Kaewkes S, Intapan PM, et al. Food-borne trematodiases in Southeast Asia epidemiology, pathology, clinical manifestation, and control. Adv Parasitol 2011; 72:305-50.

[16]   Choi MS, Choi D, Choi MH, et al. Correlation between sonographic findings and infection intensity in clonorchiasis. Am J Trop Med Hyg 2005;73(6):1139-44.

[17]   Soukhathammavong P, Odermatt P, Sayasone S, et al. Efficacy and safety of mefloquine, artesunate, mefloquine-artesunate, tribendimidine, and praziquantel in patients with Opisthorchis viverrini: a randomised, exploratory, open-label, phase 2 trial. Lancet Infect Dis 2011;11(2):110-8.

[18]   Gomez-Seco J, Rodriguez-Guzman MJ, Rodriguez-Nieto MJ, et al. Pulmonary paragonimiasis. Arch Bronconeumologia 2011;11:22-8.

[19]   Lemos AC, Coelho JC, Matos ED, et al. Paragonimiasis: first case reported in Brazil. Braz J Infect Dis 2007;11(1):153-6.

[20]   Aka NA, Adoubryn K, Rondelaud D, Dreyfuss G. Human paragonimiasis in Africa. Ann African Med 2008;7(4):153-62.

[21]   Chen J, Chen Z, Li F, et al. Cerebral paragonimiasis that manifested as intracranial hemorrhage. J Neurosurg 1992;6:572-8.

[22]   Nkouawa A, Okamoto M, Mabou AK, Edinga E, Yamasaki H, Sako Y, et al. Paragonimiasis in Cameroon: molecular identification, serodiagnosis and clinical manifestations. Trans R Soc Trop Med Hyg 2009;103(3):255-61.

[23]   Ming-gang C, Zheng-shan C, Xiang-yuan S, et al. Paragonimiasis in Yongjia County, Zhejiang Province, China: clinical, parasitological and karyotypic studies on Paragonimus westermani. Southeast Asian J Trop Med Public Health. 2001;32(4):760-9.

[24]   Cabrera BD. Paragonimiasis in the Philippines: current status. Arzneimittel-Forschung. 1984;34(9B):1188-92.

Submitted: September 04, 2011. *Revised:* November 02, 2011. *Accepted:* November 11, 2011.

In: Public Health Yearbook 2012
Editor: Joav Merrick

ISBN: 978-1-62808-078-0
© 2013 Nova Science Publishers, Inc.

Chapter 17

SNAKEBITES

Richard R Roach*, MD, FACP and Jishu Das, MD

Internal Medicine Department, Michigan State University/Kalamazoo Center for Medical
Studies, Kalamazoo, Michigan, United States of America

ABSTRACT

Snakes bite children in tropical countries at play, during family activities, and in
agricultural communities when children start to perform adult activities. They cause a
significant morbidity of limb loss as well as mortality. When the snake is identified
correctly and specific anti-venom is available, these bites can be treated specifically;
however, this is often not the case and the clinician is left to treat symptomatically or
provide management based on the most common venom in the patient's geographic area.
This article presents the types of snakes by geography and clinical manifestations to
allow the clinician to appropriately treat the patient even when specific identification is
not possible. We review the anti-venoms available and where they can be obtained.

Keywords: Snake bites, tropical medicine, public health

INTRODUCTION

Of the three thousand species of snakes on earth only an estimated 15% are considered
venomous. All snakes have venom, but snakes that are considered 'non-poisonous' have
venom that is either non-toxic to humans or too dilute to be harmful. Some snakes with toxic
venom are considered non-venomous, because their mouth and fang anatomy does not allow
them to envenomate humans. Most venomous snakes live in tropical areas. India, for
example, reports more than 50,000 deaths annually from snakebites. Most of these victims
never reach the hospital (1).

---

* Correspondence: Richard R Roach, MD, FACP, Assistant Professor, Internal Medicine Department, Michigan
State University/ Kalamazoo Center for Medical Studies, 1000 Oakland Drive, Kalamazoo, Michigan 49008,
United States. E-mail: roach@ kcms.msu.edu

Children tend to come in contact with snakes during play and family activities, whereas adults usually come in contact with snakes during agricultural activity. Inamdar described a series of consecutive admissions for snakebites, 34% of which occurred in children under 15 years of age, two thirds of whom were boys (2). Other studies have shown similar ratios. Thus, venomous snakes are a major health problem for children living in tropical areas.

VENOMOUS SNAKES

There are three families of venomous snakes: Atractaspididae, Elapidae (which includes sea snakes), and Viperidae. Although the Colubridae family includes snakes that are mildly venomous, many of the snakes in this family are either too small or lack sufficient venom to be harmful to humans. Venomous snakes have one or more pairs of fangs in their upper jaws, which are enlarged teeth that have grooves or channels through which venom is injected when the victim is bitten. The fangs are found in different locations in different snakes so the mechanics of envenomation vary from snake to snake. Some snakes "spit" their venom in a spray at the victim's face or rhythmically across the facial plane seeking mucosa (eyes or mouth) for effective absorption. See table 1 for a geographic distribution of venomous snakes.

Table 1.

AREA	Venom Type	COMMON NAME
North America	Viperid Viperid Elapid	Rattlesnakes Copperheads/Cottonmouths Coral snakes
Central America	Viperid	Central American Rattlesnakes Terciopelos
South America	Viperid	Fer-De-Lance, Barba Amarillas Jararacas South American Rattlesnakes
Africa	Viperid Elapid Atractaspid	Saw-Scaled /Carpet Vipers Puff Adders African Spitting Cobras Egyptian Cobra Mole viper/ Burrowing Asp/ Stilettos
Asia, Middle East	Viperid Elapid Atractaspid	Saw-Scaled /Carpet Vipers Levantine Vipers Palestine Vipers Oxus Cobras Stilettos
Indian Sub Continent Southeast Asia	Elapid Viperid Elapid	Asian Cobras Kraits Russell's Vipers Malayan Pit Vipers Asian Cobras King Cobra

AREA	Venom Type	COMMON NAME
Far East Asia	Elapid	Asian Cobras
		Chinese Kraits
	Viperid	Japanese Habus
		Chinese Habus
		Mamushis
Australasia	Elapid	Death Adders
		Brown Snakes
		Tiger Snakes
		Taipans
Europe	Viperid	Vipers, Adders
		Long Nosed Vipers

Atractaspid: mole vipers, stiletto snakes and burrowing asps [many are too small to effectively bite humans

Elapidaes: cobras, kraits, mambas, Australian copperheads, sea snakes and coral snakes.

Viperidaes: vipers, rattlesnakes, copperheads/cottonmouths, adders and bushmasters.

Colubridaes: boomslangs, tree/vine/mangrove snakes [many are non-venomous].

Not all bites lead to envenomation. For reasons related to the mechanics of the jaw and venom apparatus, a snake may not be able to bite and envenomate a human victim as easily as its natural prey. A dry bite (i.e., a bite that does not envenomate the victim), often occurs if the snake is surprised or bites in self-defense. For many snakes, the first bite is the most potent, so if the snake bites another victim soon after, the second bite may not deliver any venom if the venom glands are depleted. Some snakes, however, are capable of multiple sequential toxic envenomations.

Venom composition

Snake venom is modified saliva (ninety percent water) but contains proteins, usually polypeptides that produce toxic, allergic or irritant effects when injected in or squirted on the victim. Venom of snakes considered "poisonous" contains enzymes, non-enzymatic polypeptide toxins, and biogenic amines. The composition varies by species, yet even within the same species, venom varies by age of the snake, geographical location, and season of the year. It may even vary depending on the snake's diet, since some venom incorporates toxins from frogs or other prey. All snake venoms, even those considered "non-poisonous", contain hyaluronidase, an enzyme which can cause local inflammation. Comments are now provided on these three venom components: enzymes, neurotoxins, and biogenic amines.

Enzymes

Enzymes in snake venom digest and denature amino acids, nucleotides, phospholipids, and even DNA. Eighty-nine to 95% of viperid and 25-70% of elapid venoms consist of hydrolases (i.e., proteinases, peptidases, phosphodiesterases, and phospholipases). The ubiquitous hyaluronidase disrupts tissue planes to spread the venom. Other proteins activate or inactivate the prey's homeostatic mechanisms.

Richard R Roach and Jishu Das

Elapid venom contains acetylcholinesterase, phospholipases B, phospholipases A_2 and glycerophosphatase which damage membranes of mitochondria, red blood cells and leucocytes. Under experimental conditions these enzymes damage peripheral nerve endings, skeletal muscle, and endothelium, resulting in pre-synaptic neurotoxicity and endorphin release. This toxicity explains the clinical neuropathy, encephalopathy, and myopathy.

In addition to the membrane digesting enzymes, viperid venom contains endopeptidases and kininogenases which affect the clotting system with thrombin-like serine proteases and activating enzymes of factor X and prothrombin. Endopeptidases and hydrolases cause edema, blistering, bruising, and necrosis. Metalloproteinases cause local and systemic hemorrhage in muscle.

Neurotoxins

Polypeptide toxins are almost exclusive to elapids and include α-bungarotoxin, and cobrotoxin which are α-neurotoxins and act post-synaptically, binding to $α_1$ component of nicotinic ACh receptors at the neuromuscular junction; this causes flaccid muscle paralysis. Death ensues from generalized bulbar or respiratory paralysis. β-neurotoxins such as β-bungarotoxin, crotoxin, and taipoxin target pre-synaptic nerve endings at the neuromuscular junction and act on the voltage gated potassium channels blocking acetylcholine release. This paralysis is reversible with the anticholinesterase blocker neostigmine.

Mamba venom has unusual neurotoxins. Its dendrotoxins bind to voltage gated potassium channels at nerve endings and cause acetylcholine release; in addition, calcicludine blocks calcium channels and fasciculins inhibit acetylcholinesterase causing persistent muscle fasciculations.

Krait venoms contain both pre-synaptic and post-synaptic neurotoxins as well as neurotoxic phospholipases, which attack the acetylcholine receptors in the brain and ganglia. Some neurotoxic phospholipases have direct myotoxicity.

Biogenic amines

Biogenic amines, such as histamine and serotonin, are most commonly found in viper venoms leading to local pain, swelling, and permeation of the venom. Biogenic amines also stimulate endogenous histamine release.

PATHOPHYSIOLOGY OF ENVENOMATION

Local injury

Snakebites cause minimal mechanical injury; however, the enzymes and biogenic amines cause local tissue inflammation, permeability, vascular injury, extravasation, thrombosis, and myonecrosis. Tissue swelling, local hemorrhage, and vascular injury cause ischemia, necrosis of skin, and sloughing of deep tissues. Amputation is the most important morbidity associated with survival, with approximately 5000-14,000 reported annually in Sub-Saharan Africa (3).

Local swelling develops rapidly after rattlesnake bites but may be delayed for 2-4 hours after other vipers and cytotoxic cobra bites.

Swelling then increases for two or three days but resolution may take months because of vascular and lymphatic damage. Regional lymphadenopathy follows the trauma and tissue necrosis. Tissue necrosis then provides an environment for superimposed infection. If swelling does not occur within 4 hours, the bite was dry, meaning that no envenomation occurred.

Systemic injury

Venoms of *Vipera berus, Daboia spp, Bothrops spp*, and the *Lachesis* species produce a reaction similar to anaphylaxis within minutes of a bite. This is mediated by biogenic amines: endogenous eicosanoids, angiotensins, kinins, nitric oxide, and endothelins. The venom of the *Bothrops* species releases angiotensin-converting enzyme inhibitors and oligopeptides that potentiate kinins.

This results in hypotension and shock secondary to capillary leakage and vasodilatation. Pulmonary edema and serous effusions develop in severe cases. Hemorrhage from venom induced-coagulopathy contributes to shock and hemorrhage in internal organs often parallels hemorrhage in the bitten limb.

Bleeding and clotting disturbances

Anti- hemostatic effects are a feature of envenoming by vipers, pit vipers, Australian elapids, and colubrids as a result of consumptive coagulopathy, thrombocytopenia, and vessel wall damage. Pro-coagulant enzymes in venoms of Colubridae, *Echis spp*, and Australian tiger snakes activate prothrombin. *Daboia* venom contains factor V and X activators, and many pit viper venoms have a direct thrombin-like effect on fibrinogen. Venom of rattlesnakes activates the endogenous fibrinolytic system. Phospholipases also have anticoagulant action.

Platelet dysfunction

Mocarhagin (Naja mossambica), jararaca (Bothrops jararaca) venoms contain metalloproteinases that cleave GPIbα and GPIa-IIa, inhibiting platelet endothelium interaction. *Rhodocetin (Calloselasma rhodostoma)* inhibits platelets via interaction with GPIa-IIa. Venom peptides such as trigramin and echistatin are powerful inhibitors of GPIIb-IIIa and impair platelet-fibrinogen interaction. Malayan and green pit viper venoms initially inhibit platelet agglutination and then activate clumping of platelets.

Complement activation and inhibition

Elapid and some colubrid venoms activate the alternative complement pathway. Cobra venoms have Cobra C3b. Viperid venoms activate the classic complement pathway. Mojave desert rattlesnakes and South Pacific rim rattlesnakes inactivate both pathways.

Intravascular hemolysis

Bothrops and Russell's vipers in India and Sri Lanka, some Australasian elapids, and members of Colubridae cause massive intravascular hemolysis leading to renal failure. Spontaneous systemic bleeding is attributable to hemorrhagins which damage vascular endothelium. Australian brown snake and *Bothrops* venoms cause hemolysis leading to severe anemia, hemoglobinuria and renal failure.

Rhabdomyolysis

Generalized rhabdomyolysis is an effect of phospholipase A_2 which is present in the venoms of most sea snakes, the terrestrial Australasian tiger snake, King Browns, Taipans, krait (Bungurus niger), several species of *Viperidae*, tropical rattlesnake, Mojave rattlesnake, and Sri Lankan Russell's viper. Rhabdomyolysis precipitates hyperkalemia resulting in muscle weakness. The muscle weakness maybe severe enough to cause respiratory paralysis; myoglobinuria, and acute tubular necrosis. The hyperkalemia, if severe, can cause cardiac arrhythmias.

Renal failure

Renal failure is a common complication of Russell's viper, tropical rattlesnake, and sea snake envenomation. However, it may occur with mild envenomation by *Vipera berus* and hump-nosed viper because acute tubular necrosis results from the direct toxic effect of the venom on the renal tubule. Hemoglobinuria, myoglobinuria, hyperkalemia, disseminated intravascular coagulation (DIC), and shock all contribute to renal insult. Histopathology varies from proliferative glomerulonephritis to toxic mesangiolysis with platelet aggregation. Fibrin deposition, ischemic changes, tubular necrosis, and renal cortical necrosis all occur. Renal failure is the main cause of the late deaths (4).

Neurotoxicity

Paralytic symptoms are characteristic of envenomation by elapids such as cobras, kraits, coral snakes, mambas, terrestrial Australian snakes, sea snakes, Sri Lankan Russell's vipers, and a few other species of Viperidae in China,. Severe muscle paralysis leads to respiratory failure and upper airway obstruction. Respiratory paralysis may last as long as 10 weeks. Some patients become pathologically drowsy due to endorphin release triggered by elapid or viper venom. The African spitting cobras, in contrast to other elapids, do not cause neurotoxicity.

Death

Death can occur as rapidly as a few minutes after a King Cobra bite. With most elapid bites, death occurs within hours and most sea snakes' bites cause death within 12 to 24 hours. Viper bites usually kill within days. Initial mortality is caused by neuromuscular paralysis and necrosis. Later mortality is related to coagulopathy and hemorrhage. Late death is related to renal failure and secondary infection.

DISTINCTIVE CLINICAL FEATURES

The clinician's task, i.e., to identify the exact species of snake and thereby know the specific venom constituents, is often impossible. Snakebites typically occur in inconspicuous situations: snakes bite in the dark, when tread upon, when accidentally handled, in rice fields, underwater or in dense foliage, then, they retreat quickly so they are difficult to identify. Bite marks are not characteristic of any snake. Geographical as well as seasonal prevalence and previous sightings provide the best speculation of the snake species involved.

In places where a single venomous species is prevalent or the snake has peculiar characteristics, it is easier to identify the specific snake and to characterize the venom toxicity.

Since symptoms vary with venom composition, close observation may determine the species of the snake or at least the toxin type. Often the patient or an accompanying person kills the snake and brings it to the health care facility. Proper identification can categorize the venom and expected toxicity. At times the snake is brought to the clinician alive.

Curious local customs sometimes dictate that the killed snake should be used as a tourniquet around the bitten limb. The physician and care providers should be aware that a dead snake may still envenomate if the glands reflexively contract during examination.

ATRACTASPIDS

Stiletto snakes, mole vipers, and asps have venom that is primarily cytotoxic and causes severe local swelling as well as tissue necrosis. They cause high morbidity but low mortality (5). Tissue necrosis can lead to myoglobin in serum as well as urine and hyperkalemia; thus, careful attention to renal function is important. Compartment syndrome and amputation are also common.

ELAPIDS

Local injury

Asian Cobras and African Spitting Cobras cause extensive local injury at the site of the bite. Painful swelling leads to extensive loss of skin and subcutaneous tissue. Blistering surrounds a demarcated pale or blackened anesthetic area of skin. Regional lymph nodes swell and in extreme cases, gangrene develops. King cobra bites cause severe swelling and bullae formation but no necrosis. Kraits, mambas, coral snakes, sea snakes, and Australasian elapids cause minimal local injury.

Neurotoxic effects

Descending flaccid paralysis is characteristic of patients bitten by Asian cobras, king cobras, and most other elapids, but not African Spitting Cobras. The earliest symptom of systemic envenoming is uncontrolled vomiting but this clinical feature can be obscured by the use of emetics or local traditional herbs. Early pre-paralytic symptoms include contraction of the frontalis muscle, followed by ptosis, blurred vision, peri-oral paresthesia, loss of smell as well as taste, headache, dizziness, and vertigo. Autonomic hyper-stimulation manifests as hypersalivation and pilo-erection.

Paralysis is first detectable as ptosis and external opthalmoplegia, which occurs as rapidly as 15 minutes after the bite of cobras and mambas; however, this is delayed by as much as 10 hours following krait bites. Later, facial muscles, palette, jaws, vocal cords, neck muscles, and muscles of deglutition become paralyzed. Respiratory arrest occurs from paralysis of the upper airway muscles, intercostals, and diaphragm. Patients become drowsy from endorphin release.

Neurotoxic effects are completely reversible in response to antivenom for Asian Cobras, South American Coral snakes, and Australian Death Adders. The paralysis may respond to anticholinesterases even if snake- specific antivenom is not available. Even without appropriate antivenom, paralysis dissipates in 1 to 4 days sufficiently for the patient to breathe adequately. Ocular muscles recover in 2 to 4 days and full recovery of motor function typically occurs in 3 to 7 days.

AUSTRALIAN ELAPIDS

Australian elapids include those found in Australia as well as the surrounding countries of Southeast Asia. Their bites cause mild local injury and lymphadenopathy but severe rhabdomyolysis and hemostatic disturbances have been reported. Early symptoms include vomiting, headache, and syncopal attacks. Electrocardiographic changes are common in taipan bites in Papua New Guinea but do not cause much myocardial injury as evident by minimal rise in cardiac enzymes. Persistent bleeding from wounds and spontaneous systemic bleeding from the gums and the gastrointestinal tract occurs due to coagulopathy following bites by many Australian species. Hemostatic abnormalities are common and serious in patients bitten by tiger snakes, taipans, and brown snakes but are rare with death adders or black snakes. Hemoglobinuria and myoglobinuria can cause renal failure.

SEA SNAKES

Bites are painless and may not be noticed at the time of the bite, but the teeth may be left in the wound. Sea snake bites cause minimal local inflammation as generalized rhabdomyolysis is the dominant effect. Early symptoms include headache, a thick feeling of the tongue, thirst, sweating, and vomiting. Generalized aching, stiffness, and tenderness of the muscles occur between 30 minutes to 4 hours after the bite. Trismus is common and passive muscle stretching is painful. Progressive flaccid paralysis starts with ptosis and respiratory failure follows. Myoglobin in serum and urine are seen 3 to 8 hours after the bite.

SPITTING ELAPIDS

Venoms of spitting Cobras are intensely irritating and cause cell destruction on contact with mucous membranes or conjunctiva. Spitting elapid bites cause intense local pain, blepharospasm, and palpebral edema. Corneal erosions from the toxicity of the venom can lead to blindness in addition to secondary infection from anaerobic bacteria in the snake's saliva. However, coagulation, platelet effects, and hepatic pathology contribute to mortality and morbidity (6).

VIPERS

Local injury

Venoms of vipers and pit vipers cause intense local reaction. Absence of detectable local swelling two hours after a viper bite means that no venom was injected, since swelling generally appears within 15 minutes and spreads rapidly involving the whole limb and the adjacent trunk. Intense pain results and persistent bleeding from the fang marks occurs. The swollen limb third-spaces liters of extravasated blood and serum leading to hypovolemic shock. Blisters occur within 12 hours and contain bloody fluid. Necrosis of skin, soft tissue, and muscles develops in 10% of hospitalized patients. Compartment syndrome compromises limb integrity as vessels thrombose and cause subsequent gangrene. Myanmar Russell's vipers and tropical rattlesnakes are exceptions in that they cause severe systemic effects with minimal local response.

Hemostasis

Hemostatic abnormalities are characteristic of viper venom, though this is not true for smaller European varieties while some rattlesnakes and coagulation abnormalities rarely occur with *Bothrops* envenomation. Coagulopathy is due to the disseminated intravascular coagulation, fibrinolysis, and coagulation factor inactivation. It manifests as persistent bleeding from the fang site, spontaneous hemorrhage into skin, nasal as well as oral mucosa and conjunctiva followed by systemic bleeding of gastrointestinal and genitourinary tracts. Intracranial bleeding rarely occurs. Earliest bleeding occurs from the gingiva. Russell's viper and *Bothrops* bites may cause bleeding into the pituitary gland leading to pituitary insufficiency and secondary adrenal insufficiency. Retro- and intraperitoneal hemorrhage cause enough blood loss to precipitate shock. Arterial thrombosis is characteristic of bites from the Fer de lance of Martinique and *Bothrops caribbaeus* of St Lucia. Spontaneous systemic bleeding is also due to hemorrhage of the endothelium.

Intravascular hemolysis

Indian and Sri Lankan Russell's viper and South American *Bothrops* species cause intravascular hemolysis. Patients present with hemoglobinuria, anemia, and renal failure.

Circulatory shock

Hypotension and shock are the serious venom effects of old world vipers such as Russell's viper, *Daboia palastinae*, *Bitis gabonica*, and North American rattlesnakes.

The mechanism involves an anaphylaxis-like reaction, increased capillary permeability, and external and internal hemorrhage. Some viper bites cause toxin induced bradycardia and other arrhythmias (7-9). However, toxins from various snakes have failed to show direct cardiac muscle toxicity although animal studies have demonstrated decreased contractility and toxin induced pulmonary artery hypertension. Repeated and transient syncope is related to neurologic toxicity. Vomiting, colic, diarrhea, bronchospasm, urticaria, and angioedema may occur as early as 5 minutes or as late as several hours after the bite.

Renal failure

Renal failure can occur from envenomation by any venomous snake but is the most common cause of death in victims of Russell's viper, tropical rattlesnakes, and some species of Bothrops. Back pain and tenderness experienced within the first 24 hours progresses to acute renal failure in 3 to 4 days. The mechanisms of renal failure include direct glomerular or tubular toxicity, myoglobinuria, and renal failure from shock and hemorrhage. Mortality from renal failure in some series is 32% and two-thirds of survivors still had renal impairment at ten year follow-up (10).

Neurotoxicity

Neurotoxicity is most common with elapid envenomation because of oligopeptides. Sri Lankan Russell's viper, *Vipera aspis*, and *Bitis atropos* (puff adder) venoms contain neurotoxic phospholipases A_2 that cause generalized paralysis and respiratory failure similar to elapid venom. Pupillary dilatation is a feature of tropical rattlesnakes and small *Bitis* species. Severe envenoming by Mojave rattlesnakes causes weakness and fasciculations involving muscles enervated by cranial nerves. This manifests as ptosis, diplopia, dysphagia, dysphonia, and respiratory failure.

LABORATORY INVESTIGATION

Systemic envenoming is usually associated with leukocytosis. Hematocrit increases from capillary leakage but later falls due to hemolysis; in addition, thrombocytopenia is common. Non-coagulable blood is a cardinal sign of systemic envenomation by Viperidae, many of the Australasian elapids, and venomous Colubridae. A bedside clinical test for coagulation is adequate: a few milliliters of blood taken by venipuncture in a glass vial and left to stand for 20 minutes is then tilted to look for clotting. If it has not clotted, there is significant coagulation dysfunction.

Prothrombin time [PT], activated patial thromboplastin time [PTT], fibrin degradation products, and D-dimer tests are more precise if available where the patient presents. Creatinine kinase rises dramatically with rhabdomyolysis from Sri Lankan Russell's viper, sea snake, tropical rattlesnake, and Australian elapid bites. Myoglobin is present in the plasma if a spun specimen is pink. Hemoglobinuria manifests as black urine, and myoglobinuria manifests as brown urine. Increased blood urea nitrogen (BUN), increased creatinine, and metabolic acidosis define the degree of renal failure. Patients with severe neurotoxicity, generalized paralysis, and respiratory failure develop respiratory acidosis.

Chest radiographs may reveal evidence of pulmonary edema. The electrocardiographic abnormalities include sinus bradycardia, ST-T changes, and various degrees of conduction block in addition to effects of hyperkalemia.

IMMUNODIAGNOSIS

Enzyme immunoassay (EIA) is a rapid and sensitive test to accurately diagnose snake envenomation and is specific to snake species; however, it does not distinguish between past and present venom exposure. False-positive EIA is common in rural tropical populations. The sensitivity increases if it is performed on swabs or aspirates from the wound. Results are available within 15 to 30 minutes. Unfortunately availability and cost clearly limit their practical application. Commercial venom detection kits are available only in Australia.

MANAGEMENT OF SNAKE BITES

First aid

Several studies have demonstrated that first aid should never interfere with transporting the victim to a health care facility. In Papua New Guinea the main cause of mortality is the country's lack of roads, which limits access to medical care. In addition, morbidity is increased with more frequent amputation, tissue necrosis, and secondary infection (11). Once transport is arranged the following measures are recommended:

1. Reassure the victim as their distress causes increased heart rate and blood pressure, which increases venom systemic circulation. In addition, a thorn prick, a rodent bite or a dry bite, which are more benign, may be the actual injury.
2. Immobilize the limb, and keep the victim still because movement increases venom dissemination.
3. Do not tamper with the wound. Incision of the wound followed by suction is commonly taught and practiced, but multiple studies have shown increased damage to nerves, blood vessels, and tissues without any benefit. Introduction of infection causes unnecessary loss of limb and tissue. Cauterization, instillation of chemicals like potassium permanganate, application of "venom-ex" vacuum apparatus, and tight tourniquets are useless and harmful.
4. Pressure immobilization is a judicious form of tourniquet and has been advocated in Australia. This involves application of bandages with sufficient pressure to occlude venous and lymphatic flow without compromising arterial supply. Pressure should not cause ischemic pain. A traditional tight tourniquet causes ischemic injury, compartment syndrome, and loss of limb (12). One study reported from Myanmar

showed application of a foam rubber pad directly over a bite wound delays systemic envenoming (13). Preliminary trials suggest possible benefit with no increased morbidity.

5. Pain is intense in viper bites and one can treat with paracetamol/acetaminophen or opioids. NSAIDs should not be used because they increase the hemostatic abnormalities of the venom.

6. Vomiting is a common early systemic symptom and can be treated with anti-emetics.

7. Syncope due to vagal hyper-stimulation is common. Keep the patient prone. Hypotension due to anaphylaxis should be treated with epinephrine followed by an H_1 blocker.

8. Airway protection and ventilatory support with endotracheal intubation may be needed. Ambu bag ventilation should be used for patients with respiratory compromise.

9. If the snake has been "killed", make sure that it is definitely dead before transporting it to the health care facility for species identification. Do not touch the head of the snake, because passive bites from dead snakes can still envenomate.

TREATMENT AT THE HEALTH CARE FACILITY

Initial assessment and resuscitation of the patient should be started immediately. Unfortunately most snake bites occur in rural areas, while medical facilities capable of managing the complex problems are located in urban areas.

One study demonstrated that a nurse-run clinic with personnel knowledgeable of appropriate treatment is effective at decreasing morbidity and mortality (14). If the snake accompanies the patient, identification should be attempted. If the snake is identified as non-venomous and the patient shows no signs of venom toxicity, the patient may be discharged after local wound care and tetanus toxoid injection.

Management of envenomated patients involves administration of appropriate antivenom if the snake can be identified or if geography dictates a specific prevalence.

Attention should be directed to specific venom toxicity and administration should focus on systemic effects of the venom, not the local effects (15). Various studies have shown that only a minority of snake bite patients require antivenom (16). Antivenom is often in short supply and specific antivenom for all snakes is not available (17) (see table 2).

It is very important to use appropriate antivenom because use of the wrong antivenom is not only useless but can be hazardous (18). Antivenom is derived from horse serum and is relatively contraindicated in patients allergic to horse serum. Even without a history of reaction, as many as 10% of patients may develop serum sickness.

Table 2.

COMMON NAME	ANTIVENOM	MANUFACTURER	INITIAL DOSE
Death Adder	Monovalent	CSL	3000-6000 units
Puff Adder	Polyvalent	Sanofi-Pasteur SAVP	80 ml
Jararaca	Bothrops Polyvalent	Brazil	20 ml
Common Krait	Polyvalent ASVS	Bharat Serum	100 ml

COMMON NAME	ANTIVENOM	MANUFACTURER	INITIAL DOSE
Malayan Pit Viper	Monovalent	Thai Red Cross	100 ml
Russells's Viper	Polyvalent ASVS	India	100 ml
	Monovalent	Myanmar	40 ml
		Thailand	50 ml
Indian Cobra	Polyvalent ASVS	India	100 ml
Saw-Scaled Viper	Polyvalent ASVS	India	100 ml
Carpet Viper	Monovalent	Sanofi-Pasteur	100 ml
	Monovalent	SAVP	20 ml
Thai Cobra	Monovalent	Thai Red Cross	100 ml
Green Pit Viper	Monovalent,	Thai Red Cross	100 ml
Sea Snakes	Monovalent	CSL	1000 units
Tiger Snake	Monovalent	CSL	3000-6000 units
Taipan	Monovalent,	CSL	12,000 units
E. Diamondback W. Diamondback W.Rattlesnakes	Co-Fab	Protherics	7-15 vials
Palestine Viper	Monovalent	RMRI	50-80 ml

CSL=Commonwealth Serum Laboratories, Australia.
ASVS= Polyvalent Anti Snake Venom Serum.
SAVP=South African Vaccine Producers.
RMRI=Rogoff Medical Research Institute, Tel Aviv.

Table Indications for antivenom

1. Neurotoxicity manifested by paralysis and fasciculations.   2. Haemostatic abnormalities including DIC and other coagulopathies.   3. Cardiovascular abnormalities including cardiac arrhythmia and conduction disorder.   4. Generalized rhabdomyolysis   5. Severe local envenoming: extensive blistering / bruising of the affected limb   6. Rapid spread of local swelling.

In life-threatening cases, patients who are allergic to horse serum and have severe systemic envenomation, may be given antivenom after pretreatment with intramuscular 0.01% epinephrine injection, an H_1 blocker, and corticosteroid injections. Rapid desensitization is not recommended.

Antivenoms are monovalent or polyvalent depending on whether they contain antibodies to venom of one or more species. When the snake is accurately identified, monovalent antivenom should be used if it is available. In India, monovalent antivenom is not available, and the available antivenom contains antibodies to the most common venomous snakes including cobra (*Naja naja*), common krait (*Bungarus ceruleans*), Russell's viper (*Vipera russelii*), and saw scaled viper (*Echis carinatus*). If the polyvalent antivenom does not address the snake involved, administration of polyvalent antivenom is useless and hazardous.

Antivenom is generally a lyophilized powder, which is reconstituted and given intravenously as a bolus or infusion. Intramuscular injection is acceptable but not as effective if intravenous access is not possible. Local infiltration into the bite wound is not helpful. Antivenom should be given as early as possible but can be given as long as systemic signs persist. These signs can persist for 2 days for sea snake bites to days or weeks in cases of prolonged defibrination from viper bites. Local effects of the bite are only reversible if antivenom is given early. The dose depends upon the preparation (See Table 2). The dose for children is usually the same as for adults, but some children require more than the adult dose to treat the systemic effects. Large doses are required for bites by king cobra, black mambas, and diamondback rattlesnakes since these snakes inject large volumes of venom.

Neurotoxic signs may improve within 30 minutes of antivenom administration but generally require hours to subside. Hypotension, sinus bradycardia, and spontaneous systemic bleeding respond within 10 to 20 minutes. Blood coagulability is usually restored within 1 to 6 hours provided that sufficient antivenom is given and coagulation factors, synthesized by the liver, return to normal. Coagulation function can be monitored by performing the 20 min whole blood clotting test, previously described, every six hours if more sophisticated testing is not available.

The half-life of antivenom ranges from 26 to 95 hours depending on which IgG fragment it contains. Preparations containing Fab fragments only are short lived. Following antiserum administration and initial reversal, re-envenomation may occur due to clearance of antivenom and continued release of venom from the wound into the circulation. The initial positive response to antivenom determines the need for further doses. A second dose should be given if shock persists for more than 30 min and if coagulation defects persist for more than six hours.

Early antivenom reactions are complement mediated and cannot be predicted by hypersensitivity skin tests. Reactions develop between 10 minutes to 2 hours and are characterized by itching, urticaria, fever, tachycardia, palpitations, nausea, vomiting, bronchospasm, and angioedema. These are difficult to identify as they can be mistaken for effects of the venom. Isolated fever is due to presence of endotoxin-like compounds in the antiserum. Late serum sickness reactions develop approximately 7 days after treatment and include: fever, itching, urticaria, arthralgia, arthritis, albuminuria, and rarely, encephalopathy. Symptomatic treatment is appropriate.

SUPPORTIVE TREATMENT

Neuromuscular paralysis and respiratory failure are common causes of early mortality. Antivenom does not reverse bulbar and respiratory paralysis. Anticholinesterase drugs, such as neostigmine, can be useful in this regard (19). Before starting neostigmine, assess the therapeutic benefit by performing a "Tensilon test". Tensilon (edrophonium) is administered and the patient is observed for improvement. If there is improvement, neostigmine can be used for maintenance at the dose of 0.5 to 2.5 mg every 1 to 3 hours. This is not standard practice and mechanical ventilation may still be needed to prevent respiratory failure from neuromuscular paralysis. Respiratory failure also occurs from toxin-induced pulmonary hypertension and pulmonary cellular membrane damage.

Shock should be treated aggressively. Copious fluid resuscitation and vasopressors are often required immediately, even though pulmonary edema may result later in the clinical course due to pulmonary tissue damage and re-absorption of the fluid, complicated by compromised renal function. If renal failure results from rhabdomyolysis treatment should include bicarbonate intravenous infusion. Severe renal failure compounded by electrolyte abnormalities and pulmonary edema may require dialysis.

Hemostatic abnormalities, platelet dysfunction, and clotting abnormalities respond to antivenom. Replacement of clotting factors or platelets may be needed if hepatic function is compromised. Severe anemia from hemolysis may require transfusions.

The use of steroids is controversial, and studies with green pit vipers, demonstrated no benefit. Steroids were hypothesized to limit the inflammatory component of limb edema, but blinded, placebo controlled trials in Thailand showed no objective improvement (20).

LOCAL WOUND CARE

A booster dose of tetanus toxoid should be given in order to prevent subsequent tetanus. Prophylactic antibiotics are not indicated in attempts to prevent local infection; however, if the wound becomes infected, antibiotic should be directed against the bacterial flora of the snake's buccal cavity, which is generally anaerobic. Blisters should not be lanced and wounds should be aseptically dressed to prevent nosocomial infection.

Snake bites are at risk for developing compartmental syndrome in the affected limb which can lead to amputation. A fasciotomy early in the clinical course can save the limb, but this requires frequent assessment of limb musculature and compartment pressure and then appropriate surgical intervention.

For snake venom exposure to eyes, wash immediately. The African spitting cobra (*naja nigricollis*) venom causes severe pain and may lead to edema, conjunctivitis, and corneal erosions. Antivenom directly into the eye has been reported to resolve the pain (21), but local anesthesia is also effective. Antibiotic ointments have been recommended but there are no clinical trials to support their use. Ciliary spasm can be treated with local topical cycloplegics, but steroids are contraindicated (22). Antihistamines may be of some value while atropine eye drops treat the blepharospasm. In a rabbit model, heparin was effective at preventing corneal scarring, while tetracycline and steroids worsened the results (23).

CONCLUSION

Snakebites in children are common and not well recognized for the profound annual mortality and morbidity they cause. The lack of available medical care in rural areas, where most snakebites occur, is a major health problem. Specific antivenoms are extremely valuable but much can be done to prevent unnecessary mortality and morbidity even without antivenom. Increased understanding of proper first aid procedures has put to rest a number of useless and dangerous practices that often delay transport to proper medical care. In developing countries, lack of roads continues to be the single greatest infrastructural impairment to saving children's lives.

REFERENCES

[1]   Bawaskar HS. Profile of snakebite envenoming in rural Maharashtra, India. J Assoc Physicians India 2008;56: 88-95.

[2]   Inamdar F. Snakebite: Admissions at a tertiary health care centre in Maharashtra, India. S Afr Med J 2010;100(7):456-8.

[3]   Chippaux JP. Estimate of the burden of snakebites in sub-Saharan Africa: a meta-analytic approach. Toxicon 2011;57(4): 586-99.

[4]   Athappan G. Acute renal failure in snake envenomation: a large prospective study. Saudi J Kidney Dis Transplant 2008;19(3):404-10.

[5]   Leisewitz AL. The diagnosis and management of snakebite in dogs--a southern African perspective. J S Afr Vet Assoc 2004;75(1): 7-13.

[6]   Warrell DA. Necrosis, haemorrhage and complement depletion following bites by the spitting cobra (Naja nigricollis). Q J Med 1976;45:1-22.

[7]   Marsh NA, Whaler BC, The Gaboon viper (Bitis gabonica): its biology, venom components and toxinology. Toxicon 1984;22(5):669-94.

[8]   Tibballs J. Cardiovascular, haematological and neurological effects of the venom of the Papua New Guinean small-eyed snake (Micropechis ikaheka) and their neutralisation with CSL polyvalent and black snake antivenoms. Toxicon 2003; 42(6):647-55.

[9]   Lalloo DG. Electrocardiographic abnormalities in patients bitten by taipans (Oxyuranus scutellatus canni) and other elapid snakes in Papua New Guinea. Trans R Soc Trop Med Hyg 1997;91(1): 53-6.

[10]   Sinha R. Ten-year follow-up of children after acute renal failure from a developing country. Nephrol Dial Transplant 2009;24(3): 829-33.

[11]   Michael GC, Thacher TD, Shehu MI, The effect of pre-hospital care for venomous snake bite on outcome in Nigeria. Trans R Soc Trop Med Hyg 2011; 105(2): 95-101.

[12]   Bandyopadhyay SK. Prognostic factors in haemotoxic viper bite: analysis of data from a referral hospital. J Indian Med Assoc 2009;107(1):12-3.

[13]   Pe T. Field trial of efficacy of local compression immobilization first-aid technique in Russell's viper (Daboia russelii siamensis) bite patients. Southeast Asian J Trop Med Public Health 2000;31(2): 346-8.

[14]   Yates VM. Management of snakebites by the staff of a rural clinic: the impact of providing free antivenom in a nurse-led clinic in Meserani, Tanzania. Ann Trop Med Parasitol 2010;104(5):439-48.

[15]   Warrell DA. Researching nature's venoms and poisons. Trans R Soc Trop Med Hyg 2009;103(9):860-6.

[16]   Campbell BT. Pediatric snakebites: lessons learned from 114 cases. J Pediatr Surg 2008;43(7):1338-41.

[17]   Casewell NR. Pre-clinical assays predict pan-African Echis viper efficacy for a species-specific antivenom. PLoS Negl Trop Dis 2010;4(10):e851.

[18]   Warrell DA. Unscrupulous marketing of snake bite antivenoms in Africa and Papua New Guinea: choosing the right product--'what's in a name?' Trans R Soc Trop Med Hyg 2008;102(5):397-9.

[19]   Watt G. Positive response to edrophonium in patients with neurotoxic envenoming by cobras (Naja naja philippinensis). A placebo-controlled study. N Engl J Med 1986;315(23):1444-8.

[20]   Nuchprayoon I, Pongpan CN, Sripaiboonkij N. The role of prednisolone in reducing limb oedema in children bitten by green pit vipers: a randomized, controlled trial. Ann Trop Med Parasitol 2008;102(7):643-9.

[21]   Fung HT. Local antivenom treatment for ophthalmic injuries caused by a Naja atra. J Med Toxicol 2003;6(2):147-9.

[22]   Chu ER.. Venom ophthalmia caused by venoms of spitting elapid and other snakes: Report of ten cases with review of epidemiology, clinical features, pathophysiology and management. Toxicon. 2011;56(3):259-72.

[23]   Cham G. Effects of topical heparin, antivenom, tetracycline and dexamethasone treatment in corneal injury resulting from the venom of the black

[24]   spitting cobra (Naja sumatrana), in a rabbit model. Clin Toxicol (Phila) 2006; 44(3):287-92.

Submitted: September 04, 2011. *Revised:* November 02, 2011. *Accepted:* November 11, 2011.

In: Public Health Yearbook 2012
Editor: Joav Merrick

ISBN: 978-1-62808-078-0
© 2013 Nova Science Publishers, Inc.

Chapter 18

CHAGAS DISEASE

Richard R Roach, MD, FACP and Joanne Monterroso, MD*

Internal Medicine Department, Michigan State University/Kalamazoo Center for Medical Studies, Kalamazoo, Michigan, United States of America

ABSTRACT

Although Chagas disease only infects children in the American hemisphere, and though children do not suffer the morbidity and mortality of the disease, it is a disease of children. The acute form of the infection, though self-limited, is a harbinger of the most common cause of heart failure in the world. The treatment has moderate benefit and thus, identifying the infection in children and preventing the disease has a profound impact on the goal of reducing some of the millions of deaths from heart failure.

Keywords: Public health, tropical medicine, Dengue virus infection

INTRODUCTION

Although Carlos Chagas first described the disease that carries his name in 1909, there is still no cure. Recently there has been an increased interest in the condition because globalization has made it an emergent health problem in non endemic areas (1-4). Although the common disabling symptom complexes occur in adults, primary infection usually occurs in children. Without solving childhood infection, adult morbidity and mortality will never be resolved.

ETIOLOGY

Chagas disease is caused by the protozoan parasite *Trypanosoma cruzi*., whose genome parasite was described in 2005. The life cycle of T cruzi is complex. A triatomine bug takes

---

* Correspondence: Richard R Roach, MD, FACP, Internal Medicine Department, 1000 Oakland Drive, Kalamazoo, Michigan 49008 United States. E-mail: roach@ kcms.msu.edu

blood from an infected source (a human with chronic Chagas disease, for example) and ingests trypomastigotes, which transform into epigmastigoes and replicate by binary fission in the insect's midgut. The epimastigotes migrate to the hindgut as well as rectum and differentiate into metacylic trypomastigotes; they are then released by defecation onto the skin of a mammalian host. The metacyclic trypomastigotes enter the host through the host's rubbing or scratching the bite wound or by contamining mucosal or conjunctival tissues. Trypomastigotes are recruited and fused with lysosomes to penetrate local cells and differentiate into amastigotes, which replicate by binary fission and then transform into trypomastigotes. [1-4].

TRANSMISSION

Chagas disease is transmitted to humans by large blood sucking reduviid bugs of the subfamily Triatominae. The most important *T cruzi* vectors in the transmission to man are *Triatoma infestans*, *Rhodnius prolixus*, and *Triatoma dimidiata*. (1). Other documented forms of transmission are blood transfusion, vertically transmission from mother to infant (5), and organ or bone marrow transplantation (6-8).

The risk of acquiring Chagas disease by blood transfusion from an infected donor depends on the concentration of parasites in the blood product, the blood component transfused, and the parasite strain. Blood transfusions carry a transmission risk of approximately 10 to 20% depending on the parasite load. The risk appears to be higher with transfusion of platelets (2).

Vertical transmission from chronically infected women studied in endemic areas of South America occurs in 5% of pregnancies (1,2). Several investigators describe the prevalence of mother to child transmission in endemic areas to be the same as in non-endemic areas where the child has no environmental risk (2,5,9).

According to Buekens, in 2008, there were 944,993 Hispanic live births per year to an estimated 3,780 seropositive mothers in the United States; assuming a 0.4% seropositivity, there is thus an estimated 189 newborns who were infected, based on a 5% mother to child transmission rate (5). Verani estimated that there are 300 congenital infections annually in the United States (10).

PATHOGENESIS

Chagas disease is caused by the parasite and by the host immune-inflammatory response. Rodriguez describes several determinant factors of disease such as the quantity of parasites in the initial infection, infective forms in the initial inoculation, lineage of inoculated *T cruzi* (Tcl-TcVI), re-infection, quality of the strains and clones, specific clonal histotropic receptors of the host, and the patient's initial immune response (11). The detailed biological interactions between *T cruzi* and its host have been extensively described in recent articles but go beyond the scope of this discussion (1,12).

The parasites deposited in the skin of the host create a local inflammatory reaction, specifically a lymphoreticular response. Clinically this is described as the Romana's sign or inoculation Chagoma (1). Trypomastigotes are taken up by macrophages and circulate to the liver, spleen, ganglia, and muscles, where they form pseudocysts of amastigotes. The parasite creates an immune response led by T-helper 1 and both CD4 and CD8 cells. The immune response leads to production of interferon γ, tumor necrosis factor α and interleukin 12, and an inflammatory reaction that causes cell destruction. The balance between the immune mediated parasite containment and inflammation determines the course of the disease. In chronic Chagas heart disease there is a depressed T cell response (1,2,11).

EPIDEMIOLOGY

Chagas disease was originally confined to Latin-American countries in areas where poverty encouraged transmission from the vector to human. In the past 20 years there has been improved vector control in Latin America which has reduced the burden of Chagas disease (2).

According the World Health Organization's (WHO) epidemiological record published in 2010, there are 10 million people infected with *T cruzi* worldwide, mostly in Latin America (13).

Latin American countries with high prevalence include Argentina, Bolivia, Brazil, Chile, Colombia, Costa Rica, Ecuador, El Salvador, Honduras, Mexico, Paraguay, Panama, Peru, Uruguay, Venezuela, and Guatemala (14). Some authors group the epidemiological characteristics of Chagas disease in 5 sets of countries (11). Mocayo reported that the incidence of Chagas disease has decreased from 700,000 to 800,000 new cases per year in 1991 to 41,200 in 2006. The annual death toll has fallen from more than 45,000 to 12,500 (14).

The transmission of Chagas disease by the main domiciliary vector *T infestans,* was halted in Uruguay in 1997, Chile in 1999, Brazil in 2006, and in Guatemala in 2009 (1,2)

The vector has been eliminated in parts of Argentina and Paraguay (1). However, due to an influx of immigrants from endemic countries, Chagas disease has become an important health issue for countries such as the United States, Canada, Spain, France, Switzerland, Japan, some Asian countries, and Australia (2,11,15).

The estimated number of cases imported into the United States in 2006 was 30,000 to 300,000 (1). The prevalence of *T. cruzi* antibodies in blood donors in the United States is about 1 in 27,800 with the prevalence varying depending on the location. In Los Angeles, for example, the prevalence of antibodies in donors has increased to 1 in each 2000 blood donations (1,16). However, there have been only seven reported cases of post transfusion transmission in the United States as well as Canada and five cases of transmission through organ transplantation (1).

Regulations in countries where the disease is endemic require analyzing blood donations for *T.cruzi* antibodies. In 2006 the ELISA screening test for *T.cruzi* was approved by the United States Food and Drug Administration (US FDA)

Since January 2007 both the American Red Cross and Blood Systems, Inc., together responsible for approximately 65% of the American blood supply began screening all blood donations for *T. cruzi*.

CLINICAL MANIFESTATIONS

The clinical manifestations of Chagas disease can be described according the phase (acute or chronic) of the natural history of the disease.

Acute Chagas disease

Acute infection is asymptomatic in most individuals secondary to a low parasitic load. A minority of patients develop fever, malaise, splenomegaly, hepatomegaly, lymphadenopathy, edema, morbiliform rash or diarrhea. Vector transmission leaves signs at the portal of entry such an indurated erythematous skin lesion (i.e., Chagoma) and a painless unilateral bipalpebral edema (i.e., Romana sign). Severe forms of the initial disease can present with myocarditis and meningoencephalitis (1,2). Diagnostic testing is reviewed for acute disease in Table 1.

Table 1. Diagnostic testing in acute Chagas disease

Laboratory Results	Imaging	EKG	Other
Normo- or microcytic anemia Elevated AST, ALT Hypergammaglobulinemia Proteinuria	CXR:cardiomegaly Echocardiogram: dysfunctional ventricle.	Sinus tachycardia 1° AV block Low QRS voltage T wave changes.	Parasite by Giemsa stained thick/thin blood film Microhematocrit PCR Indirect methods: xenodiagnosis, blood culture

AST= aspartate aminotransferase.
ALT = alanine aminotransferase.
CXR= chest x ray.
AV = atrioventricular.
PCR= polymerase chain reaction.

Congenital Chagas disease

Symptoms manifested at birth or weeks after delivery of the infected infant include hypotonicity, fever, hepatosplenomegaly, anemia, prematurity, low birthweight, jaundice, and low Apgar score. Life threatening presentations include myocarditis, meningoencephalitis, and pneumonitis. Only 10 to 30% of infected newborns have symptoms and 10% will die within 2 days if not treated. The severity of congenital infection correlates with neonatal and maternal parasitemia as well as maternal re-infection. *In utero*, infections manifest as abortion and neonatal death. The best diagnostic test is microhematocrit from cord blood. Peripheral blood is diagnostic if taken from 2 or more samples in the first month of life. If negative IgG serology is diagnostic at 6 to 9 months of age. Other diagnostic methods include polymerase chain reaction analysis (PCR) (1,2).

Chronic Chagas disease

Clinical manifestations of chronic Chagas disease appear 5 to 15 years after initial infection. The percentage of infected hosts that remain asymptomatic varies from 40% to 90% depending on the region. Despite lack of symptoms, infected people have positive serologic reactions, xenodiagnosis, and a positive PCR (11). The clinical manifestations appear in organs such as the heart or gastrointestinal tract. There are subpopulations at increased risk, such as patients who have undergone transplantation or have HIV/AIDS and these subpopulations have characteristic manifestations of Chagas disease.

Cardiomyopathy

Chagas cardiomyopathy presents early with non-specific malaise; electrical disturbances with palpitations, and syncope; signs of heart failure (such as right upper quadrant abdominal pain, jugular venous distention, and peripheral edema), and embolic phenomenon such as stroke. Cardiac pathology is the most frequent manifestations of chronic Chagas disease and develops in 20% to 30% of infected individuals.

Late manifestations of progressive disease include atypical chest pain, syncopal episodes, sudden cardiac death, dyspnea, orthopnea, fatigue, heart murmur, and stroke. The predominant symptoms correlate with right heart failure during the advanced stages; left-sided manifestations include increased risk for systemic and pulmonary thrombi. According to Rassi, the major cause of mortality is sudden death, followed by refractory heart failure in 25% to 30% and thrombo-embolism in 15% to 30% (2). Diagnostic studies are noted in Table 2. The combination of right bundle branch block and left anterior fascicular block is typical of Chagas heart disease. Another hallmark is sustained ventricular tachycardia.

Gastrointestinal chronic Chagas disease

Gastrointestinal disease is secondary to dysperistalsis of the esophagus and colon, which itself results from destruction of the myenteric plexi, presenting as megaesopagus and megacolon (11). Esophageal disease presents with dysphagia, odynophagia, regurgitation, cough, weight loss, and aspiration pneumonia. Colonic disease presents with chronic abdominal pain, constipation, fecaloma, volvulus, and peritonitis. The small intestine disease presents with abdominal pain, bacterial overgrowth syndrome, malabsorption, and pseudo-obstruction (1).

Evaluation includes a barium esophagogram to demonstrate a dilated esophagus, manometry to document impaired peristalsis and inability to relax lower esophageal sphincter, endoscopy to identify mucosal lesions, and a barium enema to illuminate a megacolon. The diagnosis of infection associated with the gastrointestinal manifestations can be made by serology (1).

Chagas disease in HIV

Patients with HIV reactivate Chagas disease when their CD4 count falls below 200 cells/μL. According to Cordova, the most common manifestations are mass lesions in the central nervous system or acute diffuse meningoencephalitis in 75% to 90% of cases

Table 2. Diagnostic testing for Chagas disease with cardiac disease

Laboratory Results	Imaging	EKG	Other
Non-specific	Echocardiography: Early: wall motion dysfunction, segmental thinning of the wall Late: dilated cardiomyopathy, tricuspid and mitral valve regurgitation, apical aneurism. MRI: myocardiac fibrosis	Early: Right bundle branch block, fascicular block, premature ventricular ectopy, non sustained ventricular tachycardia, atrioventricular block. Late: Atrial fibrillation/flutter, low QRS voltage Holter and stress testing: frequent PVC and non sustained ventricular tachycardia.	Serology

Acute myocarditis occurs in 30% to 45% of cases (1). Reactivation of Chagas disease in this patient population has a high mortality even when treated. Parasitemia is more common and the parasite load is higher in this patient population. Meningoencephalitis manifests as fever, seizures, nuchal rigidity, paresis, and paralysis. HIV patients also develop heart failure, myelitis, and peritonitis.

Cerebrospinal fluid analysis shows pleocytosis, lymphocytosis (100 /μL), increased protein, decreased glucose, and even parasites. Imaging studies such as CT scan or MRI show white matter involvement, hemorrhagic foci single or multiple with ring enhancement, with or without mass effect. The neuroimaging findings are indistinguishable from *Toxoplasma gondii* encephalitis (1).

The diagnosis can be made with direct parasitological methods or histologic examination. Systemic serologic screening is recommended for patients with HIV who have lived or visited regions endemic for Chagas disease (1).

Chagas disease and transplantation

The increased use of immunosuppressive drugs for transplanted solid organs or bone marrow increases the risk of Chagas disease reactivation. Infection through an infected graft or bone marrow donation can cause acute disease (18). The transmission of Chagas disease after kidney transplantation occurs in 20% to 35% of cases. Descriptions after liver and hematopoietic cell transplantation have been reported but their rate of transmission is not as well understood. Reactivation after heart transplantation occurs in 20% to 75% of cases and after kidney, liver and hematopoietic cells transplants in 9% to 18% of cases.

The clinical manifestations include nodules, erythematous plaques on skin, myocarditis, and meningoencephalitis (1). Other manifestations of reactivation in this patient population include panniculitis, brain lesions, and myocarditis. The incidence of Chagas disease is higher in patients taking mycophenolate compared with patients taking cyclosporine, azatioprine or corticosteroids. Diagnosis of reactivation requires direct parasitological methods such as microhematocrit or Strout method and histologic examination (1).

Neurological manifestations of Chagas disease

Central nervous system involvement in the acute phase is usually limited to children under 2 years of age. Meningoencephalitis manifests as confusion, headache, hypertonia, seizures, and meningismus. The frequency in this age group is 0.8%. In chronic Chagas disease, the involvement of the central nervous system manifests as dementia, confusion, chronic encephalopathy, sensorial and motor deficits. Histopathology shows granulomatous encephalitis.

Stroke has been described in Chagas disease. This is associated with heart failure, mural thrombus, left ventricular apical aneurysm, left ventricular systolic disfunction, female gender, hypertension, and cardiac arrhythmias. The prevalence of cardioembolism is reportedly as high as 56 %. According to Lima-Costa, the risk of stroke in *T cruzi* infected patients in a recent published cohort study was twice that of the uninfected population (20). Peripheral nervous system involvement includes paresthesias, decreased muscle reflexes, impaired vibration, and positional sense. Ten percent of patients with chronic Chagas disease develop mixed peripheral neuropathy (1).

DIAGNOSIS

Acute phase

The diagnosis can be made by direct observation of the parasites in the blood. The Strout method or microhematocrits are the reference methods of diagnosis (1). In congenital infection, the microhematocrit is the method of choice. Blood from the cord or periphery can be analyzed during the first month of life (2). If the results are negative or are performed later, anti *T cruzi* IgG antibodies can be tested for at 6 to 9 months of age after maternal antibodies are no longer present in the infant. Other methods available are DNA analysis by polymerase chain reaction (PCR) technology.

Chronic phase

In the chronic phase the diagnosis is made by serology. The WHO recommends at least two positive techniques to establish a diagnosis of Chagas disease and this has subsequently been validated (1,2). The serological methods used are ELISA, indirect immunofluorescence or indirect hemagglutination. DNA by PCR is used as a research tool and not widely available, but this testing can confirm infection if the serology is inconclusive or as an auxiliary method to monitor treatment. PCR analysis has increased sensitivity compared to other parasitological methods (2).

PROGNOSIS

Cardiac complications are the main prognostic factor (1). Fifty percent of deaths are due to sudden electrical arrhythmias followed by heart failure in 37% of cases. Rassi proposed risk stratification for mortality (Table 3). The strongest predictors of mortality are New York Heart Association functional classes III or IV. Cardiomegaly on chest radiography, impaired left ventricular function on echocardiogram or non sustained ventricular tachycardia on Holter monitoring suggests additional risk (2).

TREATMENT

Treatment is strongly recommended for all cases of acute, congenital, and reactivated infection as well as for all children with infection and for patients up to 18 years old who have chronic disease. Evidence suggests that early treatment may prevent the chronic morbidity and mortality that adults experience. Treatment of adults, 19 to 50 years old, can be prescribed if they do not have advanced heart disease and there seems to be a benefit. Treatment of adults more than 50 years of age remains controversial because it has dubious benefit (1,2). Contraindications for treatment include pregnancy as well as severe renal and hepatic disease. Once megaesopagus or advanced heart disease has developed, the patient should not be treated (2).

The drugs recommended for treating Chagas disease are nifurtimox and benznidazole (See Table 4) (1,3). The treatment for acute cases is nifurtimox 10mg/kg/day in children for 90 days and 8mg/kg/day for 60 to 90 days in adults. The total daily dosage should be divided in 3 doses and taken with food. In some countries such as Brazil, where nifurtimox is not available; benznidazole is used. The dose of benznidazole is 5 to 10mg/kg/day for 60 days in children and 5mg/kg/day for 60 days in adults, divided in 2 or 3 doses and taken after meals (3). Rassi concludes that benznidazole has the best safety and efficacy profile and should be the first line treatment (2). The most common side effects from nifurtamox and benznidazole include weight loss, nausea, vomiting, dyspepsia, leucopenia, thrombocytopenia, agranulocytosis, rash, atopic dermatitis and polyneuropathy (3).

The BENEFIT trial, currently in progress in several cities in Latin America, will evaluate whether etiologic treatment is beneficial for patients presenting with clinical manifestations of Chagas heart disease (4). Patients with chronic heart disease who have sustained ventricular tachycardias, non-sustained ventricular tachycardia, and myocardial dysfunction can be treated with amiodarone.

Some observational trials have suggested improved survival from amiodarone treatment. Other treatments under investigation include implantable cardioverter defibrillator (ICD) placement, cardiac transplantation, and bone marrow cell transplantation; however, there are no guidelines established at this time (2). Rassi recommends anticoagulation therapy for patients with atrial fibrillation, previous embolism, and apical aneurysm with thrombus (2).

The treatment of megaesophagus is aimed at palliation. The lower esophageal sphincter is usually achalasic. Treatment with sublingual nitrates and nifedipine have shown some symptomatic efficacy. Endoscopic botulinum toxin injection or pneumatic balloon dilatation are temporary management measures. Definitive treatments include laparoscopic Heller's myotomy (2).

Table 3. Rassi Score for Prediction of Total Mortality in Chagas Heart Disease

Risk Factor		Points
New York Heart Association class III or IV		5
Cardiomegaly (chest radiograph)		5
Segmental or global wall motion abnormality (2D echocardiogram)		3
Non-sustained ventricular tachycardia (24 hour Holter)		3
Low QRS voltage (ECG)		2
Male sex		2
Total Points	Total Mortality 5 years 10 years	Risk
0-6	2% 10%	Low
7-11	18% 44%	Intermediate
12-20	63% 84%	High

Table 4. Treatment regimen for Chagas disease

Acute Chagas Disease	Nifurtimox 8mg/kg/day for 60 to 90 days in adults and 10mg/kg/day for 90 days in children.* Benznidazole 5mg/kg/day for 60 days in adults and 5-10mg/kg/day for 60 days in children
Congenital Chagas Disease	Nifurtamox 8-10mg/kg/day for 60 days* Benznidazole 5-7mg/kg/day for 60 days. May also use phenobarbital in therapeutic doses for first 15 days of treatment.
Organ Transplants	Solid organ: Nifurtamox 8mg/kg/day in adults and 10mg/kg/day in children for 60 days or Benznidazole 5mg/kg/day in adults and 5-8mg/kg/day in children for 60 days. Bone marrow: Same dose as above but given for 2 years
Reactivation and Immunosupressed Patients with HIV/AIDS	Doses as stated for acute infection. Treatment for 60 days or until CD4/CD8 counts increase after that the schedule can be changed to every 3 days for maintenance treatment.

*Total daily dosages of nifurtamox and benznidazole should be divided into 3 equal doses and taken with food.

Colonic dysfunction can be treated symptomatically with a fiber rich diet, increased fluid intake, enemas, and laxatives. Fecal impaction may require manual disimpactation under anesthesia. If the patients fail conservative treatment and have recurrent fecalomas or volvulus, they may require surgical resection of the dyskinetic colon (2).

CONCLUSION

Measures that prevent Chagas disease remain paramount to its control. Changing the environment in which the vector is comfortable has shown benefit. Treating children with congenital and acute infections is the next step in diminishing the profound effect this disease has later on adults. Treating adults after the disease manifests itself with heart failure and dyskinesis of the gastrointestinal system is only palliative.

REFERENCES

[1] Lescure FX, Le Loup G, Freilij H, Develoux M, Paris L, Brutus L, et al. Chagas disease: changes in knowledge and management. Lancet Infect Dis; 2010; 10(8):556-70.

[2] Rassi A, Jr., Rassi A, Marin-Neto JA. Chagas disease. Lancet. 2010 ;375(9723):1388-402.

[3] Apt W. Current and developing therapeutic agents in the treatment of Chagas disease. Drug Design, Develop and Ther' 2010; 4:243-53.

[4] Muratore CA, Baranchuk A. Current and emerging therapeutic options for the treatment of chronic chagasic cardiomyopathy. Vascular health and risk management. 2010; 6:593-601.

[5] Buekens P, Almendares O, Carlier Y, et al. Mother-to-child transmission of Chagas' disease in North America: why don't we do more? Maternal and Child Health J. 2008; 12(3):283-6.

[6] Villalba R, Fornes G, Alvarez MA, et al. Acute Chagas' disease in a recipient of a bone marrow transplant in Spain: case report. Clin Infect Dis. 1992;14(2):594-5.

[7] Barcan L, Luna C, Clara L, et al. Transmission of T. cruzi infection via liver transplantation to a nonreactive recipient for Chagas' disease. Liver Transpl. 2005; 11(9):1112-6.

[8] Souza FF, Castro ESO, Marin Neto JA, et al. Acute chagasic myocardiopathy after orthotopic liver transplantation with donor and recipient serologically negative for *Trypanosoma cruzi*: a case report. Transplan Proc. 2008;40(3):875-8.

[9] Brutus L, Santalla JA, Salas NA, et al. Screening for congenital infection by *Trypanosoma cruzi* in France. Bulletin de la Societe de pathologie exotique (1990). 2009;102(5):300-9.

[10] Verani JR, Montgomery SP, Schulkin J, et al. Survey of obstetrician-gynecologists in the United States about Chagas disease. Amer J Trop Med and Hygiene. 2010;83(4):891-5.

[11] Coura JR, Borges-Pereira J. Chagas disease: 100 years after its discovery. A systemic review. Acta Tropica. 2010;115(1-2):5-13.

[12] de Souza W, de Carvalho TM, Barrias ES. Review on *Trypanosoma cruzi*: host cell interaction. Int J Cell Biol.2010; 295394.

[13] Chagas disease (American trypanosomiasis) fact sheet (revised in June 2010). Releve epidemiologique hebdomadaire / Section d'hygiene du Secretariat de la Societe des Nations = Weekly epidemiological record / Health Section of the Secretariat of the League of Nations. 2010 Aug 20;85(34):334-6.

[14] Moncayo A. Chagas disease: current epidemiological trends after the interruption of vectorial and transfusional transmission in the Southern Cone countries. Memorias do Instituto Oswaldo Cruz. 2003; 98(5):577-91.

[15] Develoux M, Lescure FX, Jaureguiberry S, et al. Emergence of Chagas' disease in Europe: description of the first cases observed in Latin American immigrants in mainland France. Med Trop (Mars). 2010; 70(1):38-42.

Submitted: September 03, 2011. *Revised:* November 05, 2011. *Accepted:* November 10, 2011.

In: Public Health Yearbook 2012
Editor: Joav Merrick

ISBN: 978-1-62808-078-0
© 2013 Nova Science Publishers, Inc.

Chapter 19

SCORPION ENVENOMATION

Joav Merrick, MD, MMedSc, DMSc[*,1,2,3,4]
and Mohammed Morad, MD[1,4,5,6]

[1]National Institute of Child Health and Human Development, Jerusalem,
[2]Division of Pediatrics, Hadassah Hebrew University Medical Center,
Mt Scopus Campus, Jerusalem,
[3]Office of the Medical Director, Health Services, Division for Intellectual and
Developmental Disabilities, Ministry of Social Affairs and Social Services,
Jerusalem, Israel,
[4]Kentucky Children's Hospital, University of Kentucky, Lexington,
United States of America,
[5]NHS Lanarkshire, Law House, Carluke, United Kingdom and
[6]Clalit Health Services, South Region, Beer-Sheva, Israel

ABSTRACT

Scorpion sting is a common event in tropical and subtropical regions, especially Africa, South India, the Middle East, Mexico and South Latin America. Out of about 1,500 scorpion species, 50 are dangerous to humans and it is estimated that the annual number of scorpion stings is 1.2 million with about 3,250 deaths. Humans and especially children are stinged, when scorpions are touched in their hiding places and therefore most of the stings occur on the hands and feet. The treatment of a scorpion sting is first of all to calm the victim, immobilize the affected limb (in a functional position below the level of the heart) and quick transport to a hospital. It is also advisable to put some ice on the sting. Prognosis is dependent on many factors, like the specific scorpion, patient age, health status and access to medical care. Delay in seeking medical treatment is associated with higher likelihood of mortality in children and adolescents.

Keywords: Public health, scorpion sting, epidemiology

---

[*] Correspondence: Professor Joav Merrick, MD, MMedSci, DMSc, Medical Director, Health Services, Division for Intellectual and Developmental Disabilities, Ministry of Social Affairs and Social Services, POBox 1260, IL-91012 Jerusalem, Israel. E-mail: jmerrick@zahav.net.il

INTRODUCTION

Scorpion envenomation is a common event in tropical and subtropical regions and a public health concern in many countries, especially Africa, South India, the Middle East, Mexico and South Latin America. Out of about 1,500 scorpion species, 50 are dangerous to humans and it is estimated that the annual number of scorpion stings is 1.2 million with about 3,250 deaths (0.27%) and more persons killed by scorpion than by snakes worldwide (1).

THE SCORPION AND THE FROG

One day, a scorpion looked around at the mountain where he lived and decided that he wanted a change. So he set out on a journey through the forests and hills. He climbed over rocks and under vines and kept going until he reached a river.

The river was wide and swift, and the scorpion stopped to reconsider the situation. He could not see any way across. So he ran upriver and then checked downriver, all the while thinking that he might have to turn back.

Suddenly, he saw a frog sitting in the rushes by the bank of the stream on the other side of the river. He decided to ask the frog for help getting across the stream.

"Hellooo Mr. Frog!" called the scorpion across the water, "Would you be so kind as to give me a ride on your back across the river?"

"Well now, Mr. Scorpion! How do I know that if I try to help you, you wont try to kill me?" asked the frog hesitantly.

"Because," the scorpion replied, "If I try to kill you, then I would die too, for you see I cannot swim!"

Now this seemed to make sense to the frog. But he asked. "What about when I get close to the bank? You could still try to kill me and get back to the shore!"

"This is true," agreed the scorpion, "But then I wouldn't be able to get to the other side of the river!"

"Alright then...how do I know you wont just wait till we get to the other side and THEN kill me?" said the frog.

"Ahh....," crooned the scorpion, "Because you see, once you've taken me to the other side of this river, I will be so grateful for your help, that it would hardly be fair to reward you with death, now would it?!"

So the frog agreed to take the scorpion across the river. He swam over to the bank and settled himself near the mud to pick up his passenger. The scorpion crawled onto the frog's back, his sharp claws prickling into the frog's soft hide, and the frog slid into the river. The muddy water swirled around them, but the frog stayed near the surface so the scorpion would not drown. He kicked strongly through the first half of the stream, his flippers paddling wildly against the current.

Halfway across the river, the frog suddenly felt a sharp sting in his back and, out of the corner of his eye, saw the scorpion remove his stinger from the frog's back. A deadening numbness began to creep into his limbs.

"You fool!" croaked the frog, "Now we shall both die! Why on earth did you do that?"

The scorpion shrugged, and did a little jig on the drownings frog's back.

"I could not help myself. It is my nature."

Then they both sank into the muddy waters of the swiftly flowing river.

Self destruction - "It's my Nature", said the Scorpion...

This fable is of unknown origin and author, but can be found in different variations, which include a farmer, youth, turtle or fox in place of the frog and a snake in place of the scorpion.

EPIDEMIOLOGY

In the United States only one (straw-colored Centruroides) out of 30 species is lethal (2). Less than 1% of stings from Centruroides are lethal to adults, but 25% of children younger than five years stung will die if not treated (2). The majority of cases are from rural areas and usually in the summer months.

Internationally (temperate and tropical regions) stings also occur during the summer and evening times usually outside their home. Many events are unreported and statistics therefore not accurate, but it has been estimated that there are 1.2 million scorpion stings taking place every year (1).

SCORPION BEHAVIOR

Scorpions are usually not aggressive and they do not generally hunt for prey, but instead wait for it and usually at night, where they can hide. Humans and especially children are stinged, when scorpions are touched in their hiding places and therefore most of the stings occur on the hands and feet.

Almost all of the lethal scorpions, except the Hemiscorpius species, belong to the scorpion family called the Buthidae. The Buthidae family is characterized by a triangular-shaped sternum, as opposed to the pentagonal-shaped sternum found in the other five scorpion families.

SCORPION STINGS

The venom of the scorpion has an effect on the nervous system, heart and blood vessels and the sting in itself is very painful. When a fair amount of venom is injected, the effects on the body will be seen very quickly. The reaction to the venom is restlessness, muscle cramps, lots of sweating and tearing of the eyes, faster pulse rate, and increasing damage to the heart, until failure is possible.

Scorpion stings can cause a wide range of conditions, from severe local skin reactions to neurologic, respiratory and cardiovascular collapse. Envenomation from most scorpions results in a simple, painful, local reaction that can be treated with analgesics, antihistamines, and symptomatic/supportive care.

A recent retrospective study over 13 years (1990-2002) in the intensive care unit of a university hospital in Tunisia (3) included 685 children aged less than 16 years who were admitted for a scorpion sting. There were 558 patients (81.5%) in the grade III group (with cardiogenic shock and/or pulmonary edema or severe neurological manifestation [coma and/or convulsion]) and 127 patients (18.5%) in the grade II group (with systemic manifestations). In this study, 434 patients (63.4%) had pulmonary edema, and 80 patients had cardiogenic shock; neurological manifestations were observed in 580 patients (84.7%), 555 patients (81%) developed systemic inflammatory response syndrome (SIRS), and 552 patients (80.6%) developed multi-organ failure. 61 patients (8.9%) died. Most deaths occur during the first 24 hours after the sting and are secondary to respiratory or cardiovascular failure.

In children admitted for severe scorpion envenomation, coma with Glasgow coma score = 8/15, pulmonary edema, and cardiogenic shock were associated with a poor outcome (3).

The clinical manifestations are very similar despite the diversity of species and toxins (4). The signs are determined by the scorpion species, venom composition and the victim's physiological reaction to the venom. Almost 2.5% of envenomated patients exhibit systemic manifestations severe enough to require hospital or intensive care admission and overall about 10% ultimately die. Cardiogenic shock and pulmonary edema account for the 1-2% overall mortality of scorpion envenomation (2).

Usually the weakest, children and the elderly, are at the greatest risk for morbidity and mortality. A smaller child with a lower body weight and therefore a larger ratio of venom to the weight will lead to a more severe reaction. A mortality rate of 20% is reported in untreated babies, 10% in untreated school-aged children and 1% in untreated adults (2).

In patients presenting with scorpion stings it should be important to know (2):

- Time of envenomation
- Nature of the incident
- Description of the scorpion or if possible the scorpion (dead or alive) to verify the classification of the scorpion
- Local and systemic symptoms: Pain and paresthesias often are present. Nausea and vomiting are common.
- Age of the victim
- General health of the victim
- Presence of comorbidities

The most dangerous of all scorpions in Israel is the yellow scorpion, which is prevalent in almost all parts of the country. The southern scorpion is found in northern Africa and in the southern Sinai, while the Tunisian fat-tail scorpion is prevalent in the all areas of Israel, and its sting is almost as bad as the sting of the yellow scorpion.

Scorpion stings hurt. The less dangerous are the Black fat-tail scorpion, prevalent mainly in central Israel and in the south, and the bicolor scorpion, prevalent from the sandy coastal plain to the Negev and also in Sinai. While the Black Judea scorpion, is prevalent in the country from Beit Guvrin to the northern border, is less dangerous than those previously mentioned.

TREATMENT

The treatment of a scorpion sting is first of all to calm the victim, immobilize the affected limb (in a functional position below the level of the heart) and quick transport to a hospital. It is also advisable to put some ice on the sting, which will alleviate the pain and slow the progress of the venom.

Antivenom is the only available specific treatment for scorpion envenomation, but controversies among professionals about its use has resulted in unclear guidelines. Symptomatic treatment with steroids, nonsteroidal antiinflammatory agents, aspirin, and vasodilators are commonly used. In the emergency room the patient is treated according to symptoms and when the sting is serious, antivenom is administered.

Inpatient care is dictated by the severity of the envenomation and consists of stabilizing the patient, neutralizing the venom, providing supportive therapies, and preventing complications. Intensive care unit (ICU) setting is preferred, because of the unpredictability of the symptomology, the risks associated with antivenin administration and the need for airway or blood pressure support.

PREVENTION

The best thing to do is prevent the sting in the first place. Be careful when approaching places where venomous animals like to hide, such as underbrush, inside corners of buildings and piles of wood or stones.

Avoid putting your hands in these places, and if you need to move a pile of wood or stones, use a rod or pole to shift the materials before picking them up.

When you are out camping in the wilderness, take great care when you wake up, to check the tent and the sleeping bag and shake clothes and shoes (outside the tent) before putting them on. Protective clothing, such as shoes or gloves, may prevent some scorpion envenomations.

In your house keep yards free of debris, which can serve as a place for scorpions to hide. Make sure windows and doors fit tightly to prevent scorpions from entering the house. Avoid walking barefoot, especially at night when scorpions are active.

PROGNOSIS

Prognosis is dependent on many factors, like the specific scorpion, patient age, health status and access to medical care. Delay in seeking medical treatment is associated with higher likelihood of mortality in children and adolescents. Most patients recover fully after scorpion envenomation. Symptoms generally persist for 10-48 hours. If the victim survives the first few hours without severe cardiorespiratory or neurologic symptoms, the prognosis is usually good. Furthermore, surviving the first 24 hours after a scorpion sting also carries a good prognosis.

A worse prognosis can be expected with the presence of systemic symptoms such as cardiovascular collapse, respiratory failure, seizures, and coma.

REFERENCES

[1]   Chippaux JP, Goyffon M. Epidemiology of scorpionism: A global apprasial. Acta Trop 2010;107:71-9.

[2]   Cheng D, Dattaro JA, Yakobi R, Bush SP, Gerardo CJ. Scorpion envenomation. Medscape 2011. Accessed 2011 Sep 15. URL: http://emedicine.medscape.com/article/168230-overview.

[3]   Bahloul M, Chabchoub I, Chaari A, Chtara K, Kallel H, Dammak H, et al. Scorpion envenomation among children: clinical manifestations and outcome (analysis of 685 cases). Am J Trop Med Hyg 2010;83(5):1084-92.

[4]   Singhal A, Mannan R, Rampal U. Epidemiology, clinical presentation and final outcome of patients with scorpion bite. J Clin Diagnostic Res 2009;(3)1523-8.

Submitted: September 18, 2011. *Revised:* November 10, 2011. *Accepted:* November 23, 2011.

In: Public Health Yearbook 2012
Editor: Joav Merrick

ISBN: 978-1-62808-078-0
© 2013 Nova Science Publishers, Inc.

Chapter 20

BURKITT LYMPHOMA

Renuka Gera, MD[*]*, Elna Saah, MD*
and Ajovi Scott-Emuakpor, MD, PhD

Michigan State University, College of Human Medicine, Department of Pediatrics and
Human Development, Division of Hematology/Oncology, East Lansing Campus, East
Lansing, Michigan, United States of America

ABSTRACT

Burkitt lymphoma is a very aggressive childhood cancer. C-Myc translocation is the
hallmark of all forms of Burkitt lymphoma. Three distinct types of Burkitt lymphoma are
morphologically identical but have a distinct geographical distribution and clinical
course. Endemic Burkitt lymphoma affects children from equatorial Africa and accounts
for most cases of childhood cancers from the region. Epstein-Barr virus and malaria seem
to play a significant role in the pathogenesis of endemic form and have been the focus of
research worldwide. The tumor is extremely sensitive to chemotherapy. With aggressive
chemotherapy and supportive care 80-90% of patients with Burkitt lymphoma may be
cured. This chapter reviews current understanding regarding this cancer.

Keywords: Tropical pediatrics, public health, cancer, lymphoma, Burkitt lymphoma

INTRODUCTION

Burkitt lymphoma is an aggressive and unique cancer seen in children all over the world. It is
unique in its geographic distribution, clinical presentation, and its association with two
infectious agents, Epstein-Barr virus and malaria. The relationship with malaria and EBV has

[*] Correspondence: Professor Renuka Gera MD, Professor and Associate Chair, Department of Pediatrics/Human
Development, Division of Pediatric and Adolescent Hematology/Oncology. Michigan State University
College of Human Medicine, B220 Clinical Center, 138 Service Road, East Lansing, MI 48824-1313 United
States. E-mail: gera@msu.edu Renuka.Gera@hc.msu.edu

resulted in extensive research to understand the pathogenesis of this tumor. It will not be an exaggeration to say that this tumor has become a paradigm for cancer biology research.

Burkitt lymphoma was first described as tumor of the jaw in children from central Africa by the British surgeon Denis Parsons Burkitt (1911–1993) in 1958, while he was in Uganda (1). Within Africa, the tumor affected children from low lands with tropical climate more often than children living in high land with dry climate. This observation directed the attention towards finding an association with malaria and arthropod born viruses, resulting in the establishment of a link between Burkitt lymphoma and Epstein-Barr virus (EBV) in 1961 (2).

Since that time, three distinct types of Burkitt lymphoma, namely, "endemic" Burkitt lymphoma (eBL), "sporadic" Burkitt Lymphoma (sBL) and "immunodeficiency associated" Burkitt lymphoma (ID-BL), have been described. Thus, Burkitt lymphoma was the first cancer to be linked to a virus, the Epstein Barr virus, and this virus is present in a majority of eBL, though its relationship with sBL and ID-BL is variable.

This observation has prompted extensive research aimed at understanding the role of EBV in the pathogenesis of Burkitt lymphoma and has earned this tumor the title of "Rosetta Stone" of oncology (3). In terms of histology, all three forms of Burkitt lymphoma are indistinguishable, yet the clinical presentation and outcome of these three forms is very different.

Epidemiology

Burkitt lymphoma is the most common type of non-Hodgkin lymphoma in children and, as stated earlier, there are three forms of the disease: *Sporadic Burkitt Lymphoma (sBL)*, *Endemic Burkitt Lymphoma*, and *Immunodeficiency Associated Burkitt Lymphoma*.

Sporadic Burkitt lymphoma (sBL)

Most cases of sBL are reported from developed countries such as Europe and the United States. More recently, cases of sBL are being reported from developing countries, including Africa (4). In the United States Burkitt lymphoma is the most common type of non-Hodgkin lymphoma and third most common lymphoid malignancy seen in children younger than 15 years.

The incidence of "sporadic" Burkitt lymphoma in the United States has remained stable at 2.5/million (5). "Sporadic" Burkitt Lymphoma shares some of the same characteristics as eBL, such as early age of onset (3-5 years) and male preponderance (79% (6). However, sBL is more common in Whites (81%).

Endemic Burkitt lymphoma

eBL is the most common childhood cancer in equatorial African countries with tropical climate and low socioeconomic status. The incidence of endemic Burkitt lymphoma in Africa is much higher ranging between 4.7- 25/ million (7,8) to as high as 6-7 cases/100, 000 annually from central Africa and New Guinea (9). The age of onset is between 6-7 years and there is male preponderance.

Immunodeficiency associated Burkitt lymphoma

ID-BL has been reported from all over the world. It affects patients infected with HIV (HIV-BL) more often and hence the name HIV-BL. Rarely, patients who have undergone organ transplantation also develop ID-BL (10). The recent increase in the incidence of lymphoma in Africa in due in large part to increases in the incidence of HIV related Burkitt Lymphoma.

PATHOLOGY AND PATHOGENESIS OF BURKITT LYMPHOMA

Burkitt lymphoma is one of the most rapidly growing cancers with a very high rate of mitosis and apoptosis. The tumor consists of monomorphic lymphoblasts with basophilic cytoplasm with large nuclei and multiple nucleoli.

BL have high mitotic index but are very prone to apoptosis (11). A high rate of apoptosis results in macrophage infiltration giving the tumor a characteristic "starry sky" appearance. The histology of all three types is almost identical.

The lymphoma cells are positive for B cell markers CD10, CD19, CD20 and BCL6 and surface immunoglobulins. This immunophenotype suggests that the tumor most likely arises from germinal center B cells. However, clinical presentation of Burkitt Lymphoma, most of the times, is in extra-nodal sites.

MOLECULAR BIOLOGY

The hallmark of Burkitt lymphoma is the unique chromosome translocation that involves chromosomes 8 and 14. The translocation breakpoint on chromosome 8 is at band q24 and coincides with the c-Myc proto-oncogene, whereas the breakpoint on chromosome 14 is at band q32 coinciding with the gene for the immunoglobulin heavy chain. c-Myc is a 64 kd protein that regulates growth signals and is expressed in all eukaryotic cells; c-Myc is required for cells to enter S-phase from G1 phase of the cell cycle (12).

Most cases of Burkitt lymphoma show a balance translocation of c-Myc from chromosome 8 and the immunoglobin heavy chain locus on the short arm of Chromosome 14. In small number of cases, there are variant translocations between the c-Myc locus on chromosome 8 the immunoglobulin kappa light chain locus on chromosome 2 or the lambda light chain locus on chromosome 22. Such translocations result in the positioning of the c-Myc gene next to the immunoglobulin genes, which function as enhancers of c-Myc expression. When this occurs, it results in the over-expression of c-Myc proliferative function. This also results in the removal of the internal negative regulatory function (apoptosis) of c-Myc gene (13). As a result of over-expression of c-Myc protein the cell may enter S phase from G1 phase of cell cycle without any mitogenic stimuli and continue to divide and proliferate.

Also, c-Myc over-expression is associated with genomic instability and other features of cancer, such as reduced cell-cell adhesion, aberrant protein synthesis, and increased angiogenesis (14-16). In addition, t(8;14)(q24:q32) is seen 80% of cases with Burkitt lymphoma regardless of its geographic location of origin. However, there is a correlation between the site of breakpoint on chromosome 8 and the geographic origin of the tumor (17). In 75% of the "endemic" form of Burkitt lymphoma, the breakpoint on chromosome 8 occurs some distance upstream of the gene and, in this case, there appears to be a mutation in the first exon of the c-Myc gene, whereas the breakpoint on chromosome 14 usually occurs in the immunoglobulin heavy chain joining regions (J_H). In the "sporadic" and "AIDS-associated" Burkitt lymphoma, the t(8:14) breakpoints tend to fall between exons 1 and 2 of the c-Myc gene on chromosome 8 and within the immunoglobulin heavy chain switch region on chromosome 14 (18). This molecular diversity suggests that Burkitt lymphomas are mixtures of molecular sub-types, similar yet distinct and susceptible to different environmental factors.

EPSTEIN-BARR VIRUS

Burkitt lymphoma is one of the very few cancers where association of cancer with viral infection was first recognized. The geographic distribution within equatorial Africa, where we see a higher incidence in low land with tropical climate and lower incidence in high lands with dry climate, brought an arthropod born infection to the center of the quest for establishing the etiology of the disease. Anthony Epstein identified a herpes virus in a small proportion of tumor cells in the suspensions prepared from Burkitt lymphoma frozen tumor and hypothesized that the virus played an important role in the pathogenesis of this cancer. Subsequently EBV genome was identified in "endemic" Burkitt lymphoma cells (18), making the virus the prime suspect for causing the disease.

EBV is a γ herpes virus that infects B-lymphocytes and cohabitates with the B lymphocyte for the rest of its life. B cells infected with EBV in vitro may activate and transform into blast forms (19). All children who are infected with EBV do not develop "endemic" Burkitt lymphoma. Virologists Gertrude and Henle analyzed the frozen sera of HIV negative patients with eBL and patients without eBL using an immunofluorescence technique (20). Their analysis showed that 95% of the sera from both patients with and without Burkitt lymphoma from central Africa were positive for Epstein Barr virus antibodies. Children from central Africa acquire EBV early and 95% become seropositive by age 2-3 years. EBV infection occurs later in the western world and manifests as infectious mononucleosis. EBV gene products can inhibit a variety of pathways that lead to apoptosis and senescence and thus, EBV probably enhances the proliferation activities of deregulated c-Myc. This facilitates the development of Burkitt Lymphoma (21).

MALARIA AND ENDEMIC BURKITT LYMPHOMA

Endemic Burkitt lymphoma is the most common cancer in children from equatorial Africa and Papua New Guinea/Irianjaya in Asia where *Plasmodium falciparum* malaria is holo-endemic or hyper-endemic. Immunity to falciparum malaria develops in a step-wise manner. Some children infected with *P. falciparum* develop a state of chronic infection characterized by chronic splenomegaly and hypergammaglobinemia. This hypergammaglobinemia is not due to specific antibodies against *P. falciparum* but represents a polyclonal B-cell activation. Endemic Burkitt lymphoma develops in the context of uninterrupted parasitemia, immune system activation, and concurrent infection by viruses, bacteria, and other parasites.

Malaria is known to cause immune suppression. The number of B cells carrying EBV viral protein increases during an acute episode of malaria (22). Viral reactivation and increased viral burden are common during malaria infection (23). High levels of EBV-DNA may be indicative of EBV reactivation as well as indicative of an increased number of EBV infected B cells (24). Proliferation of B cells due to reactivation of EBV caused by *Plasmodium falciparum* may make them susceptible to acquire and/or maintain c-Myc translocations. The evidence to support the role of malaria as a cofactor is indirect and continues to be an area of ongoing research.

EXPOSURE TO HERBAL PLANTS AND ENDEMIC BURKITT LYMPHOMA

The parent compound of 12-0-tetradecanoylphorphol-13-acetate (TPA), a tumor promoter, is present in the extract of Chinese and African Euphorbiacae plants and it is capable of enhancing EBV induced transformation of lymphocytes. *Euphorbia tirucalli* (milk bush) and other Euphorbiacae plants are used for various religious as well as for ceremonial activities, and as an herbal remedy for some illnesses in Africa. Often children play with rubber like sap from these plants (25). The role of Euphorbiacae plants in the pathogenesis of eBL was suggested by a study from Malawi that showed that homes of patients with eBL were more likely to have the plant when compared to controls (26). These observations suggest that exposure to carcinogens, such as these plants, may also play a role in the pathogenesis of "endemic Burkitt lymphoma" (eBL).

HUMAN IMMUNODEFICIENCY VIRUS (HIV) AND BURKITT LYMPHOMA

Burkitt lymphoma is the most common malignancy seen in children with HIV infection (27). Interesting features of HIV associated BL are:

1. There is a stronger association of HIV with Burkitt lymphoma in the Western world than in Africa (28). Shorter survival of African children with HIV may be responsible for this difference.
2. About 30-40% of cases of "HIV associated" Burkitt lymphoma are EBV positive (29).
3. c-Myc translocation in HIV-BL structurally resembles that of "sporadic" Burkitt lymphoma (sBL).

While EBV, malaria, and exposure to other environmental factors may help explain part of the pathogenesis of "endemic" Burkitt lymphoma, it raises more questions than it provides answers and does not explain the evolution of "sporadic" Burkitt lymphoma and immunodeficiency associated" Burkitt lymphoma.

CLINICAL PRESENTATION OF BURKITT LYMPHOMA

Although Burkitt Lymphoma occurs everywhere in the world, the relative frequency of the disease has a marked geographical variation. In tropical Africa, lymphomas make up about half of all childhood cancers, of which about 90% are Burkitt's lymphoma (30). Because of this concentration of the disease in tropical Africa, it is referred to as "endemic" Burkitt lymphoma, as opposed to the "sporadic" form found elsewhere in the world. Whereas about 95% of all endemic form of the disease is associated with Epstein Barr viral (EBV) infection, only about 15 % of the "sporadic" form has EBV association.

Most individuals with Burkitt lymphoma present with a limited number of clinical symptoms. About 80% of the "sporadic" form present with abdominal tumors. Consequently, their symptoms are related to abdominal discomfort, such as pain, distention, obstruction, ascites, and vomiting at the time of presentation. In a few cases patients have presented with intussusceptions, nausea, and vomiting. Evidence of gastrointestinal bleeding and, rarely, bowel perforation, has been reported as part of the presenting signs (31). When the disease arises in the terminal ileal area, ileo-cecal junction or the right ileac fossa, they may create inflammatory changes that resemble appendicitis. In such cases, they will present with fever, nausea, guarding, and abdominal pain with rebound tenderness. This is the case in about 25% of the "sporadic" form of Burkitt lymphoma, which may be mistaken for appendicitis.

In the "endemic" Burkitt, the disease occurs predominantly in any of the jaw quadrants. It appears that the frequency of jaw involvement is age-dependent. The tumor occurs in the jaws of 70% of children younger than 5 years, but only in about 25% of children older than 14 years (32). There is a decreasing frequency of jaw involvement with increasing age at diagnosis. In a small percentage of the "endemic" form, orbital involvement without jaw disease exist and is found particularly in very young children. In the "sporadic" form, about one-fifth of them will have jaw tumors at presentation (33).

Bone marrow involvement has been reported in <10% of patients with the "endemic" form of the disease, while in the "sporadic" form it is found in >50% of patients. Involvement of the central nervous system (CNS) at the time of diagnosis is very rare in the "sporadic" form of Burkitt, but does occur mostly when there is also bone marrow disease. In the "endemic' Burkitt, CNS involvement, particularly para-spinal disease, is very common. Paraplegia or extremity weakness is the presenting symptom in 15% of patients (34). Although it has been rare, Burkitt lymphoma may have gonads as a primary presenting site. Table 1 shows symptoms to look for when evaluating a patient with this disease.

STAGING

The staging system used for the "endemic" form of Burkitt lymphoma essentially reflect the volume of the tumor that is present. The United States National Cancer Institute (NCI) staging system was devised for the "endemic" form, but was not sufficiently adequate for the "sporadic" form. Using the NCI system of staging, there are five stages (Table 2), namely, A, AR, B, C, and D. Stage A is a single extra-abdominal tumor; Stage AR is a completely resected intra-abdominal tumor without extra-abdominal disease; Stage B is multiple extra-abdominal tumor; Stage C is Intra-abdominal tumor with or without a single jaw tumor; Stage D is Intra-abdominal tumor with extra-abdominal sites other than a single jaw site. Because these tumors are very sensitive to chemotherapy, surgical resection is not usually advocated which makes this staging in today's cancer care suboptimal.

Table 1. Expected Symptoms of Burkitt Lymphoma in Relation to Site of Disease

Disease Location	Symptoms
1. ABDOMEN	Pain; Bowel obstruction; Abdominal Distention; Vomiting; Ascites; Symptoms of appendicitis if in the right iliac fossa
2. JAW	Dental malocclusion; Facial pain; Facial deformity; Facial nerve paralysis; Pain related anorexia; dysphagia and stridor if jaw tumor extends to the pharynx and neck.
3. BONE MARROW	Symptoms of bone marrow failure; Pancytopenia and Leukemia
4. ORBITS	Proptosis; Visual disturbance; Abnormal extra-ocular movements
5. CENTRAL NERVOUS SYSTEM	Headaches; Vomiting; Ataxia; Paraplegia; Other lateralizing signs
6. GONADS	Swelling (mostly painless) +-and Testicular pain in boys; Pelvic pain in girls

Table 2. NCI Staging System for Burkitt Lymphoma

STAGE	DEFINITION
A	is a single extra-abdominal tumor
AR	completely resected intra-abdominal tumor without extra-abdominal disease
B	multiple extra-abdominal tumor
C	intra-abdominal tumor with or without a single jaw tumor
D	intra-abdominal tumor with extra-abdominal sites other than a single jaw site

Table 3. St Jude's System of Staging non-Hodgkin's Lymphoma

STAGE	DEFINITION
I	single tumor (extranodal) or single anatomic area (nodal), excluding mediastinal or abdomen
II	single tumor (extranodal) with regional node involvement on the same side of the diaphragm; two or more nodal areas; two or more extranodal tumors with or without regional node involvement; primary GI tumor with or without mesenteric node involvement, completely resected
III	Tumor on both sides of the diaphragm, two single extranodal tumors, two or more nodal areas, all primary intrathoracic tumors, All unresectable extensive intra-abdominal tumors, all primary paraspinal or epidural tumors regardless of other sites
IV	any of the above with CNS or bone marrow involvement

The St. Jude's system for non-Hodgkin's lymphoma has been used in the staging of the "sporadic' form of Burkitt. There are four stages in this system, namely, I, II, III, and IV, presented in Table 3. Stage I is a single tumor (extranodal) or single anatomic area (nodal), excluding mediastinal or abdomen; Stage II is single tumor (extranodal) with regional node involvement on the same side of the diaphragm, two or more nodal areas, two or more extranodal tumors with or without regional node involvement, primary GI tumor with or without mesenteric node involvement, completely resected; Stage III is tumor on both sides of the diaphragm, two single extranodal tumors, two or more nodal areas, all primary intrathoracic tumors, all unresectable extensive intra-abdominal tumors, all primary paraspinal or epidural tumor intra-abdominal tumor with extra-abdominal sites other than a single jaw site regardless of other sites; Stage IV is any of the above with CNS or bone marrow involvement.

PROGNOSIS

Several attempts have been made to determine the prognosis of this disease. The available evidence shows that the main determinant of outcome is the burden of tumor at the time of presentation (35). Even then, with current treatment, remission can be attained in close to 94 % of all cases and event free survivals of 80% are attainable for Stage III and IV disease (36).

Because of the importance of tumor burden on treatment outcome, it is essential to investigate the patients thoroughly before commencing treatment.

The following minimum requirements are essential for accurate staging

1. A good physical examination, paying attention to lymph nodes and masses
2. Complete blood count, to enable a good assessment of the presence or absence of blasts.
3. A comprehensive metabolic panel, including serum lactic dehydrogenase and uric acid.
4. Imaging studies, such as chest X-ray, CT scan of the chest, abdomen, and pelvis, abdominal ultra sound where CT is not available, Gallium scan. PET scan has replaced Gallium in most centers
5. Bone marrow examination
6. Cerebrospinal fluid cytology

These studies are important in assessing the degree of tumor burden in the individual patient.

Treatment of Burkitt lymphoma

Following completion of staging as described above, risk adapted therapy is administered. The therapy is intensified with advanced stages of the disease. Most chemotherapy protocols use Society of French Pediatric Oncology LMB-89 regimen back bone. Remission can be attained in close to 94 % of the cases and event free survivals of 80% are attainable for Stage III and IV disease (36).

Because these tumors are very highly chemosensitive, *surgical resection* is very rarely indicated. In some situations, total resection or excisional biopsy may be done in order to establish the diagnosis, as is the case with tonsillar tumors presenting with symptoms of obstructions. Although these tumors are radiosensitive, *radiation* is seldom used in their management. The tumors are considered to be systemic diseases and long-term disease-free survival rate for even localized tumors are not optimal with radiation alone.

Chemo responsiveness to cyclophosphamide was demonstrated early. However, more recent studies have shown that combination chemotherapy is superior to cyclophosphamide alone. As a result, multiple agents are currently being used in various combinations with appropriate intensification based on disease stage. The most commonly used agents include cyclophosphamide, vincristine, methotrexate, Adriamycin, and prednisone (Table 4). Treatment regimens that require intensification usually add to the combination chemotherapy, high-dose methotrexate, and high-dose cytarabine (36).

Table 4. Drugs used for treatment of Burkitt lymphoma

Regimen Acronym	Chemotherapeutic Agents
C	Cyclophosphamide
COP	Cyclophosphamide, Oncovin, Prednisone
COPADM	Cyclophosphamide, Oncovin, Prednisone, Adriamycin, Methotrexate
CYM	Cytarabine , Methotrexate

The phases of therapy generally include a reduction and induction phase, based on a steroid (prednisone) backbone, which yield remission rates as high as 94%. This is usually followed by a short consolidation phase for duration of 3-4 months. For high stage (III and IV) disease, maintenance phase is added in some regimens, utilizing most of the same agents listed above in varying combinations for 2-4 more cycles, giving total treatment duration from 6-8 months (36). Combination chemotherapy with monoclonal antibody (anti-CD 20) has been used.

CNS prophylaxis: presently, chemoprophylaxis is utilized with the intrathecal administration of methotrexate, with or without the addition of cytarabine and hydrocortisone.

Tumor Lysis Syndrome (TLS)

Burkitt lymphoma is very sensitive to chemotherapy. As a result, the risk of tumor lysis syndrome is very high. The management of life threatening metabolic derangements caused by tumor lysis syndrome must be aggressive. These tumors are both rapidly dividing and highly chemo-sensitive; therefore, the majority of patients present with laboratory derangements which only escalate with the initiation of chemotherapy.

Tumor Lysis Syndrome is a metabolic syndrome defined by both laboratory and clinical parameters. These metabolic derangements result from a high tumor burden releasing its intracellular contents. These include nucleic acids, proteins, potassium, and phosphorus. There is a resultant hyperkalemia, huperuricemia, and hyperphosphatemia which shifts the homeostatic balance leading to hypocalcemia and acidosis. If these metabolic abnormalities go unmanaged, uric acid and calcium/phosphate crystals get deposited in the renal tubules impairing renal function and further complicating management. The ultimate result is increased morbidity and mortality for these patients (37).

Anticipation and prevention of TLS complication is the most important factor in effective management of Burkitt lymphoma. This is the reason why many regimens employ "reduction phase" prior to starting intense chemotherapy. The management of TLS consists of vigorous hydration as well as monitoring of urine output and uric acid. Allopurinol is used to decrease the uric acid. Where available, patients may be treated with the recently approved recombinant urate oxidase (38). This drug should be given sooner rather than later as it rapidly breaks down the uric acid. The uric acid should be monitored closely and additional doses given if uric acid increments occur with chemotherapy.

Supportive care such as effective control of nausea and vomiting, early treatment for neutropenia, fever, and infections in addition to appropriate use of granulocyte colony stimulating factor (G-CSF) and blood component therapy are the keys to success of the aggressive chemotherapy.

Children with endemic lymphoma may not have excellent outcomes because of such factors as having poor access to care, the high cost of treatment, and/or lack of timely access to supportive care. In order to overcome such barriers modified treatment protocols that utilize high dose cyclphosphamide and methotrexate have been tried (39).

SUMMARY

This article reviews the current status of Burkitt lymphoma, a very aggressive childhood cancer. Three forms of Burkitt's lymphoma are considered which are morphologically identical but have a distinct geographical distribution and clinical course. Endemic Burkitt lymphoma affects children from equatorial Africa and accounts for most cases of childhood cancers from the region. Epstein-Barr virus and malaria seem to play a significant role in the pathogenesis of endemic form and have been the focus of research worldwide. The tumor is extremely sensitive to chemotherapy. With aggressive chemotherapy and supportive care 80-90% of patients with Burkitt lymphoma may be cured. Unfortunately some do not have excellent outcomes because of lack of access to quality care.

REFERENCES

[1]   Burkitt D. A sarcoma involving the jaws in African children Br J Surg 1958;46:218-23.
[2]   Epstein MA, Achong BG, Barr YM. Viral particles in cultured lymphoblasts from Burkitt's lymphoma. Lancet 1964;1:702-3.
[3]   Martin R, Gemma KL, Bell I, Rickinson AB. Burkitt's lymphoma: The Rosetta Stone deciphering Epstein-Barr virus biology. Semin Cancer Biol 2009;19: 377-88.
[4]   Biggar RJ, Gardiner C, Lennette ET, Collins WE, Nkrumah FK, Henle W. Malaria, sex, and place of residence as factors in antibody response to Epstein-Barr virus in Ghana, West Africa. Lancet 1981;2:115-8.
[5]   Cancer topics. Accessed 2011 Sep 15. URL: http://www.cancer.gov/cancertopics/pdq/treatment/child-nonhodgkins/HealthProfessional/page1
[6]   Mbulaiteye SM, Biggar RJ, Bhatia K, Linet MS, Devesa S. Sporadic childhood Burkitt lymphoma incidence in the United States during 1992–2005. Pediatr Blood Cancer 2009;53:366-70.

[7]   Ogwang MD, Bhatia K, Biggar RJ, et al. Incidence and geographic distribution of endemic Burkitt lymphoma in northern Uganda revisited. Int J Cancer 2008;123:2658-63.

[8]   Vaccine. Accessed 2011 Sep 15. URL: http://www.who.int/vaccine_research/diseases /viral_cancers /en/index1.html

[9]   Gong JZ, Stenzel TT, Bennett ER, et al. Burkitt lymphoma arising in organ transplant recipients: a clinicopathologic study of five cases. Am J Surg Pathol 2003;27(6):818-27.

[10]   Magrath I. The pathogenesis of Burkitt Lymphoma. Adv cancer Res 1990; 55:133-70.

[11]   Patel JH. Analysis of genomic targets reveals complex function of MYC. Nat Rev Cancer 2004;4:562.

[12]   Hayday AC, Gillies SD, Saito H, et al. Activation of a translocated human c-myc gene by an enhancer in the immunoglobin heavy- chain locus. Nature 1984;307:334-40.

[13]   Ar-Rushdi A, Nishikura K, Erikson J, et al. Differential expression of translocated and untranslocated c-myc oncogene in Burkitt lymphoma. Science 1983;222:390-3.

[14]   Adhikary S, Eilers M. Transcriptional regulation and transformation by Myc proteins. Nat Rev Mol Cell Biol 2005;6:635-45.

[15]   Shiramizu B, Barriga F, Neequaye J, et al. Patterns of chromosomal breakpoint location on Burkitt's lymphoma: relevance to geography and Epstein-Barr association. Blood 1991;77:1516–26.

[16]   Gutierrez MI, Bhatia K, Barriga F, et al. Molecular epidemiology of Burkitt's lymphoma from South America: Differences in breakpoint location and Epstein-Barr virus association from tumors in other world regions. Blood 1992;79:3261-6.

[17]   Hecht JL, Aster JC. Molecular biology of Burkitt lymphoma. *J Clin Oncol 2000;18: 3707-21.*

[18]   Borkman GW. Epstein-Barr virus and pathogenesis of Burkitt lymphoma: more questions than answers. Int J Cancer 2009;124(8):1745-55.

[19]   Counter CM, Botelho FM, Wang P, Harley CB, Bacchetti S. Stabilization of short telomeres and telomerase activity accompany immortalization of Epstein-Barr virus-transformed human B lymphocytes. J Virol 1994;68:3410–4.

[20]   Henle G, Henle W, Clifford P, Diehl V, Kafuko GW, Kirya BG, et al. Antibodies to Epstein-Barr virus in Burkitt's lymphoma and control groups. J Natl Cancer Inst 1969;43:1147–57.

[21]   Allday MJ. How does Epstein-Barr complement the activation of Myc in the pathogenesis of Burkitt lymphoma? Sem Cancer Biol 2009;19:366–76.

[22]   Carpenter LM, Newton R, Casabonne D, Ziegler J, Mbulaiteve S, Mbidde E, et al. Antibodies against malaria and Epstein-Barr virus in childhood Burkitt lymphoma: a case control study in Uganda. Int J Cancer 2008;122:1319-23.

[23]   Donati D, Espmark E, Kironde F, Mbidde EK, Kamya M, Lundkvist A, et al. Clearance of circulating EBV DNA in children with acute malaria after antimalaria treatment. J Infect Dis 2006;193(7):971-7.

[24]   Rasti N, Falk KI, Donati D, Gyan BA, Goka BQ, Troye-Blomberg M, et al. Epstein-Barr virus in children living in malaria endemic areas. Scand J Immunol 2005;61(5):461-5.

[25]   Orem J, Mbidde EK, Lambert B, Sanjose S de, Weiderpass E. Burkitt's lymphoma in Africa, a review of the epidemiology and etiology. Afr Health Sci 2007;7:166-75.

[26]   Van den Bosch C, Griffin BE, Kazembe P, Dziwani C, Kadzamira L. Are plant factors a missing link in the evolution of Burkitt's lymphoma? Br J Cancer 1993;68(6):1232-5.

[27]   Pollock BH, Jenson HB, Leach CT, McClain KL, Hutchison RE, Garzarella L, et al. Risk factors for pediatric human immunodeficiency virus-related malignancy. *JAMA* 2003; 289(18):2393–9.

[28]   Orem J, Maganda A, Mbidde EK, Weiderpass E. Clinical characteristics and outcomes in children with Burkitt lymphoma in Uganda according to HIV infection. Pediatr Blood Cancer 2009;52(4):455-8.

[29]   Bower M. Acquired immunodeficiency related systemic Non-Hodgkin's lymphoma. Br J Haematol 001;112(4):863-73.

[30]   Scott-Emuakpor AB, Saah E. Pediatric Neoplasms in Nigeria. Arch Ibadan Med 2007; 8:38-44.

[31]   Meyers PA, Potter VP, Wollner N, Exelby P. Bowel perforation during initial treatment for childhood non-Hodgkin's Lymphoma. Cancer 1985;56:259.

[32]   Burkitt DP. General features of facial tumors. In: Burkitt DP, Wright DH, eds. Burkitt's lymphoma. Edinburgh: Livingstone, 1970:6.

[33]   Sariban E, Donahue A, Magrath IT. Jaw involvement in American Burkitt's lymphoma. Cancer 1984:53:141.

[34]   Magrath IT. African Burkitt's lymphoma: history, biology, clinical features, and treatment. Am J Pediatr Hematol Oncol 1991;13:22.

[35]   Magrath IT, Lee YJ, Anderson T, et al. Prognostic factors in Burkitt's lymphoma: importance of total tumor burden. Cancer 1980;45:1507.

[36]   Okebe JU, Skoetz N, Meremikwu MM, Richards S. Therapeutic interventions for Burkitt lymphoma in children. Cochrane Database Syst Rev 2011;7:CD005198.

[37]   Coiffer B, Altman A, Pui CH, Younes A, Cairo MS. Guidelines for the management of pediatric and adult tumor lysis syndrome: An evidence based review. J Clin Oncol 2008; 26:2767-78.

[38]   Pui CH, Mahmoud HH, Wiley JM, et al. Recombinant urate oxidase for the prophylaxis or treatment of hyperuricemia in patients with leukemia or lymphoma. J Clin Oncol 2001; 19:697-704.

[39]   Hessling P, Molvneux E, Kamiza S, Israel T, Broadhead R. Endemic Burkitt lymphoma: a 28-day treatment schedule with cyclophosphamide and intrathecal methotrexate. Ann Trop Paediatr 2009;29(1):29-34.

Submitted: October 02, 2011. *Revised:* November 10, 2011. *Accepted:* November 26, 2011.

SECTION THREE - BUILDING COMMUNITY CAPACITY

In: Public Health Yearbook 2012
Editor: Joav Merrick

ISBN: 978-1-62808-078-0
© 2013 Nova Science Publishers, Inc.

Chapter 21

POLICY AND COMMUNITY PARTNERSHIPS AS PUBLIC HEALTH MANAGEMENT TOOLS FOR CHILDHOOD LEAD POISONING

Rosemary M Caron, PhD, MPH[*]
and Jessica D Ulrich, MA

Department of Health Management and Policy,
College of Health and Human Services and Department of Sociology,
College of Liberal Arts, University of New Hampshire,
Durham, New Hampshire, United States of America

ABSTRACT

The gradual decline in childhood lead poisoning in the United States is widely regarded as a public health accomplishment. Yet, a significant number of children under the age of six years in the United States continue to be poisoned by lead paint each year. New England residents face a greater risk of lead poisoning due to the area's older housing stock containing lead paint. Primary prevention methods which eliminate the potential risk for disease or disability have focused on addressing housing as the main source of lead exposure. However, primary prevention methods with respect to housing, such as lead abatement, although cost-effective in the long-term, are often prohibitively expensive in the short-term. We highlight health policy and academic-community partnerships as two potential complementary tools to assist in the management of this persistent, complex public health issue that affects numerous, diverse communities across the country. The former tool may integrate educational policy, housing policy, and occupational policy to achieve protection of a vulnerable population. The latter tool calls upon the knowledge, expertise, and resources of academic and community partners to develop interventions that are tailored to the community's identified needs. Previous work and issues for consideration regarding each of these approaches is presented. Furthermore, although the public health management tools described are based in work

---

[*] Correspondence: Rosemary M Caron, PhD, MPH, University of New Hampshire, College of Health and Human Services, Department of Health Management and Policy, #319 Hewitt Hall, Durham, New Hampshire, USA. E-mail: Rosemary.Caron@unh.edu

conducted in New England, we propose that they can serve as models for other communities who are working to address childhood lead poisoning, especially in a time of budget and resource constraints.

Keywords: Public health policy, academic-community partnership, childhood lead poisoning, primary prevention, community-based, New England

INTRODUCTION

The environmental causes, toxic neurocognitive and physiological effects, and clinical management of lead poisoning have been well documented in the peer-reviewed literature (1-3). Briefly, lead poisoning dates back to the time of the Romans (and some believe earlier) who documented its effects (4). The discovery of lead poisoning in children was first identified over a century ago in 1892 in Australia (5). It was not until 1914 that the first case of childhood lead poisoning was diagnosed in the United States in Baltimore, Maryland by Thomas and Blackfan (6).

The primary sources of lead poisoning in the United States are from past uses of lead including dust and paint chips from deteriorating lead-based paint used on the interior and exterior of older housing stock; dust and soil which contain lead from gasoline and paint; folk remedies and products imported from countries without regulation on the use of lead-based paint (7,8). The clinical identification of lead poisoning in children, as a result of the above-mentioned exposures, can be challenging since the signs and symptoms can be non-specific and may include gastrointestinal effects, growth retardation, and neurological issues (2). Yet, young children are extremely susceptible to the effects of lead due to their low body weight, hand-to-mouth activity, developmental stage, and in many cases, their iron deficiency and poor nutritional status (9,10). Epidemiologic studies have found that children's intellectual functioning decreases at low blood lead concentrations, thus prompting the Centers for Disease Control and Prevention (CDC) to repeatedly lower its action level of concern. The CDC's current screening guidelines for lead exposure in children is 10 micrograms of lead per deciliter of blood (10μg/dl) (9). Bellinger (2004) states that this screening guideline "is a risk management tool and should not be interpreted as a threshold for toxicity. No threshold has been identified, and some data are consistent with effects well below 10."

SOURCE OF EXPOSURE - HOUSING

Regardless of the public health advances associated with removing lead from gasoline, household paint, food canning, industrial emissions and drinking water, exposure to lead is a persistent environmental hazard for children in many regions of the United States (9,10). Sargent et al. (1999) stated "Despite these gains, hazards to children from exposure to lead paint in older, deteriorating housing continue to be a problem, especially in the Northeast and the Midwest."

Most elevated blood lead levels (EBLLs) in children are a result of exposure to deteriorating lead-based paint in older housing. Children in New Hampshire, as in other areas of the Northeast, are at particular risk for lead poisoning due to this region's prevalence of older housing (12).

New Hampshire has some of the oldest housing stock in the nation. For example, approximately 77 percent of housing units in the state's largest city, Manchester, were built prior to the 1978 federal ban on lead paint and in some areas the quality of the housing stock is extremely poor (13, 14).

PRIMARY PREVENTION

An estimated 2.2% (434,000) children, ages one to five years, in the United States have an EBLL (15). Yet, childhood lead poisoning prevention in the United States is regarded by many local health departments and federal health agencies, including the CDC and Environmental Protection Agency, as a public health success story (16,17). Jacobs, Kelly, and Sobolewski (18) state that "Although this progress is substantial, it should be tempered by the realization that it took nearly a century to develop the necessary infrastructure to begin to solve the problem, and that far too many children will be poisoned unnecessarily by lead in the coming years unless additional action is taken." Needleman argues that this additional action should be in the form of primary prevention which involves acting before harm occurs in a population (1,14).

Many efforts in primary prevention have focused on addressing the major source of lead exposure for many – housing – via establishing, implementing, and evaluating housing policy that reduces or eliminates children's lead exposure. Much work in this area has been conducted in New England due to its historical use of lead paint and older housing stock.

Several articles have studied the relationship between sociodemographic and housing characteristics and housing policies on childhood lead poisoning. Sargent et al. (19) examined childhood lead poisoning data in urban, suburban, and rural communities in Massachusetts. The authors found childhood lead poisoning cases in all types of communities but concluded that "those children living in communities with high rates of poverty, single-parent families, and pre-1950s housing and low rates of home ownership were 7 to 10 times more likely to have lead poisoning." Based on this work, the authors "suggest that legislative efforts requiring abatement of lead-based paint directed towards pre-1950s houses that are not owner occupied would confer the greatest benefit to children in terms of lead poisoning prevention." Sargent et al. (11) also examined the effectiveness of household lead abatement policies in Massachusetts and Rhode Island in reducing childhood lead exposure. The authors' findings were that the policy in Massachusetts which places the liability for childhood lead poisoning on property owners and requires the abatement of lead in children's homes was effective in reducing cases of childhood lead poisoning in the state compared to Rhode Island, which lacked a similar policy (11). Additional work in this area by Brown, Gardner, Sargent, et al. (20), examined the effectiveness of housing policies in reducing children's lead exposure in two Northeastern states. The authors found that the enforcement of housing policies can mitigate repeated lead exposure from housing units (20).

Lead abatement, a form of primary prevention, from at-risk housing units has been demonstrated to lower the risk of childhood lead exposure (11, 14-16). Although lead abatement programs are quite costly, the benefits are estimated to outweigh the costs. For example, "the cost of lead hazard control was estimated to be $253 million, but the benefits were estimated to be $1.1 billion" in subsidized housing in the United States (18). Needleman (14) stated "that the reduction of exposure yields huge economic as well as health benefits are strong warrants for a systematic program of abatement of lead from the single remaining major source: lead in older homes." The expense of this primary prevention method may result in reducing and potentially eliminating this persistent public health problem.

NEW ENGLAND: HEALTH POLICY
TO PREVENT CHILDHOOD LEAD POISONING

As a region with a disproportionate amount of its population at risk of exposure to lead poisoning, New England is an important place to examine health policies with the goal of reducing lead exposure (11,12). In this section, we outline national and state policies aimed at the primary prevention of childhood lead poisoning (see Table 1). On top of those required at the national level, each state has additional policies that vary in focus and requirements. New England states also have policies in place considered secondary or tertiary prevention strategies such as screening children for lead poisoning, conducting property inspections, or introducing safety standards for children's products. Thus, unlike primary prevention strategies, these strategies do not actively try to prevent lead poisoning from occurring, rather they address the problem after realizing its existence.

NATIONAL PRIMARY PREVENTION POLICY

In 1992, Congress passed the Residential Lead-Based Paint Hazard Reduction Act (also known as Title X). Although lead-based paint legislation has existed since the 1970s, Title X represents the first national policy aimed at preventing lead-based paint hazards. Recognizing the need for a comprehensive strategy aimed at reducing exposure to lead, and in particular, preventing childhood lead poisoning, this law directed the Environmental Protection Agency (EPA) and the Department of Housing and Urban Development (HUD) to require disclosure of information concerning lead upon the transfer of residential property. As required by Title X, the EPA and HUD jointly issued the Lead Based Disclosure Rule (or Lead Safe Housing Rule) in 1996. his rule ensured that renters and buyers would have the proper information about lead hazards in their housing unit before agreeing to purchase or rent pre-1978 housing. In 2008, the EPA issued the Repair, Renovation, and Painting Rule (RRP). This rule acknowledged the risks associated with common renovation activities (e.g., sanding, cutting, demolition) in exposing children and adults to hazardous lead dust and chips. The RRP Rule requires that paid renovation work be done by EPA certified renovators in pre-1978 housing, childcare facilities, and schools. Notably missing from federal policy are rules and regulations aimed at addressing lead exposure in public or commercial buildings.

Table 1. National and New England Policies on Primary Prevention of Childhood Lead Poisoning

	Policy/Law	Goal/ Aim	Requirements	Implemented
National	Lead-Based Disclosure Rule (or the Lead Safe Housing Rule)	Ensure that potential tenants and home buyers have adequate information necessary to protect themselves and their families from lead-based paint hazards prior to their purchase or rental of pre-1978 housing.	Landlords, property managers, real estate agents, and sellers must inform potential lessees and purchasers of the presence of lead-based paint and lead-based paint hazards in pre-1978 housing. (www.epa.gov; www.hud.gov)	1996
	EPA Renovation, Repair and Painting Rule (RRP)	Reduce the risk of lead poisoning in common renovation activities in pre-1978 housing, childcare facilities, and schools.	Requires that paid renovation work be done by EPA certified renovators in pre-1978 housing, childcare facilities, and schools. (www.epa.gov)	2008
Connecticut	Lead Poisoning Prevention and Control Regulations	Prevention of lead poisoning by giving increased authority and power to the state and local health authorities to enforce investigation and abatement standards.	Requires the proper abatement of defective interior and exterior surfaces which contain toxic levels of lead in residential dwellings with children <6 years old and child day care facilities. The regulations do not require that a child be diagnosed with an elevated blood lead level in order for the regulations to be applicable. (www.ct.gov)	1992
	Lead Licensure and Certification Regulations	Ensure that the removal of lead from homes and child day care facilities is done effectively.	Requires licensing of lead abatement contractors and lead consultant contractors and certification for lead activities professionals. (www.ct.gov)	1995
Maine	Act to Ensure Safe Abatement of Lead Hazards (Lead Management Regulations, Chapter 424)	Safely and permanently eliminate lead hazards.	Directs the Department of Environmental Protection to adopt regulations establishing procedures and requirements for the certification and licensing of persons engaged in residential lead-based paint activities, work practice standards for performing such activities, and the licensing of lead training providers and accreditation of lead training programs. (www.maine.gov)	1997
	Lead Poisoning Prevention Fund (LPPF)	This fund is meant to increase state resources dedicated to the primary prevention of lead poisoning (specifically education and outreach efforts).	The fund is supported by requiring paint manufacturers to annually pay $0.25 for every gallon of paint they sell in Maine. (www.maine.gov)	2005

Table 1. (Continued)

	Policy/Law	Goal/ Aim	Requirements	Implemented
Massachusetts	Massachusetts Lead Law	The lead law is meant to protect a child's right to a lead-safe home. One of the first national state laws aimed at primary prevention.	The Lead Law requires the removal or covering of lead paint hazards in homes built before 1978 where any children under six live. Owners are responsible with complying with the law. This includes owners of rental property as well as owners living in their own single family home. (www.mass.gov)	1971
New Hampshire	Lead Paint Poisoning Prevention and Control Act (RSA 130-A)	Control childhood lead poisoning in New Hampshire.	Requires that all lead inspectors and abatement professionals be certified or licensed, that any laboratory performing blood lead analysis report the test results to the Childhood Lead Poisoning Prevention Program (CLPPP), and that requires that the CLPPP investigate all cases of lead poisoning in children under the age of six whose venous blood lead level is ≥20 µg/dL. (www.nhlgc.org)	1993
	Air Pollution Control Regulation #24	Sets forth standards for the removal of lead based paint from exterior surfaces.	Sets forth regulations for all people involved in the removal of lead based paint from exterior surfaces of buildings or other structures. (www.dem.ri.gov)	1993
Rhode Island	The Lead Hazard Mitigation Law	Provide all Rhode Island residents with access to housing that is adequately maintained and enable the primary prevention of childhood lead poisoning.	Requires that property owners of rental housing constructed prior to 1978 mitigate or abate lead hazards in housing units, premises and associated common areas. (www.hrc.ri.gov)	2005
Vermont	Vermont Lead Law (Includes Essential Maintenance Practices)	Prevent childhood lead poisoning in rental housing and child care facilities by establishing a standard of care in older rental housing (pre-1978) that includes property maintenance activities as well as safe practices when disturbing lead paint.	Requires sellers to provide lead disclosure information and educational materials approved by the Vermont Department of Health during real estate transactions for all pre-1978 housing, whether owner occupied or rental. Also requires owners of residential rental units built before 1978 to perform or have performed "Essential Maintenance Practices" (EMPs) to reduce lead paint poisoning hazards. (www.leadsafevermont.org;www.cvoeo.org)	1996

Table 2. Community-Based Childhood Lead Poisoning Prevention Initiatives in New England

	Initiative	Operating Principle
New England	New England Lead Coordinating Committee (NELCC)	"A regional consortium of state and tribal agencies that are working to eliminate lead poisoning, especially in children. NELCC develops regional projects and promotes the exchange of information, ideas, materials, and programs among its member agencies, federal agencies, and other organizations working to eliminate lead poisoning throughout New England." (www.nelcc.uconn.edu)
	Healthy Homes Promotion Project (H2P2) (Part of the New England Asthma Regional Council) Initiative	"The broad vision of ARC's H2P2 is to promote healthier housing across New England, focusing on the environmental health and safety of low income populations. The New England Asthma Regional Council (ARC) is a coalition of public agencies, private organizations, and researchers working to address the environmental contributors to asthma. Part of ARC's new action plan includes promoting an integrated and broad-based healthy homes agenda." (www.asthmaregionalcouncil.org) Operating Principle
Connecticut	Lead Poisoning Prevention and Control Program (LPPCP)*	"A diverse group of experts from housing, medical, social service, public health, legal, and media sectors assembled the Childhood Lead Poisoning Elimination Task Force with the goal to eliminate childhood lead poisoning in Connecticut by the year 2010. Underlying objectives are to protect the health and safety of the people of Connecticut, to prevent lead poisoning and to promote wellness through a wide range of lead poisoning prevention strategies." (www.ct.gov.dph.cwp)
	Coalition for a Safe and Healthy Connecticut	The coalition is "comprised of citizens, health professionals, workers, environmental justice groups, educators, and others seeking preventive action on toxic hazards." (www.safehealthyct.org/)
	Lead Action for Medicaid Primary Prevention (LAMPP) Project	"An early intervention and prevention program working to reduce lead hazards in homes in fourteen cities and towns in Connecticut. The goal is to protect children before they get lead poisoned, intervene at lower blood lead levels, and prevent exposure to children who will move into the same housing in the future. Through collaboration with partners and participating state agencies LAMPP educates the public to the dangers of lead poisoning and turns apartments and homes with lead hazards into lead safe homes." (www.connecticutchildrens.org)
Maine	Childhood Lead Poisoning Prevention Program (CLPPP)*	Primarily provides secondary prevention through blood screening and treatment; however, also works to educate the public, parents, and professionals about lead issues. (www.maine.gov)
	Healthy Maine Partnerships (HMP)*	"At the State level, the Healthy Maine Partnerships are programs and organizations dedicated to promoting health all over Maine. These statewide partners support the 28 local HMPs with training, technical assistance, evaluation, program development, and media help in order to reach the communities at the local level." Some, but not all, of the 28 state partners are involved in lead issues. Some funding provided by the Lead Poisoning Prevention Fund. (www.healthymainepartnerships.org)
Massachusetts	Childhood Lead Poisoning Prevention Program (CLPPP)*	"Established for the prevention, screening, diagnosis, and treatment of lead poisoning, including the elimination of sources of poisoning through research and educational, epidemiologic, and clinical activities as may be necessary. CLPPP provides a range of both primary and secondary prevention services to the children of the Commonwealth of Massachusetts, their families and others with an interest in the prevention of lead poisoning. In order to accomplish the fundamental goals of identifying lead poisoned children and ensuring that they receive medical and environmental services as well as preventing further cases of lead poisoning, CLPPP has developed linkages with a wide array of professionals and programs that provide services to children." (www.mass.gov)

Table 2. (Continued)

	Initiative	Operating Principle
	Boston Healthy Homes and School Collaborative (BHHSC)	The LAC is "a partnership of non-profit organizations, foundations, and government agencies that has been working to substantially reduce the incidence of childhood lead poisoning in Boston's highest risk neighborhoods since 1993. Our multifaceted approach to combating lead poisoning includes increasing visibility, ensuring the effectiveness of related policies and regulations through advocacy and coalition building, and training community groups to develop and sustain their own outreach programs at the grassroots level." (www.leadactioncollaborative.org)
New Hampshire	Healthy Homes Lead Poisoning Prevention Program (HHLPPP)*	"The Healthy Homes and Lead Poisoning Prevention Program (HHLPPP) is a resource for New Hampshire residents who need help addressing the hazards of lead in their children's environment. The HHLPPP is committed to eliminating elevated BLLs among New Hampshire children." Includes the creation of local lead action committees in five areas that have been determined to be at high risk for childhood lead poisoning. (www.dhhs.nh.gov)
	Greater Manchester Partners Against Lead Poisoning (GMPALP)	"GMPALP is an open organization representing the Manchester community, including, but not limited to: private citizens, public health and private care agencies, property owners, tenants, businesses and other agencies. This coalition has been established to comprehensively address and prevent lead poisoning in the children of Manchester." (www.manchesternh.gov)
Rhode Island	Healthy Homes and Childhood Lead Poisoning Prevention Program (CLPPP)*	"Coordinates statewide efforts to eliminate lead poisoning; reduce lead exposure in children; develop and implement policies to enforce healthy housing practices; and create a safer living environment for all Rhode Islanders." (www.health.ri.gov)
	Childhood Lead Action Project (includes the Get Out the Lead Coalition (GLOC))	"The Childhood Lead Action Project is a non-profit organization dedicated to eliminating childhood lead poisoning in Rhode Island through education, parent support and advocacy. The Project is the only organization in Rhode Island devoted exclusively to this critical issue." Includes the Get Out the Lead Coalition. (www.leadsafekids.org/)
Vermont	Lead Poisoning Prevention and Surveillance Program*	"Provides information for parents, home owners, realtors, child care providers, schools, renovation contractors, and lead professionals -- including resources for protecting children from lead, lead-safe work practices, essential maintenance practices for landlords, and guidelines for blood lead screening for health care providers." (www.healthvermont.gov)
	Lead Safe Vermont	"Part of a comprehensive lead awareness program administered by the Vermont Housing & Conservation Board. " Includes the Lead-based Paint Hazard Reduction Program (www.leadsafevermont.org)
	Burlington Lead Program	"Conducts public education to raise awareness about lead paint hazards and provides information, technical services, and financial assistance for Burlington and Winooski residents to address lead-based paint hazards." (www.cedoburlington.org)

Note: Financial programs solely meant to help people do repairs/renovations were not included in this table.

*Housed in state health and human services department.

PRIMARY PREVENTION POLICIES IN NEW ENGLAND STATES

Connecticut - In 1992, the state of Connecticut enacted the Lead Poisoning and Prevention Control Regulations giving increased authority and power to the state and local health authorities to enforce investigation and abatement standards. For instance, these regulations require that residential units with children under the age of six that contain toxic levels of lead be properly abated. Connecticut also requires licensing and certification for lead abatement contractors and lead activities professionals, in order to ensure that the removal of lead from homes is completed effectively and safely.

Maine - The Act to Ensure Safe Abatement of Lead Hazards was enacted in Maine in 1997 to ensure the safe and permanent removal of lead hazards in residential buildings and child occupied facilities. The act requires that the state's Department of Environmental Protection adopt more stringent procedures and requirements for the certification and licensing of people engaged in lead-based activities. Additionally, in order to increase state resources dedicated to the primary prevention of lead poisoning, in 2009, the Maine State Legislature established the Lead Poisoning Prevention Fund which requires that paint manufacturers pay $0.25 for every gallon of paint that they sell in the state.

Massachusetts - The Commonwealth of Massachusetts enacted one of the nation's first state laws geared toward the primary prevention of lead poisoning in 1971. The Massachusetts Lead Law requires that property owners update housing units to be lead-safe when children under the age of 6 reside in the unit. Since 1971, a number of updates to the law – including, upgrading requirements regarding the training and licensing of contractors, expanding the number of units in compliance by providing financial assistance for owners, and universal blood lead screening – have made the Massachusetts Lead Law an effective tool at preventing childhood lead poisoning.

New Hampshire - The state of New Hampshire enacted the Lead Paint Poisoning and Prevention and Control Act in 1993. This law requires that all lead inspectors and abatement professionals be certified or licensed, that any laboratory performing blood lead analysis report the test results to the Childhood Lead Poisoning Prevention Program (CLPPP), and that requires that the CLPPP investigate all cases of lead poisoning in children under the age of six whose venous blood lead level is $\geq 20\mu g/dl$.

Rhode Island - In 1993, Rhode Island enacted the Air Pollution Control Regulation No. 24. Although only setting forth standards for the removal of lead-based paint from exterior surfaces, these regulations were a step forward for the state in primary prevention. In effect since 2005, the Lead Hazard Mitigation Law is an effort to give all Rhode Islanders access to housing that is uncontaminated by lead. This law requires that property owners of units built before 1978 meet a number of requirements including taking lead awareness classes, fixing lead hazards on their rental properties, and getting their properties regularly inspected.

Vermont - Vermont enacted the Lead Law in 1996 to prevent childhood lead poisoning in rental housing and childcare facilities. The Vermont Lead Law requires that sellers disclose lead information and provide state-approved educational materials when conducting real estate transactions for all pre-1978 housing. It also requires that owners of residential rental units built before 1978 perform or have performed "Essential Maintenance Practices" (EMPs). EMPS are approved work safety practices conducted by trained persons which aim to safely remove lead hazards from residential units and childcare facilities.

With the exception of the Massachusetts Lead Law enacted in 1971, the majority of New England states implemented primary prevention policies during the 1990s, around the same time national policies were coming into effect. Today, most policies in New England focus on the disclosure of lead information for housing units, the proper certification and training of people working with lead-based paint, and the abatement of lead-based paint in housing units with children under the age of six. Although progress has been made in lowering the incidence of childhood lead poisoning in New England, more comprehensive strategies such as universal abatement could alleviate this public health issue altogether. The funding of such strategies, however, are often controversial – particularly in times of constrained federal, state, and household budgets. One New England state – Maine – has developed a strategy to shift some of the monetary burden to the producers of paint in order to help keep their primary prevention programs funded.

COMMUNITY-BASED LEAD POISONING INITIATIVES IN NEW ENGLAND

A variety of community-based groups across New England have sought to raise public awareness and come up with solutions for the persistent public health risk of childhood lead poisoning (see Table 2). While the reach of some initiatives span the entire region, each state –and some cities – has also developed its own initiatives to address lead risks. Many groups are associated with their states' department of public health, while some are independent initiatives bringing together various stakeholders. In this section, we focus on community-based initiatives using primary prevention strategies to address childhood lead poisoning in their communities. The tools and resources that groups have at their disposal vary, as do the collaborators involved, and the overall effectiveness and reach of their initiatives. The community-based lead poisoning initiatives across New England will be discussed followed by a discussion of some the programs that individual states have initiated to address their concerns about lead safety throughout communities in their states.

NEW ENGLAND INITIATIVES

In 1992, the New England Lead Coordinating Committee (NELCC) was formed to promote "the exchange of information, ideas, materials, and programs among its member agencies, federal agencies, and other organizations working to eliminate lead poisoning throughout New England" (21). One primary function of the NELCC has been to educate New Englanders about the lead risks involved in pre-1978 housing unit improvements. As homeowners are not governed by the EPA's RRP Rule, the New England Don't Spread Lead Campaign (formerly the Keep it Clean Campaign) works to educate do-it-yourself homeowners about lead-safe practices before they begin home improvement projects. As part of the Asthma Regional Council of New England (ARC), the goal of the Healthy Homes Promotion Project (H2P2) is to "promote health and safety of New England residents by increasing: a) availability of green, healthier, affordable housing; and b) eliminating exposures to home-based environmental toxins through the promotion of evidence-based policy and practice, and improved program coordination" (22).

Particular attention is given to high-risk neighborhoods and populations. Recognizing that the "underlying causes of these home health hazards often overlap, as do the interventions that correct those causes" the H2P2 is a collaboration of multiple interest groups that aim to improve the quality homes and thus overall health (22).

NEW ENGLAND STATE INITIATIVES

Connecticut - Comprised of a diverse group of experts, the Connecticut Lead Poisoning Prevention and Control Program (LPPCP) emerged out of a union of other state lead poisoning prevention initiatives in 2005 (23). The primary goal of the LPPCP was to eliminate lead poisoning in Connecticut by 2010. The LPPCP accomplished their goal in 2009 by setting forth recommendations aimed at eliminating lead poisoning over the short term (4-6 years) and recognizing the need for innovative funding mechanisms. Another early intervention and primary prevention program in the state of Connecticut is the Lead Action for Medicaid Primary Prevention (LAMPP) project. Since beginning in 2003, LAMPP has abated lead hazards in 1,300 housing units since its inception in 2003 in 14 different communities (24). Along with addressing lead hazards in homes, LAMPP also educates the public about the dangers of lead poisoning. Finally, the Coalition for a Safe and Healthy Connecticut is comprised of a diverse group of stakeholders (e.g., citizens, health professionals, workers, and environmental justice groups) which seek to change policies that allow toxic hazards (including lead) to harm residents' health and the environment (25).

Maine - The Maine Childhood Lead Poisoning Prevention Program (MCLPPP) is primarily focused on secondary lead poisoning prevention strategies such as blood screening and treatment; however, it also works to educate the public, parents, and professionals about the public health risks of lead (26). With the overall goal of making Maine a healthier place to live and work, the Healthy Maine Partnership (HMP) includes 28 local HMPs dedicated to promoting health all over Maine (27). Some, but not all, of the 28 state organizations are involved in lead issues. In 2010, the Maine Center for Disease Control announced that it was awarding more than $300,000 in contracts to HMPs for childhood lead poisoning prevention programs with funds generated from the Lead Poisoning Prevention Fund (28).

Massachusetts - The Childhood Lead Poisoning Prevention Program (CLPPP) of Massachusetts "was established for the prevention, screening, diagnosis, and treatment of lead poisoning, including the elimination of sources of poisoning through research and educational, epidemiologic, and clinical activities as may be necessary" (29). The CLPPP provides both primary and secondary prevention services through a diverse group of professionals and programs. The Boston Healthy Homes and School Collaborative (BHHSC) is the result of a recent merger between the Lead Action Collaborative (LAC) and Boston Urban Asthma Coalition. The mission of the BHHSC is to "promote healthy homes, schools, and childcare centers in Boston, and enhance the well-being of individuals who live, work, and play in them, working to reduce health disparities and promote the health of low-income and minority populations" (30). Since 1993 the LAC has been working to reduce the incidence of lead poisoning in Boston's high-risk neighborhoods through a collaboration of non-profits, foundations, and government agencies. With volunteers and a detailed tracking system, the LAC developed a Community Assessment Tool (CAT) which has enabled them to target the neighborhoods at highest risk for lead contamination.

New Hampshire - The Healthy Homes and Lead Poisoning Prevention Program (HHLPPP) in New Hampshire was created to be a resource for residents to address lead hazards (31). Focusing on both primary and secondary prevention, the HHLPPP's goal is to eliminate EBLLs among New Hampshire Children. The HHLPPP created local lead action committees in five areas across New Hampshire that were determined to have the highest risk for childhood lead poisoning (Berlin, Claremont/Newport, Franklin/Laconia, Manchester, and Nashua). The hope is that the five lead action committees will become the "leaders in bringing about stronger community capacity for eliminating childhood lead poisoning" in particularly vulnerable New Hampshire communities (32). The creation of these committees reflects the need for local investment in combating this persistent health problem. In reaction to the death of a refugee child to lead poisoning in 2001, the Greater Manchester Partners Against Lead Poisoning (GMPALP) has also brought together diverse stakeholders to address the issue of childhood lead poisoning (33). The GMPALP recognized the need for a community action plan to address lead and set forth their recommendations for future lead poisoning prevention initiatives.

Rhode Island - The Rhode Island Healthy Homes and Childhood Lead Poisoning Prevention Program (CLPPP) "coordinates statewide efforts to eliminate lead poisoning; reduce lead exposure in children; develop and implement policies to enforce healthy housing practices; and create a safer living environment for all Rhode Islanders" (34). In terms of primary prevention, the CLPPP conducts public outreach and education, does lead training of people in the building and renovation industries, and is in charge of compliance and enforcement of lead policies. As the only organization dedicated solely to eliminating childhood lead poisoning in Rhode Island, the Childhood Lead Action Project (CLAP) has been working to solve the problem through education, parent support, and advocacy since 1992 (35). The CLAP coordinated the Get the Lead Out Coalition (GLOC), which is "a network of groups and individuals advocating for state and local policies that protect children from lead exposure" (35). Through the GLOC, the state has been able to make progress in preventing childhood lead poisoning through pushing for innovative public policy.

Vermont - Finally, the Vermont Lead Poisoning Prevention and Surveillance Program provides information for stakeholders enabling them to be knowledgeable about protecting children and practice lead-safe work. Lead Safe Vermont, "is part of a comprehensive lead awareness program administered by the Vermont Housing & Conservation Board" (36). As part of Lead Safe Vermont, the Lead Paint Hazard Reduction Program "provides financial and technical assistance to income-eligible landlords and homeowners to reduce the risk of lead poisoning caused by lead-based paint hazards" (37). The City of Burlington also has the Burlington Lead Program which aims to prevent childhood lead poisoning by reducing hazards and increasing lead awareness. Since 2004, this initiative has reduced lead hazards in over 100 homes with the goal of reaching even more of the more than 10,000 homes built before 1978 estimated to contain lead-based paint hazards (38).

In summary, while every state in New England has a program housed in their health department addressing lead related issues, not all focus solely on primary prevention. Many programs housed within health departments focus their efforts on blood screening and treating those with EBLLs. Additionally, not all agencies collaborate effectively with other stakeholders. Initiatives outside of health departments tend to focus more on primary prevention and have a more diverse group of collaborators. Realizing that their interests overlap, some initiatives are moving towards collaboration with other public health groups, particularly those focused on healthy homes and living environments. As government and privates funds become increasingly tight, this may be a smart move for all involved in order to holistically address public health issues like lead poisoning, asthma, and exposure to toxic hazards. Finally, although not discussed in this section, many of the initiatives discussed also provide various forms of financial assistance, such as low-interest loans or grants for homeowners or businesses to address lead problems.

UNIVERSITY AND COMMUNITY: PARTNERSHIPS WITH THE POTENTIAL TO PREVENT CHILDHOOD LEAD POISONING

As the previous section on health policy and community-based initiatives outlined, childhood lead poisoning is a persistent public health problem that involves multiple stakeholders, for example, local health departments, housing authority, building inspectors, property owners, refugee resettlement agencies, and the residents of poor quality housing. Considering the various missions of these organizations and agencies, we propose that many of these stakeholders view the responsibility for this persistent public health problem, as well as its solutions, differently. In addition to policy development, we propose that partnerships also be considered as part of the prevention solution. Green et al. (39) state that partnerships to address community-based public health issues are essential. "Partnerships and coalitions are necessary in developing prevention and health promotion programs or research today because no one agency has the resources, access, and trust relationships to address the wide range of community determinants of public health problems" (39). Green et al. (39) further describe the benefits of community-based partnerships as offering their varied resources to address the public health issue; distributing the burden of the issue across multiple stakeholders; creating broad public awareness; and providing varied perspectives regarding the challenges and approaches to addressing the public health problem. The principles of good community partnerships as outlined by Green et al. (39) include: trust, respect, commitment, clear communication, transparency in decision-making, governance structure, equal voice among all partners, to name a few. "Successful partnerships begin with principles of community self-determination and ownership of problems, which are essential before building consensus on priorities, resources, and specific actions. Successful partnerships focus on commonplace, easily identifiable, solvable, and publicly owned problems that citizens feel competent in resolving" (39).

We propose that there is value in including academia as a partner to address community-based public health issues, such as childhood lead poisoning. Academicians can provide knowledge, expertise, and resources, in terms of grant dollars and the necessary workforce to supplement a community initiative. Maurana and Goldenberg (40), Baker et al. (41) and Wells et al. (42) have presented the principles for academic-community partnerships, which include the following selected examples: sharing responsibility, building trust, teamwork and mutual respect, compromise, active listening, consideration of multi-disciplinary approaches, capacity development, and the implementation of evaluation strategies. An overarching theme for academic-community partnerships that mirrors the partnership principles previously presented by Green et al. (39) is that the development of such a relationship is a process and requires time, respect, and dedication to the issue, as well as the transparency of the process.

Caron and Serrell (43) reported an academic-community partnership that they developed to address childhood lead poisoning which facilitated change in an urban community through a collaboration that utilized a "doing with" approach as opposed to a "doing to" approach. The importance of partners working together in a collaborative relationship grounded in a framework of trust, respect, adaptability, and shared authority cannot be underestimated (43). The community "owns" the public health issue of concern to them and academia is the "visitor" who has to earn their seat at the community's work table. This relationship building can take time and the process should not be rushed. Additional successful examples of academic-community partnerships that have implemented these participatory principles to address persistent public health issues, such as HIV/AIDS, obesity, and diabetes have been documented (42,44,45).

BARRIERS TO ACADEMIC-COMMUNITY PARTNERSHIPS

It is important to consider the barriers to such collaborations since they will vary by the composition of the academic and community partnership and will depend on the public health issue being addressed. In general, Maurana and Goldenberg (40) identify the following selected barriers to academic-community partnerships: community feeling "used", community's needs identified by academicians and not the community, sustainability of the work, value of community-engaged scholarship as part of the promotion and tenure process for faculty, etc. Regarding these issues, Baker et al. (41) emphasized that partners in such collaborations need to be willing to engage in work that they may not otherwise conduct. "For example, community members may need to take time to share in the tasks associated with writing papers, and academicians may need to take time to share in the tasks associated with organizational planning" (41). The partners may need to leave their "comfort zone" to get the work done. However, an important theme evident in these identified barriers is that of "time." It will take time to not only develop the partnership and its operating principles but the barriers will take time to emerge and it will take time to develop and implement the solutions to adequately address these challenges.

ACADEMIC-COMMUNITY PARTNERSHIPS AND CHILDHOOD LEAD POISONING

Previous work by Serrell et al. (44) demonstrated that although academic partnerships with community organizations can be challenging, such partnerships can translate science and evidence-based practices into social action and policy change to address childhood lead poisoning. Additional work by Caron and Serrell (43) not only highlighted the value in utilizing academic-community partnerships to address childhood lead poisoning but also demonstrated the importance of considering a community's ecology and the social context of risk as it pertains to building the community's capacity to address this persistent public health problem. We propose that academic and community partners should view the childhood lead poisoning problem through their own lens of knowledge and experience but strive to embark on the challenging yet productive and effective work of partnering to address community-based public health issues. For such a partnership to be effective, all partners must be "involved" in each step of the process, as opposed to just providing "input" intermittently. We propose that academic-community partnerships are well-poised to expand their utility in preventing childhood lead poisoning via primary methods, including education and policy initiatives.

CONCLUSION

One of the CDC's *Healthy People 2020* goals is to reduce mean blood lead levels in children aged one to five years and to eliminate elevated blood lead levels in children by the year 2020 (46). This is an ambitious challenge to the nation's public health system. We propose that the tools to manage this persistent public health issue must come from the communities that live with this problem. We have outlined representative health policies implemented in New England, a geographic region that is disproportionately affected by the childhood lead poisoning problem due to the prevalence of older housing stock with lead paint. It is important to note that the policies highlighted are specific public health management tools tailored to the affected communities that incorporate educational policies, home inspection policies, lead abatement policies, etc., all of which influence the health policy for that community. Secondly, we present academic-community partnerships as another tool to manage this community-specific public health issue. Although these partnerships are time-intensive in their development and maintenance, the potential exists for them to provide varied perspectives, resources, and innovative approaches to prevention methods that are based in policy and consider the constraints of the varied stakeholders. Furthermore, these public health management tools can serve as models for other communities who are working to address childhood lead poisoning, a persistent public health issue in numerous, diverse communities across the country.

REFERENCES

[1]   Needleman H. Lead poisoning. Annu Rev Med. 2004;55:209-222.

[2]   Warnimet C, Tsang K, Galazka SS. Lead poisoning in children. Am Fam Physician 2010;81(6):751-7.

[3]   Bellinger DC. Lead. Pediatrics 2004;113(4):1016-22.

[4]   Gilfillan SC. Lead poisoning and the fall of Rome. J Occup Med 1965;7:53-60.

[5]   Gibson JL. Notes on lead-poisoning as observed among children in Brisbane. Proc Intercolonial Med Congr Austr 1892;3:76-83.

[6]   Thomas H, Blackfan, K. Recurrent meningitis due to lead in a child of five years. Am J Dis Child 1914;8:377-80.

[7]   American Academy of Pediatrics Committee on Environmental Health. Lead exposure in children: prevention, detection, and management. Pediatrics 2005;116(4):1036-46.

[8]   Levin R, Brown MJ, Kashtock ME, Jacobs DE, Whelan, EA, Rodman, J, et al. Lead exposures in U.S. children, 2008: Implications for prevention. Environ Health Perspect 2008;116(10):1285-93.

[9]   Centers for Disease Control and Prevention (CDC), National Center for Environmental Health. Preventing Lead Poisoning in Young Children. Accessed. 2011 September 20. URL: http://www.cdc.gov/nceh/lead/publications/books/plpyc/contents.htm.

[10]   Agency for Toxic Substances Disease Registry (ATSDR). Toxicological Profile for Lead. Accessed 2011 September 20. URL: http://www.atsdr.cdc.gov/toxprofiles/tp13.html .

[11]   Sargent JD, Dalton M, Demidenko E, Simon P, Klein RZ. The association between state housing policy and lead poisoning in children. Am J Public Health 1999;89(11):1690-5.

[12]   Bailey AJ, Sargent JD, Blake MK. A tale of two counties: Childhood lead poisoning. Econ Geography 1998;74:96-111.

[13]   City of Manchester, New Hampshire Health Department (MHD). Public Health Report Cards. Accessed 2011 September 20. Accessed URL: http://www.manchesternh.gov/website/Departments /Health/PublicHealthData/ArchivedHealthData/tabid/1696/Default.aspx   .14.   Needleman   HL. Childhood lead poisoning: The promise and abandonment of primary prevention. Am J Public Health 1998;88(12):1871-7.

[14]   Needleman HL. Childhood lead poisoning: The promise and abandonment of primary prevention. Am J Public Health. 1998;88(12):1871-1877.

[15]   Centers for Disease Control and Prevention (CDC). Preventing lead exposure in young children: A housing-based approach to primary prevention of lead poisoning. Atlanta, GA: CDC, 2004.

[16]   Centers for Disease Control and Prevention (CDC). Lead. Accessed 2011 September 20. URL: http://www.cdc.gov/nceh/lead/.

[17]   Environmental Protection Agency (EPA). Lead in paint, dust, and soil. Accessed 2011 September 20. URL: http://www.epa.gov/lead/

[18]   Jacobs DE, Kelly T, Sobolewski J. Linking public health, housing, and indoor environmental policy: Successes and challenges at local and federal agencies in the United States. Environ Health Perspect 2007;115(6):976-82.

[19]   Sargent JD, Brown MJ, Freeman JL, Bailey A, Goodman D, Freeman DH. Childhood lead poisoning in Massachusetts communities: Its association with sociodemographic and housing characteristics. Am J Public Health 1995;85(4):528-34.

[20]   Brown MJ, Gardner J, Sargent JD, Swartz K, Hu H, Timperi R. The effectiveness of housing policies in reducing children's lead exposure. Am J Public Health 2001;91(4):621-4.

[21]   New   England   Lead   Coordinating   Committee.   Accessed   2011   Nov   9.   URL: http://www.nelcc.uconn.edu/.

[22]   Asthma Regional Council of New England. Accessed 2011 Nov 9. URL: http://www.asthmaregional council.org/.

[23]   Connecticut Lead Poisoning Prevention and Control Program. Accessed 2011 Nov 9. URL: http://www.ct.gov/dph/cwp.

[24]   Lead Action for Medicaid Primary Prevention Project. Accessed 2011 Nov 9. URL: http://www. connecticutchildrens.org.

[25]   Coalition for a Safe and Healthy Connecticut. Accessed 2011 Nov 9. URL: http://www. safehealthyct.org/.

[26]   Maine Childhood Lead Poisoning Prevention Program. Accessed 2011 Nov 9. URL: http://www. maine.gov/dhhs/eohp/lead/.

[27]   Healthy Maine Partnerships. Access 2011 Nov 9. URL: http://www.healthymainepartnerships.org/.

[28]   Maine Center for Disease Control and Prevention. State Announces More Than $300,000 in Contracts To   Prevent   Lead   Poisoning.   Accessed   2011   Nov   9.   URL: http://www.maine.gov/dhhs/boh/press_release.shtml?id=124705.

[29]   Childhood Lead Poisoning Prevention Program of Massachusetts. Accessed 2011 Nov 9. URL: http://www.mass.gov/eohhs.

[30]   Lead Action Collaborative. Accessed 2011 Nov 9. URL: http://leadactioncollaborative.org/.

[31]   Healthy Homes and Lead Poisoning Prevention Program in New Hampshire. Accessed 2011 Nov 9. URL: http://www.dhhs.nh.gov/dphs/bchs/clpp/index.htm.

[32]   Childhood Lead Poisoning Prevention Program. Eliminating Childhood Lead Poisoning in New Hampshire. New Hampshire Department of Health and Human Services, Division of Public Health Services, 2004. Accessed 2011 Nov 9. URL: http://www.cdc.gov/nceh/lead/StrategicElimPlans /NH%20Elimination%20Plan.pdf.

[33]   Caron, RM, DiPenitma R, Alvarado C, Alexakos P, Filiano J, Gilson T, et al. Fatal pediatric lead poisoning – New Hampshire. MMWR 2000;50:457-9.

[34]   Rhode Island Healthy Homes and Childhood Lead Poisoning Prevention Program. Accessed 2011 Nov 9. URL: http://www.health.ri.gov/programs/childhoodleadpoisoningprevention/.

[35]   Childhood Lead Action Project. Accessed 2011 Nov 9. URL: http://www.leadsafekids.org/

[36]   Lead Safe Vermont. Access 2011 Nov 9. URL: http://www.leadsafevermont.org/home.html.
[37]   Vermont Lead-Based Paint Hazard Reduction Program. Accessed 2011 Nov 9. URL: http://www.vhcb.org/lead.html.
[38]   Burlington Lead Program. Accessed 2011 Nov 9. URL: http://www.cedoburlington.org/housing/programs_and_services/lead_paint/lead_program_main.htm.
[39]   Green L, Daniel M, Novick L. Partnerships and coalitions for community-based research. Public Health Rep 2001;116(S1):20-31.
[40]   Maurana, CA, Goldenberg, K. A successful academic-community partnership to improve the public's health. Acad Med 1996;71(5):425-31.
[41]   Baker EA, Homan S, Schonhoff R, Kreuter M. Principles of practice for academic/practice/community research partnerships. Am J Prev Med 1999;16(3S):86-93.
[42]   Wells KB, Staunton A, Norris KC, CHIC Council, Bluthenthal R, Chung B, et al. Building an academic-community partnered network for clinical services research: The community health improvement collaborative (CHIC). Ethnicity Dis 2006;16:S1-17.
[43]   Caron RM, Serrell N. Community ecology and capacity: Keys to progressing the environmental communication of wicked problems. Appl Environ Educ Commun 2009;8:195-203.
[44]   Serrell N, Caron RM, Fleishman B, Robbins ED. An academic-community outreach partnership: Building relationships and capacity to address childhood lead poisoning. Progr Commun Health Partnerships 2009;3(1):53-9.
[45]   Baldwin J, Johnson JL, Benally CC. Building partnerships between indigenous communities and universities: Lessons learned in HIV/AIDS and substance abuse prevention research. Am J Public Health. 2009;99(S1):S77-S82.
[46]   Healthy People 2020. Accessed 2011 September 20. URL: http://www.healthypeople.gov/2020/topics objectives2020/objectiveslist.aspx?topicid=12

Submitted: November 15, 2011. *Revised:* December 20, 2011. *Accepted:* December 30, 2011.

In: Public Health Yearbook 2012
Editor: Joav Merrick

ISBN: 978-1-62808-078-0
© 2013 Nova Science Publishers, Inc.

Chapter 22

TRIBAL CAPACITY BUILDING AS A COMPLEX ADAPTIVE SYSTEM: NEW INSIGHTS, NEW LESSONS LEARNED

Michelle Chino, PhD[*]

Department of Environmental and Occupational Health, School of Community Health
Sciences, University of Nevada Las Vegas, Las Vegas, Nevada, United States of America

ABSTRACT

American Indians face severe cancer disparities including high mortality rates and limited access to prevention and treatment resources. The Southwest American Indian Collaborative Network (SAICN) was established to build the capacity of tribal communities in the southwestern United States to address gaps in cancer education, access to services and policy and to promote community based participatory research. A comprehensive evaluation of the five-year project identified numerous successes and struggles faced by the project but was challenged to fully describe and measure the cultural and community dynamics of capacity building in the participating Tribal communities. A complex adaptive systems framework was employed to more fully understand and describe project outcomes. Adapted from the biological sciences, complex adaptive systems theory offers a non-linear, non-mechanistic approach to understanding how individuals act and respond within a larger system. This framework revealed important understandings about the project and identified important lessons learned for future programs, particularly with regard to the cultural context and cross-cultural learning.

Keywords: Tribal capacity building, cancer disparities, complex adaptive systems

[*] Correspondence: Michelle Chino, PhD, Associate Professor, Department of Environmental and Occupational Health, School of Community Health Sciences University of Nevada Las Vegas, 4505 Maryland Parkway Box 453064, Las Vegas, Nevada 89154-3064 United States. E-mail: Michelle.chino@unlv.edu

INTRODUCTION

American Indians face significant health problems and are at increasingly high risk for cancer and other chronic diseases (1,2). In the last half of the 20th century, cancer has become a leading cause of death for American Indians over age 45 and the 3rd frequent reason for hospital stays (3). Further, cancer is responsible for more deaths among American Indians than alcoholism or diabetes, which are the major health priorities in most tribal communities. Despite some positive changes in cancer rates in recent years, disparities between American Indians and Non-Hispanic Whites persist in healthcare access, health status indicators, cancer risk factors, and use of cancer screening tests. Protective behaviors such as fruit and vegetable consumption are low and risk factors such as limited physical activity, obesity, alcohol and tobacco use are high (4).

Cancer disparities arise from the interplay of socio-economic factors that influence health behaviors leading to poorer health outcomes such as tobacco use, poor nutrition, inactivity and obesity. These factors further impact access to early detection, treatment, and palliative care (5). American Indian tribes are more likely than the general U.S. population to suffer greater poverty, lower levels of education, and poorer housing conditions. Social disparities are strongly reflected in disparate patterns of cancer occurrence and cancer survival among American Indians. When compared to other US populations, American Indians tend to be poorer and less educated and often share a suite of cancer risk factors such as tobacco and alcohol use, obesity, and exposure to harmful environmental agents (6). Even when income is controlled, the cancer survival gradient seen for other US populations is not seen for American Indians, due, in part, to the lowest use of mammography and Pap tests (7). Although American Indian communities have repeatedly described their need for improved health services, cancer care for American Indians is fragmented and not connected to the historical patterns of health care found within their communities.

Cultural factors, particularly for American Indians, impact attitudes towards illness, and belief in the role of western medicine versus alternative forms of healing impact (5). For many American Indians cancer is considered a "white man's disease" and thus is not discussed and may even be considered a form of punishment, shame or guilt (3). Identified major barriers for cancer care are often poverty related (life priorities, transportation, child care, no insurance or reliance on the Indian Health Service). Psychosocial barriers such as low literacy, cancer equating to death, mammogram fears, denial, and fatalism also complicate prevention and treatment. Among the most challenging however, may be socio-cultural barriers. There is no word for cancer in Native languages and there are assumptions that since no Indian specific materials exist, cancer does not occur among Indian people. Culturally, there is a great deal of shame associate with diagnosis and culturally ingrained opposition to losing body parts. Further, traditional medicine is rarely included in cancer care plans.

To address this salient public health issue and in response to a Request for Proposals from the National Cancer Institute (NCI), the Inter Tribal Council of Arizona (ITCA) along with health care and academic partners from the Phoenix Indian Medical Center (PIMC), the Arizona Cancer Center (ACC) at the University of Arizona (UA), and the University of Nevada, Las Vegas (UNLV) established a Community Network Program (CNP) entitled the Southwest American Indian Collaborative Network (SAICN). The charge of the SAICN was to build local capacity to eliminate cancer disparities through research, education and policy development. To achieve this goal a system of core teams concentrated efforts and provided direction, synergy and coordination to support Community Based Participatory Research (CBPR) and the development of effective system-community partnerships and the utilization of culturally appropriate interventions to reduce cancer (8).

Interest in, and funding for the SAICN initiative grew out of a growing national focus on effective ways to build a community's capacity to eliminate health disparities (9). Various models of community capacity building have been integrated into American Indian and Alaska Native programs designs over the past decade, many of which have helped involve the community in responding to health disparities. However, as with other strategies and best practices, these concepts have been brought to Tribal communities primarily by mainstream researchers and practitioners. These models and their resultant programs are based on imported Western frameworks rather than on indigenous "ways of knowing" (10), and frequently have limited application in meeting the needs and realities of tribal communities (11).

As with any collaborative network such as the SAICN, elements such as consensus building and other forms of collaborative planning are useful for dealing with social, cultural and political fragmentation, shared power, and conflicting values evident in the system of cancer care for American Indians. Consensus building processes are not only about producing agreements and plans but also serve to promote experimentation, learning, change, and build shared meaning. To evaluate this emergent set of practices, however, a framework modeled on a view of self-organizing, complex adaptive systems rather than a more linear, structured approach, was needed.

A complex adaptive system is a group of diverse but interdependent actors whose actions impact the organization of the system even without centralized control. Individuals gather information from the external environment then apply simple local rules to develop responses that work their way through the interconnected system components. New properties emerge while others are constrained or eliminated allowing the system to adapt and the components to co-evolve (12).

Complex adaptive systems (CAS) are non linear perspectives on time, space, and construct (13) that recognize the dynamic nature of human interaction and learning. In fact, its very nature defies the mechanistic approach that prevails in most fields of study (14). CAS perspectives grew out of the biological sciences and have since been applied to a diversity of fields. These perspectives also parallel a Native world-view. Traditional Western approaches tend to be more mechanistic, deterministic, and linear, as are the expectations for results. Not only was a CAS framework recognizable and appropriate to a Native world-view, it allowed for an expanded and perhaps more accurate understanding of actual and potential outcomes of the SAICN project.

METHODS

The goal of the SAICN was to eliminate cancer health disparities by building the capacity of tribes to understand and respond to cancer risks and treatment gaps and build capacity for community-based research. Participants included local tribes, tribal health professionals, community health educators, health care partners from the Indian Health Service, academic partners – both Native and non-Native, and mainstream organizations providing cancer services and information in the local area. The project was unique in that it employed an Indigenous framework for working with tribal communities on issues related directly to American Indians and cancer.

The scope and complexity of the SAICN project and its unique tribal context provided many challenges for assessment and evaluation. Initially, the evaluation process relied on traditional mainstream methods including process and outcome assessments and use of a RE-AIM framework (15), for considering the longer-term impact of the project and its activities. The revelation that the SAICN could effectively be viewed as a complex adaptive system quickly led to an entirely new set of evaluation criteria.

According to Plesk, (16) a complex adaptive system has a number of important properties that reveal ways to rethink and better understand system dynamics. These include several seemingly disparate yet integrally related constructs:

- *Adaptable elements*. The agents and elements of the system can learn, adapt and change themselves. Change happens from within. It is not imposed as in a mechanical system. This is the very essence of community capacity building.
- *Simple rules*. Plesk notes that a few simple rules, applied locally, can result in complex outcomes. This concept is manifested, repeatedly, in the biological sciences and reminds us that conditions for community change can be understandable and repeatable.
- *Nonlinearity*. Change often comes from small, unexpected actions and may have more influence on behavioral outcomes than a large structured program. In many examples of capacity building it is often one individual who or one idea that serves as a catalyst for change.
- *Emergent behavior*. In proscribed mechanistic systems novelty and creativity are rare. In a CAS, continual creativity, new ideas and the opportunity to explore them are inherent properties of the system. Community capacity depends on the willingness of agents to think outside the box and be willing and able to bring new ideas forward.
- *Not predictable in detail*. Despite our desire to predict, measure, and quantify people and programs, in a CAS relations are nonlinear and behaviors are creative. According to Plesk "the only way to know what a CAS will do is to observe it". So much of process evaluation examines programs adherence to or deviation from a predefined baseline. This limited a focus may obscure the more innovative and serendipitous elements of change.
- *Inherent order*. A system does not need rigid internal framework to function effectively. Self- organization is an effective strategy for group behavior, recognized by biological, social, and even computer sciences. Individual actors do not need to know what everyone else is doing. Subgroups can act independently and self-regulate while still being an essential component of the system. This is often how community change occurs, with different segments of the community contributing different element to the larger collective goal.
- *Context and connectedness*. The context is an agent of the system and what happens within one part of the system will impact the other parts. This would seem to be an essential understand for program evaluation and community capacity yet it is often

overlooked in the push for a more tradition linear and mechanistic approach. Fortunately, communities are increasingly insisting that context matters.

- *Co-evolution*. Change, tension, and uncertainly are healthy states in a CAS. But since they are uncomfortable states, programs often seek a more mechanistic and predictable approach. A mechanical system, however, does not grow, adapt, or evolve. An essential part of capacity building must be acknowledgement of "growing pains" and the skills to work through them.

These properties provided a mechanism for the project team to see the project in a new way, re-examine key components of community capacity - leadership, training and education, research, policy, and self-assessment and identify success and lessons learned.

Lessons learned

In five years, the SAICN project accomplished a great deal. The more traditional evaluation methods identified tangible results such as the various products, toolkits, publications, and partnerships. More important perhaps for tribal communities (if not for the funding agency), however, were the less tangible but more world-changing results illuminated by the CAS framework. The evidence suggests that while the project was disseminating the more quantifiable elements of the project, a great deal of thought and effort went into affirming the validity of project strategies, developing coordinated approaches, and working with communities in culturally appropriate ways. The lessons learned are best summed up through the CAS properties in which they were recognized.

Project components need to be adaptable

Adaptability within the SAICN came by necessity and by design. The project fostered innovative solutions by creating opportunities for small changes at multiple levels as opposed to structuring relationships from the top down (8). Throughout the project process, this approach created interplay between clinicians, cancer patients, researchers, administrators, community members, tribal leadership, and academia.

Simple rules promote understanding

The indigenous, capacity-building framework (11) employed by the project incorporated Western concepts of community capacity building and paralleled the values of community-based participatory research (8). Both the philosophy and method, however, went beyond the assumptions and methods of most mainstream approaches. There were four simple rules for building capacity: 1) build relationships, 2) build skills, 3) promote inter-dependence, and 4) promote commitment. As personal and professional relationships developed, they led to the development of individual and group skills. These skills in turn led to effective working partnerships, ultimately promoting a commitment to the issue, the network, and the process. The SAICN process created an interest in new relationships, the need for new skills, and new opportunities for collaboration and a long-term commitment to positive change. Rooted in indigenous ideology, this model exemplified the type of capacity-building framework that can work well in tribal communities.

Native reality is not linear

A Native world-view and indigenous approaches were essential to engaging the tribal communities. A more linear or more rigid process would not have fared well. Tribal practitioners needed a process that would engage tribal communities on their own terms. The project had to be flexible enough to take advantage of individual skills and collective assets. It had to be willing to shift gears in order to focus on issues appropriate to local Indian people. The project also needed to create a web of effective linkages between existing community initiatives and mainstream resources and efforts (17).

An important example is the legal and political issues that arise when working with sovereign Tribal nations. Tribal leaders dictate the direction and use of tribal resources and health disparities is only one of hundreds of issues with which they must deal. Personnel changes within tribal programs are another reality for tribal projects. People come and go, often taking project and institutional knowledge with them. New expertise is often needed and new people must be informed and brought into the communication loop. Projects such as the SAICN take small steps forward with many compromises along the way.

Let originality and creativity emerge

The communities often adopted and modified existing concepts and products to fit their needs and world view. The Native health educators developed products such as the Gathering Basket, a web-based and CD-ROM to educate tribal health educators and community members about cancer reflected an intimate knowledge of tribal culture and community partnerships (http://www.gatheringbasket.org/). One creative endeavor led to another. The funding agency's agenda was more limited in its scope and focused primarily on the research elements. But the research context is unique and even a CBPR approach to research was thought to be mainstream. From a Native perspective, research historically means a lack of local involvement, limited local interpretation, nothing given back to community, a failure to incorporate the cultural context, and limited attention paid to community consent issues. Community-based participatory research became tribally driven participatory research, leading some tension with the funding agency despite the recognition of the need for Native ownership of the project and the process. Tribal leaders and communities wanted and needed the project activities to work. Health care providers from the Indian Health Service wanted and needed a better way to meet the needs of patients and their families. Novel ideas and creative strategies were essential.

Predictability hinders progress

This project was novel in many ways and often went in unpredictable directions. Allowing the process to unfold in a way appropriate to the tribal communities was an essential part of the process. This often meant that a definite point of arrival where one could identify a completed objective was often lacking. Rather, it was the evolution of the partnerships, the undertaking and support of continued discourse between the network partnership and the tribal communities that was viewed as success. The key players, the topics, and the framework for on-going dialog about cancer changed throughout each year of the project. Input of energy and resources helped maintain continuity and effectiveness, resulting in a productive interchange between the network partnership and the tribal communities that continues to this day.

A simple underlying framework is sufficient to ensure forward progress

The project established a system of core teams focused on participatory education, training, policy, and research, with an underlying administrative foundation. The core teams were designed to concentrate efforts and provided direction, synergy and coordination as a way to support CBPR and the development of effective system-community partnerships and increase the utilization of culturally appropriate interventions to reduce cancer disparities. Teams cycled between work on independent projects and coming together to work as a larger group. It was not unusual for the activities to change dramatically as a result. The core teams served as framework for structure and guidance as well as a foundation for creativity and experimentation.

Context is everything

The tribal context is unique. For the SAICN project, context included community perspectives about cancer, the nature of American Indian cancer disparities, the knowledge, skills, and abilities of project partners, and the realities of life in Tribal communities. In tribal communities, knowledge of the cultural, historical, political and economic context is essential to understanding community dynamics. The project process had to reflect indigenous reality. It needed to integrate the past, the present, and the community's vision for the future. It needed to allow communities to build a commitment to identifying and resolving health concerns and issues on their terms. Fortunately, funding agencies are increasingly recognizing the importance of the cultural and community context. In addition, more and more researchers and evaluators are members of these cultural groups and are changing the way evaluation is conceptualized and the way research is conducted.

Co-evolve

Capacity building is a participatory process where mutual learning must take place. This means transcending the more linear, static, time-oriented format tendencies of the mainstream scientific community, which may only impede involvement, and a sense of ownership. Tribal initiatives however, must also incorporate strategies for non-Native partners to raise their awareness of tribal sovereignty and community issues, ensure adherence to appropriate tribal guidelines and protocols, and become effective allies of indigenous people.

Even when there is a great deal of cultural knowledge and experience, bridging cultural gaps can be challenging. Agreements on how to get things done, how to approach problems, and how to engage participants, relied on the extent of cross-cultural understanding between the various project partners. One of the first critical issues was the perception of cancer itself. Some project partners weren't aware that cancer was a taboo subject for many community people. It was easier for community leaders to focus on external environmental problems. Fear, misconceptions, and a lack of specific cancer focused services in most communities were early barriers to the project's progress. Through the hard work of the SAICN project communities become more involved, gained awareness and a working vocabulary of a complex set of diseases, and connected over shared ideas and experiences.

DISCUSSION

The elimination of cancer disparities is one of the overarching themes of the American Cancer Society 2015 challenge goals (18). However, few resources have been and are currently available to address this salient public health issue among American Indians especially when compared with other prevention and health promotion issues such as diabetes and obesity (18), (4). For these reasons, there is a continuing and pressing need for education, problem definition, resource sharing, systems change within the context of a sovereign tribal nation.

The five-year SAICN project resulted in a myriad of outcomes. Tribal communities gained access to information, resources, and support for local cancer prevention and intervention. Individuals became empowered to speak about cancer in their lives. Mainstream cancer support services were able to reach remote tribal communities. Tribal leaders were given the tools they needed to better understand cancer prevalence and priorities for research and programming. Academic partners and Native student interns helped bridge the gaps between community perspectives on research and the value of a Tribally Driven approach. Health professionals gained a better understanding of the barriers faced by Indian people and their families and helped create new strategies for change. Everyone learned something about cancer and about community (19, 20).

Did the project, however, build local capacity to "close the gap" between community health needs and the systems that provide health services? The activities, partnerships, products and publications indicate that significant strides were made. Momentum was established and community leaders are already building on the foundation built by the SAICN project. Further, the experience of the SAICN project has given the project team and their partners a skill set and knowledge base that has allowed them to ask an array of new research questions. They are now able to conceptualize community based research strategies for locally identified problems. And, the promise of new research partners, a new generation of skilled Native researchers, and the ability of tribes to define, fund, and implement research will open an array of possibilities for the ITCA and the continued success of the SAICN.

What can a complex adaptive system approach tell us about project outcomes? Much of the success of the project as well as the many challenges it faced might have gone unrecognized without considering the implications of a complex adaptive system approach. Even with a rigorous evaluation, designed by an American Indian evaluator, it was clear that many of the more subtle dynamics of the project were essential to measure but hard to quantify. The project itself served as a reminder that there is a need to learn from other disciplines and together develop new and innovative strategies for understanding issues such as capacity building. The more we understand biologically rooted concepts such as complex adaptive systems and disciplines of study such as biomimicry, the more likely we are to design sustainable solutions to problems and to problem solving.

ACKNOWLEDGMENTS

The author wishes to acknowledge the primary partners of the Southwest American Indian Collaborative Network and the Inter-Tribal Council of Arizona. John Lewis, Kenton Lafoon, Alberta Tippiconic, Kathryn Coe, Naomi Lane, Agnes Attakai, Norm Peterson, Tim Mathews, Catherine Witte, and Alida Montiel.

REFERENCES

[1] Roubideaux Y. Perspectives on American Indian Health. Am J Public Health 2002 09;92(9):1401-6.

[2] Holman RC, Curns AT, Kaufman SF, Cheek JE, Pinner RW, Schonberer LB. Trends in infectious disease hospitalizations among American Indians and Alaska Natives. Am J Public Health 2001;91(3):425-31.

[3] Burhansstipanov L, Olsen SJ. Cancer prevention and early detection in American Indian and Alaska Native populations. Clin J Oncol Nurs 2004;8(2):182-6.

[4] Steele CB, Cardinez CJ, Richardson LC, Tom-Orme L, Shaw KM. Surveillance for health behaviors of American Indians and Alaska Natives. Findings from the behavioral risk factor surveillance system, 2000-2006. Cancer 2008;113(5):1131-41.

[5] Smedley BD, Stith AY, Nelson AR, Ebrary I. Unequal treatment. Washington, DC: National Academy Press, 2003.

[6] Cobb N, Wingo PA, Edwards BK. Introduction to the supplement on cancer in the American Indian and Alaska Native populations in the United States. Cancer 2008;113(5):1113-6.

[7] Ward E, Jemal A, Cokkinides V, Singh GK, Cardinez C, Ghafoor A, et al. Cancer disparities by race/ethnicity and socioeconomic status. CA Cancer J Clin 2004;54(2):78-93.

[8] Israel BA, Shulz AJ, Parker EA, Becker AB, Allen AJ, Guzman JR. Critical issues in developing and following community-based participatory research principles. In: Minkler M, Wallerstein N, eds. Community based participatory research for health. San Francisco, CA: Jossey-Bass, 2003.

[9] Goodman RM, Speers MA, McLeroy K, Fawcett S, Kegler M, Parker E, et al. Identifying and defining the dimensions of community capacity to provide a basis for measurement. Health Educ Behav 1998;25(3):258-78.

[10] LaFrance J. Culturally competent evaluation in Indian Country. New Direct Evaluat 2004;102:39-50.

[11] Chino M, DeBruyn L. Building true capacity: Indigenous models for indigenous communities. Am J Public Health 2006;96(4):596-9.

[12] Eidelson RJ. Complex adaptive systems in the behavioral and social sciences. Rev Gen Psychol 1997;1(1):42-71.

[13] Begun J, Zimmerman B, Dooley K. Health care organizations as complex adaptive systems. In: Mick SS, Wyttenbach ME, eds. Advances in health care organization theory. 1st ed. San Francisco, CA: Jossey-Bass, 2003.

[14] Dooley KJ. A complex adaptive systems model of organization change. Nonlinear Dynamics Psychol Life Sci 1997;1(1):69-97.

[15] Glasgow RE, Vogt TM, Boles SM. Evaluating the public health impact of health promotion interventions: The RE-AIM framework. Am J Public Health 1999;89(9):1322-7.

[16] Institute of Medicine. Committee on Quality of Health Care in America, ebrary I. Crossing the quality chasm. Washington, DC: National Academy Press, 2001.

[17] McNeely J. Community building. J Commun Psychol 1999;27(6):741-50.

[18] Byers T, Mouchawar J, Marks J, Cady B, Lins N, Swanson GM, et al. The American Cancer Society challenge goals. How far can cancer rates decline in the U.S. by the year 2015? Cancer 1999;86(4):715-27.

[19] Evans K, Attakai A, Witte C, Riding In-Warne M, Coe K. Responding to American Indian communities: Southwest American Indian Collaborative Network (SAICN) Cancer Educational Activities. J Health Disparities Res Pract 2011;4(3):18-33.

[20] Peterson NJ, Sujata J, Flood T, Coe K. Prioritizing interventions and research to address the cancer disparities of Arizona's American Indian population. J Health Disparities Res Pract 2010;4(1):70-6.

Submitted: September 11, 2011. *Revised:* November 11, 2011. *Accepted:* November 21, 2011.

In: Public Health Yearbook 2012
Editor: Joav Merrick

ISBN: 978-1-62808-078-0
© 2013 Nova Science Publishers, Inc.

Chapter 23

AGAINST THE CURRENT: STRATEGIES FOR ADDRESSING PUBLIC HEALTH CONCERNS IN A NATIVE AMERICAN COMMUNITY THROUGH PARTNERSHIP

Joy Doll*, OTD, OTR/L, Linda Ohri, RP, BS, PharmD, MPH, Teresa Cochran, PT, DPT, GCS, MA, Caroline Goulet, PT, PhD, Ann Ryan Haddad, PharmD and Wehnona Stabler, MPH

Department of Occupational Therapy, Department of Pharmacy Practice, Department of Physical Therapy and Department of Pharmacy Practice, School of Pharmacy and Health Professions, Creighton University, Omaha, Nebraska, University of the Incarnate Word, San Antonio, Texas and Tribal Member, Omaha Nation, United States of America

ABSTRACT

The Ten Essential Services of Public Health offer a framework for developing and analyzing academic community partnerships. This manuscript will identify how the Ten Essential Services provided this framework for implementation and analysis of a partnership between an academic institution and a Native American community in order to meet identified public health needs. A reflective analysis was completed using the ten essential services that identified lessons learned from the partnership. These lessons learned provide an exemplar for identifying and addressing the public health needs of the Native American community through an academic-community partnership model. A thorough discussion of the lessons learned and the partnership model will be discussed as a framework for addressing public health needs in a Native community.

Keywords: academic-community partnership, ten essential services of public health, Native American community

---

* Correspondence: Joy Doll, OTD, OTR/L, Assistant Professor, Director, Post Professional OTD Program, Core Faculty, Office of Interprofessional Scholarship, Service and Education (OISSE), Department of Occupational Therapy, School of Pharmacy and Health Professions, Creighton University, 2500 California Plaza, Omaha, Nebraska 68178 United States. E-mail: joydoll@creighton.edu

INTRODUCTION

With the economic downturn and the disturbing persistence of health care disparities, community-academic partnerships offer a critical strategy to maximize scarce resources and address health needs in underserved communities. If carefully coordinated, such partnerships may concurrently help academic institutions prepare health professions students for the realities of practice and learn skills to address public health issues (1,2). Community-academic partnerships have been demonstrated as a successful approach to addressing health concerns (3,4). Many examples of partnerships between academic institutions and minority communities exist in the research literature, providing a natural fit for combining resources to aid both the community and the academic institution. Furthermore, these partnerships maximize the expertise of a diverse group of stakeholders to address a problem or issue (3). These partnerships, however, are riddled with challenges as minority communities are already disadvantaged and academic institutions tend to leverage power in the relationship. Challenges, such as each partner's unique cultural context, impact the ability to develop and maintain a successful academic-community partnership. This holds especially true in Native American communities where trust in institutions is often limited, due to a long history of oppression and abuse, including exploitation by institutions of higher education (5).

Public health issues remain a significant concern in Native American communities. Specific examples to Native American communities include domestic violence, suicide, obesity and substance use and abuse (6-8). Native American communities struggle to address these issues due to lack of support, trained staff, and funding (8). To be effective, public health initiatives in Native communities need to be culturally appropriate, recognizing not only the cultural values of Native Americans as a whole, but also each unique Native community (9). Chino and DeBruyn argue that current partnerships and capacity building efforts with Native American communities frequently neglect the "culture, language, issues of identity and place, and the need for tribal people to operate in both traditional and dominant cultures" (5). Academic institutions must make a concerted effort to support and recognize the unique needs of each tribal community with which they forge a partnership. Institutions of higher education must seek awareness of Native historical context and community values in order to develop and maintain effective partnerships to address targeted public health problems.

Public health, as a discipline, has historically addressed the needs of populations, but more importantly, communities. In an effort to identify the core functions of public health for addressing community health issues, the National Public Health Performance Standards Program (NPHPSP) (10) developed and published ten essential services of public health, which include:

1. "Monitor health status to identify and solve community health problems.
2. Diagnose and investigate health problems and health hazards in the community.
3. Inform, educate, and empower people about health issues.
4. Mobilize community partnerships and action to identify and solve health problems.
5. Develop policies and plans that support individual and community health efforts.
6. Enforce laws and regulations that protect health and ensure safety.

7. Link people to needed personal health services and assure the provision of health care when otherwise unavailable.
8. Assure competent public and personal health care workforce.
9. Evaluate effectiveness, accessibility, and quality of personal and population-based health services.
10. Research for new insights and innovative solutions to health problems" (10).

Each essential service of public health is important to consider in implementing an academic-community partnership to ensure equity and success in approaching public health needs in a culturally appropriate and community-focused manner.

The purpose of these essential services is to provide a framework to help communities understand health status; raise community awareness of health issues and their impact; and engage community members in developing relevant health care policies and regulations to address identified needs. Furthermore, these essential services of public health attempt to ensure community members are able to access necessary health care from a trained workforce.

Evaluation and ongoing improvement are also critical aspects of the essential services ensuring that innovation and best practices are identified and maintained to meet community public health needs (10).

The purpose of this manuscript is to reflectively analyze an academic-community partnership between a Midwestern University and a Native American tribe by applying the framework of the ten essential services. This framework illustrates guidelines that help ensure equitable and culturally appropriate care to address public health needs for the benefit of both partners. The ten essential services allow reflective analysis of the partnership to identify and describe how each essential service was implemented; lessons learned and challenges faced will be discussed.

THE OMAHA TRIBE

The word "Omaha" translates from "Umonhon", the language of the Omaha Tribe, to "against the current" in English. This metaphor also describes the challenges the Omaha Tribe faces in addressing multiple public health issues. Compared to the general population, Native Americans face significant health and education disparities, in addition to conditions of poverty and unemployment (11). According to the Centers for Disease Control and Prevention (12), the rate of diabetes among Native Americans doubled from 1994 to 2004, posing a significant threat to the wellness of Native people. Mortality rates for Native Americans are significantly higher than those for the general population, and across the diagnoses of heart disease, accidents, alcoholism, suicide and tuberculosis, mortality rates are the highest of any minority group (6,7,13,14). The Omahas are no exception to these challenges.

The Omaha Tribe of Nebraska resides on a reservation located in northeast Nebraska, 70 miles from Omaha, Nebraska, on a small portion of the Tribe's original land base. Macy, Nebraska is the Tribal Headquarters of the Omaha Tribe, which has an enrolled population of around 6,000 members and a Reservation population of a little over 4,200 people. The economy of the Tribe is tied closely to Tribal government, with the largest employers including the Tribe and the Carl T. Curtis Health Education Center, the Tribal-operated health facility (15).

Today, the Omaha Tribe maintains rich cultural traditions still used to promote health and wellness. Common practices among Omahas include Native American Church services, sweat lodges, sundance, smoking sacred tobacco and burning cedar as methods for purification of the mind, body and soul. Historically, the Tribe followed a clan system for family organization with each clan representing a significant role within the community. In current times, Omahas may still identify with their clan identities, based on the sacred circle or the Huthuga, which divided the ten original clans into the Earth and Sky. Traditionally, the Huthuga offered a mechanism to maintain order and provided each Omaha with a specific place in the circle.

ANALYSIS OF THE PARTNERSHIP

Around 17 years ago, leaders of the Omaha Tribe recognized the need for collaboration to address the Tribe's public health issues. The Tribal leaders approached Creighton University, a Jesuit Catholic institution located in Omaha, Nebraska, to seek assistance. Due to the mission of the University, leaders from the university responded to this call and collaborated to address public health needs of the Tribe. Leaders from both groups recognized opportunities for education, addressing health professions shortages, research and resource sharing to build the Omaha community's capacity to address the significant public health issues faced by the Tribe. A series of grants from the Health Resources and Services Administration (HRSA) were garnered to support initial planning and implementation of the partnership. These projects funded the work of interprofessional teams of health care educators and students to collaborate with Tribal members for education and health care outreach. Over time, the focus of projects maintained a community-centered approach and evolved according to the community needs identified by Tribal leaders.

LESSONS LEARNED: HISTORICAL ANALYSIS USING THE TEN ESSENTIAL SERVICES OF PUBLIC HEALTH

In this analysis, the Ten Essential Services of Public Health are used here as a basis for reflecting on the history of the partnership between the Omaha Tribe and Creighton University to identify best practices and challenges that emerged through this successful partnership exemplar. During the process, all but one of the Essential Services was fully implemented. Essential Service 1: Monitoring of Health Status - Throughout the partnership, monitoring of the health status of the Omaha Tribe has occurred on an ongoing basis through both formal and informal means. Essential Service 1 focuses on assessing community health status including risks, disparities and capacities (10,16). Early on in the partnership, the academic representatives at the University learned the importance of their presence in the community. Due to issues of trust and historical trauma, it became critical for academic representatives to visit with Tribal leaders frequently, at least monthly, to build strong, trusting relationships. Meetings were both formal and informal, allowing leaders from both entities of the partnership to learn from and about one another. These gatherings helped to establish an equitable partnership, where each entity could identify relevant health issues needing attention. As trust developed, faculty members from the University were invited to participate in selected cultural practices, which enhanced their understanding of the culture and helped ensure the development of appropriate interventions. From these encounters, significant public health issues were identified, including: 1) a shortage of qualified health professionals in the community; 2) the impact of chronic disease, including diabetes and heart disease on the community; and 3) the importance of promoting healthy living for community members, a real value held both culturally and by many community members.

Essential Service 2: Diagnosing and Investigating Problems. As relationships within the partnership strengthened, both entities centered on the importance of identifying health threats to the community. It soon became evident through meetings and community assessment that a significant issue was the shortage of health professionals to address the chronic diseases of the population. The Omaha Tribal Health Center was understaffed and faced challenges in recruiting qualified practitioners, not to mention practitioners with an interest and sensitivity towards the Omaha culture. Through the collaborative process, it became clear that this was an area where the University could assist. As this was identified by both entities in the partnership, Essential Service 7 was enacted which links people to health services to provide care that would otherwise not be available (10,16). Through the partnership, both entities were able to coordinate needed services for the underserved population.

Faculty practitioners from the health sciences began offering weekly pro bono services at the clinic to begin to address this identified concern. Since chronic disease management was a critical need, the Tribe had an interest in gaining access to rehabilitation professionals. Both physical and occupational therapy faculty began providing services to aid Tribal members in self management of chronic diseases like diabetes. These rehabilitation professionals were found to be successful in providing quality care, saving Tribal health funds normally allocated to contracted services, and serving as an adjunct to current health care services provided at the Tribal Health Center. A need emerged for full time staffing and a contract with the Indian Health Service (IHS) was acquired to achieve more stable provision of rehabilitation services. The contract is evidence of Essential Service 5, to Develop Policies and Plans that support individual and community health efforts, which focuses on the development and implementation of needed services to attend to community needs (10,16).

A secondary effort that addressed the shortage of health care professionals emerged from the University to provide student training to establish a work force for the underserved community. Through discussions with health care providers in the community, and as evidenced in the literature (17,18), it was determined that learning strategies to provide effective care in such a unique community requires direct exposure and training of students considering such practice. The University partner recognized an opportunity to provide focused education of future health professionals to pursue careers in rural, medically-underserved communities. Grant funds were garnered and a coordinator was hired to help facilitate educational opportunities in this local community. Experiential education offerings provided were interprofessional and intensive, allowing students' exposure to the local community and the local health care system (19). Surveys from alumni who participated in the training showed that 30% chose to work in a rural or vulnerable community as professionals, reporting that their experience and training in the Native American community influenced this choice (20). Furthermore, alumni from the University programs began to seek positions in this specific Native community, filling manpower gaps and also providing to the community a work force of providers familiar and sensitive to their unique cultural beliefs and health issues. This initiative fits with Essential Service 8 to Assure a Competent Health Care Workforce, which specifically focuses on educating and training health professions students through partnerships (10,16). In addition, completion of Essential Service 8, served as a catalyst to enable local efforts to accomplish Essential Service 4: Mobilize Community Partnerships and Action to identify and solve health problems, which identifies that an important aspect of public health includes adding rehabilitation as a critical service to meet public health needs (10,16).

One significant area of concern for the community that emerged through monitoring was the need to address diabetes in the youth population (Essential Service 3) (10,16). An initiative, entitled the Health Report Card Project (21), was developed to address both Essential Services 2 and 3 (Diagnose and Investigate health problems and health hazards in the community; and Inform, Educate and Empower people about health issues, respectively) (10,16). Annually, the Tribal Health Facility conducts health screenings on all youth enrolled in the two reservation schools. Historically, these screenings revealed youth exhibit high rates of, or are at high risk for, developing type 2 diabetes. Tribal leaders expressed concern that many parents did not know or understand the lifestyle factors that contribute to diabetes.

Through a joint community-University meeting, the Health Report Card Project was born. The Health Report Card resembles an academic report card that children receive during the educational experience, except that this report focused on the individual's health status. In partnership with Tribal elders, students and faculty members from the University developed a report card that identified a child's current health status, quantifying in understandable terms, their risk for obesity and diabetes, as identified through the health screenings. This report card was distributed to parents at the school's parent-teacher meetings, with concurrent on-site presence of health care providers available for questions. This project evolved to include data from multiple years of screenings so parents could monitor the changes in health status and a child's risk for developing diabetes which, in turn, addresses Essential Service 3, focusing on informing, educating and empowering people about health issues (10,16). This service concentrates on providing information that is accessible and relevant to the community, emphasizing health promotion through educational programming, all foundational to the Health Report Card Project. Through the partnership, the screenings were moved beyond isolated assessments and became a tool for educating the community on the issue of youth diabetes.

Essential Service 10: Research also emerged as a critical need identified by the community-University partners (10,16). The purpose of this service is to link communities with institutions of higher education to conduct relevant public health research. After exploration, the partners agreed that effective research in the Omaha community would be best implemented following a community-based participatory research (CBPR) approach (4). This type of participatory action research promotes a collaborative research design where the community drives the research question, agenda and design. One exemplar of a CBPR research project is Project HOPE (22). Project HOPE, a suicide prevention effort funded through a federal grant, explored how community driven and culturally appropriate interventions can reduce both suicidal ideations and discrete acts of suicide. In collaboration with the community, a professor in occupational therapy developed a curriculum for stress management using a sensory-based approach, a common intervention in occupational therapy. The grant supplied sensory equipment and teachers at the two reservation-based schools were trained in equipment use and curriculum implementation. Approval from the institutional review board at the University was acquired, and youth participants were evaluated to determine if the intervention provided any impact on stress experiences potentially related to suicide. Across the three-year project, data analysis revealed that incidence of suicidal ideations among Omaha youth decreased (22). Because the project was driven by the local culture, hundreds of evaluations were collected and analyzed, providing a testament to the success of collecting data with community support and buy-in to the research goal and design. Traditionally, collecting adequate samples of data in such communities has proven challenging, making it difficult to assess significance of any results obtained.

Essential Service 9: Evaluating Effectiveness, Accessibility, and Quality of Personal and Population-based Health Services, remains an ongoing focus of the partnership (10,16). This service identifies the importance of ongoing evaluation and program change to continue to effectively meet public health concerns. Evaluation, both formal and informal, has been a critical component of the partnership on multiple levels. On the macroscopic level, the leaders and representatives in the partnership conduct annual intensive meetings to evaluate programs and the collaboration itself. Although these meetings do not include a formal evaluation, they remain a critical activity to evaluate the partnership holistically to ensure it continues to meet the needs of all entities involved. On a microscopic level, evaluation has been a critical piece of the individual projects including the interprofessional student training as accountable to HRSA and through the health promotion projects including Project HOPE. For the student training, evaluation included assessment of student learning pre and post-experience in the Native American community along with the collection of data post-graduation (23). For Project HOPE, focus groups were utilized to assess the perceptions of the project by students, instructors and community leaders (22). Focus groups were selected due to their similarity to the cultural practice of talking circles, common in Native American communities. Focus groups data lead to the development of future evaluation tools used in the project and ensured compliance with the principles of CBPR (4). Evaluation remains a critical aspect of the partnership to ensure that all parties' needs are met and the focus of the partnership remains on the public health concerns of the community.

CONCLUSION

Partnerships can promote the public health of minority communities as evidenced in this exemplar of a partnership between an academic institution and a Native American community. The Ten Essential Services of Public Health (10,16) provide a framework for analyzing this historical partnership and its impact on the health-related interventions with the community. Generalized lessons learned through this analysis include the following:

1. The 10 Essential Services provide a holistic framework for thoroughly analyzing the partnership and provide a road map for assisting academic-community partnerships in effectively addressing complex public health needs.
2. The needs of both partners must be prioritized in order to develop effective public health initiatives, which can happen by following the ten essential services of public health. By this, the authors mean that only through partnership and focusing on the essential services can an academic-community partnership collaborate to holistically

address public health needs which are complex, especially in a Native American community riddled with health disparities.

3. Addressing public health issues is a dynamic process. Although all the essential services were identified in this analysis of the partnership except one, the process of identification and implementation of public health needs is dynamic and does not follow a linear, sequential process. The dynamic nature of the partnership is important to address needs as they arise and focus on the partnership, not the priorities of one entity. Furthermore, fluidity is important to ensure that the process of prioritizing health needs occurs based on actual need and not an academic process.

Research identifies that partnerships, especially those between academic institutions and minority communities, are complex and challenging (24). However, by following the ten essential services of public health, academic-community partnerships can maintain a public health focus and truly collaborate to tackle challenging public health needs that better the entire community and benefit both partners.

The comprehensive nature of the essential services ensure that academic-community partnerships, even when facing complicated issues and disparities, can initiate and successfully implement programs and research that attend to the public health needs of a minority community.

REFERENCES

[1]   Plowfield LA, Wheeler EC, Raymond JE. Time, tact, talent, and trust: Essential ingredients of effective academic-community parternships. Nurs Educ Perspect 2005;26:217-20.

[2]   Wolff M, Maurana CA. Building effective community-academic partnerships to improve health: A qualitative study of perspectives from communities. Acad Med 2001;76:166-72.

[3]   Becker AB, Israel BA, Allen AJ. Strategies and techniques for effective group process in CBPR partnerships. In: Israel BA, Eng E, Schulz AJ, Parker EA, eds. Methods in community-based participatory research for health. San Francisco, CA: Jossey-Bass, 2007:52-72.

[4]   Roussos ST, Fawcett SB. A review of collaborative partnerships as a strategy for improving community health. Annu Rev Public Health 2000;21:369-402.

[5]   Chino M, DeBruyn L. Building true capacity: Indigenous model for indigenous communities. Am J Public Health 2006;93:9-12.

[6]   Jones DS. The persistence of American Indian health disparities. Am J Public Health 2006;12:2122-34.

[7]   Castor ML, Smyser MS, Taualii MM, Park AN, Lawson SA, Forquera RA. A nationwide population-based study identifying health disparities between American Indians/Alaska Natives and the general populations living in select urban counties. Am J Public Health 2006;96:1478-84.

[8]   Alcantara C, Gone JP. Reviewing suicide in Native American communities: situating risk and protective factors within a transactional-ecological framework. Death Stud 2007;31:457-77.

[9]   Jackson KF, Hodge DR. Native American youth and culturally sensitive interventions: A systematic review. Res Soc Work Pract 2010;20:260-270.

[10]   Public Health Functions Steering Committee. 10 essential services of public health. Public Health Functions Steering Committee, 1994.

[11]   Warner D. Research and educational approaches to reducing health disparities among American Indians and Alaska Natives. J Transcultural Nurs 2006;17:266-71.

[12]   Center for Disease Control and Prevention. Diagnosed diabetes among American Indians and Alaska Natives Aged <35. Atlanta, GA: Center Disease Control Prevention, 2006.

[13] Doshi SR, Jiles R. Health behaviors among American Indian/Alaska Native women. J Women's Health 2006;8:919-27.

[14] Dapice A. The medicine wheel. J Transcultural Nurs 2006;17:251-60.

[15] Nebraska Department of Health and Human Services Office of Minority Health. Omaha Tribe of Nebraska in Thurston County, Nebraska. Health and Human Services, 2004.

[16] Center for Disease Control and Prevention. 10 essential public health services. Atlanta, GA: Center Disease Control Prevention, 2010.

[17] Slack, MK, Cummings, DM, Borrego, ME, Fuller, K, Cook, S. Strategies used by interdisciplinary rural health training programs to assure community responsiveness and recruit practitioners. J Interprofessional Care 2002;16:129-38.

[18] Daniels, ZM, VanLeit, BJ, Skipper, BJ, Sanders, ML, Rhyne, RL. Factors in recruiting and retaining health professionals for rural practice. J Rural Health 2007;23:62-71.

[19] Cochran, TM, Jensen, GM, Gale, JR, Voltz, JD, Coppard, BM, Haddad AR, et al. Practice and educational Innovation: Revision of rehabilitation roles to extend scarce resources in a rural community. National Rural Health Association Annual Conference; 2006, May; New Orleans, LA.

[20] Gale, JR, Cochran, TM, Wilken, M, Cross, PS, Parker, D, Voltz, JD. Community-based primary care: A model for practice. All Together Better III, London, England, 2006.

[21] Wilken MK. Health report card project: building community capacity. In: Royeen CB, Jensen JM, Harvan R. Leadership in interprofessional health education and practice. Sudbury, MA: Jones Bartlett, 2009:413-26.

[22] Doll, JD, Brady, K, Begay, J. Project HOPE: Sensory integration for suicide prevention in a Native American community. American Occupational Therapy Association Annual Conference; 2011, April; Philadelphia, PA.

[23] Mu K, Chao CC, Jensen GM, Royeen C. Effects of interprofessional rural training on students' perceptions on interprofessional health care services. J Allied Health 2004;33:125-31.

[24] Benoit C, Jansson M, Millar A, Phillips R. Community-academic research on hard to reach populations: Benefits and challenges. Qual Health Res 2005;15:263-82.

Submitted: September 15, 2011. *Revised:* November 25, 2011. *Accepted:* December 07, 2011.

In: Public Health Yearbook 2012
Editor: Joav Merrick

ISBN: 978-1-62808-078-0
© 2013 Nova Science Publishers, Inc.

Chapter 24

LESSONS LEARNED FROM ADAPTATION AND EVALUATION OF HOME VISITATION SERVICES FOR LATINO COMMUNITIES

*Arthur H Owora, MPH[1], Jane F Silovsky, PhD[*1],*
Lana O Beasley, PhD[1,2], Patty DeMoraes-Huffine, BA[3]
and Ivelisse Cruz, MA[3]

[1]Center on Child Abuse and Neglect (CCAN), Department of Pediatrics,
University of Oklahoma Health Sciences Center,
[2]Oklahoma State University and
[3]Latino Community Development Agency, Oklahoma City, Oklahoma,
United States of America

ABSTRACT

Cultural adaptation of child abuse and neglect prevention services facilitates building community's capacity to address this critical public health concern. Adapting evidence-based services and systematically examining the extent to which it enhances receptivity and responsiveness by improved cultural congruence is not straight forward due to the diversity and idiosyncrasy of the targeted at risk populations. The objective of this paper is to share the challenges and lessons learned from our collaboration with a local Latino community agency to adapt an evidence-based home visitation program. Areas of challenges and lessons learned during the feasibility phase of the project included but were not limited to: language diversity, literacy issues, recruitment of bi-lingual providers and training thereafter, lack of standardized measures, data collection, management, evaluation procedures and process issues. The lessons learned from these undertakings underscored the importance of taking time to create a culturally sensitive and congruent approach to service provision and evaluation. Our experiences and lessons learned offer some insights for program practice, implementation and research.

* Correspondence: Jane Silovsky, PhD, Professor, Center on Child Abuse and Neglect (CCAN), Department of Pediatrics, University of Oklahoma Health Sciences Center, 940 NE 13th St., Nicholson Tower Suite 4900, Oklahoma City, OK 73104, United States. E-mail: Jane-Silovsky@ouhsc.edu

Keywords: Adaptation, Latino, evaluation, lessons learned, evidence based practice, implementation, SafeCare, child maltreatment prevention program

INTRODUCTION

Child abuse and neglect is a serious public health concern (1,2). Childhood maltreatment has been found to be an important contributing factor to serious health concerns in adulthood (3). Recently, considerable efforts have been poured into preventing child abuse and neglect through home based visitation services (4,5).

In the last three decades, there has been tremendous growth in Latino population across the United States (6). This growth has also been associated with widening of racial disparities found across the board for negative health and social outcomes. The prevalence of risk factors most proximal to child maltreatment such as: poverty, substance abuse, domestic violence, and mental illnesses have been reported to be higher among minority populations (African Americans and Latinos) when compared to Caucasians (7,8). In these studies, recent immigrants tended to be overrepresented in the Latino samples (8,9). Furthermore, there has been a growing percentage of Latino children among child welfare cases with a disparity ratio above 1.5 when compared to Caucasian children (10,11). In our target community, compared to the overall Oklahoma population, Latino parents involved in the Child Welfare system tended to be younger, have lower income, have lower education levels and were less likely to speak English as a primary language (12).

Current child maltreatment prevention services/programs fail to address the challenges presented in curtailing or attenuating this trend. The adaptation of services/programs is evidently a necessity evidenced by several evaluation study reports indicating null or minimal effects at the very best when conventional prevention programs are used with Latino communities (11). The adaptation of prevention home visiting programs for minority and culturally diverse segments of the population still lags behind and does not seem to adequately address the contextual realities of the unique ethnic, cultural heritages and migration experiences (13,14). Translation of program material while necessary is not sufficient for the holistic cultural adaptation of service models. Adapting service delivery to meet cultural congruency needs while maintaining fidelity to the core components is a difficult balance to make using a home visitation approach of service delivery. Evaluation of receptivity and acceptability of services as well as short-term and long-term outcomes should be embedded in the adaptation process.

The evidence supporting the ability of home visitation programs to ameliorate child maltreatment is limited, particularly among high risk populations, such as families with parental substance use disorders, intimate partner violence (IPV), parental depression and/or other multiple risk factors (15-17). As a remedy, it has been proposed that these programs should be intensive, use skills-based services, ensure fidelity, train home visitor in recognizing and responding to imminent child maltreatment and risk factors, systematically address caregivers' motivation to change problematic behaviors, and successfully link families with services (15-21). Rigorous evaluation methods and procedures are recommended to examine adapted service models, including experimental research designs, independent data collectors, standardized measures, and responsiveness to human subjects concerns.

Thoughtful cultural adaptation of service models with subsequent planned evaluation of the process and outcomes are critical to advancing our ability to address public health concerns, such as child abuse and neglect, and address the racial disparities. Pursuing this goal in a culturally diverse Latino population is neither easy nor straightforward. The complexities and challenges faced were not unique to implementation but also extended to the evaluation of the processes involved and impact of the adapted program model.

In this article, we share the lessons learned from our efforts to culturally adapt an evidence-based home visitation program (EBHV) and evaluate the process and outcomes. First, we will give a brief overview of our adaptation and evaluation to provide context. Next, we will review a series of lessons learned related to language diversity, literacy issues, recruitment and training of providers, measurement, data collection, and evaluation procedures and issues. Each section will describe our challenges, our efforts to address the challenges, and recommendations. We conclude with summarizing our lessons learned to facilitate others pursuing this line of work. The lessons learned are not unique to this population or the topic of child maltreatment prevention, but rather they can be applied to a range of efforts to culturally adapt public health service models.

ADAPTATION AND EVALUATION METHOD

The home visitation based prevention program chosen for this project was SafeCare (SC, www.nstrc.org), which was originally designed for child welfare populations and has empirical support for reduced involvement in child welfare. SC is based on developmental-ecological theory on the etiology of physical child abuse and neglect, using an eco-behavioral model (22). The underlying principles in the eco-behavioral approach are robust and transferable across diverse populations (23). The "eco" refers the ecological approach and that interventions need to be sensitive to the different levels of the ecological system. The "behavioral" component is related to which targets are emphasized (proximal skills and behaviors), as well as technical aspects of how change is pursued (24-26) . The SC model has demonstrated support for reduced recidivism and parent behavior change across a series of studies in both intervention and prevention trials (23,27-29). The core components of SC have been considered to be robust in its use with diverse populations by home visitors (30). Individualized adaptations have been recommended by the providers, with specific suggestions regarding addressing health practices and addressing language and literacy issues to improve receptivity of the materials and handouts (30).

The adaptation process undertaken involved (a) identification of the core components of SC, both topic and procedures, (b) identification of a team of SC experts, prevention of child maltreatment researchers, and service directors and providers from the local Latino communities to guide the adaptation process, (c) review of literature on cultural considerations, (d) identification of cultures and subcultures to be served, (e) identification of factors that potentially impact service delivery, barriers, and challenges, (f) examination of areas of adaptation, (g) creation of guidelines for end products, (h) creation of adapted curriculum and training material, and (i) examination of the process and outcomes in feasibility and implementation trials. Areas of adaptation identified were language and format for learning (i.e., translation issues, reading level, illustrations, etc.), extended families and social networks, acculturation, traditional health beliefs and practices, storytelling and proverbs, racism/discrimination, spirituality/religion, immigration laws, and relationship development. Efforts to culturally adapt interventions must be sensitive to concerns of promoting stereotypes. To this end, the adaptation focused not only on the SC curriculum but also the training of the providers to deliver the curriculum in a culturally congruent and sensitive approach.

In order to adequately capture and assess the intrinsic contextual and measureable attributes of the adaptation, we used mixed research methods. Quantitative measures were used to determine how much of an impact/change the overall adapted SC modules had on the target areas of parent-child interaction, child health, improvement of home safety and healthy relationships. The data collection activities involved using questionnaire guided interviews by data collectors who were independent from the home visitors. Data was collected pre and post services to track progress and change in program target areas (child health, home safety, parenting and healthy relationships). In addition to the quantitative measures, qualitative factors were also assessed. The perceptions of the workers on training material, perceptions of the consumers on the trainings, materials and the context of the relationships formed between consumers and home providers were also sought through face to face interviews.

The feasibility results from these evaluative activities showed parents and providers found the adapted model culturally congruent and useful. Further, families served reported significant improvements in targeted parenting skills and knowledge. The objective of the current paper, however, is not to provide details of the adaptation or results from process and impact evaluation but rather to share the challenges and lessons learned from these endeavors. A detailed report describing the adaptation, process and impact evaluation results can be found elsewhere (31).

LESSONS LEARNED

While the pace, scale of the adaptations, and evaluation of the feasibility phase of the study have been successful, there were significant challenges encountered. These challenges, however, are common in the prevention field and warrant continued examination (32-34). In discussing the lessons learned, we provide some context to: (a) challenges encountered, (b) remedies explored to address the challenges, and (c) some recommendations based on our experiences.

Language is diverse. The overwhelming majority of Latino participants served as part of the feasibility study could not proficiently read or understand materials in English, therefore, the likelihood that participants would respond to training material or questionnaire assessments from their own perspective, inconsistent with the underlying intent if the training and assessments were maintained in English was high. Thus, translating the curriculum, handouts, and training materials into Spanish was a priority.

Translating parent material and measures that are readily understood by such a diverse population posed many challenges. The Latino population in many communities in the US is comprised of Spanish speaking immigrants from multiple countries and regions of the world (35, 36). In our area, these include Mexico, Central America, South America, and the Caribbean Islands. We saw distinct differences in the conceptualization and understanding of some of the program concepts and materials due to this diversity. The perception and interpretation of some training material was different when piloted among participants with varying countries of origin and Spanish dialects. Some words had distinct meanings, either in addition to the global meaning (under "standard" Spanish) or in place of it across the dialects. For example, in our community, Latinos from Mexico may use the term "Estoy endrogado" to mean that they have lots of debts, but it literally means "to be drugged out." Some will use "mueble" to mean "car" when the literal translation is "furniture". Some Puerto Ricans call the stomach "pipa" or "pipita" whereas for other Latino's "pipa" means "pipe".

The distinct meanings in the different regional dialects not only impacted the development of training materials but also the evaluation measures used to assess the trainings received by the participants. To help bridge these differences and allow for a mutual comprehension of adapted training material, we worked closely with the service director (PD) and supervisor (IC) who knew the families served well to facilitate choosing terms and words most representative for the families. Often this involved using formal Spanish also at times termed as "Neutral" or "Standard" Spanish. The formal Spanish often disregards the local grammatical and phonetic peculiarities while preserving a more commonly acknowledged canon across dialects from varying origins (37). Formal Spanish was also preferred as it was considered more respectful to the family, particularly during the initial contact with the family and measurement collection. Further, we were careful to train the data collector and providers to be aware of language differences, in order to detect and correct any misunderstandings.

Literacy issues. As a sobering backdrop to the need for appropriate material for training and evaluation, the demographic survey administered to study participants at enrollment revealed that less than 30% had a high school degree or its equivalent. To effectively communicate with the parents, training handouts had to be revised to simpler language aided with more pictures to help clarify instructions. The combination of the relatively high illiteracy rates in the community and the limitations of the text-to-speech computer programs required that questionnaire items (from risk assessment measures) be recorded for the computer interviews to provide audio assistance to address reading proficiency issues. It is important to note that while the recorded interviews have been a tremendous help in addressing literacy issues; the use of the computer for the interview has also been a bit intimidating to families unfamiliar with technology.

Our provider agency team's knowledge of and experience with the local Latino communities' was invaluable as we adapted parent training materials and evaluation measures. Their involvement ranged from piloting the original questionnaires, offering suggestions for modifications and changes, adapting materials for use with the families, to attesting of the final measures and parent training material.

Despite having literacy problems, participating families seemed eager and willing to learn and implement new ways of parenting and more appropriate behaviors that were beneficial to their children, particularly when they fit with their cultural values and practices. The SafeCare protocol was adapted in conformity with these expectations embedded in the concept of "familia" (importance of family involvement in day to day decision making process and livelihood). This in many ways was a motivating factor in by itself in fostering the learning process as a whole.

Formal versus informal language. Officially translated measures were inconsistent in regards to formality of the language used, which can be jarring when integrated into an audio computer assisted self- interview (ACASI) package. It was based on this reality that we decided to augment measures with additional background information to provide context for the assessment interviews in an effort to reasonably accommodate these realities. When we could, we used a neutral ("standard") dialect of Spanish which conformed to the formal setting (attenuating the peculiarities across dialects) intended for the administration of the measure assessments (for example, demographic questionnaires, Center for Epidemiologic Studies Depression Scale measure, etc.). For officially translated measures, we used their published form to allow for comparability and generalizability of our measure results to the norming populations used in measure development (for example, the Conflict Tactics Scale, a screening tool for domestic violence). To address the differences across measures, we trained data collectors to prepare parents (study participants) for potential differences in question formality and dialects during assessment interviews.

Hiring Providers. The pool of competent bilingual and bicultural service providers in the Latino community is relatively small. This was further compounded by the fact that bilingual profieciency was a necessary but not a sufficient attribute for employment eligibility. In addition to being bilingual, prospective providers needed to be aware of the cultural nuances in order to understand and appreciate the diversity of the families being served.

In past studies, home based providers with bachelor's degrees in social services, Early Childhood Education, or other related fields have been readily identified, hired, and trained to fidelity in SC successfully (23). However, for this project the providers needed to be bilingual. Given the intrisic challenges already elaborated upon above, we had to lower our education level requirement for home visitor positions to accommodate Associate Degree graduates and/or paraprofessionals with some college education in the related fields. Having some related community experiences or knowledge of the community and its resources was an added advantage. These accomodations were sanctioned by the SC model developers. Further, we took into account the potential effects of "machismo" (traditional roles and acceptable behavior for men) in the local community, particularly when considering hiring male home visitors and how it may impact acceptability and cultural congruence of the parenting curriculum and healthy relationships curriculum (an augmentation of the adapted SC protocol to addresses domestic violence) among young mothers who tended to form the majority of the enrolled study participants.

Providers training. Providers face multiple challenges providing services in Latino communities due to a number of unique circumstances in which they find their clients. The intersection of language differences, immigration related issues and cultural diversity can create barriers that providers may not be trained to navigate, resulting in frustration and burnout. A culture of openness and realization of these challenges was important and crucial in helping providers feel comfortable seeking help and guidance through supervision, coaching and ongoing trainings.

Although all providers recruited were bilingual, they differed in whether English or Spanish was their primary/first language. Training in both English and Spanish was important to accommodate the need to process and practice the material in different languages. Our expectations were not that the providers be proficient in both languages but rather be willing to learn and better their trade in service provision for the presumed diverse clientelle.

Furthermore, inlight of the potential differences between provider and client backgrounds, it was incumbent upon the team to offer extensive training to the providers to ensure proper understanding of potential differences in language and personalismo expectations (the need to relate in personal terms with more warmth and less clinical detachment) needed to serve our clients. The Latino Agency staff (PD and IC) provided invalauble insights in the training process and integration of the modified SC modules to fit the personalismo expectations.

There was a steep learning curve in the mastery of the the SC protocol. However, this was not unique to our SC program since similar experiences have been reported by other EBHV grantees implementing EBHV models even among experienced home visitors (38). The coaching/shadowing approach to training providers used by SC beyond the certification process proved to be an invaluable asset in achieving provider confidence and competence. Even though shadowing after a provider had received full certification was of less intensity and frequency,we found it to be an effective way to provide feedback to providers to support flexibly in adaptating the program to each families' unique circumstances while maintaining the core components and model fidelity.

Evaluation context. The additional program efficacy achieved as a direct result of adaptations of evidence based prevention programs for different cultures is not well documented (11, 32, 39). Often, external validity and generalizability of adapted program outcome across diverse cultures and populations is not possible. Furthermore, the variance in accommodations to balance fidelity and cultural responsiveness make unbiased comparisons across different population often unattainable. While a broad approach to addressing these challenges faced by the prevention field is warranted, we believe, we were better served with a set of narrow and focused evaluation objectives given the low sample size (N=28) in the feasibility phase. The broader questions were planned for the larger outcomes evaluation. We focused our feasibility study evaluation activities on three main areas: 1) acceptability of the adapted SC protocol including its augmentations (healthy relationship curriculum), 2) usefulness of the new model in addressing SC target areas (parenting, healthy relationships, home safety and child health) and the underlying co-morbid risk factors: IPV, depression and other mental disorders, and substance abuse, and 3) adherence by families served and home visitors (providers) to the new (adapted and augmented) SC protocol.

A major challenge in our evaluation planning was selection of evaluation measures and processes. It was critical to have validity weigh heavily on the chosen measures and approaches. Although issues surrounding validity have often been specific for the various outcomes targeted by prevention programs, one overarching concern was whether chosen instruments were appropriate (that is, reading level, wording, length of items, structure, format). In some cases, measurement evaluation was warranted to assess possible variations in questions or instrument interpretation and understandability. In piloting paper measures (for example, the Working Alliance Inventory), we found that providing context and assurances beyond what is provided in the standard measure instructions went a long way in clarifying intent of measures was to seek an honest opinion regarding service provision rather than a biased response seeking to portray services or home visitors (providers) based on perceived and perhaps cultural expectation. Further, items on measures that used double negatives were identified as difficult to understand and resulted in reduced accuracy of responses.

Another challenge was minimizing the quantity of data that is requested from participants while ensuring high data accuracy and validity. This was further compounded by the need to adhere to the common cultural verbal and non-verbal communication norms while showing respect and personal caring. Collaboration among evaluation and local agency staff was important in aiding the reflective decision making process with respect to who collects what type of data (independent data collectors versus home visitors) depending on the content and tact needed during the data collection process. Caution is needed in making considerations to avert or attenuate potential biases in the data collection process. For example, while the use of audio computer assisted interviews has many advantages (40), it limited a respondent's ability to clarify responses. For some questionnaire items where we felt consumers needed allowances for clarification, we found it necessary to include prompts in the ACASI (Audio Computer Assisted Self Interview) interview for consumers to consult with the data collectors. We also realized some lines of questioning needed a more sensitive approach to data collection and were best conducted by a face to face interview format outside the context of ACASI. It was a delicate balance making the trade-off between confidentiality and being able to obtain valid data. For fidelity measures, the home visitors seemed to be in a better position to obtain more valid responses because of their established relationship and time spent with the family.

It was important to be able to align the flow of the assessment processes so that participants could transition from one method to the next with limited fatigue in the evaluation processes. Involvement of providers in evaluating progress made by their clients grounded a shared sense of purpose on the part of service team as a whole, and was a motivation for reaching service goals. The use of home visitors as data collectors was not without its challenges. Not only did this require measure collection specific training (e.g. training for the collection of Ages and Stages questionnaire data) upfront. It took some getting used to for some providers to fully appreciate the importance of being objective and unbiased during assessments.

While the quantitative evaluations seemed to be exhaustive, there was a clear need for a qualitative context to all study activities through the eyes of the families served. The providers (home visitors), agency and research staff also indicated a need for more contextual feedback beyond what quantitative measures provided. Though not initially planned as part of the feasibility study, we instituted study protocol modifications to be able to use a face to face interview approach to address this need. We were not only interested in the opinions, ideas and information to inform our larger outcome study but also needed to address some inadequacies of the universally validated instruments used for quantitative assessments (33). Mindful of the diversity in Spanish dialect and given the fact that translations of written data collection measures however good often change meanings of questions (34), it was imperative to capitalize on the stimulation, refinement of thoughts and perspectives of the interactive approach offered through interviews. While the potential for interviewer bias cannot be overlooked, overall, this process enabled the research team to answer important questions about participant engagement and effectiveness of the services provided. The process also helped the team better interpret and put into perspective some of the reported field experiences during data collection and trainings with the providers.

CONCLUSION

Despite these challenges, the lessons learned from these undertakings underscored the importance of taking time to create a culturally sensitive and congruent approach to service provision and evaluation. For the providers, ongoing coaching and close supervision is necessary to ensure they feel supported and encouraged to deal with the complexities in service provision. Furthermore, a shared objective in valid and effective assessment of progress and impact of services among all parties involved is needed to achieve overall project goals. The adaptation process requires attention to issues related not only to the evaluative processes of its relevance and impact but also the cultural context in which they are perceived; these issues intersect to determine the overall validity of results obtained (35, 36, 41). In addition, aspects related to provider (home visitor) adherence and competence to deliver the adapted program with fidelity should not be overlooked.

Overall, there were many lessons learned through the feasibility study phase of the project. The extent to which such accommodations may make a difference in prevention outcomes remains to be investigated. Furthermore, assessing whether the direct and indirect costs incurred in the adaptation process and the effects of maladaptation outweigh the benefits is warranted. As we transition to the full project implementation and evaluation, we look forward to continuing to learn lessons as there is no doubt that this is an ongoing process. Future implementation efforts could explore ways of adapting other standard home visitation models locally in congruence with the unique attributes of the populations they seek to serve.

ACKNOWLEDGMENTS

This research was supported by a research grant from Children's Bureau, Administration for Children and Families, U.S. Department of Health and Human Services #90CA1764 (Principal Investigator: Jane F. Silovsky). The opinions expressed are those of the authors and do not necessarily reflect those of the OUHSC or USDHHS. The authors would like to recognize the support, input, technical assistance, and hard work on this project from our colleagues at the Latino Community Development Agency, including providers, data colletors, and Cindy Garcia, and SafeCare consultant Karla Ledesma from South Bay Community Services. We would also like to recognize the technical assistance provided by the training and research team at the Center on Child Abuse and Neglect (CCAN) at The University of Oklahoma Health Sciences Center (OUHSC): David Bard, Debra Hecht, Steve Ross, Lorena Burris, Donna Wells, La Chanda Stephens-Totimeh, Carrie Schwab, and Melissa Brown, as well as colleagues at the National SafeCare Training and Research Center (www.nstrc.org), John Lutzker and Dan Whitaker. The authors declare that they have no conflict of interest.

REFERENCES

[1]   Runyan D, Wattam C, Ikeda R, Hassan F, Ramiro L. Child abuse and neglect by parents and caregivers. In: Krug E, Dahlberg LL, Mercy JA, Zwi AB, Lozano R, editors. World report on violence and health. Geneva, Switzerland: World Health Organization, 2002: 59-86. Accessed 2011 Nov 15. Available from: www.who.int/violence_injury_prevention/violence/global_campaign/en/chap3.pdf

[2]   Foege WH. Adverse childhood experiences. A public health perspective. Am J Prev Med 1998;14(4):354-5.

[3]   Weiss MJ, Wagner SH. What explains the negative consequences of adverse childhood experiences on adult health? Insights from cognitive and neuroscience research. Am J Prev Med 1998;14(4):356-60.

[4]   White C. The Health Care Reform Legislation: An overview. The Economists' Voice 2010;7:Article 1.

[5]   United States Department of Health and Human Services Secretary Kathleen Sebelius. Sebelius Remarks: Health Reform and You: How the New Law Will Increase Your Health Security. 2010.

Accessed 2011 Nov 15. Available from: http://www.hhs.gov/news/press/2010pres/04/20100 406b.html. .

[6]   U.S. Bureau of the Census, Statistical Abstract of the United States, Washington, DC: U.S. Government Printing Office, 2010.

[7]   Braveman PA, Cubbin C, Egerter S, Williams DR, Pamuk E. Socioeconomic disparities in health in the United States: what the patterns tell us. Am J Public Health 2010;100 Suppl 1:S186-96.

[8]   Alegria M, Canino G, Shrout PE, Woo M, Duan N, Vila D, et al. Prevalence of mental illness in immigrant and non-immigrant U.S. Latino groups. Am J Psychiatry 2008;165(3):359-69.

[9]   Grant BF, Stinson FS, Hasin DS, Dawson DA, Chou SP, Anderson K. Immigration and lifetime prevalence of DSM-IV psychiatric disorders among Mexican Americans and non-Hispanic whites in the United States: results from the National Epidemiologic Survey on Alcohol and Related Conditions. Arch Gen Psychiatry 2004;61(12):1226-33. Epub 2004/12/08.

[10]   Shusterman, GR, Hollinshead, D, Fluke, JD, Yuan, Y.T Alternative responses to child maltreatment: Findings from NCANDS.Washington, DC: U.S. Department of Health and Human Services, Office of the Assistant Secretary for Planning and Evaluation, 2005.

[11]   The Workgroup on Adapting Latino Services Adaptation guidelines for serving Latino children and families affected by trauma (1st Ed.). San Diego, CA: Chadwick Center for Children and Families, 2008.

[12]   Oklahoma Department of Human Services, Children and Family Services Division. OKDHS annual report. Oklahoma, OK, 2010.

[13]   Comas-Di´az, L. Latino healing: The integration of ethnic psychology into psychotherapy. Psychology Theory Res Pract Training 2006; 436-453.

[14]   Whaley AL, Davis KE. Cultural competence and evidence-based practice in mental health services: a complementary perspective. Am Psychol 2007;62(6):563-74.

[15]   Duggan A, Fuddy, L., Burrell, L., Higman, S. M., McFarlane, E., Windham, A., Sia, C. Randomized trial of a statewide home visiting program to prevent child abuse: impact in reducing parental risk factors. Child Abuse Negl 2004;28(6):623-43.

[16]   Duggan A, McFarlane E, Fuddy L, Burrell L, Higman SM, Windham A, et al. Randomized trial of a statewide home visiting program: impact in preventing child abuse and neglect. Child Abuse Negl 2004;28(6):597-622.

[17]   Gomby DS, Culross PL, Behrman RE. Home visiting: recent program evaluations-analysis and recommendations. The Future of children/ Center for the Future of Children, the David and Lucile Packard Foundation, 1999;9(1):4-26, 195-223.

[18]   Gutterman NB. Early Prevention of Physical Child Abuse and Neglect: Existing Evidence and Future Directions. Child Maltreat 1997;2:12-34.

[19]   Gutterman NB. Enrollment strategies in early home visitation to prevent physical child abuse and neglect and the "universal versus targeted" debate: A meta-analysis of population-based and screening-based programs. Child Abuse Negl 1999; 23:863-90.

[20]   Landsverk J, Carillio T, Connelly CD, Ganer WC, Slymen DJ, Newton RR, et al. Healthy families San Diego clinical trial: Technical Report. San Diego Children's Hospital and Health Center, Child and Adolescent Services Research Center, 2002.

[21]   Tandon SD, Parillo KM,Jenkins C,Duggan A K Formative evaluation of home visitors' role in addressing poor mental health, domestic violence, and substance abuse among low-income pregnant and parenting women. Matern Child Health J 2005;9(3):273-83.

[22]   Lutzker JR, Bigelow KM. Reducing child maltreatment: A guidebook for parent services. New York: Guilford, 2002.

[23]   Silovsky JF, Bard D, Chaffin M, Hecht D, Burris L, Owora A, et al. Prevention of child maltreatment in high-risk rural families: A randomized clinical trial with child welfare outcomes. Child Youth Serv Rev 2011;33:1435-44.

[24]   Lutzker JR. Project 12-Ways: Treating child abuse and neglect from an ecobehavioral perspective. In: Dangel RF, Polster RA, eds. Parent training: Foundations of research and practice. New York: Guilford, 1984.

[25]   Belsky J. Etiology of child maltreatment: A developmental-ecological analysis. Psychol Bull 1993;114:413-34.

[26]   Bigelow KM, Lutzker JR. Using video to teach planned activities to parents reported for child abuse. Child Fam Behav Ther 1998;20:1-14.

[27]   Lutzker JR, Rice, J. M. Using recidivism data to evaluate Project 12-Ways: An ecobehavioral approach to the treatment and prevention of child abuse and neglect. J Fam Violence 1987;2:283-90.

[28]   Lutzker JR, Rice JM. Project 12-Ways: Measuring outcome of a large-scale in-home service for the treatment and prevention of child abuse and neglect. Child Abuse Negl 1984; 8:519-24.

[29]   Lutzker JR, Bigelow K M, Doctor R M, Gershater R M, Greene B F. An ecobehavioral model for the prevention and treatment of child abuse and neglect. In Lutzker JR, Handbook of Child Abuse Research and Treatment. New York: Plenum Press, 1998.

[30]   Self-Brown S, Frederick K, Binder S, Whitaker D, Lutzker J, Edwards A et al. Examining the need for cultural adaptations to an evidence-based parent training program targeting the prevention of child maltreatment. Child Youth Serv Rev 2011;33(7):1166-72.

[31]   Beasley L, Silovsky JF, Burris L, Owora, A. Preventing child maltreatment in high risk latino communities: Model adaptation, implementation and lessons learned. Unpublished Manuscript, 2011.

[32]   Bauer RM. Evidence-based practice in psychology: implications for research and research training. J Clin Psychology 2007;63(7):685-94.

[33]   Clark MJ, Cary S, Diemert G, Ceballos R, Sifuentes M, Atteberry I et al. Involving communities in community assessment. Public Health Nurs 2003;20(6):456-63.

[34]   Huer MB, Saenz TI. Challenges and strategies for conducting survey and focus group research with culturally diverse groups. Am J Speech Lang Pathol 2003;12(2):209-20.

[35]   Meeting the health promotion needs of Hispanic communities. National Coalition of Hispanic Health and Human Services Organizations (COSSMHO) Policy and Research. Am J Health Promo 1995; 9(4):300-11.

[36]   Capitman JA, Pacheco TL, Ramírez M, Gonzalez A. Promotoras: Lessons learned on improving healthcare access to latinos. Fresno, CA: Central Valley Health Policy Institute, 2009.

[37]   Cotton EG, Sharp JM. Spanish in the Americas. Georgetown University Press, 1998.

[38]   Del Grosso P, Hargreaves H, Paulsell D, Vogel C, Strong DA, Zaveri H, et al. Building infrastructure to support home visiting to prevent child maltreatment: Two-year findings from the cross-site evaluation of the supporting Evidence-Based Home Visiting Initiative.Children's Bureau, Administration for Children and Families, U.S. Department of Health and Human Services. Available from Mathematica Policy Research, Princeton, NJ , 2011.

[39]   Fontes L. Child abuse and culture: Working with diverse families. New York: Guilford, 2005.

[40]   Metzger DS, Koblin B, Turner C, Navaline H, Valenti F, Holte S, et al. . Randomized controlled trial of audio computer-assisted self-interviewing: utility and acceptability in longitudinal studies. HIVNET Vaccine Preparedness Study Protocol Team. Am J Epidemiol 2000;152(2):99-106.

[41]   Kumpfer KL, Alvarado R, Smith P, Bellamy N. Cultural sensitivity and adaptation in family-based prevention interventions. Prev Sci 2002;3(3):241-6.

Submitted: October 16, 2011. *Revised:* November 28, 2011. *Accepted:* December 04, 2011.

In: Public Health Yearbook 2012
Editor: Joav Merrick

Chapter 25

ENVIRONMENTAL PUBLIC HEALTH EDUCATION PARTNERSHIPS: SUCCESSES AND CHALLENGES

*Mary O Dereski, PhD** and Lisa Pietrantoni, BS*

Institute of Environmental Health Sciences, Wayne State University, Detroit, Michigan, United States of America

ABSTRACT

The Healthy Homes = Healthy Kids (HH=HK) program was developed at Wayne State University (WSU) in collaboration with the city of Detroit Head Start Program (DHSP). The HH=HK Program consists of six topics with a focus on the environmental health of children living in urban homes. The topics included in the program are: Heavy Metals, Poisonous Look-a-Likes, Food Safety, Indoor Water, Indoor Air, and Pest Control. The program was disseminated through Train-the-Trainer workshops with participants from DHSP and subsequently from the Childcare Coordinating Council in Detroit, Michigan. Workshop participants were provided with presentation materials, fact sheets, and posters in English, Spanish and Arabic. To assess the effectiveness of the workshops, participants were given content knowledge tests prior to (pre) and after (post) the Train-the-Trainer sessions. Follow-up surveys were mailed to participants within one year of completing the training to determine training material usage within the community. HH=HK fact sheets were also made available for download on the National Institutes of Environmental Health Sciences (NIEHS) web-based resource page. Results of the pre- and post-tests, follow-up surveys, and numbers of fact sheet downloads are presented and discussed. The successes and challenges facing partnership building for effective environmental health education programs are addressed.

Keywords: Environment, public health, train-the-trainer, university partnerships

---

* Correspondence: Mary O Dereski, PhD, Associate Professor, Oakland University William Beaumont School of Medicine, 127 O'Dowd Hall, Rochester MI, 48309. Email: mdereski@oakland.edu.

INTRODUCTION

The Healthy Homes=Healthy Kids (HH=HK) program was developed through a partnership between Wayne State University (WSU), and the City of Detroit Head Start Program (DHSP) in order to build community capacity to address indoor environmental health concerns. The program incorporated a Train-the-Trainer component with evaluation of training material usage and dissemination through follow up surveys. The successes and challenges of this health education partnership are described.

Increasing industrialization in urban cities provides areas of environmental health concerns for its residents. Progressively more of this environmental burden is borne by the youngest and oldest members of our population. As a consequence, universities are exploring mechanisms for environmental health education in an urban setting. As these programs develop, universities recognize the advantage of partnering with organizations that work directly within the community. These partnerships can involve a spectrum of activities from Community Health Educational Programs (1-3) to those recruiting participants into Community-Based Participatory Research (4). The common element underlying success of these programs is building a strong and sustainable collaboration between the partners including strong ties within the community. These types of partnerships have the potential for building community capacity for better environmental health (5). Knowledge can be gained from assessing the process whereby these partnerships are built and the subsequent programs that have developed from these collaborations (6).

The HH=HK program described here, addresses several indoor environmental health issues facing young children living in the city of Detroit, Michigan. An integrative topic approach was utilized since children are often simultaneously exposed to multiple environmental health hazards while in their homes (7).

METHODS

Funding for development of the HH=HK program was secured through a National Institutes of Environmental Health Sciences (NIEHS) Center supplement at Wayne State University (WSU). The program partnership was a collaborative effort between WSU and DHSP. Translation of materials into Spanish and Arabic was provided through a community-based program (Lead Busters) funded by the Environmental Protection Agency (Region 5).

DHSP was selected as a university partner due to its mission as a national program promoting school readiness by enhancing the social and cognitive development of children through educational, health, nutritional, social and other services to families. Additionally, significant emphasis is placed on the involvement of parents in the administration of local DHSP programs, thereby offering the potential for subsequent in-home utilization of the HH=HK training contents by trainers who are also members of the affected community.

Following a series of joint DHSP-WSU meetings, it was decided that the HH=HK program would focus on indoor environmental health hazards. This specific focus was chosen since children living in urban homes constitute a highly vulnerable population for adverse environmental exposures (8). It would also allow the community members to take ownership and action regarding one or more of their children's environmental health areas of concern. Moreover, choosing a focus that allowed direct action on the part of the participants helped allay the feeling of helplessness that is often experienced by individuals exposed to environmental hazards. The ability to act upon environmental exposures is consistent with an Environmental Health Model where value is placed on the ability to decrease environmental hazards exposure (9).

The HH=HK program consisted of information on the environmental hazards and preventative measures associated with the following topics: Heavy Metals (Lead and Mercury), Pesticides (including Integrated Pest Management), Indoor Air (asthma triggers, carbon monoxide, and tobacco smoke), Indoor Water (lead, copper, arsenic), Poisonous Look-a-Likes (in the bedroom, kitchen, bathroom, garage and garden), and Food Safety (food handling and types of bacterial contamination).

Once the topics were chosen, faculty and staff of the Institute of Environmental Health Sciences (WSU) began to develop fact sheets for each topic. A uniform format for each fact sheet was utilized and the readability level was determined to be appropriate by DHSP members.

Standardization of information on each fact sheet allowed for compatibility between training sessions covering the various environmental health topics. An example of the uniform questions answered for each topic is presented below for Mercury:

- What is Mercury?
- What is Mercury poisoning?
- What happens if someone is poisoned by Mercury?
- Where is Mercury found in and around your home?
- What should you do if mercury is spilled in your home or if you eat fish from Michigan's lakes and rivers?
- Did you know these interesting facts about Mercury?

Upon completion of the fact sheets, a graphic artist was hired to enhance the visual appeal of the program materials and to develop a colorful poster to illustrate the various topics covered by the Train-the-Trainer program (Figure 1). The poster highlighted the six environmental health topics. Subsequently, individuals from the local Arabic and Hispanic communities were hired to translate the fact sheets into the appropriate languages for their communities.

In preparation for the Train-the-Trainer sessions, WSU staff developed PowerPoint presentations and transparencies for presentation purposes. A training manual was also developed to accompany the 12 hours of instruction (2 hours for each of the 6 topics). The two hour sessions incorporated pre- and post-knowledge testing for each topic, a PowerPoint presentation, a hands-on activity and discussion of information contained on the fact sheet. Training manuals, fact sheets and posters were made available for all participants attending the Train-the-Trainer sessions. In addition, a resource manual was compiled with applicable brochures, web sites and contact information for Detroit-based organizations that would complement the content of each training session topic.

Upon completion of the manual, training workshop sessions were scheduled with DHSP program representatives from throughout the city of Detroit. DHSP leadership was asked to determine the day, time, and length of the training sessions.

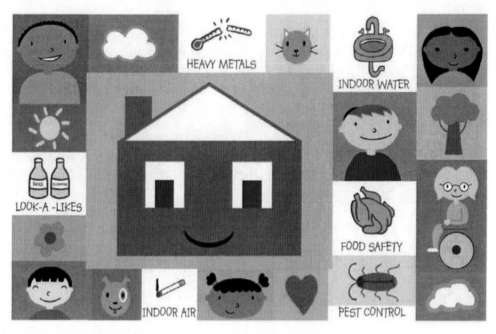

Figure 1. Healthy Homes=Healthy Kids Poster. The following poster was utilized for Train-the-Trainer and community presentation purposes. Each participant in the Train-the-Trainer programs received a poster in the language(s) requested (English, Arabic, Spanish). Artist: Mary Iverson.

An Agreement of Collaboration between WSU and the Director of DHSP describing the topics to be included in the training workshops, the time frame in which the workshops were to take place, and the use of pre- and post-tests, as well as surveys was signed by both the WSU principal investigator and DHSP leadership.

Sessions were held in the DHSP main headquarters where trainers were familiar with the surroundings and accustomed to attending training workshops as a requirement of their employment. Upon successful completion of the DHSP

Train-the-Trainer sessions, a community-based organization, the Child Care Coordinating Council of Detroit (4Cs) was contacted to participate in the trainings. The 4Cs of Detroit is a private, non-profit organization that has been providing services to families, children and child care professionals since 1970.

The mission of 4Cs Detroit/Wayne County, Inc. is to educate, support and thereby empower families, communities and service programs to provide quality care and healthy environments for all children. Leadership from the 4Cs organization was instrumental in scheduling the HH=HK training sessions with individuals from their organization.

Follow-up surveys were sent to all participants in the Train-the-Trainer workshops within one year of completion of the training. A gift card in appreciation for participation and a stamped, self-addressed envelope were enclosed with the follow-up survey.

RESULTS

Outcomes of the Train-the-Trainer workshops that were assessed:

1. Partnership building and program development;
2. Recruitment for Train-the-Trainer sessions;
3. Knowledge assessment and workshop satisfaction evaluation; and
4. Follow up usage and dissemination survey.

1. Partnership building and program development

The partnership building between WSU and the DHSP took place over several months. The leadership of DHSP was initially contacted and their interest and enthusiasm for development of the Train-the-Trainer programs was gauged by their willingness to participate in the planning process. Following several collaborative meetings, it was jointly decided that indoor environmental health topics would be the main focus of the educational programs. Six topics were identified that were of particular interest and relevance to the community. Single-sided "Fact Sheets" outlining educational and prevention measures for the six topics were the core of the program. DSHP indicated that the amount of information on a single sheet of paper in black and white could be easily copied and would contain an appropriate amount of information for the community members to understand and act upon. In addition, it was proposed by DSHP, that the accompanying fact sheets and poster should be translated into Spanish and Arabic for use by their trainers within the appropriate bilingual communities.

2. Recruitment for train-the-trainer sessions

Officials from DHSP and the 4Cs were directly responsible for recruitment of their members into the Train-the-Trainer workshops. A series of three workshops on the HH=HK program were scheduled (12 total hours of training). Trainers were provided with training manuals and fact sheets following participation in the training sessions. Requests for materials occurring after the training workshops were also honored.

Individuals from DHSP and 4Cs were recruited and participated in separate training workshops. Two of the six HH=HK topics were presented during each workshop day, with a lunch break between topics. Although, care was taken to schedule the training sessions according to the requests of the organizational leadership, attending all six topic trainings proved difficult if not impossible for each of the Train-the-Trainer workshop participants. Complete training manuals and materials covering all six topics were provided to the trainers regardless of their participation in every training workshop.

3. Knowledge assessment and workshop evaluation

Pre- and post-tests of knowledge consisting of ten questions for each of the six indoor environmental health topics. The tests were given to the Train-the-Trainer participants immediately before and after the training workshops on the particular topic. Unpaired tests were not included in the analysis. An anonymous post workshop survey was also administered to the participants at the conclusion of the Train-the-Trainer workshops to gauge satisfaction and usefulness of the content and delivery of the training.

Anonymity of the participants was maintained by suggesting that the participants utilize a false name or a numerical value on both the pre- and post-tests. The participants indicated that this option placed them at ease with regard to the fear of reporting potentially low test scores to the organizational leadership.

DHSP

There were 39 participants in total. The pre- and post-tests were paired for each participant and the change in percent correct score for each topic was analyzed using a paired student t-test. The data show a significant rise in post-test scores for each of the six topics (Figure 2, Head Start, $p<0.002$). These data indicate the workshops were effective in conveying the educational information presented during the Train-the-Trainer sessions, and that knowledge regarding these environmental topics was needed by the trainers. The largest gain in knowledge was in the area of indoor water health education covering the topics of lead, copper and arsenic contamination.

Post-training workshop surveys indicated that all participants felt confident in utilizing the HH=HK materials for community education. Forty-three percent of the Head Start trainees indicated that the training manual would be the most useful resource in presenting the information to their clients within the community. The remainder felt that the transparencies or the PowerPoint presentation would be most useful.

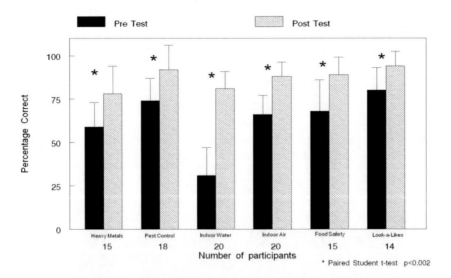

Figure 2. DHSP (Head Start) Pre- and Post-Test Scores. There was a significant increase in post-test scores for participants from Head Start trainings. The greatest increase in percent correct score involved the materials that covered the Indoor Water topics (lead, copper and arsenic). Paired student t-test scores indicated a significant increase in percentage correct answers for all topics ($p<0.002$).

4Cs

Pre- and post-tests of knowledge on the various topics were given to the 4Cs Train-the-Trainer participants immediately before and after the training sessions on each of the six topics (n=14). These tests were paired for each participant and evaluated using a paired student t-test. The data show a significant rise in post-test scores for each of the six topics (Figure 3, p<0.05) indicating the workshops were effective in conveying the educational information. The largest gain in knowledge was again in the area of indoor water health education.

The program was enthusiastically received by the attendees from both organizations. Participants stated that they planned to use the materials with the families they counsel and that all six indoor environmental health topics were informative and useful. All trainers felt that the material was covered thoroughly and presented at a level that could easily be understood and conveyed to their clients within the community. Trainers stated they would recommend the HH=HK program to other personnel from their organizations.

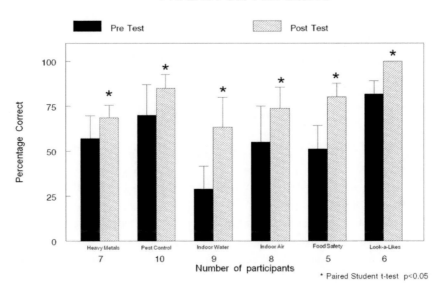

Figure 3. 4Cs (Childcare Coordinating Council) Pre- and Post-Test Scores. There was a significant increase in post-test scores for participants from 4Cs trainings. The greatest increase in percent correct score involved the materials that covered the Indoor Water topics (lead, copper and arsenic). Paired student t-test scores indicated a significant increase in percentage correct answers for all topics (p<0.05).

4. Follow up usage and dissemination survey

DHSP

A follow up survey was sent within one year of the training to the participants in the DHSP Train-the-Trainer workshops. Twenty participants responded to the follow up survey (51% response rate).

Those who responded were asked to report how many families attended the training sessions and received the educational materials. Respondents indicated that the materials were used in: counseling sessions with families as a whole, one-on-one family workshops, parent workshops, healthcare review sessions, support meetings, new employee trainings, teachers, childcare directors, and church family meetings.

Sixty-five percent of those who responded to the survey stated that in addition to the families (parents, caregivers, extended family members) with whom they used the materials, they plan to train co-workers, parents and community members in using the materials to present to others. Materials were requested only in English.

The total number of families that received the information was 4,273 (the average dissemination was 200 families per trainer). The topics for the community training sessions were selected by the trainers and consisted of the following:

616	Families----Heavy Metals
66	Families----Indoor Air
1,274	Families----Poisonous Look-A-Likes
754	Families----Pesticides
659	Families----Indoor Water
904	Families----Food Safety

In addition, DHSP workshop participants made the following comments about the HH=HK materials:

- "[The] material is very informative, especially the heavy metal material. We have had workshops for both parents and staff."
- "The parents seemed interested. Parents have followed up with lead cleaning in the homes."
- "The materials seem to be very informative. Many of the families learn quite a bit from the information we give them."
- "Parents want to be informed. They were very receptive. Thank you for giving me the opportunity to participate."
- "Parents are glad to be made aware of dangers [in their home] and [the] preventative resources [available]."

4Cs

Only five participants of the fourteen who attended the training workshops, responded to the follow up survey (37%). Of these responses, 80% of the participants indicated that they utilized the training workshop materials with individual community members and not with families as was the case with DHSP. The topics chosen by the 4Cs trainers for dissemination in the community were as follows:

45 individuals--- Heavy Metals
50 individuals---Indoor Air
40 individuals---Poisonous Look-A-Likes
40 individuals---Pesticides
40 individuals---Indoor Water

50 individuals---Food safety

A total of 265 community members attended the Trainer's workshops and received materials (average dissemination was one trainer reaching 20 community members). 4Cs trainers did not request materials in any language other than English. Additional comments:

- "[The materials were] useful for understanding Heavy Metals"
- "Very good material, learn[ed] something new."
- "Clients found the information very useful and informative."

National availability on the NIEHS resource web site

In addition to the locally held Train-the-Trainer sessions, fact sheets for all topics and languages were made available on the NIEHS Resources web page. The number of fact sheet downloads from the NIEHS Resources page was 25,507 during a three year period (Figure 4). The materials that were downloaded most frequently were the Heavy Metal fact sheets. These materials were downloaded primarily in Arabic. The Indoor Water fact sheets showed a similar download pattern. Food Safety and Pest Control were requested at a slightly lower frequency than the Indoor Water and Heavy Metal fact sheets. Materials with the least number of downloads were fact sheets on Poisonous Look-a-Likes.

DISCUSSION

Workshop results

A summary of the challenges and successes of the HH=HK program are listed below. The source for the observation is in parentheses next to the comments. Challenges included:

- Flexibility in training times and schedules for community trainers (end of training survey)
- Consistency in leadership and trainers (trainer follow-up surveys)
- Availability of trainers for comprehensive Train-the-Trainer workshops involving all six environmental health topics (end of training survey)
- Low use of materials in Arabic and Spanish (follow-up survey)
- Low return rate on follow-up survey for 4Cs trainees (37.5% follow-up surveys returned)

Successes included:

- Interest in all six topic programs (end of training survey results)
- Effectiveness of the training (pre- and post-test scores)
- Education was needed in all of the topic areas (pre- and post-tests)
- Interest in materials available (number of fact sheets and posters requested)

- All topics covered were useful and informative to the participants (end of training survey)
- High intended use of all the presentation materials after the training workshops (end of training survey)
- High return rate on follow-up survey for Head Start trainees (51% follow up surveys returned)
- Utilization of the materials with community members was high for the Head Start Trainees (follow-up survey)
- Arabic and Spanish material utilization through Internet downloads from the NIEHS Resource Center Web site.

There were many challenges as well as successes in the HH=HK Train-the-Trainer program. Overall, the program was able to reach thousands of individuals with the prevention measures necessary to avoid environmental health hazards in the homes of young urban children.

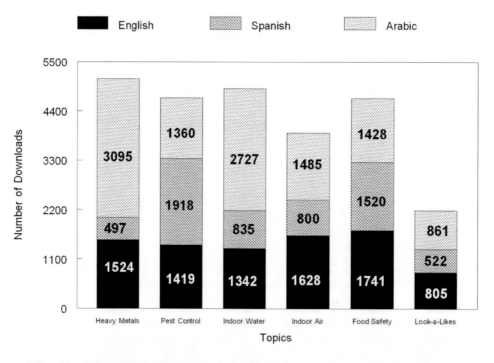

Figure 4. Downloads from NIEHS Resources Page. The greatest number of downloads over a three year period for fact sheets from the NIEHS Resource Page were for the topic of "Heavy Metals", with the largest number of downloads in Arabic for the same topic.

The learning process of building a meaningful relationship with the community through well-established partners cannot be trivialized. Building bonds and trust is a lengthy process and requires a clear understanding of expectations on both sides of the partnership. In addition, both the WSU program principal investigator and DHSP leadership brought extensive expertise to collaboration. The WSU Institute of Environmental Health Sciences brought the necessary monetary resources from grant funding and the expertise on preventative measures for environmental health exposures, and the DHSP leadership brought the training personnel and the knowledge of the needs and concerns of the families that reside in Detroit. Partnership with a well-established organization, who is a trusted member of that community, should be recognized as the foundation for a successful and sustainable university initiated environmental health program.

Families living in an urban environment often have an inherent mistrust of university faculty and staff. There is often a negative connotation associated with "research" being conducted within the community. This perception may be due to potential conflicts of interest with funding sources (10), or as we have observed, a sense of university researchers entering the community, conducting research and retrieving data without subsequent dissemination of the results to the individuals most affected by the outcome.

By working with an organization (e.g. DHSP) that is recognized and trusted by community members, an excellent foundation upon which to breakdown these barriers can be built. In the case of the HH=HK program, there was the common goal of WSU program principal investigator and DHSP leadership to achieve the health and safety of young children living in urban homes.

A strength of the HH=HK program was development and dissemination to meet the needs of the people that it was intended to serve.

The greatest challenge to implementation of the HH=HK program was the availability of time for the trainers to attending the workshops. Although the schedule for the training programs was arranged by the organizational leadership, the trainers often ran into scheduling conflicts. Both organizations (DHSP and 4Cs) were also severely understaffed, which led to the unavailability of the trainers for the amount of time required (12 hours) to attend all six topic trainings. Due to these challenges, flexibility was required for the trainers. They were allowed to attend as many or as few of the training workshops as possible in order to participate in the program at some level. Additional trainer challenges became apparent with the 4Cs program. There was substantial turnover in the leadership and trainers within this organization.

This ultimately led to low participation rate in the training workshops and a low return rate on the follow-up surveys when compared to the more stable employee base within the DHSP. DHSP recruits employees from within the community that it serves, thereby contributing to a more stable employee base upon which to build and sustain the HH=HK program.

With a firm foundation of individuals upon which to build a partnership, the HH=HK program was successful and led to a productive collaboration for all partners. A cautionary note is provided to university program faculty and staff is to predetermine if possible, the stability of your external organizational partners before entering into a potentially long lasting collaboration.

Additionally, involvement of the organization throughout the formative phases of program development is also a strong contributing factor to the success of any Train-the-Trainer educational program. A common goal between partners also allows the program to reflect the needs and interests of the affected communities (1,11).

Although both DHSP and 4Cs had trainers in ethnically diverse and minority represented communities throughout the city of Detroit, the fact sheets in Arabic and Spanish were not requested by these workshop participants.

The reason for lack of trainer utilization of these culturally sensitive resources was not apparent. However, the downloading of literally thousands of copies of the translated fact sheets through the NIEHS Center web-based Resource Resources pages indicated that materials in various languages should be made readily available whenever possible to meet the needs of communities beyond those initially targeted.

Subsequent additional positive outcomes

The program exceeded its initial objectives and provided the HH=HK materials to additional community groups and forums. As a result of the DHSP partnership, the WSU principal investigator was invited to participate as an advisor, planner and collaborator with other agencies and organizations including: the Detroit Alliance for Asthma Awareness, City of Detroit Head Start Disabilities Advisory Board, Detroit Lead Partnership, the Detroit Asthma Coalition and the Child Care Coordinating Council Advisory Board.

Further dissemination of HH=HK materials occurred through requests from the City of Detroit Department of Health and Wellness Promotion (DHWP) and additional development of a one-page fact sheet addressing the dangers of lead poisoning during home repair. This renovation and repair handout, along with the HH=HK Heavy Metal fact sheets were distributed to 1,000 families in urban Detroit neighborhoods through the DHWP.

An additional collaboration with the Henry Ford Health System-Detroit Public School-Based Health Initiative and WSU Physician Assistant Studies Program, disseminated the HH=HK information as patient education materials in Detroit Public School clinics. HH=HK indoor air fact sheets were also made available at an asthma education conference where they were distributed to over 125 Detroit Public School staff, nurses, parents and students.

CONCLUSION

Partnerships aimed at achieving an understanding of environmental health issues can be extremely productive when the approach is not "top down" (university driven) or "bottom up" (driven by the community without a sound research design) but a true partnership where both parties invest at every stage of the process and contribute to the success of the program (12). With combined expertise provided by these partnerships, and meaningful evaluation of the programs, the potential for impact on environmental health becomes maximized (9).

By involving leadership from a well-recognized and trusted organization with a presence within the community, the success of an environmental health program is increased. In addition, ideally the organization should have stable leadership and employee base upon which the foundation for sustainability can be built. It is also apparent that if the organization takes an active role in development of a "needs-based" environmental health educational program, it contributes to the success and sustainability of the initiative.

Additionally, although not all communities readily utilize technology and Internet-accessible materials, web accessible materials can be regarded as a useful resource for communities and health care providers across the country. The success of dissemination nationally, was largely due to access through NIEHS as a recognizable leader in the field of environmental health.

ACKNOWLEDGMENTS

The authors are grateful to Sue Charette (Lead Busters, Detroit) for assistance with Integrated Pest Management information and funding resources for translations; Lisa Nelson, P.A. (Physician Assistant Program, WSU) for delivery of program materials to Detroit Public Schools; and Sheila O'Brien for delivery of information subsequent to the Train-the-Trainer sessions. This project was supported by NIEHS Grant P30ES06639.

REFERENCES

[1]   Gaetke L, Gaetke K, Bowen C. Challenges to superfund community nutrition programs in Kentucky. Environ Toxicol Pharmacol 2008;25:277-81.

[2]   Primono J, Johnston S, DiBiase F, Nodolf J, Noren, L. Evaluation of a community-based outreach worker program for children with asthma. Public Health Nurs 2006;23:234-41.

[3]   Mir DF, Finkelstein Y, Tulipano GD. Impact of integrated pest management (IPM) training on reducing pesticide exposure in Illinois childcare centers. NeuroToxicology 2010;31:621-6.

[4]   Parker EA, Baldwin GT, Israel B, Salinas M. Application of health promotion theories and models for environmental health. Health Educ Behav 2004;31:491-509.

[5]   Freudenberg N. Community capacity for environmental health promotion: determinants and implications for practice. Health Educ Behav 2004;31:472-90.

[6]   O'Fallon L, Dearry A. Community-based participatory research as a tool to advance environmental health sciences. Environ Health Perspect 2002;110(2):155-9.

[7]   Pronczuk J, Surdu S. Children's environmental health in the twenty-first century. Ann NY Acad Sci 2008;1140:143-54.

[8]   Brenner BL, Markowitz S, Rivera M, Romero H, Weeks M, Sanchez E, et al. Integrated pest management in an urban community: a successful partnership for prevention. Environ Health Perspect 2003;111:1649-53.

[9]   Wing, S, Horton, RA, Muhammad, N, Grant, GR, Tajik, M, Thu, K. Integrating epidemiology, education, and organizing for environmental justice: community health effects of industrial hog operations. Am J Public Health 2008;98:1390.

[10]   Kegler MC, Miner K. Environmental health promotion interventions: considerations for preparation and practice. Health Educ Behav 2004;31:510-25.

[11]   Goodman RM, Yoo S, Jack L. Applying comprehensive community-based approaches in diabetes prevention: rationale, principles, and models. J Public Health Manage Pract 2006;12:545-55.

[12]   Roussos ST, Fawcett, SB. A review of collaborative partnerships as a strategy for improving community health. Annu Rev Public Health 2000;21:369-402.

Submitted: August 26, 2011. *Revised:* October 20, 2011. *Accepted:* November 03, 2011.

In: Public Health Yearbook 2012
Editor: Joav Merrick

ISBN: 978-1-62808-078-0
© 2013 Nova Science Publishers, Inc.

Chapter 26

LESSONS LEARNED FROM THE PROTECCIÓN EN CONSTRUCCIÓN (PENC) COMMUNITY RESEARCH PARTNERSHIP

Linda Sprague Martinez, PhD[*], *Uchenna J Ndulue, MPH* and *Maria J Brunette, PhD*

Community Health Program, School of Arts and Sciences, Tufts University, Medford and Department of Work Environment, University of Massachusetts, Lowell, Massachusetts, United States of America

ABSTRACT

PenC (Protección en Construcción) seeks to build community-university-labor partnership in order to design, implement and evaluate an intervention aimed at preventing falls and silica exposure among Latino construction workers. This study evaluated the PenC partnership process. Semi-structured partner interviews and surveys were used. Thematic, univariate and bivariate analyses were conducted; results were presented back to partners who then provided data context. Although all partners report increased capacity including new connections and knowledge, resident researchers, here promotores, are much more likely to share information with their neighbors and other local residents. Engaging residents can lead to deeper community penetration.

Keywords: Community, occupational health, Latino health, public health

INTRODUCTION

The contributions of community-based participatory research (CBPR) approaches to the development of sustainable public health interventions aimed at tackling health disparities have been well documented (1,2). Essential to the CBPR process is collaboration between

---

[*] Correspondence: Linda Sprague Martinez, Ph.D., Tufts University School of Arts and Sciences, Community Health Program, 112 Packard Avenue, Medford MA 02155, United States. E-mail: linda.martinez@tufts.edu.

multiple stakeholders. However, the diverse interests and perspectives represented by CBPR collaborations require an intentional and continual attention to the partnership process. Evaluation of the various dimensions of collaboration, including communication, trust, and capacity building, are central to effective CBPR interventions.

CBPR strategies may be of particular utility in promoting occupational health and safety. Since CBPR partnerships require the participation of multiple sectors of community life including industry, labor, and government, CBPR interventions are uniquely positioned to address occupational morbidity and mortality. Additionally, as over a quarter of all construction workers in the United States (US) are of Latino heritage, effective CBPR interventions may reduce health disparities among Latino Americans in the construction trades (3). Appropriately designed CBPR partnerships can integrate Latino-Americans and Latino immigrants into the design and implementation of effective health promotion interventions. However, few CBPR studies have examined the development processes of partnerships focused on promoting worker health and safety among the Latino population (4).

The purpose of this study is to present a partnership evaluation of Protección en Construcción: The Lawrence Latino Safety Partnership (PenC), a CBPR project focused on promoting Latino construction worker health and safety. This external evaluation set out to 1) explore the ways in which employing a CBPR approach has contributed to participation, capacity building and empowerment among a multi-ethnic/multilingual group of partners (5) and 2) identify relationships between group dynamics and preliminary project outcomes (6).

BACKGROUND

Latinos are disproportionately impacted by occupational health disparities and experience more hazardous working conditions than their non-Hispanic peers; the fatality rate for Latinos is approximately 20% higher than that of Caucasians or African-Americans (3,7). Particularly in the building trades, Latinos are concentrated in high risk job categories such as laborers, helpers, roofers, and, concrete workers; all positions where workers are likely to be exposed to hazards.

Occupational health and safety concerns among Latinos are a priority for the city of Lawrence, MA due to the large proportion of Latinos residents in the construction trades (8,9). In an attempt to tackle occupational health disparities among Latino construction workers in Lawrence, researchers from the University of Massachusetts Lowell, Department of Work Environment in partnership with the City of Lawrence Mayor's Health Task Force, the Laborers International Union of North America Local 175 and a team of community residents under the direction of John Snow Inc. formed Protección en Construcción (PenC): The Lawrence Latino Safety Partnership in 2006. Funded by the National Institute for Occupational Safety and Health (NIOSH), the group set out to build a community-university-labor partnership to design, implement and evaluate strategies to reduce falls and silica dust exposure among Latino construction workers in the City of Lawrence Massachusetts.

In keeping with a CBPR approach, PenC uses a committee structure that allows members from partner organizations to be integrated and take leadership roles in various aspects of the research planning, implementation, and dissemination processes. The work of PenC is guided by a steering committee or management team with representation from each of the four partner organizations. Additional teams include: 1) outreach (which focuses on local marketing); 2) dissemination; and 3) intervention planning, each with mixed representation. Finally, a networking committee that brings together members of the broader community such as small contractors, construction workers, residents and staff from non profit and governmental organizations, provides a mechanism by which researchers can share project developments and received feedback on the development and implementation of the intervention.

This project structure, anchored in the community, also allows partners to take the lead on different aspects of the research and ensures that diverse perspectives are represented each step of the way.

Although the partnership was formally established in 2006, the group coalesced as result of previous collaborations and pre-existing relationships.

As seen in figure 1, The Partnership Timeline, initial collaborations began in 2003 when a University-Labor partnership led to an Occupational Safety and Health Administration (OSHA) training program for over 400 Latino construction workers (10). Having the structure in place, and most importantly, the commitment to continue working with the Latino working community to address issues of importance to the community, the labor and the research group planned on sustaining efforts on a major safety (falls from working at heights) and health (silica exposure) aspect of the Latino population they served.

The partnership evaluation set out to explore whether employing a CBPR approach contributes to participation, capacity building and empowerment among partners (5) and to identify relationships between certain group dynamics processes and preliminary project outcomes (6).

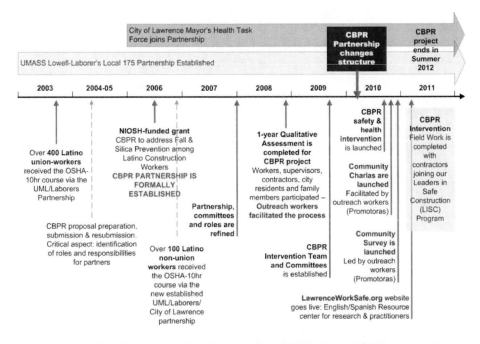

PROTECCIÓN EN CONSTRUCCIÓN: TIMELINE OF OUR PARTNERSHIP ESTABLISHMENT AND RESEARCH ACTIVITIES
"Participation, Capacity Building and Empowerment: Lessons learned from the Protección en Construcción (PenC) community research partnership"

Figure 1. Partnership Timeline.

Moving beyond traditional evaluation, the work described here was formative, in that research findings were reported back to partners and used to develop team-building activities aimed at enhancing relationships and fostering communication.

This is significant as it is often the case that once a study is underway the focus shifts from the interactions between partners to the business of research. Using a formative approach to evaluating the process brought the focus back to the relationships, interactions and coordination among partners.

METHODS

The evaluation process utilized a participatory approach. Participatory evaluation allows partners to take an active role in the evaluation process (11). Research partners determined their goals for the evaluation, informed key research questions and methods, and identified the study sample. When initial data collection and analyses were completed, study findings were shared with participants to inform the partnership process. Throughout the evaluation, findings were reported back to project partners who then incorporated lessons learned to develop strategies aimed at strengthening the partnership.

Design

The study design was longitudinal and employed both qualitative and quantitative methods. Qualitative methods included an annual semi-structured partner interview, which captured CBPR outcomes including participation, capacity building and empowerment. Quantitative methods, meanwhile, involved yearly a partner survey based on the Eastside Village Health Worker Survey (12), which was designed to explore group dynamics.

Measures

Participation, capacity building and empowerment were examined. Participation was explored through self report on 1) how often partners attended and helped to plan meeting, programs and activities, 2) the number of committees partners reported serving on, and 3) by examining the extent to which partners provided information, expressed opinions, pulled ideas and opinions together and provided direction at meetings. Capacity building was assessed qualitatively by asking partners to describe the ways in which participation influenced their individual and organizational capacity. In addition, capacity building was explored by measuring 1) partner reports of increased knowledge about partner organizations and the role they serve in the community, 2) increased knowledge related to family and community health issues, and 3) the extent to which partners believed their organizations use information garnered via PenC.

Finally, empowerment was conceptualized as the extent to which partners felt they had the ability to make change. Perceived influence over decision-making, sense of ownership, and the extent to which partners reported sharing project-related knowledge in the community were examined. In addition, partners were asked to describe ways in which participation in PenC has led to feelings of empowerment.

Group dynamics were examined as group dynamics may have a direct effect on partnership programs and interventions (6).

Working relationships, satisfaction with decision making, mutual respect, and power over the decision-making process were included as measures of group dynamics. Each was measured using a 5 point Likert scale.

Sample

The sample was defined by the steering committee. All personnel, representing the partnership organizations and outreach team members, were included. As such the sample consisted of university researchers (n=5), union staff members (n=2), city representatives (n=2), and promotores (n=5).

Procedures

Prior to implementation, research protocols were approved by the University of Massachusetts Institutional Review Board (IRB). Qualitative interview respondents were contacted via telephone and invited to participate in the study. At the onset of the telephone conversation, the purpose of the evaluation, evaluation procedures, and the interview process were explained in detail. Respondents were given the option of scheduling a telephone or in person interview with the researcher that could be conducted in either English or Spanish. A total of 11 individuals were interviewed over the phone. Nine of the interviews were conducted in English and two were conducted in Spanish. Prior to the initiation of the survey, consent was verbally obtained from each respondent. Once consent was received, respondents were asked a series of semi-structured qualitative items. The average duration of the interviews was thirty minutes.

Quantitative partner surveys were announced during a PenC project meeting and the procedures were explained. Surveys were then sent to project partners (n=14) via U.S. mail. Three were sent in Spanish and eleven were sent in English. Respondents were also given the option to complete the survey electronically.

Analysis

Qualitative interview notes were recorded by hand and typed in a Microsoft word file. Qualitative data was then coded thematically. Quantitative data was entered into a Microsoft Excel 2007® file and then exported to SPSS. Respondents were categorized by partner type (university researcher, organizational researcher, or promotore) to explore variation in responses. Bivariate and univariate analyses were conducted. Once analyzed, all data were presented back to project partners. Key themes and initial findings were shared with steering committee members and feedback was elicited to help contextualize the data.

RESULTS

Eleven of fourteen participants (79 %) completed the qualitative telephone interviews and thirteen (93 %) participated in the partner survey. The findings here are divided into two sections; the first section describes the CBPR outcomes while the second highlights the group dynamics.

CBPR outcomes

Participation: Most of the participants (92%) attended more than nine project related events per year. Similarly, 85% of partners had participated in the planning of more than nine events. When asked to describe participation on one of the four established committees, all partners reported serving on a least one committee, while the mean number of committees served on was two. Beyond actual events attended and committees served on, partners were asked to describe their participation at meetings. Specifically, they were asked how often they provided information, expressed their opinions, pulled together ideas and opinions, and pointed out ways to proceed when the group was stuck. Responses were measured on a four point Likert-type scale and were overwhelmingly skewed positive across the board. All participants consistently reported a high degree of participation. A relationship between partner type and committee service was not evident.

When asked to describe the factors that contributed to their participation, participants described that having clearly defined roles and responsibilities was essential. In addition, partners reported that the meeting structure, which involved rotating facilitation and structured opportunities for partners to share their expertise and experience, encouraged a higher degree of participation as it allowed them to provide direction to the group. It was stated that such leadership experiences "encouraged information sharing, and promoted ownership". Ice breakers and group activities were also described as "encouraging partner participation" indirectly by strengthening relationships which was described as increasing one's comfort in expressing opinions. Furthermore, the high level of co-learning that occurred at the various meetings was described as a contributor to active participation. Such learning was not only about occupational safety and health concerns but also each partner's culture, environment, opportunities and struggles, and strategies for affecting change. Finally, a key activity that was cited by nearly all partners as improving their comfort participating was the "buddy system". This system involved assigning individuals a "buddy", which was generally a member of the UML research team, giving community partners a point person to go to if issues came up or if they had a specific idea to convey.

Capacity building: As seen in Table 1: Individual and organizational capacity, partners reported that participating in the collaboration increased their knowledge and understanding of partner organizations and the work each partner does in the community, as well as their general knowledge of "community health issues experienced by Latino construction workers". Furthermore, participants reported that their organizations utilized information generated by the PenC partnership. With respect to utilizing information there was a relationship between partner type and organizational use of new information.

Participants described the benefits of participation as "Bettering their understanding of the Lawrence community and local resources available in the city"; "Strengthening their knowledge related to construction workers, their needs and rights"; and "Increasing their comfort in the community, working with diverse groups, and negotiating multiple interests". Partners also described a number of activities aimed at building partner capacity. Such activities included trainings related to worker rights and occupational safety.

Beyond increased knowledge, participants provided accounts of increased capacity which resulted from new connections made through partner organizations.

Table 1. Individual and organizational capacity

	Strongly Agree	Agree	Neutral	Disagree	Strongly Disagree
Knowledge of partner organizations	70%,	15%	15%	0.0%	0.0%
Knowledge of family community health issues	46%	31%	23%	0.0%	0.0%
New information gained by organization	31%	38%,	31%	0.0%	0.0%

Table 2. Information sharing

	Often	Sometimes	Rarely	Never
Friends	46 %	31%	0.0%	15%
Family	46%	23%	8%	8%
Neighbors	31%	8%	23%	23%

Finally, partners shared that being part of PenC exposed them to diverse perspectives representing multiple sectors of the community and such exposure contributed to increasing their overall comfort in engaging with the community. In sum, participation in PenC was generally described in ways consistent with increasing human, social and cultural capital for of the partners and their members.

Empowerment: The extent to which participants felt they had influenced others had an increased sense of ownership over the project was also explored. 76% reported having been influenced by other participants and 92% reported a sense of ownership over the project. When examined by partner-type there were no differences among responses.

Finally, data indicated that partners were sharing the knowledge that they gained as a result of their participation in PenC with friends, family and neighbors. As illustrated in Table 2, partners were more likely to share information with friends and family than with neighbors. There was a relationship between partner-type and information sharing related to sharing information with friends and neighbors and to sharing information with family. Promotores were more likely to report sharing information with family, friends and neighbors.

In terms of activities that contributed to empowerment, participants described participation as well as opportunities for capacity building, specifically trainings as contributing to feelings of empowerment. Participants reported that the information they received at meetings and trainings gave them "more power to make change in the community"; while others reported feeling empowered "to collaborate and to share information". Participants further described feeling empowered "to share what they were learning by way of their participation with family, friends and the greater Lawrence community". Finally, partners reported that being part of PenC left them feeling empowered to "facilitate groups and to serve as a leader".

Group dynamics

Initial data indicates that the PenC partnership has a positive group dynamic. Most respondents (92%) agreed that the partnership works well together, while 85% reported being satisfied with the decision making process. Improvement areas that were suggested for the group to work on included mutual respect and shared decision making. When asked about respect, 69% of respondents agreed that partner members expressed respect for one another's points.

Lessons learned

This evaluation aimed to explore the PenC CBPR process as well as the group dynamics between partners. Using evaluation findings the partnership was able to assess successes and work through challenges as they emerged via a continuous improvement process that fed the results to the partnership. During the course of the program evaluation 3 key lessons emerged 1) there are benefits to engaging multiple levels of community, 2) engagement increases capacity, knowledge and cultural sensitivity, and 3) "community" is complex and poses a number of challenges.

Engaging community: The literature indicates that there are benefits to engaging residents in research (13-15). PenC engages organization partners from the community as well as residents, who served as promotores. The residents involved with PenC are both monolingual Spanish and bilingual. In addition, half the residents involved are community elders. During the course of the project it became clear that engaging residents gave PenC the ability to penetrate deeper into the community reaching a population that was less likely to be connected to organizational partners. Evaluation findings indicate that both mono and bilingual promotores enjoyed taking on leadership roles, such as presenting at meetings and sharing their experiences in the community with other community organizations. Monolingual Spanish promotores were also were most likely to share information they were learning with friends and neighbors and reported feeling empowered to share new information and resources with others in the community. This finding has led the partnership to incorporate promotores across committees and finding places for them to take on leadership roles. For example, PenC now holds Charlas (community talks) where promotores along with other members of the outreach committee provide trainings and disseminate health and safety information for state and local organizations.

Building Capacity: Partners reported gaining knowledge by way of their participation. It is well documented that new ties (social capital) can produce new knowledge particularly in places where the ties are weak-such as those between promotores and university researchers (16,17). Community partnerships can lead to new thinking by exposing team members to multiple perspectives. Findings here highlight how a CBPR approach can not only provide researchers with an understanding of contextual community level factors that influence occupational safety, but can also increase their comfort level engaging in intercultural exchanges with the community. This was facilitated by the committee structure, the personnel meetings, the use of the buddy system, and ultimately, the continuous improvement derived from the evaluation process.

The challenges of "community": The literature indicates that communities are complex, shaped by historical, economic and political events. Social ties, comprised of multiple sectors, are adaptive and constantly evolving both within and across sectors (18,19). Furthermore, being sensitive to the cultural values of immigrant communities constitutes a challenge for partner members that are newly exposed to these populations. Working in partnership with communities also requires a level of flexibility that is not always innate to the academy. An early challenge in the PenC project represented this obstacle. The city of Lawrence was an important PenC partner; more specifically a member of the community development department was a named investigator representing the city. During the second year of the evaluation municipal leadership changed leading to a major reorganization which led to the "city investigator" no longer working for the city. This change was complicated in that it was important for the city as well as the investigator to remain partners discord. Communities are not static and there is always the possibility that organizations will change staffing or lose funding altogether. Thus partnerships need contingency plans. What happens if there is a change? Who is the partner the organization or the individual? These things need to be clearly delineated from the start. In the case of PenC, both the individual and the city were key players in the project and as such both remained, but this led to an interruption that involved time and additional planning and paperwork, on the part of the steering committee and principal investigator.

Beyond the evolving nature of community are historical relationships which can be both positive and negative. It cannot be assumed that everyone gets along just because they are in the same community, are committed to improving the health of a given population, or share cultural or linguistic ties. During the course of the evaluation a history of conflict between partners community partners consistently emerged, which may account for why only 70 percent of partners reported that partners expressed respect for one another. In order to try to work through historical conflict between partners team building and communication starter activities aimed at improving communication and building relationships were implemented at all personnel meetings. Here research partners worked to ease historical conflicts in order to engage in collective action.

Also, it should be noted that the socio-cultural and economic background of the Latino immigrant population, the target group of this study, added another layer of complexity to the investigation. However, the process by which the project evolved generated a certain level of commitment among the partners that was unique in a sense that it led to additional activities conducive to the improvement of the quality of life and the provision of decent and safe conditions of work for all.

Overall, a general feeling of being committed to a critical and current social justice issue and the belief in the research intervention as a mechanism to improve worker conditions became an attribute to the PenC partnership.

CONCLUSION

Process evaluation is an important component of CBPR in that it allows partners to both identify group dynamics that may serve to hinder or facilitate research outcomes and document factors that contribute to partnership goals.

As reported here there are many benefits to partnership, however it is important to keep in mind the threat poor group dynamics can pose, all partners need to feel as though they have some level of power over the decision making process. Here process evaluation revealed a story about how engaging community resident leaders can result in deeper community penetration by university based researchers and grassroots advocates, the ways in which partnership builds capacity, and the challenges partnering with "community" can pose.

This is significant as "community partners" are often one step removed from the "community" --organizational representatives serving as community gatekeepers. The PenC partnership provides a valuable model for engaging residents in public health research.

ACKNOWLEDGMENTS

This work is supported by funding from National Institutes for Health (NIH), National Institute for Occupational Safety and Health (NIOSH) (Grant # R01-OH-008750). We would like to offer many thanks to the PenC community research partners and to the University of Massachusetts, Lowell (UML) researchers for their willingness to engage in critical self reflection throughout the research process. The content is solely the responsibility of the authors and does not necessarily represent the official views of NIOSH or NIH.

REFERENCES

[1]   Schulz AJ, Parker EA, Israel BA, Allen A, Decarlo M, Lockett M. Addressing social determinants of health through community-based participatory research: The east side village health worker partnership. Health Educ Behav 2002;29(3):326-41.

[2]   Wallerstein N, Duran B. Using community-based participatory research to address health disparities. Health Promot Pract 2006;7(3):312-23.

[3]   CPWR. The Center for Construction Research and Training: The construction chart book: The US construction industry and its workers. Silver Spring, MD: Center Construction Research Training, 2008.

[4]   Azaroff L, Nguyen H, Do T, Gore R, Goldstein-Gelb M. Results of a community-university partnership to reduce deadly hazards in hardwood floor finishing. J Community Health 2011;36(4):658-68.

[5]   Chrisman NJ, Senturia K, Tang G, Gheisar B. Qualitative process evaluation of urban community work: A preliminary view. Health Educ Behav 2002;29(2):232-48.

[6]   Schulz AJ, Israel BA, Lantz P. Instrument for evaluating dimensions of group dynamics within community-based participatory research partnerships. Evaluat Program Plann 2003;26(3):249-62.

[7]   2005-2007 American Community Survey 3-year Estimates [database on the Internet]. US Census Bureau. 2007. Accessed 2009 Jun 05. URL: www.census.gov

[8]   Cole DB. Immigrant city: Lawrence, Massachusetts, 1845-1921. Chapell Hill, NC: Chapell Hill: University North Carolina University Press, 1963.

[9]   The City of Lawrence Massachusetts: About Lawrence. Accessed 2011 March 24. URL: http://www.cityoflawrence.com/about-the-city.aspx.

[10] Brunette MJ. Development of educational and training materials on safety and health: Targeting Hispanic workers in the construction industry. Fam Community Health 2005;28(3):253-66.

[11] Cousins JB, Earl LM. The case for participatory evaluation. Educ Evaluat Policy Analysis 1992;14(4):397-418.

[12] Parker EA, Schulz AJ, Israel BA, Hollis R. Detroit's east side village health worker partnership: Community-based lay health advisor intervention in an urban area. Health Educ Behav 1998;25(1):24-45.

[13] Viswanathan M, Ammerman A, Eng E, Gartlehner G, Lohr KN, Griffith D, et al. Community-based participatory research: Assessing the evidence. Rockville, MD: Agency Healthcare Research Quality, Rep 99, 2004.

[14] Minkler M, Vasquez VB, Chang C, Miller J. Promoting healthy public policy through community-based participatory research: Ten case studies. Berkeley, CA: University California, School Public Health Policy, 2008.

[15] Wallerstein NB, Duran B. Using community-based participatory research to address health disparities. Health Promot Pract 2006;7(3):312-23.

[16] Burt RS. Structural holes: The social structure of competition. Cambridge: Harvard University Press, 1992.

[17] Nahapiet J, Ghoshal S. Social capital, intellectual capital, and the organizational advantage. Acad Manage Rev 1998;23(2):242-66.

[18] Manson SM. Simplifying complexity: A review of complexity theory. Geoforum 2001;32(3):405-14.

[19] Miller WL, McDaniel RRJ, Crabtree BF, Stange KC. Practice jazz: Understanding variation in family practices using complexity science. J Fam Pract 2001;50(10):872.

Submitted: September 08, 2011. *Revised:* October 09, 2011. *Accepted:* November 03, 2011.

In: Public Health Yearbook 2012
Editor: Joav Merrick

ISBN: 978-1-62808-078-0
© 2013 Nova Science Publishers, Inc.

Chapter 27

ISSUES TO CONSIDER WHEN ADAPTING EVIDENCE-BASED PHYSICAL ACTIVITY INTERVENTIONS WITH AND WITHIN RACIAL/ETHNIC MINORITY COMMUNITIES

Elizabeth A Baker, PhD, MPH[*],
Freda Motton, MPH and E Yvonne Lewis
Saint Louis University and Faith Access to Community and Economic Development, Saint Louis, Missouri, United States of America

ABSTRACT

There is a growing demand for utilizing evidence-based approaches to increase physical activity. While systematic reviews have recommended strategies, researchers have cautioned that these strategies must be adapted to fit the needs of specific populations and the community context. The purpose of our work was to use a community-based participatory research approach to identify issues to consider when adapting evidence-based physical activity interventions with and within racial/ethnic minority communities. Concept mapping was used to enable members of racial/ethnic minority communities who were engaged in prevention research to identify issues to consider when adapting physical activity recommendations for use with and within racial and ethnic minority communities. Concept mapping resulted in ten issues to consider when adapting physical activity interventions. Areas of similarity and difference in how these issues were ranked among racial/ethnic groups were reviewed. The issues to consider when adapting evidence-based physical activity interventions with and within racial/ethnic minority communities were similar to those discussed in previous literature, however, the operationalization of many of these issues was seen as unique.

Keywords: Physical activity, evidence-based approaches, community-academic partnership, concept mapping, practice considerations

[*] Correspondence: Elizabeth A Baker, PhD, MPH, Saint Louis University, 3545 Lafayette Ave, Saint Louis MO 63130 United States. E-mail: bakerpa@slu.edu

INTRODUCTION

Physical inactivity is an important public health issue that has received increased attention over the past few decades (1-4). A review of studies on physical activity and the incidence of coronary heart disease found that those with sedentary lifestyles were almost twice as likely to have heart disease as those who were not sedentary (3). In addition to contributing to reduced risk of heart disease, physical activity contributes to lower risk for a variety of other chronic diseases including hypertension, non-insulin dependent diabetes, colon cancer, osteoarthritis, and osteoporosis (4). It is estimated that as many as 250,000 US deaths per year, or 12% of the total number of deaths, are attributable to physical inactivity (5,6). In 1996, the US Surgeon General released a landmark report recommending that all adults participate in at least 30 minutes of moderate-intensity physical activity on most, and preferably, all days of the week (4).

Despite these recommendations, according to the most recent Behavioral Risk Factor Surveillance System (BRFSS) data, only 49% of the population meets recommended levels of physical activity (7). Similarly, recent data from BRFSS show that 36% of Hispanics and 31% of African Americans get no leisure time activity, in comparison to 20% of whites (7).

The Healthy People 2010 target is to reduce this proportion of inactive adults to 20 percent for all population groups, and using this reduction in disparities in physical activity as a way of reducing health disparities overall.

Over ten years ago, the Institute of Medicine (IOM) identified several factors associated with the success of public health interventions. Most notably, the IOM found that public health efforts are most likely to be successful if they used an intervention approach whose effectiveness has been established in the scientific literature (8). In response to this and similar calls for defining evidence-based approaches within public health, the Task Force on Community Preventive Services supported by the Centers for Disease Control and Prevention, published The Guide to Community Preventive Services: What Works to Promote Health? (i.e., the Community Guide) to provide guidance on evidence-based approaches across various ecological levels (9). The Community Guide points to the benefits of intervening on multiple levels to increase physical activity by working to enhance access through environmental and policy change while also providing cues to action through point of decision prompts, social support for interventions, and/or creating individually-adapted educational programs to increase physical activity. The six specific physical activity strategies that the Community Guide recommends are: community-wide campaigns, point-of-decision prompts (e.g., signs to use the stairs), school-based physical education, individually-adapted health behavior change programs, social support interventions in community settings, and creation of (or enhanced) access to places for physical activity combined with informational outreach activities.

PURPOSE

While the Community Guide review suggests that these are useful strategies to increase rates of physical activity, researchers have cautioned that strategies must be modified or adapted to fit the needs of specific populations and the community context (10). The best intervention strategy to use will depend on the community context, population of interest, and history of previous work conducted within the community. This is particularly important in working with racial/ethnic minority communities because many of the studies reviewed by the Community Guide did not include, or did not focus on, these populations. The question, for these communities, is what specifically should be considered when adapting these interventions in terms of context, population and history?

This article describes how a national community-academic partnership worked with local community members who were engaged in prevention research (from white and racial/ethnic minority communities) to create a set of "issues to consider" when adapting physical activity interventions with and within racial/ethnic minority communities.

METHODS

The funding for this project came from a special interest project from the Center for Disease Control and Prevention's Prevention Research Centers (PRC) and the Division of Nutrition Physical Activity and Obesity. The idea to apply for this grant was generated by a member of the Prevention Research Center National Community Committee (PRCNCC) leadership team, and the grant was designed, written, and implemented by an academic partner at one of the PRCs and the NCC leadership team. A protocol was submitted and approved by the Saint Louis University Institutional Review Board.

EBPH Course

The PRCNCC is comprised of community partners from the Center for Disease Control and Prevention's Prevention Research Centers. The NCC includes representatives from geographically and economically diverse communities including African American, Latino, Asian, Native American, and Caucasian communities across 26 states. All of the Prevention Research Centers (33 centers) were invited to send community partners to an EBPH course. Twenty-nine community representatives gathered in St. Louis, Missouri, for this EBPH course. Each of the course participants had previous experience in and a commitment to prevention research as well as formal and informal ties to their respective communities.

The EBPH course incorporated material from previous courses (initially organized by Dr. Ross Brownson, Saint Louis University School of Public Health) but was modified by our community-academic partnership to highlight the importance of community-academic partnerships and to focus on the adaptation of evidence-based physical activity interventions for racial/ethnic minority communities (11).

The Leadership Team of the PRCNCC participated in the course development, instruction, and group facilitation. The planning and implementation of the course formed the foundation for common language and understanding and allowed for co-learning among participants and facilitators.

After learning about evidence-based public health, the participants were asked to take part in a concept mapping process to develop a list of issues to be considered when implementing physical activity interventions with and within racial/ethnic minority communities.

Concept mapping is a process whereby qualitative data are elicited, sorted, and ranked. Concept Systems Software (Concept Systems Software, 2006) was used to visually depict and analyze the results. The process involved several steps, outlined below.

Brainstorm sessions

The first step involved brainstorming sessions. The sessions were led by two facilitators, one academic and one member from the NCC leadership team. Participants were given a prompt and asked to respond to it as facilitators recorded their statements. The focus prompt asked, "What is important to consider when implementing physical activity interventions in racial and ethnic minority communities?" This process took approximately one hour.

A total of 204 statements were produced at these sessions. The statements were reviewed by one academic partner to identify duplicates. These duplicates were then discussed and eliminated as appropriate after conversation among community and academic partners. This process resulted in a 175 individual statements. These statements were then entered into the Concept Systems program.

Sorting and rating

The participants were provided with these 175 statements and asked to evaluate the individual statements in two ways: how the statements "hung together" (sorting), and importance of the statement (rating). During sorting, each participant was given cards with a single statement listed on each. The participants were asked to create piles of cards with statements that seemed similar. The participants were then asked to name their piles. For example, one participant may have created a pile with ten statements such as, "Consider the importance of cultural norms" and "Provide cultural competency training for staff", and may have named this pile "Culture".

Finally, each participant rated each individual statement on its importance, from 1 to 5 (with 1 being the least important and 5 being the most important). Each participant put this information in a separate envelope along with a brief demographic survey. This process of sorting and rating each statement took approximately two hours.

Data entry

After the participants finished sorting, information about each participant was entered into the Concept Systems software program. The demographic information (i.e. racial/ethnic group, gender, and urban/rural location), sort piles, and ratings developed by each member were created in separate files.

Map creation

The concept map is a visual representation of how participants sorted the statements into piles. The concept mapping software (Concept Systems, 2006) utilizes multidimensional scaling and cluster analysis to create the concept maps and pattern matches. The software program also generates an automatic title based on the titles the participants gave to each of their piles. The software program provides information on how many statements are in each cluster, the degree to which the statements were consistently placed together as opposed to being placed in another pile, and the average ranking of importance for each of the statements.

In developing the maps, the Concept System software allows the user to modify the number of clusters to the most appropriate fit. The objective is to find the number of unique clusters that represented the participants' sorting process. By examining the concept maps with between five and 20 clusters, the most parsimonious number of clusters was chosen. This involved starting with 20 clusters and having discussions among community and academic partners to review maps as one cluster at a time was removed, reflecting when a theme was lost or when removing a cluster unnecessarily broke another theme apart.

Pattern matching

Once a map was determined to adequately and parsimoniously reflect the concepts raised, a pattern match was conducted. The sorting and ranking data were used to create the pattern match, specifically comparing ranking of statements within each cluster by group (i.e., racial/ethnic group).

The pattern match is a visual way to compare two groups and see where there is agreement or disagreement regarding their ranking of clusters. On each side of the pattern match, the cluster titles and their average ranking within a sub-group are displayed vertically in order of highest rank. A line connects each title from left to right visually representing the two groups' level of agreement.

RESULTS

Twenty-nine individuals participated in the concept mapping process. All individuals took part in the brainstorming sessions, the sorting session, and rating of statement importance. The group consisted of 26 females and thre 3 males. The two largest groups were African American, with 12 participants (41.4%) and White Non-Hispanic, with 10 participants (34.5%). The remaining 7 participants were Hispanic (3 participants, 10.3%), Asian (2 participants, 6.9%), and Native American (2 participants, 6.9%). The majority of participants were from urban areas (20 participants, 68.9%) rather than rural areas.

Final concept map

As illustrated in figure 1, participants sorted and categorized the statements into the following issues to consider when adapting physical activity interventions with and within racial/ethnic minority communities: culture, gender issues, tailoring the intervention, engaging the community in intervention planning and implementation, previous studies, intervention resources, community infrastructures to support the intervention, safety, community support, and community assessment.

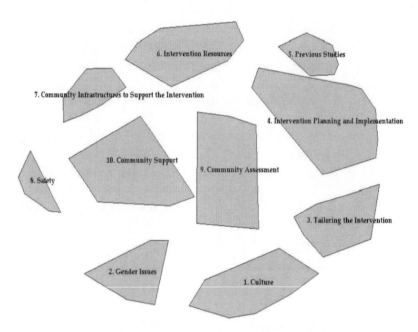

Figure 1. Considerations for adapting physical activity interventions with and within racial/ethnic minority communities (generated by racial/ethnic minority participants).

Pattern matching

After creating the concept map, a pattern match was used to compare the participants' statement ratings. The pattern match allowed the comparison of the importance of the statements' rankings within each cluster between the two subgroups, with 1 being least important and 5 being the most important: racial/ethnic minorities (REM) (n=19) and White non-Hispanics (WNH) (n=10). In the pattern match, horizontal lines represent closer agreement regarding the importance of the statements in that cluster and as they trend vertically so does the discordance among the groups. The pattern match is useful for revealing where differences exist. The pattern created indicated that there was a correlation or agreement of 0.66. The pattern match also indicated where the specific differences were the greatest. Figure 2 is the pattern match comparing racial/ethnic minority groups (REM) and white non-Hispanic participants (WNH).

Similarities

In looking at the pattern match there were a number of important similarities between the REM and WNH participants. Overall, the range of ratings did not vary much between the two groups. The REM group's rating was between 3.78 and 4.31 and the WNH group between 3.61 and 4.23, respectively.

    There were a number of clusters that were ranked exactly the same or very close by both groups. Gender Issues was rated similarly by both groups of participants. The cluster had the same rating of 3.78; both groups rated it as the least important cluster. Of the total statements included for sorting and ranking, 17 were similar to those used by the Community Guide to identify characteristics of successful programs including items addressing program planning, design, and evaluation (9). This cluster, Previous Studies, was ranked as the second most important by both groups. Engaging the Community in Intervention Planning and Implementation was ranked fourth by both groups. The average rating for the clusters varies only by 0.02. This cluster included statements regarding how information will be shared, who should be involved in intervention planning and implementation, and highlighted the importance of community involvement.

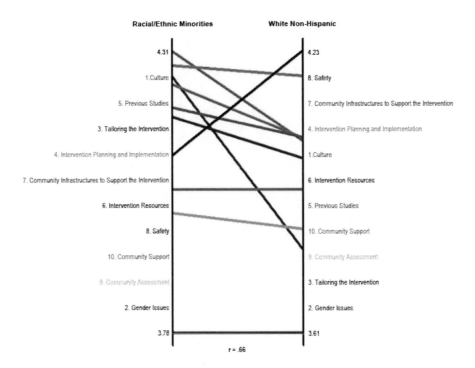

Figure 2. Pattern Match Comparing Participant Groups.

Differences

The findings also reveal important differences between the groups of participants. The REM participants ranked Culture as the most important issue to consider when adapting physical activity interventions, with an average rating of 4.31; Tailoring the Intervention to the Community was ranked third. However, the WNH group ranked Culture fifth, with an average rating of 3.79; Tailoring the Intervention was ranked ninth. The most important topic for the WNH group was safety, with an average rating of 4.43. The REM group gave safety an average rating of 4.11 falling to seventh of the ten clusters.

Moving from generation of issues to practice considerations

The information gathered from the concept mapping process was used to create a list of considerations for adapting physical activity interventions within racial/ethnic minority communities. To accomplish this, the NCC leadership team worked with academic partners to convert the list of issues into actionable items. For instance, "culture" was changed to "attend to culture". The practice considerations generated were: Attend to Culture, Build Upon Previous Studies, Tailor the Intervention to the Population you Intend to Serve, Engage the Community in the Planning and Implementation of the Intervention, Create or use Existing Community Infrastructures to Support the Intervention, Ensure Appropriate Intervention Resources, Ensure Personal and Environmental Safety, Create Community Support, Conduct a Full Community Assessment, and Recognize the Importance of Gender Issues. The clusters are listed in Table 1 in order of importance, as ranked by the racial/ethnic minority participants in the concept mapping process. See Table 1 for definitions and operationalizations of each consideration.

Table 1. Operationalization of practice considerations based on statements sorted into each cluster

1. Attend to Culture
−   Consider the importance of cultural norms
o   Incorporate spirituality
o   Consider discomfort from treatment by others
o   Consider how physical activity is valued and understood in the community (e.g. is time for physical activity considered a luxury?)
−   Develop culturally appropriate intervention materials and approaches. Consider:language and communication style; provide ongoing cultural competency training for all partners
−   Avoid stereotyping
−   Create policies for improved infrastructure attentive to cultural differences (e.g. translation services)
−   Consider community history and reason for migration to the United States
−   Develop an intervention that enhances culture of the community you intend to work with
2. Build on Previous Studies
−   Consider strategies that the Community Guide has recommended. An overview of these is provided below. For additional information please check their website (http://www.thecommunityguide.org/pa/)
−   People and places · Start with interventions from other communities and learn from their experiences
3. Tailor the Intervention to the Population or Community You Intend to Serve
−   Develop a plan that matches community readiness to change in the level of the intervention (individual, social, environmental)
−   Create materials and messages that are appropriate for the education level in the population you intend to work with; use plain language in all communications
−   Assess the knowledge and attitudes of your targeted community
−   Evaluate how community members associate physical activity and disease, and what is considered physical activity
−   Evaluate population characteristics in the area you intend to serve:

     o   Physical and mental abilities of community members
     o   Single mothers
     o   Work/ occupation of community members
     o   Healthy v. less healthy
     o   Disabilities
     o   Age group

4. Engage the Community in the Planning and Implementation of the Intervention
- Evaluate what is necessary to implement the intervention (e.g. who, what, when, where):
- Take into account who should be brought to the table in developing the intervention: use familiar people and consider bringing together people from unusual places (e.g. individuals/
organizations not normally engaged in health activities)
- Take into account necessary skills and education: increase the training and certification in order to develop the amount of skilled people of that community that can be instructors
- Engage community to ensure you provide clear and consistent messages about physical activity and to ensure that you include appropriate and essential elements of the intervention
- Maintain the importance of community involvement through all phases of planning, implementation and evaluation
- Consider how information will be shared

5. Create Community Infrastructures to Support the Intervention
- Evaluate what level of medical care is available, the costs involved and the availability of sliding scales and insurance options
- Consider the availability and number of recreational facilities: audit the condition and quality of parks, green space, and sidewalks (curb cuts) in the community
- Consider the availability of flexible childcare options
- Involve local business as a financial resource
- Locate current workplace support of physical activity and promote similar activities in other locations
- Assess transportation options available to the community, specifically thinking about: availability of public transportation and distance between locations (e.g. medical facilities, physical activity facilities, locations where interventions will be conducted, and the neighborhood you intend to serve)

6. Ensure Appropriate Intervention Resources
- Assess the existing resources in the community, specifically in terms of: money, in-kind support, other groups or programs to piggy-back on (e.g. school systems)
- Explore the option of renting space
- Consider potential incentives for participants
- Investigate the need for/ current level of liability coverage
- Include the need for long-term funding in your plans
- Investigate funding restrictions that may apply

7. Ensure Personal and Environmental Safety
- Investigate crime rates in the neighborhood where you intend to work

Table 1. (Continued)

–   Assess availability of streetlights
–   Find applicable leash and poop-scoop laws that pertain to stray dogs
Consider the personal concern for safety if body gets smaller in some communities
8. Create Community Support
–   Assess the level of trust among the groups who will implement the program
–   Consider the level of buy-in and trust among the community leaders and stakeholders in the community
9. Recognize the Importance of Gender Issues
–   Take into account male expectations of the traditional roles of women
–   Consider female's own expectations of themselves (e.g., feeling guilty for taking time to do physical activity)
–   Consider the way men and women interact in developing intervention strategies
10. Conduct a Full Community Assessment
–   Investigate the socio-economic status of community members you intend to work with
–   Review the density of the community (number of people in small area)
–   Assess community capacity, for example, by evaluating the relationship of the community to local, state, and federal entitites, and/or the level of trust within the community
Consider whether the community is rural or urban and how that affects your intervention strategies

DISCUSSION

The purpose of this article was to describe a community-academic collaborative process used to create a list of issues to consider in adapting evidence-based physical activity interventions with and within racial and ethnic minority communities, and the development of practice considerations. In doing so, we found that the types of things that representatives of racial/ethnic minority communities think are important are often, but not always, the same as what white non-Hispanic representatives think are important.

The community members who took part in this process were individuals who were committed to prevention research and engaged members of their respective communities. Our findings suggest that what was considered most important when implementing interventions within racial/ethnic minority communities depended on who was asked. Attending to Culture and Tailoring the Intervention were seen as critical features of adapting interventions by racial/ethnic minority community participants, but not as much so by white-non Hispanic community participants. This finding reinforces what other behavioral science researchers have promoted, namely the importance of involving those affected by the research in intervention planning and implementation. In other words, it is important to work not only within community, but also with community members. By including community members from the beginning, interventions can be framed, developed, implemented and evaluated in ways that address issues of culture and tailor the intervention to the community, thereby maximizing the community benefit.

Another important finding from our work is that both groups considered the findings from previous studies to be important in developing interventions. This signals that our findings do not counter the Community Guide or the recent support of evidence-based approaches.

The fact that these statements were rated highly and placed together consistently by the overall group and the subgroups demonstrates their importance. It is important to note however, that this process was conducted as part of an EBPH course focusing on evidence-based physical activity interventions, as defined by the Community Guide. The fact that participants felt that these criteria were important could be a bias related to this process being conducted during an EBPH class.

Another important consideration is that while many of the issues for consideration are similar to actions already taken in the field (e.g., attend to culture), we see the operationalization of these as unique when considering conducting collaborative approaches with and within racial/ethnic minority communities. For example, attending to culture is not just a photograph that illustrates the community of interest or cultural competency training of professional staff.

It actually requires ongoing cultural competency of all partnership members to learn about the cultures of all partners and recognizing the influence of community sites chosen for the location of the intervention.

The process of engaging in this project, from the inception of the idea to the dissemination of the findings (including the writing of this manuscript), has occurred in a community-academic partnership. This partnership has facilitated a process that ensured that participants and researchers had common understanding of the intention of the research and the language used. Moreover, the outcomes have been interpreted through a collective lens.

This collaboration has been critical to the conduct of this research. The findings from this research have been presented to community and academic partners at conferences and at the NCC annual retreat.

Limitations

While this work builds upon and reinforces previous findings there are also limitations to this work. Although the participants represented a diverse group of geographic locations, their racial and ethnic composition was not equally representative. Most of the 29 participants were either White (n=10) or African American (n=12), with the remaining participants comprised of Native American, Asian American, and Hispanic decent (n=7). The racial/ethnic minority participants comprised the majority of participants, and African Americans composed the largest part of the entire group. It is likely that different racial and ethnic minorities would have produced somewhat different statements or concept maps, creating different themes for future implementation in physical activity interventions. Moreover, the most important issues may vary globally. Future work might focus on obtaining information from a broader range of racial and ethnic minorities and highlight differences among these groups. Similarly, there was a far greater representation of urban, in comparison to rural, participants. Future efforts might attempt to obtain more information on the unique characteristics of rural communities and how interventions might adapt to these contexts.

There is also a limitation in this work in that while it is critical to understand how to translate evidence-based physical activity recommendations within racial/ethnic minority communities, it is also important to recognize that disparities in physical activity and subsequent health outcomes are also evident in other communities that experience health disparities (e.g., by sexual orientation, ability status). This work does not provide insight into the issues that should be considered in translating evidence-based interventions into these other communities. It is also important to note that while the clusters were ranked by order of importance and are presented as such, the difference between the mean values of each was not always statistically significant. As a result one can not necessarily conclude, for example, that safety is significantly more important than conducting a full community assessment. The differences in ranking illustrate that what is most important differs among community partners.

Building capacity to improve physical activity

The capacity to adapt evidence-based physical activity interventions with and within racial/ethnic minority communities requires consideration of a number of issues. Our work suggests that it may be helpful to consider culture, tailoring the intervention, community infrastructures and support, engaging the community, intervention resources, safety, community assessment, and gender issues. In doing so, it is important to work with the community of interest to operationalize these issues in ways that are locally relevant and meaningful. Future efforts to evaluate this work will benefit from tracking the specific impact that adhering to these considerations has on intervention outcomes.

ACKNOWLEDGMENTS

The authors would like to thank Refilwe Moeti, Catherine Morrison, Ralph Faccillo, Ella Green Motton as well as the National Community Committee membership and Cheryl Kelly for their contributions to our work. We would also like to acknowledge financial support from the Centers for Disease Control and Preventions' Prevention Research Center and the Division of Nutrition Physical Activity and Obesity. Funding from: CDC Prevention Research Center and the Division of Nutrition Physical Activity and Obesity.

REFERENCES

[1]   Brownson R, Boehmer T, Luke D. Declining rates of physical activity in the United States: What are the contributors? Annu Rev Public Health 2005;26:421-43.

[2]   Pate R, Pratt M, Blair S. Physical activity and public health: A recommendation from the Centers for Disease Control and Prevention and the American College of Sports Medicine. JAMA 1995;273(5):402-7.

[3]   Powell KE, Blair SN. The public health burdens of sedentary living habits: theoretical but realistic estimates. Med Sci Sports Exerc 1994;26(7):851-6.

[4]   US Department of Health and Human Services. Physical activity and health. A report of the surgeon general. Atlanta, GA: US Department Health Human Services, Centers Disease Control Prevention, 1996.

[5]   Hahn R, Teutsch SM, Rothenberg RB, Marks JS. Excess deaths from nine chronic diseases in the United States, 1986. JAMA 1990;264: 2654-9.

[6]   McGinnis J. The public health burden of a sedentary lifestyle. Med Sci Sports Exerc 1992;6(Suppl): S196-S200.

[7]   Centers for Disease Control and Prevention (CDC), Behavioral Risk Factor Surveillance System Survey Data. Atlanta, GA: US Department Health Human Services, Centers Disease Control Prevention, 2007.

[8]   National Academy of Sciences. The Future of the Public's Health in the 21st Century. Washington, DC: Natl Acad Sci, 2003.

[9]   Truman B, Smith-Akin C, Hinman A. Developing the guide to community preventive services - overview and rationale. Am J Prev Med 2000;18(1S):18-26.

[10]   Rychetnik L, Hawe P, Waters E, Barratt A, Frommer M. A glossary for evidence based public health. J Epidemiol Commun Health 2004;58(7): 538-45.

[11]   Brownson RC, Baker EA, Leet TL, Gillespie KN. Evidence-based public health. New York: Oxford University Press, 2003.

Submitted: September 02, 2011. *Revised:* November 11, 2011. *Accepted:* November 21, 2011.

In: Public Health Yearbook 2012   ISBN: 978-1-62808-078-0

Editor: Joav Merrick   © 2013 Nova Science Publishers, Inc.

Chapter 28

ROLES OF HISPANIC SERVICE ORGANIZATIONS IN TUBERCULOSIS EDUCATION AND HEALTH PROMOTION

Sue Gena Lurie, PhD[*], Stephen Weis and Guadalupe Munguia

Department of Behavioral and Community Health, School of Public Health,
University of North Texas Health Science Center, Fort Worth, Texas, Tarrant County
Public Health, Fort Worth, Texas and
University of Illinois at Chicago, Chicago, Illinois, United States of America

ABSTRACT

Tuberculosis risk and prevention, treatment and drug resistance remain problematic for recent immigrants to urban areas in the United States, including those from Mexico, Central and South America. This research on health and social agency staff serving Hispanics (Latinos) in selected urban areas with relatively high incidence of tuberculosis was designed to develop culturally-appropriate educational materials with the Centers of Disease Control and Prevention - Division of Tuberculosis Elimination. Qualitative research methods were applied in bilingual focus groups and interviews with Hispanic agency directors and staff representing health and social service organizations in eleven cities, from 2003 to 2007. Tuberculosis was found to be socially constructed in Hispanic/Latino communities as a "hidden" chronic disease in interpretations of risk and potential for recovery. Social isolation, cultural, legal and economic barriers, and limited prevention resources were identified as affecting health education, prevention and disease management with patients and clients. The majority of Hispanic organizational leaders and staff responded positively to collaboration in tuberculosis education, and modified messages to communicate disease risk and prevention effectively and reduce potential for stigmatization.

[*] Correspondence: Sue Gena Lurie, PhD, assistant professor, Department of Behavioral and Community Health, School of Public Health, University of North Texas Health Science Center at Fort Worth, 3500 Camp Bowie Boulevard, Fort Worth, Texas 76107, United States. E-mail: sue.lurie@unthsc.edu and sglurie@att.net

Keywords: Tuberculosis education, health promotion, risk communication, Hispanic/Latino
health

INTRODUCTION

Community health interventions range from those that focus on particular diseases and health problems, to those that address community awareness and capacity, social determinants of health, environmental health risks, or access to care and delivery of health services. The "health in cities" approach recognizes that the interaction of multiple groups with diverse health needs and interests requires addressing the vulnerabilities of particular populations to develop effective interventions (1). For recent immigrants in the urban United States, protection from tuberculosis risk, disease management and appropriate treatment remain crucial issues.

This research compared the context of community health and illness for Hispanics and Latinos in the urban United States, and the role of culturally-appropriate health education in reducing the risk of tuberculosis (TB), as interpreted by health and social agency leaders and staff in the communities they serve. The study was designed to develop and assess the effectiveness of culturally-appropriate educational materials for national distribution by the Centers for Disease Control (CDC) - Division of Tuberculosis Elimination in selected urban areas with high tuberculosis prevalence, from 2003-2007.

This study followed previous national studies by CDC on TB control with diverse communities and ethnic groups. National needs assessments with state and local professional stakeholders analyzed the roles of communication and public-private service collaboration in addressing barriers to TB elimination (2). Risk, prevention, treatment and drug resistance remain problematic for recent immigrants in the United States. From 1993-2006, there were 202,436 confirmed tuberculosis cases (3). In 2006, 57% of all reported cases were among foreign-born persons (4). Research on TB prevalence in the United States found that Mexico, the Philippines and Vietnam were the top three countries of origin for foreign-born cases (5, 6). Moreover, recent epidemiological research found that local spatial distribution of unique strains of tuberculosis in immigrant neighborhoods differed from the distribution in native-born neighborhoods in a north Texas county, indicating that immigrant health profiles resembled those of their communities of origin (7).

Tuberculosis remains a major health problem for Hispanics or Latinos in the United States. In 2004, TB was reported in 4,186 Hispanic or Latino persons - 29% of all persons with TB nationally. The rate of TB in Hispanic or Latino persons in 2004 was 10.1 cases per 100,000 population - more than seven times higher than the rate of TB in white, non-Hispanic persons (1.3 cases per 100,000 population). In 2004 and 2005, more tuberculosis cases were reported among Hispanics than among any other racial or ethnic population in the nation (8).

The rationale for promotion of effective partnerships with community agencies for health education was based on CDC's response in 2002 (9) to a proposal by the Institute of Medicine:

> ...given the cultural and linguistic barriers that confront individuals who have newly arrived in the United States, much might be ...attained by engaging the cooperation of community-based organizations that provide services to distinct ethnic immigrant

communities. Certainly such organizations will have much to offer local tuberculosis control programs that may be called upon to provide treatment of newly arrived immigrants for latent infections (10, p. 96)

Health promotion and communication with Hispanic service organizations

In October, 2003, the Communications, Education, and Behavioral Studies Branch in the CDC Division of Tuberculosis Elimination initiated this participatory research project (11) in health communication, to develop educational materials for, and with, local leaders and staff in urban Hispanic or Latino health and social service organizations. The study was reviewed by the Tuberculosis Epidemiologic Studies Consortium (TBESC). The purpose of the research was to provide health and social service organizations with essential information to address health needs of Hispanic or Latino patients and clients, and to evaluate the effectiveness of culturally-appropriate educational materials in English and Spanish. The ultimate goal of the project was to promote local collaboration to reduce risk and/or eliminate tuberculosis in urban communities. This study was implemented with Tarrant County Public Health TB Clinic and University of North Texas Health Science Center, on approval by both the University of North Texas Health Science Center and CDC Institutional Review Boards.

METHODS

Qualitative research methods were applied for data collection and analysis (12). The study began with formative research that included comprehensive literature review of current tuberculosis educational programs and materials primarily targeted to patients, followed by focus groups to identify local health concerns and use of health information channels by agency leaders and staff in diverse regions across the United States. Urban study sites were selected and a series of bilingual focus groups and interviews with agency directors and staff was conducted, in each study phase. For each focus group, meeting sites were located and from six to nine participants were recruited, with assistance of contact persons in each city.

As focus groups convened, participants completed a demographic information form without personal identifiers, and read and signed informed consent forms. Interviews and focus groups were conducted by facilitators in English and Spanish using a discussion guide designed for each study phase. All responses were tape-recorded, transcribed and translated; written notes by research assistants complemented recordings. One or more observers were present during each focus group to answer questions and contribute to process evaluation, after each session.

In Phase I, five bilingual focus groups were conducted from the end of 2003 to 2004 in urban areas: San Francisco, California; Fort Worth, Texas; Fort Lauderdale, Florida; Harlem and Queens, New York. Participants in these groups included Mexican-, Puerto Rican-, Venezuelan-, Ecuadoran- and Haitian-Americans, as well as indigenous persons from Latin America. Community health concerns and use of health information channels were elicited; participants' knowledge of TB symptoms, transmission and treatment processes were also assessed.

In Phase II (2005), written messages on TB risk, prevalence and treatment were pre-tested in two regions with sizeable Hispanic populations, using interviews with agency leaders and staff in Houston, Texas, and a focus group in San Diego, California. Participants included assimilated and recent immigrants from Africa and Mexico, in agencies serving Hispanics and indigenous persons from Oaxaca, and Caucasian clinical and bilingual communication staff. Culturally-appropriate tuberculosis educational messages were developed and tested, using bilingual messages and graphs. These messages were based on findings from Phase I on the perceptions of tuberculosis exposure and infection, the disease process, testing and treatment, barriers to prevention and control, and reducing risk for individual clients and communities.

In Phase III (2005-2006), an educational brochure with graphics was developed and field-tested in seven focus groups with Hispanic service organizations in the following cities: Chicago, Illinois; Los Angeles, California (two groups); El Paso, Texas (two groups); Washington, D.C.; and Phoenix, Arizona. Focus group participants in these cities included Mexican-, African-, and Caucasian- Americans. The brochure presented the prevalence of TB among Hispanics in the United States, the risk of latent TB infection and active TB disease, the importance of completing treatment and Directly Observed Therapy, and the Bi-National TB Project. Recommendations of CDC resources to support local agencies in reducing TB among "high-risk" clients were also included.

Data analysis

For this study of perceptions of tuberculosis by Hispanic organizational leaders and staff, qualitative data analysis was applied to identify themes and evaluate effectiveness of specific messages, by comparing the responses to questions for discussion, across focus groups. Since the goal was to compare group rather than individual responses, not to apply quantitative data analysis techniques or measures of statistical significance, numbers were not compiled for individual responses, but group consensus and divergence were analyzed. Preliminary reports on each study phase and a comprehensive final report with conclusions and recommendations for revisions of brochure messages and graphics were submitted by the authors to CDC for review and approval.

RESULTS

Current health promotion programs for tuberculosis (TB), designed to change interpretations of the disease to one that can be eliminated by effective treatment, emphasize risk communication to persuade community members to obtain health screening and care. Perceptions of disease affect community responses to risk, prevention and treatment. In epidemiology, tuberculosis is defined temporally as a chronic communicable disease, since it has symptoms that persist three months or longer (13). The distinction between chronic and acute diseases is also socially and culturally constructed: diseases that are perceived as difficult to treat or incurable are labeled as chronic by laypersons; those that are amenable to effective treatment are perceived as acute.

In Phase I focus groups, multi-ethnic leaders and staff in public and non-profit agencies for Hispanic advocacy, social, legal and immigration services, community health education and care, and community volunteers (promatoras de salud) voiced their priorities for reducing social, cultural, legal and economic barriers to tuberculosis prevention and care, and concerns about stigma, isolation and fear of illness. Venezuelan immigration staff in Fort Lauderdale recommended a national TB screening program, like that in their home country. Participants in various groups affirmed the need for collaboration in Hispanic community education on tuberculosis risk, latent TB infection, active TB disease, transmission, symptoms, treatment and drug resistance. Health education media, including brochures, videos, graphics, and direct communication among staff and clients were compared, but use was not specifically evaluated. Participants responded that clear messages on latent infection, active disease, TB symptoms and risk associated with HIV/AIDS, TB testing and completing treatment were essential.

Phase II focus group participants expressed the need to know how to use educational information to reduce social or environmental factors in tuberculosis risk, and perceived barriers to be culture, language, immigration, stigma, lack of resources, and access to treatment and care. While they tended to be familiar with the TB transmission processes, the response by a Mexican social service provider, "It's in our blood", could have implied a genetic "explanatory model" (14), misunderstanding of TB pathogenesis and/or confusion with the HIV infection process. There was general recognition of the need for further education on tuberculosis exposure and transmission, on screening, testing, latent and active TB, MDR-TB, and association of TB with HIV. Treatment by Directly Observed Therapy and diagnosis by QuantaFERON-Gold assay tended to be unfamiliar to most participants. The Bi-National TB Project with Mexico was primarily of interest to those from border regions in California and Texas.

Phase III focus group participants in Chicago, Los Angeles, El Paso, Washington and Phoenix responded positively to messages for tuberculosis prevention, CDC and local health department contact information, and bi-lingual information on TB symptoms. However, they cautioned health educators to avoid stigmatizing community members of minority, immigrant and undocumented groups by emphasizing their elevated risk. They did recommend information on prevention for families and risk factors for specific age and social groups, including pregnant women. Some social agency leaders and staff expressed concern about the adequacy of their resources for tuberculosis prevention.

DISCUSSION

For the majority of urban communities represented in all phases of the study, a range of chronic diseases - diabetes, cancer, cardiovascular disease, hypertension, high cholesterol, obesity, asthma, allergies, Chronic Obstructive Pulmonary Disease (COPD), lead-related illnesses, Parkinson's and Alzheimer's diseases, and low birth weight - were major concerns. Other health and social problems ranged from STD's and HIV/AIDS to domestic violence, alcoholism, drug use, poverty and occupational risks. Tuberculosis tends to be seen by service providers as declining, although it may be tabooed or considered a "hidden" disease by Hispanics or Latinos, and the general public. TB was perceived by clinic staff in Washington, D.C. as a health problem that affects different occupational groups unequally, and by social agency staff in Phoenix as an increasing risk for Native Americans.

Hispanic service organizational leaders and staff were interested in collaborating with health care agencies to improve social and economic environments for Latino immigrants and low-income clients, and to increase resources and reduce barriers to tuberculosis control. The bi-lingual educational brochures depicting multi-ethnic, age and occupational diversity, clear messages and contact information appeared to be effective in health communication. However, the selection and use of facial photographs to represent inter-ethnic diversity or unity among "Hispanics" of various ages, gender and national origins was debated among participants.

Public health terms such as "burden of disease", "minority", and epidemiological comparisons of ethnic groups were found to convey negative meanings about Hispanics. Linguistic recommendations to modify messages included use of "tuberculosis" rather than "TB" to avoid confusion. The use of both "Hispanic" and "Latino" was also supported, since the latter encompasses both Spanish and Portuguese-speakers from Latin America. Specific suggestions for brochure graphics were to add diagrams depicting potential physical effects of tuberculosis in the lungs and elsewhere in the human body, to enhance the effectiveness of risk communication.

While focus group participants tended to respond positively to health education on tuberculosis risk and the need for testing and treatment, the biomedical concept and practice of treatment as primary prevention was considered too restrictive, if not disavowed by those who sought more positive or pro-active approaches.

Major concerns expressed by Hispanic health and social service leaders and staff were: (a) the focus of health policy on reducing disease risk for particular ethnic groups and on treatment for individuals who are diagnosed with TB, rather than on primary prevention by improving overall social and economic conditions for health; (b) potential stigmatization of minority and immigrant groups as unhealthy; and (c) lack of health service resources for social agencies. Service providers in the study did support and advocate prevention through community health education to reduce potential disease risk, increasing resources for low-cost, accessible testing and treatment, and integrating staff and client health education to promote risk awareness. Specific recommendations for design of the TB educational brochure are now under review by CDC - Division of Tuberculosis Elimination and Control.

Tuberculosis tends to be socially and culturally constructed as a chronic communicable disease by health and social service providers for Hispanic and Latino communities in urban areas.

This was expressed in their concerns about the potential for stigmatizing immigrant ethnic groups, and exacerbating the social isolation of persons diagnosed with TB, despite local variations in interpretations of TB risk and prevention methods. In contrast, health education and promotion efforts by public health and medical agencies and practitioners seek to change this image of TB to that of a treatable disease that can be prevented and eliminated by screening and treating latent and active TB infections effectively.

To support this effort, raising community and professional awareness through communication and public-private agency collaboration is promoted as a means of reducing TB disease incidence, morbidity and mortality.

Community health education is oriented toward reducing TB risk for the local population, from exposure through environmental transmission, and expanding screening and effective treatment. These goals can be reached with the collaboration of community-based organizations that provide health and social services to vulnerable urban ethnic and immigrant populations.

This approach supports current national public health research goals (15) and efforts to reduce health inequity in tuberculosis (16). Through their leaders and staff, local health and social service organizations can serve as informed liaisons with communities for tuberculosis control and elimination programs, to improve the health of newly-arrived immigrants and local residents.

Effective communication using culturally- and socially-appropriate health education on tuberculosis risk, symptoms, testing and treatment is an essential component of inter-agency collaboration (17), to ensure the health of local clients and that of the larger urban community.

ACKNOWLEDGMENTS

The study was sponsored by a grant from the Centers of Disease Control and Prevention - Division of Tuberculosis Elimination (Task Order #14).

REFERENCES

[1]   Glouberman S, Gemar M, Campsie P, et al. A framework for improving health in cities: a discussion paper. J Urban Health 2006;83(2):325-38.

[2]   Communication Sciences Group. CDC/NCHSTP/TB Communications project: key informant interviews and market analysis. Final Report. San Francisco, California, July 23rd, 1999.

[3]   Tarrant County Public Health. Tuberculosis overview and extensive drug resistant tuberculosis. Eye Epidemiol 2007;9(3):1-5.

[4]   Cain K, Benoit S, Winston K, et al. Tuberculosis among foreign-born persons in the United States. JAMA 2008;300(4):405-12.

[5]   Analytic Sciences, Inc. Culturally appropriate tuberculosis patient education materials project: focus group findings report. Durham, North Carolina, 2003.

[6]   Analytic Sciences, Inc. Culturally appropriate tuberculosis patient education materials project: focus group findings report: Los Angeles, California. Durham, North Carolina, 2003.

[7]   Oppong J, Denton C, Moonan P, Weis S. Foreign-born status and geographic patterns of tuberculosis genotypes in Tarrant County, Texas. Professional Geographer 2007;59(4):478-91.

[8]   Centers for Disease Control-Division of Tuberculosis Elimination and Control unpublished report. Atlanta, GA: CDC, 2005.

[9]   Centers for Disease Control. Response to Ending neglect: the elimination of tuberculosis in the United States. Atlanta, GA: CDC, 2002.

[10]   Institute of Medicine. Ending neglect: the elimination of tuberculosis in the United States. Institute of Medicine Report. Washington, DC: IOM, 2000.

[11]   Minkler M, Wallerstein N, eds. Community-based participatory research for health. San Francisco: Jossey-Bass. 2003.

[12]   Green J, Thorogood N. Qualitative methods for health research. Second ed. Thousand Oaks, CA: Sage, 2009.

[13]   McKenzie J, Pinger R, Kotecki J. Introduction to community health, 6th ed. Sudbury, A: Jones Bartlett, 2008.

[14]   Kleinman A. Patients and healers in the context of culture. Berkeley, CA: University California Press. 1980.

[15]   Centers for Disease Control: Advancing the nation's health: a guide to public health research needs. Atlanta, GA: CDC, 2006.

[16]   Centers for Disease Control: Establishing a holistic framework to reduce inequities in HIV, Viral Hepatitis, STD's, and tuberculosis in the United States. National Center for HIV, Viral Hepatitis,

STD's, and Tuberculosis Prevention White Paper on Social Determinants of Health. Atlanta, GA: CDC, 2010.

[17]　Waisboard S. Beyond the medical informational model: recasting the role of communication in tuberculosis control. Soc Sci Med 2007; 65:2130-4.

Submitted: September 8, 2011. *Revised:* November 08, 2011. *Accepted:* November 21, 2011.

In: Public Health Yearbook 2012
Editor: Joav Merrick

ISBN: 978-1-62808-078-0
© 2013 Nova Science Publishers, Inc.

Chapter 29

PROJECT SALUD: USING COMMUNITY-BASED PARTICIPATORY RESEARCH TO CULTURALLY ADAPT AN HIV PREVENTION INTERVENTION IN THE LATINO MIGRANT WORKER COMMUNITY

Jesús Sánchez, PhD[*1],
Claudia A Serna, DDS[2]
and Mario de La Rosa, PhD[3]

[1]Department of Sociobehavioral and Administrative Pharmacy, College of Pharmacy, Nova Southeastern University, Fort Lauderdale, Florida,
[2]Department of Health Promotion and Disease Prevention and
[3]Center for Research on US Latinos, HIV/AIDS and Drug Abuse, Robert Stempel College of Public Health and Social Work, Florida International University, Miami, Florida

ABSTRACT

Despite the unique and challenging circumstances confronting Latino migrant worker communities in the U.S., debate still exists as to the need to culturally adapt evidence-based interventions for dissemination with this population. Project Salud adopted a community-based participatory research model and utilized focus group methodology with 83 Latino migrant workers to explore the relevance of culturally adapting an evidence-based HIV prevention intervention to be disseminated within this population. Findings from this study indicate that, despite early reservations, Latino migrant workers wanted to participate in the cultural adaptation that would result in an intervention that was culturally relevant, respectful, responsive to their life experiences, and aligned with their needs. This study contributes to the cultural adaptation/fidelity debate by highlighting the necessity of exploring ways to develop culturally adapted

* Correspondence: Professor Jesús Sánchez, Ph.D. Associate Professor, Department of Sociobehavioral and Administrative Pharmacy, College of Pharmacy, Nova Southeastern University, 3200 South University Drive, Fort Lauderdale, FL 33328-2018. E-mail: js2769@nova.edu

interventions characterized by high cultural relevance without sacrificing high fidelity to the core components that have established efficacy for evidence-based HIV prevention interventions.

Keywords: Latino, migrants, HIV/AIDS prevention, cultural adaptation, CBPR

INTRODUCTION

Understanding and addressing the causes of HIV related health disparities among Latinos in the U.S. is increasingly relevant as the magnitude of immigrant and migrant populations from Latin America and the Caribbean continue to grow (1). The Latino community living in the United States has been disproportionally impacted by the HIV/AIDS epidemic (2), while the development, implementation, and evaluation of HIV prevention interventions designed to reduce the risk of infection among Latinos lags behind prevention efforts targeting other communities (3). This public health gap is particularly apparent when considering the sparse attention received by Latino migrant workers in the United States despite their high risk for HIV infection. Research indicates that most Latino migrant workers (LMWs) become infected while in the U.S., underlining the importance of enhancing both HIV prevention and treatment efforts (4).

Research has specifically linked migration to increased HIV incidence and vulnerability in a variety of contexts and places. A greater risk for poor health and limited access to health services, low socioeconomic status, low levels of formal education, and marginalization are among the main reasons why LMWs are particularly vulnerable to HIV infection (5-6). The few available studies on HIV transmission and prevention specifically conducted among Latino migrant workers highlight the role played by many complex and interrelated factors. These include social norms, health-related beliefs, attitudes and behaviors related to sex and drug use, and social and environmental factors such as housing and employment (7-11). LMWs bring with them an assortment of beliefs, attitudes, and practices that vary from country to country of origin and that—when put into practice in their new communities— often result in a sense of cultural shock, stress, and alienation that may impact health-risk behaviors, in general, and HIV related risk behaviors in particular. The development of effective HIV prevention interventions for the Latino migrant worker community requires that we address the cultural and societal issues that put LMWs at risk as well as focus on the cultural strengths that might assist members of this community to stay safe.

While the existing studies have made a critical contribution to advance our understanding of the Latino migrant worker population in the US and highlight numerous potential differences between this and other populations, their HIV prevention interventions have demonstrated only limited effectiveness (12-14) and documented a critical need for tailoring effective HIV prevention interventions for the Latino migrant worker population. These adaptations, however, cannot be limited to the cultural translation of existing interventions based on cultural generalizations or preconceptions associated with Latinos (15-16). A pervasive limitation of many of these cultural translations involves the use of the umbrella category "Latino" (or "Hispanic") which presents an obfuscated description that pretends to capture the characteristics of a large group of national and ethnic populations. Another important limitation is the imposition of the term "Latino" on different subgroups with different characteristics, backgrounds, and migration experiences without asking members of these groups for their opinion. These limitations contribute to the traditional mistrust among LMWs of conventional research which they view as paternalistic, misguided, and irrelevant to their needs. As a result, conventional prevention strategies are likely to fail to adequately help Latino migrant workers to adopt and maintain HIV risk reduction behaviors in a constantly shifting personal and social environment (17-19).

Culturally adapted interventions must prompt community engagement and participation at every phase of the program if they do not want to remain culturally blind. Latino migrant workers are most likely to benefit from HIV prevention efforts when these efforts are supported at the community level, sustained over time, and the overall needs of the community are addressed (20-22).

Community based participatory research (CBPR) has emerged as a research paradigm that addresses the limitations of conventional research models and offers a "collaborative approach to research that equitably involves all partners in the research process and recognizes the unique strengths that each brings. The ultimate goal is to promote social change to improve community health and reduce health disparities" (23). Advantages of CBPR include that it is a participatory and cooperative approach, requires equitable power and mutual ownership, is framed in a co-learning experience, and seeks the balance between research and action. Furthermore, it is an empowering process that involves capacity building among all partners involved.

In this paper, we describe (a) Project Salud, a growing CBPR partnership between the Latino migrant worker community in South Florida and researchers at Nova Southeastern University and Florida International University; and (b) the value of using focus groups with the Latino migrant community in South Florida to culturally adapt an evidence-based HIV prevention intervention before implementation in the community.

METHODS

Project Salud--officially entitled "HIV Risk Reduction among High Risk Latino Migrant Workers in South Florida"--was a 4-year major study funded by the National Institute on Minority Health and Health Disparities (NIMHD) as part of C-Salud, a P20 Exploratory Center of Excellence at Florida International University. The main objective of Project Salud was to assess the differential effectiveness of an Adapted Stage-Enhanced Motivational Interviewing (A-SEMI) compared to a Health Promotion Comparison (HPC) condition for producing long-term reductions in HIV risk and increased health behaviors among LMWs. The design of the A-SEMI intervention is considered to be an enhancement over existing cognitive behavioral risk reduction approaches because A-SEMI integrates key contextual components from effective HIV prevention interventions (i.e., peer counseling) linked to maintenance of risk reduction effects. As described in this paper, the A-SEMI intervention was culturally adapted in collaboration with the LMW community.

Project Salud was conceived as a CBPR project with the goal of engaging the Latino migrant worker community in Homestead in the implementation of an HIV prevention intervention. By framing Project Salud within the CBPR approach, this study responded to the NIH priority on establishing equitable partnerships between community members and researchers with the final goal of increasing community participation in the research process, improving community health, and reducing HIV-related health disparities.

Design

At the early stages of Project Salud, we set off a plan to address the issue of cultural adaptation while reinforcing trust in the community and creating community capacity as a key building block in the development of our partnership with the Latino migrant worker community. We initiated a dialogue with key community partners and community members with the goal of identifying what type of strategies would be adequate to address the issue of HIV prevention among Latino migrant workers. The ultimate goal of this dialogue was to juxtapose the views of both the community and the researchers. Based on this exchange of ideas and using other researchers' experiences as a learning framework (24-26), we decided that focus group methodology was the appropriate approach. Researchers who work with migrant populations have reported on the complexities of working with these populations and how a unique sensitivity is required to understand how particular phenomena are experienced and expressed (27). Focus groups provide several advantages over the conventional methods in instrument development. First, focus groups are useful for developing insights into the perceptions and points of view of persons who have some common characteristics related to the research topic and for appreciating the variation in people's experiences (28). The resulting intervention is more likely to be grounded in the experiences of the population under study. Generating knowledge from focus groups can provide reasonable assurance that the instrument is culturally anchored. Second, focus groups inform researchers about the language and terminology that particular groups of people use regarding the construct under study (28). By preserving the terminology from the focus group, items included in the intervention may reflect the language of the population of interest. Third, the focus group's social nature often stimulates stories and insights that would be missed otherwise (29).

Focus groups were conducted at the early stages of Project Salud when both the project and the researchers involved in it were still unknown to many community members. We undertook a series of preparatory activities prior to conducting the focus groups to better inform the Latino migrant worker community in Homestead about who we were, the goals of the project, and our desire to establish a true partnership with the community. As part of these preparatory steps, we conducted several town hall meetings at venues such as churches, street markets, a community center, and the offices of the Farmworker Association of Florida in Homestead. We expanded our partnership with professionals in health and social services, advocates, religious leaders, AIDS educators and, more importantly, nursery and agricultural workers. As our partnership grew larger and stronger, Project Salud started being recognized in the community.

Another positive outcome of our increasing presence and recognition in the community resulted in the implementation of strategies that increased recruitment rates and representativeness. Community members' concerns about becoming involved in a focus group began to dissipate during town hall meetings and the different activities conducted at the early stages of the project. The support of community partners was crucial at a time when the current anti-immigration climate and policies in the U.S. have negatively impacted the lives of migrant workers. We addressed this issue by validating such concerns and extensively reviewing the standards of confidentiality and the rights of each participant (i.e., right to withdraw from the study at any time, right to refuse to answer questions). We also adopted community members' suggestions regarding the locations where we could meet and conduct the focus groups. The suggested sites--unlike some of the locations we had originally preselected--were considered by the community as safer and less likely to be raided by immigration authorities.

To be selected for the focus groups, participants had to (a) be 18 years old or older; (b) be a first generation immigrant; (c) be a member of the Latino migrant worker community in the Homestead area; and (d) express an interest to participate in the focus group interview.

A total of eight focus groups were conducted with a range of 6 to 12 participants per focus group. A maximum number of 12 participants per group was established in order to better facilitate group discussions. Each focus group interview lasted between 120 and 180 minutes and was held in the evening and/or weekend. All focus groups started with a dinner, an overview of Project Salud, completion of a consent form, and brief demographic questionnaire. Each participant received a $40 stipend for their participation. Participants were required by IRB policy to complete a form documenting their receipt of the participant payment; however, no personal identifiers were requested.

Eighty-three members of the Latino migrant worker community participated in the focus groups. Although it was planned in the original research protocol to organize focus groups according to a set of criteria (i.e., gender, nationality, age), the design was modified in response to the contextual challenges associated with recruitment. In particular, participants were encouraged to join whichever focus group was possible for them to attend.

Focus groups were consistent in their delivery and draw upon the same protocol guidelines. Each session was facilitated by a project member with experience in focus group facilitation while another project member was present at each session as a note-taker. Focus groups were conducted in Spanish and the discussions were audio recorded and then transcribed for purposes of data analysis. Prior to conducting the focus groups, we hired two members from the LMW community to be trained on the project, assist with the development of the focus group protocol, and support focus group sessions.

Project Salud members introduced themselves and provided a five to ten minute overview of the project. Project members made this presentation highly interactive as a means to warm up the focus group participants. For instance, they included a trivia or guessing game as part of the presentation. Group members introduced themselves and were invited to briefly express an opinion on the impact of the HIV/AIDS epidemic on their community. This initial discussion provided a context for the group from which to proceed. Participants were told that focus groups were being held in order to learn from the Latino migrant worker community about their knowledge, behaviors, and attitudes towards the HIV/AIDS epidemic. They were also inquired about their interest in participating in a study that would utilize the information learned from the focus groups to determine how the different intervention components should be adapted and implemented in order to increase community members' motivation to participate in this initiative and establish a sustainable strategy for implementing the adapted intervention in the community.

Project Salud members explained that the research team sought to offer an existing evidence-based HIV prevention intervention to the LMW community that had proven beneficial to other communities. Therefore, the focus group sessions were a key step toward clarifying how relevant LMWs find the specific core components (i.e., skills) covered in the original intervention, exploring if the intervention was responsive to their life experiences and cultural background, and making the necessary cultural adaptations. The ensuing discussion followed the protocol guidelines tailored to explore and discuss the core components of the evidence-based intervention.

RESULTS

Using focus groups proved to be a challenging but successful experience that provided many insights into culturally shaping the A-SEMI intervention. In this section, a few examples are offered on the type of knowledge that was gathered through the implementation of the focus groups as well as how that information was utilized towards the cultural adaptation of the intervention.

Talking about HIV-related behaviors, attitudes, and beliefs in a group setting can be extremely difficult for Latino men and women who view topics such as sexual behaviors as very personal. Because of this, we found that some participants would talk about these issues as if they were happening to a friend or relative. On the other hand, we also concluded that— although less private—the use of oral and group-centered strategies were more reflective of the dominant learning styles, orientations, values and educational levels of participants. As a result, although an interventionist would typically encourage participants to talk about their own experiences and opinions, we agreed that when working with the LMW community, we needed to be aware that—in some instances—one strategy to cope with the discomfort of talking about personal issues is to frame it as the experience of someone else.

The focus groups also revealed the need for a more dynamic understanding of the cultural milieu that characterizes Latino migrant worker communities. An example of how sweeping assertions about Latino culture fail to capture the shifting cultural dynamics of this community is reflected in the impact of changing gender roles on sexual relations. Traditional gender roles are often associated with Latino culture. Machismo and marianismo are presented as playing a crucial role in shaping sexual communication and relations between Latino men and women (30). Because of the apparent power imbalance that characterizes these relationships, some scholars suggest that theories that emphasize sexual division of labor and power may be an appropriate intervention framework. However, our focus groups revealed that—although often times this power imbalance may have characterized participants' sexual relations in their countries of origin—as LMWs spend more time away from their countries of origin, they begin to reconsider those gender role expectations. This trend was particularly salient among the women who participated in the focus groups. Having to endure the same harsh working and housing conditions as their male counterparts, Latina migrant workers question the traditional idea of the submissive Latina who centers her life around her family and is generally obedient to the men in her life. As a result, sexual culture in the LMW community can be characterized as the coexistence of traditional and modern values. In light of this finding, it was crucial to culturally adapt the A-SEMI intervention to reflect the coexisting cultural expectations and rules of sexual interaction among LMWs.

Another salient value associated with traditional Latino culture is familismo, which places the multigenerational extended family at the core of the culture. Familismo promotes closeness and interconnectedness among extended family members and provides a sense of responsibility to care for all members of the family (30). Most of the participants in the focus groups had few or no relatives living with them in the U.S. Many of the male participants indicated that they came to the U.S. by themselves and would not risk bringing their families over because of the risks associated with getting smuggled into the U.S. Other participants indicated that their spouses or significant others had been deported back to their countries of origin and, in most cases, were trying to cross the border again. As a result, the positive impact provided by familismo in terms of social support, knowledge, and material resources is lacking in the LMW community. In its absence, participants stressed the importance of developing a sense of community. Participants highlighted the importance of facilitating learning experiences by promoting a sense of community among those who would participate in the intervention. Specifically, rather than limiting group interventions to didactic sessions focused exclusively on disseminating knowledge and teaching skills, participants affirmed that interventions should also promote group cohesion and supportive relationships among intervention participants. Many participants in the focus groups commented on how valuable the focus group session was to them, as well as their desire to extend the same type of dynamic into the intervention. Participants expressed that the intervention groups should constitute a resource for empowering participants. Consequently, the A-SEMI intervention was culturally adapted to enhance empowerment as a multilayered process beyond the cultural domains directly related to HIV prevention (i.e., sexual relations).

Conducting project salud

A network-based sample of 278 Latino migrant workers was recruited from November 2008 to December 2010 from migrant communities in the Homestead area in Miami-Dade County, Florida. Homestead is part of a predominantly rural area in the South of Miami-Dade County, Florida. Official census data indicate that most of the population in Homestead (51.8%) is Hispanic/Latino, more than one-third (36%) is foreign born, and a majority (57.3%) speaks a language other than English at home (31). Agriculture and nursery constitute an important business in the Homestead area allowing for access to seasonal farm work. Homestead's Latino migrant worker population is composed primarily of recently arrived, young, single or married men that are in the United States alone. They live in small crowded apartments with family or friends. Most are Mexican and Central American arriving in this area with little or no English language skills and very limited resources.

After screening for eligibility, participants were administered a structured baseline questionnaire using A-CASI that included basic socio-demographic information, alcohol and other drug use history, sexual behaviors, acculturation, and behavioral intentionality. Study participants were then randomly assigned to the A-SEMI and HPC intervention groups. Two follow-up assessments were administered at 3 and 9 months after the baseline questionnaire. This study was approved by the IRB of Florida International University. Data analysis is being conducted at the present time to assess the differential effectiveness of the A-SEMI compared to the HPC condition for producing short and long-term reductions in HIV risk and increased health behaviors among LMWs.

DISCUSSION

This study contributes to the existing literature in relevant ways. For instance, the narratives shared by members of the Latino migrant worker community provide additional evidence of their resistance to participate in conventional research which they perceive as paternalistic, abusive, and irrelevant to their needs. Overcoming their traditional mistrust and engaging the LMW community was paramount for the success of Project Salud.

Culturally adapted interventions must prompt community engagement and participation at every phase of the program if they do not want to remain culturally blind. Findings from this study underscore the strong desire of LMWs in the Homestead community to participate in HIV prevention interventions and highlight the importance for interventions to be culturally relevant, respectful, and responsive to their life experiences. In particular, it is important to adapt interventions according to relevant Latino cultural values and experiences specific to the Latino group under consideration instead of just relying on sweeping generalizations about Latino culture. Participants in this study emphasized that interventionists needed to communicate to community members a genuine understanding of the contextual challenges that impact their lives, help them to address barriers to participation, and constantly promote a dialogue aimed at examining the cultural relevance of the intervention. For instance, participants conveyed the importance of promoting a sense of empowerment and community among participants taking part in the intervention and emphasized the important role this could play given that many of the participants were not living with their families. Thus, interventions that rely primarily on dyadic instruction between the interventionist and community member may be of limited appeal to the LMW community. Instead, culturally relevant interventions for LMWs should facilitate a group learning experience that promotes trust, social support, and empowerment.

We also believe that present findings also contribute in a significant way to the cultural adaptation/fidelity debate. While cultural adaptation scholars argue that evidence-based interventions should be culturally adapted before dissemination (32), fidelity advocates consider that the need for cultural adaptation has been overstated (33). Researchers have also expressed that modifying existing interventions may reduce or eliminate the impact of the core components of original interventions (33). While Project Salud recognizes the need to respect the core components of the original intervention that proved to be efficacious, we agree with those who underscore the importance of attending to the cultural values and traditions that target populations consider to be most relevant in their lives without relying on theoretical preconceptions associated with specific ethnic minority populations (34). Focus group participants understood the need to balance the cultural relevance of the intervention with the need for intervention fidelity. As a result, we believe A-SEMI can be considered what some researchers (35) refer to as a hybrid model that bridges the need for rigorous scientific research with the needs for cultural relevance in terms of intervention content and delivery.

CONCLUSION

Statistical analyses are being conducted on the effects of the A-SEMI intervention on HIV prevention in the LMW community. Consequently, we cannot evaluate whether the culturally adapted components and delivery of the A-SEMI intervention increased efficacy. However, we can attest to the positive impact of engaging the LMW community in a CBPR process in which the beneficiaries of the proposed intervention can identify the values, traditions, and cultural experiences that are most relevant to their lives.

Community members participating in the focus groups that led to the cultural adaptation of the A-SEMI intervention recognized the significance of being invited to help with the design of an HIV prevention intervention. They expressed a sense of being empowered with a voice in the design of a science-based prevention program that also fits the LMW community's traditions, values, and needs. We have also observed an increase in community awareness and in the number of members of the Latino migrant worker community who have approached Project Salud staff or any of our community partners asking about testing, resources, and referrals as a result of coming in contact with Project Salud. As evidence of the added benefit of their contribution to health promotion and disease prevention in their community continues to mount, Latino migrant workers can and should become key players toward the implementation of any CBPR-based project in the Latino migrant population of South Florida.

ACKNOWLEDGMENT

This research was funded by the National Institute on Minority Health and Health Disparities (Award # P20MD002288). The authors thank the Latino migrant worker community in Homestead, South Florida. This study could not have been conducted without their generous support and collaboration. The content is solely the responsibility of the authors and does not necessarily represent the official views of the National Institute on Minority Health and Health Disparities or the National Institutes of Health. The authors express no conflict of interest.

REFERENCES

[1]   The Hispanic population: 2010. 2010 Census Briefs. Accessed 2011 November 14. URL: http://www.census.gov/prod/cen2010/briefs/c2010br-04.pdf

[2]   HIV among Hispanic/Latino. Center for Disease Control and Prevention. Accessed 2011 August 22. URL: http://www.cdc.gov/hiv/hispanics/index.htm

[3]   HIV Behavioral Interventions for Hispanics/Latinos in the US: A Meta-Analytic Review. Center for Disease Control and Prevention. Accessed 2011 August 22URL: http://www.cdcnpin.org /scripts/HispanicLatino/files/herbst_latinoconsult.pdf

[4]   Deren S, Sheldin M, Decena CU, Mino M. Research challenges to the study of HIV/AIDS among migrant and immigrant Hispanic populations in the United States. J Urban Health 2005;82(2):iii13-25.

[5]   Soskolne V, Shtarkshall RA. Migration and HIV prevention programmes: Linking structural factors, culture, and individual behaviour--an Israeli experience. Soc Sci Med 2002;55(8):1297-1307.

[6]   Shtarkshall, R., & Soskolne, V. Migrant populations and HIV/AIDS: The development and implementation of programmes: theory, methodology and practice. UNESCO UNAIDS, 2000.

[7]   Organista PB, Organista KC, Soloff PR. Exploring AIDS-related knowledge, attitudes, and behaviors of female Mexican migrant workers. Health Soc Work 1998;23(2):96-103.

[8]   Aranda-Naranjo B, Gaskins S. HIV/AIDS in migrant and seasonal farm workers. J Assoc Nurses AIDS Care 1998;9(5):80-3.

[9]   Fernandez MI, Collazo JB, Hernandez N, et al. Predictors of HIV risk among Hispanic farm workers in South Florida: women are at higher risk than men. AIDS Behav 2004;8(2):165-74.

[10]   Hernandez MT, Lemp GF, Castañeda X, et al. HIV/AIDS among Mexican migrants and recent immigrants in California and Mexico. J Acquir Immune Defic Syndr 2004; 37(4):s203-17.

[11]   Sanchez MA, Lemp GF, Rodriguez-Magis C, Bravo-Garcia W, Carter S, Ruiz JD. The epidemiology of HIV among Mexican Migrants and recent immigrants in California and Mexico. J Acquir Immune Defic Syndr 2004;37(4):s204-14.

[12]   Mishra SI, Conner RF. Evaluation of an HIV prevention program among Latino farmworkers. In Mishra SI, Conner RF, Magaña JR, eds. AIDS crossing borders: The spread among migrant Latino. Colorado: Westview Press, 1996.

[13]   Weatherby NL, McCoy HV, Bletzer KV, et al. Sexual activity and HIV among drug users: Migrant workers and their sexual partners in southern Florida. Florida Journal of Public Health 1995:7(1):22-6.

[14]   McCoy HV, McCoy CB, Lai S. Effectiveness of HIV interventions among women drug users. Women Health 1998:27(1-2):49-69.

[15]   Kumpfer KL, Alvarado R, Smith P, Bellamy N. Cultural sensitivity in universal family-based prevention interventions. Prev Sci 2002;3:241-4.

[16]   Bernal G, Saez-Santiago. Culturally centered psychosocial interventions. J Comm Psych 2006;34: 121-32.

[17]   McCoy HV, McCoy CB, Lai S, et al. Behavior changes among crack-using rural and urban women. Subst Use Misuse 1999:34(4-5):667-84.

[18]   Weatherby NL, McCoy HV, Bletzer KV, et al. Immigration and HIV among migrant workers in rural southern Florida. J Drug Issues 1997;27(1):155-72.

[19]   Rao P, Hancy K, Velez M, et al. HIV/AIDS and farmworkers in the US. Farmworker Justice, 2008.

[20]   Organista KC, Carrillo H, Ayala G. HIV prevention with Mexican migrants. Review, critique and recommendations. J Acquir Immune Defic Syndr 2004;37(4):S227-39.

[21]   Vega WA, Rodriguez MA, Gruskin, E. Health disparities in the Latino population. Epidemiol Rev 2009;31:99-112.

[22]   Arcury TA, Austin CK, Quandt SA, et al. Enhancing community participation in intervention research: farmworkers and agricultural chemicals in North Carolina. Health Educ Behav 1999; 26(4):563-78.

[23]   Minkler M, Wallerstein N. eds. Community-based participatory research for health: From process to outcomes. 2nd Ed. San Francisco, CA: Jossey-Bass, 2008.

[24]   Rhodes SD, Hergenrather KC, Montaño J, et al. Using community-based participatory research to develop an intervention to reduce HIV and STD infections among Latino men. AIDS Educ Prev 2006;18(5):375-89.

[25]   Andrews OJ, Newman DS, Meadows O, et al. Partnership readiness for community-based participatory research. Health Educ Res 2010; PMID: 20837654.

[26]   Eisinger A, Senturia KD. Doing community-driven research: A description of Seattle partners for healthy communities. J Urban Health 2001;78(3): 519-34.

[27]   Hughes D, DuMont K. Using focus groups to facilitate culturally anchored research. American J Comm Psych 1993;21:775-806.

[28]   Morgan, DL. The focus group guidebook. Thousand Oaks, CA: Sage, 1993.

[29]   Asbury, J. Overview of focus group research. Qual Health Res 1995;5:414-20.

[30]   Vanoss Marin, B. HIV prevention in the Hispanic community: Sex, culture, and empowerment. J. Transcultural Nursing 2003;14(3):186-92.

[31]   U.S. Census Bureau. State and county quick facts, Homestead, Florida. Data derived from Population Estimates. Accesed 2011 August 22. URL: http://quickfacts.census.gov/qfd/states/12/1232275.html

[32]   Castro FG, Barrera M. Martinez CR. The cultural adaptation of prevention interventions: Resolving tensions between fidelity and fit. Prev Sci 2004;5:41-5.

[33]   Elliot DS, Mihalic S. Issues in disseminating and replicating effective prevention programs. Prev Sci 2004;5:47-53.

[34]   Griner D, Smith TB. Culturally adapted mental health interventions: A meta-analytic review. Psychother 2006;43:531-48.

[35]   Castro FG, Hernandez-Aaron E. Integrating cultural values into drug abuse prevention and treatment with racial/ethnic minorities. J Drug Issues 2002;32:783-810.

*Submitted:*September 02, 2011. *Revised:* November 15, 2011. *Accepted:* November 30, 2011.

In: Public Health Yearbook 2012
Editor: Joav Merrick

ISBN: 978-1-62808-078-0
© 2013 Nova Science Publishers, Inc.

Chapter 30

THE RELATIONSHIP BETWEEN DIABETES, OBESITY AND IRIS MARKINGS IN AFRICAN AMERICANS IN MONTGOMERY COUNTY, ALABAMA

Peggy Valentine, EdD[*], Jiangmin Xu, PhD, Tatiana Jones, MPT, Laila Haile, MPT, Myrtle Goore, MD, Jane Smolnik, ND and Marceline Egnin, PhD

Department of Healthcare Management AND Department of Physical Therapy, School of Health Sciences, Winston-Salem State University, Winston-Salem, North Carolina, Private practice, Montgomery, Alabama, Wellness Lifestyles Center, Asheville, North Carolina, College of Agricultural, Environmental and Natural Sciences, Center for Plant Biotechnology Research, Tuskegee University, Tuskegee, Alabama, United States of America

ABSTRACT

Diabetes mellitus is a common health problem in the United States and African Americans are disproportionately affected, especially among those who are overweight and obese. Health professionals are aware that obesity and a family history of diabetes increase one's risk for acquiring the disease. Therefore, the field of genetics offers insight into future risks based on the polygenic nature of inheritance and environmental components. Iridology analysis could be used as a diagnostic tool to predict and evaluate the possibility of developing type 2 diabetes for those obese individuals based on their iris markings with associated genetic inheritance. This study examined 43 African American residents in Montgomery, Alabama, where the prevalence rates of diabetes and obesity are among the highest in the nation. Comparisons of iris markings were made between individuals in different groups. The findings revealed that extremely obese group had more iris markings in the pituitary and pancreatic regions than the obese and normal weight groups. Further, the diabetic obese group had more iris markings in the

[*] Correspondence: Dr. Peggy Valentine, Dean and Professor and Dr. Jiangmin Xu, Associate Professor, School of Health Sciences, Winston-Salem State University, 601 S. Martin Luther King Jr. Drive, Winston-Salem, NC, 27104, USA. Phone: 336-750-2570 and emails: pvalentine@wssu.edu and xuji@wssu.edu.

pancreatic region than the non-diabetic obese and normal groups. The findings not only highlight the importance of iridology analysis in diabetes research but also may suggest the possibility of adding iris markers as a genetic identifier to public health strategies aimed at detecting and preventing diabetes.

Keywords: African American, diabetes, genetics, iridology, iris markings, obesity

INTRODUCTION

Diabetes mellitus is a chronic metabolic disease known to affect millions of ethnically and geographically diverse people and it is one of the leading causes of morbidity and mortality in the United States, resulting in premature deaths and disability of many patients with obesity and cardiovascular diseases. The two types of diabetes are type 1 and type 2. Type 1 is thought to be caused by an autoimmune disease or a virus that attacks the pancreas, resulting in insufficient insulin production by the body. It affects youth more often and one must inject insulin daily for proper metabolic function. Type 2 diabetes mellitus is the most common form of diabetes and is prevalent in 80–90% of all diabetes patients. It results from insulin resistance wherein the body does not produce enough insulin or the cells cannot manage its insulin effectively. The rise in prevalence rate is often attributed to and develops as the result of obesity, high blood pressure, lack of regular exercise, and family history (1,2). These individuals tend to be physically inactive and have excess body fat, especially around the waistline (3-5). Therefore, compared with type 1, type 2 diabetes is generally thought to be preventable although it may also be genetic.

African Americans are at very high risk for type 2 diabetes and its complications (6-9). It is estimated that 14.7 percent of all African Americans ages 20 years or older have diabetes (10). In addition, African-Americans have higher incidence and prevalence rates, higher rates of diabetic complications, and worse control of diabetes and co-morbid conditions than Caucasians (11-13). Some studies on African Americans have found that the chance of getting type 2 diabetes increases with age and 25 percent of African Americans between the ages of 65 -74 years are diabetic (14,15). It is estimated that as many as 33% of African Americans with diabetes are unaware that they are diabetic. Given the health consequences of untreated diabetes, early diagnosis to reduce risk is important.

Obesity is a major risk factor for type 2 diabetes. Overweight and obesity increase the risks for diabetes, heart disease, high blood pressure, and other health problems (9, 16). Obesity is increasing in the United States, particularly among the African American population. For example, the prevalence rate of obesity increased from 13.4% to 35.1% in U.S. adults aged 20 to 74 from 1960 to 2005 (17, 18). Over two-thirds of U.S. adults are overweight or obese and over one-third of U.S. adults are obese (19). This study also found that the age-adjusted prevalence of obesity (BMI $\geq$ 30) in racial and ethnic groups is higher among African American women (49.6%) and Hispanic women (43%) than among Caucasian women (33.3%). But, there are not significant differences in prevalence rates for obesity among the men's groups.

DIABETES, GENETICS AND IRIS ANALYSIS

Iridology is a study of the colored part of the eye that provides insight into one's systemic health and health problems in his/her internal organs. Patterns, colors, and other characteristics of the iris can be examined to determine and identify information about one's health problems. Iridologists see the eyes as "windows" into the body's state of health in which the right half of the body is represented in the right iris and the left half in the left iris (20). Iridologists divide the iris into zones corresponding to specific parts of the human body and they believe that certain markings or discolorations indicate potential weaknesses in those specific areas. Gunter Jarosych in Germany is credited for describing the location of the pancreas on the iridology chart in the 1960s (21). The iridology chart developed by Bernard Jensen, one of America's foremost pioneering iridologists, with revisions by Ellen Jensen (22).

Iridologists in the field believe that one is born with certain genetic disorders/ markers/ defects and one can receive useful information to promote health through consultations with an iridologist. By matching their observations to iris charts, iridologists can examine the medical conditions through irregularities of the pigmentation in the iris. By locating markings in the iris of the eye, iris analysis can reveal information about the site of strengths, disorders, and deficiencies in one's body, and some pre-clinical conditions prior to the appearance of any disease symptoms. Sometimes, iris analyses can provide clinical information that blood & urine tests, X-rays, etc., will not necessarily reveal. Many clinical practitioners and iridologists in Europe and Asia utilized this non-invasive technique as the first tool to diagnose the symptoms of disease, identify potential and existing health problems and imbalances in the body; and predict and evaluate the possibility of developing disease in the future.

On diabetes research, iridology analysis is also used to interpret genetic patterns and identify inherited disorders of various organ systems, like the pancreas, which may increase the risk factor for onset of diabetes, especially type 2 diabetes. For example, brown pigment in the iris indicates diabetes or a pancreas problem. This pigment is as a result of inadequate production of trypsinogen by the pancreas. Wibawa and Purnomo used the biological inspired computing technology to examine the presence of broken tissues in the iris in the area of the pancreas and to detect the pancreas condition according to the chart of the iris (23). After comparison with the result of insulin normality test, they found that the early detection system can effectively detect the abnormality of the pancreas and point to the existence of diabetes mellitus. Scientists at Karolinska Institutet and the University of Miami have developed a revolutionary research method for diabetes research by which a tiny part of the pancreas was translated onto the iris of mice to cure diabetes; the research result shows that diabetic mice were completely cured after pancreatic beta cells were transplanted onto the eyes (24).

Compared with Europe and Asia, relative few clinical practitioners and iridologists in US have utilized iris analysis as a tool to diagnose and detect the disease and relative few iridology studies have examined the relationships between iris, obesity and the genetic risk for diabetes; however, more and more clinical practitioners and iridologists find the important value of iris analysis in disease diagnosis and prevention, especially for diabetes (25).

Research purpose

The purpose of this research was to investigate relationships between risk factors for diabetes, obesity, and pituitary and pancreatic markings of the iris among a group of African Americans. Specifically, this study investigated the relationships between iridological variations in the pancreas and pituitary with the presence of different levels of obesity and diabetes mellitus. The hypothesis in this study is that African-Americans who are genetically predisposed to obesity and diabetes may have higher chances of prominent presentation of abnormalities of the pancreas and pituitary regions in the iris.

Iridology analysis and its application on diabetic research have received limited attention. To date, research on the topic has been limited both by sample and design features and therefore has not adequately addressed these questions. Few controlled research studies have been done and the benefits have not been well documented. Based on the above literature, this proposed research addresses two gaps in the current iridology and diabetes research. First, although iridology has been practiced in Europe and other countries with scientific studies, these studies have been done on Caucasian population, rather than African American population. Research on African Americans would provide more insight on the value of iridology and genetic predispositions. Second, although iridology has been practiced widely in Europe and other countries, it has not been widely accepted in the US. Through research studies, some intervention and prevention measures might be developed to address obesity and diabetes if a person's color, texture and location of markings on the iris indicate the possibility of developing type 2 diabetes. In other words, these imbalances may be treatable with homeopathic remedies and nutrition, such as vitamins, minerals, herbs, and other products, or with lifestyle change, such as having a well-balanced diet, increasing activity, setting health goals for weight, exercise and work.

METHODS

The selected study site was located in Montgomery, Alabama. Montgomery County ranks in the top 10% of Alabama counties with high diabetes death rates and about 24% of adults are overweight or obese (26). Research subjects were recruited by Dr. Myrtle Goore and a research team of Winston-Salem State University from Dr. Goore's practice. Dr. Goore is a bariatric physician in private practice in Montgomery, Alabama and her patients include obese and morbidly obese individuals. Dr. Goore's previous study involved genetic testing of 120 minority subjects who were obese and had risks for diabetes under NIH funded Tuskegee University Project Export.

In this study, Dr. Goore was responsible for identifying and recruiting possible subjects to participate in the study. Recruitment letters were sent to her clients for the iridology intervention study on December 18, 2009 and letters were resent a month later. A sample of 43 subjects (age ≥18) from rural Black Belt counties from Montgomery was recruited in this study and these subjects were examined and irises were photographed in 2 days. Data collection and interview of each subject occurred in two sessions. The first session was used to obtain informed consent and to collect data on demographic characteristics, family health history, fasting blood glucose (FBG), waist circumference, and blood pressure (BP). The second session was used to conduct an iridology exam and photographs. The study participants received an incentive of $20 in cash for their participation in the study. This study was funded by the Forsyth Medical Center Foundation in Winston-Salem, North Carolina.

Measures

The study was designed to explore the relationship between diabetes, obesity and iris markings in an African American population. Data such as obesity levels, diabetes status, glucose testing, body weight, waist circumference, and blood pressure (BP) measurements were collected for this specific population.

Iris exams were conducted followed by the photographs of the iris performed by a trained iridologist, Dr. Jane Smolnik. Dr. Smolnik is a naturopath and iridologist in a private Wellness Lifestyles Center in Asheville, North Carolina. She used a macro digital camera to document the color of the iris, visible pigments on the iris, structure of fibers, and fiber separation. These data of the electronic images of the iris were then viewed and analyzed to identify functioning capabilities of different organ systems, revealing predispositions, tendencies, strengths, and deficiencies.

The International Iridology Practitioners Association provided standard protocols to conduct the iris analysis using Ellen Jensen's updated full color Iridology Chart. Iris analysis includes separation of iris fibers, pigments and other descriptors of "eye signs": Orange pigment (Central heterochromia and topostable) and Irregularities in pancreatic areas (pigment, lacuna, crypts, defect signs, radial furrows, reflexives, and rarefaction).

Iridology classifies lacunae through noting irregularities of the pigmentation in the iris. These lacunae were evaluated by dimensions, depth, color, location, edges, and angles.

Pancreatic and pituitary markers are two of the most well studied genetic markers of diabetes in iridology. In this study, the iris of each eye was examined for pancreatic and pituitary markers. In both eyes, the trained iridologist looked for markers in the head and the tail of the pancreas, and examined the pituitary gland for pigments and separation of fibers.

The total number of pancreatic or pituitary markers were counted by adding both left-eye and right-eye markers.

Figure 1 is pancreatic and pituitary marker picture photographed by Dr. Smolnik (Figure 1).

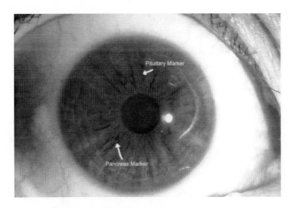

Figure 1. Picture of Pancreatic and Pituitary Markings.

Body Mass Index (BMI) was used for determining overweight and obesity, measuring body fat based on height and weight. In this study, the BMI risk levels were calculated according to the American Society of Bariatric Physicians (ASBP) Body Mass Index Chart for Overweight & Obesity: (1) BMI 25 to 29.9 – Overweight, (2) BMI 30 to 34.9- Obesity I (moderate obesity), (3) BMI 35 to 39.9- Obesity II (severe obesity), and (4) BMI > 40 – Obesity III (extreme obesity).

Blood Pressure (BP) was measured by a licensed nurse in Dr. Goore's practice using a calibrated sphygmomanometer.

Waist circumference was measured by an office staff member using a tape measure with inches and centimeters. *Weight* was measured with electronic floor scale for each study subject by office staff.

Research design

This study used comparative analyses to investigate and examine the relationships between specific structure and color variations in the iris with the presence of overweight and the genetic risks and markers for diabetes between two different group structures.

Two group structures were developed to compare the group differences. The first group structure (A) used American Society of Bariatric Physicians (ASBP) Body Mass Index (BMI) Chart to divide the subjects into four BMI subgroups based on BMI risk levels: normal, overweight, obesity, and extreme obesity.

The second group structure (B) used the current coexisting status of obesity and diabetes to divide the research subjects into 3 subgroups: subjects who are non-diabetics with normal weight, subjects who are non-diabetics with obesity, and subjects who are diabetics with obesity.

Statistical analysis

The data collected from the study was cleaned and entered into the SPSS database. Information about health histories, blood glucose data, genetic testing results, waist circumference, height, body weight, and social demographic factors were entered into the computer for each subject.

In this study, frequency and correlation analyses were conducted using SPSS software to examine the distribution and correlation of each group's clinical characteristics, genetic markers, BMI risk levels, social demographic factors and health history. For example, a series of frequency analyses were conducted to examine the distribution of BMI risk levels, the number of iris markers, and characteristics of social demographic factors.

The T-test was used to compare the group mean differences based on four categories of waist and weight. Furthermore, a correlation analysis was used to find the relationships among BMI levels, the color variations, the current coexisting status of obesity and diabetes, and the total number of pancreatic or pituitary markers.

RESULTS

The mean age was 50.35 years with the minimum age of 20 and maximum age of 81. Among 43 subjects, there were 13 (30.2%) males and 30 (69.8%) females. In addition, 15 (34.9%) subjects were diagnosed with high cholesterol and 5 (11.6%) subjects were diagnosed on site with diabetes.

The results in table 1 revealed individual characteristics of subjects' BMI levels. The results showed that female subjects were at risk of developing obesity.

There were no significant differences between obese group and non-obese group in terms of gender, age, and education because of relatively small sample size. The results also showed that subjects with the high cholesterol levels were significantly at risk with obesity. In addition, waist circumference and weight were significantly different between obese group and non-obese group.

BMI categories, iris markings and risk for diabetes

Iris markings in the pancreatic and pancreas regions were compared between the obese group and non-obese group. Table 2 indicates the different percentage rates in genetic iris markings between obesity and non-obesity groups.

Table 1. Selected Sample Characteristics by Obesity Status (N=43)

	Total N=43	%	Non-Overweight N=12	%	Overweight N=31	%	Overweight vs non-overweight p (x2 or t)
Gender							.085
Male	13	30.2	6	50.0	7	22.6	
Female	30	69.8	6	50.0	24	77.4	
Age groups (in years)							.758
18-35	7	16.3	2	16.7	5	16.1	
36-55	18	41.9	6	50.0	12	38.7	
>56	18	41.9	4	33.3	14	45.2	
Education (highest grade completed)							.141
High School	5	12.2	1	8.3	4	13.8	
Some college	15	36.6	2	16.7	13	44.8	
College Graduate	12	51.2	9	75.0	12	41.4	
High Cholesterol Level							.02**
No	27	64.3	11	91.7	16	53.3	
Yes	15	35.7	1	8.3	14	46.7	
Blood Pressure (BP)							
The systolic pressure	Mean=129	SD=17.3	Mean=160	SD=17.3	Mean=158	SD=23.3	.910
The diastolic pressure	Mean=76	SD=11.5	Mean=82	SD=12.8	Mean=81	SD=12.9	.748
Waist	Mean=37	SD=6.3	Mean=31	SD=4.3	Mean=39	SD=5.5	.000***
Weight	Mean=190	SD=44.2	Mean=147	SD=20.1	Mean=207	SD=38.9	.000***

*p< .05; ** p< .01; ***p< .001.

Relationships between Different BMI Groups and Genetic Iris Markings --- Comparative Analyses based on the First Group Structure (A)

The first group structure (A) used American Society of Bariatric Physicians (ASBP) Body Mass Index (BMI) Chart to divide the subjects into four BMI subgroups based on BMI risk levels: normal, overweight, obesity, and extreme obesity. Among all subjects, 12 (27.9%) subjects were normal, 9 (20.9%) subject were overweight, 14 (32.6%) were obese, and 8 (18.6%) were extremely obese. Figures 2-3 indicate the different percentage rates in BMI risk levels and genetic markers of iris for diabetes among different BMI groups.

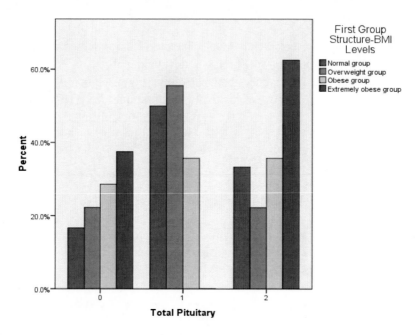

Figure 2. Total pituitary markers and BMI risk levels.

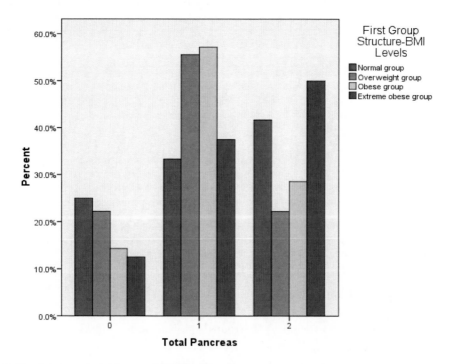

Figure 3. Total pancreatic markers and BMI risk levels.

The results showed that 50.0 % of individuals in the normal group had 1 pituitary marker and 33.3% had 2 pituitary markers. About 55.6% of individuals in the overweight group had 1 pituitary marker and 22.2% had 2 pituitary markers. Of the obese group, 35.7% had 1 pituitary marker and 35.7% had 2 pituitary markers. Of extremely obesity group, 62.5% had 2 pituitary markers.

The results also showed that 33.3 % of individuals in the normal group had 1 pancreatic marker and 41.7% had 2 pancreatic markers. Of the overweight and obese groups, 55.6% and 57.1% of individuals had 1 pancreatic marker and only 22.2% and 28.6% had 2 pancreatic markers. Of the extremely obese group, 37.5% of individuals had 1 pancreatic marker and 50.0% had 2 pancreatic markers.

Relationships between BMI categories and genetic markers. Comparative analyses based on the second group structure (B)

The second group structure (B) used the current coexisting status of obesity and diabetes to divide the research subjects into 3 subgroups: subjects who are non-diabetics with normal weight, subjects who are non-diabetics with obesity, and subjects who are diabetics with obesity. Among our samples, there were 12 (27.9%) subjects in normal group without DMI and obesity, 26 (60.5%) in non-diabetic group, and 5 (11.6%) in diabetic obese group.

Figures 4-5 indicate the different percentage rates in obesity categories and genetic markers of iris for diabetes based on the current coexisting status of obesity and diabetes.

Of the normal group, 50.0 % had 1 pituitary marker and 33.3% had 2 pituitary markers. Of the non-diabetic obese group, 30.8 % had 1 pituitary marker and 34.6% had 2 pituitary markers. Of the diabetic obese group, 40.0% had 1 pituitary marker and 60.0% had 2 pituitary markers.

The individuals in the diabetic obese group are more likely to have high pituitary makers than individuals in the other two groups.

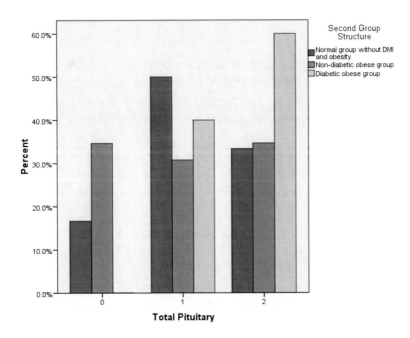

Figure 4. Total pituitary markers and the *coexisting* status of *obesity* and *diabetes*.

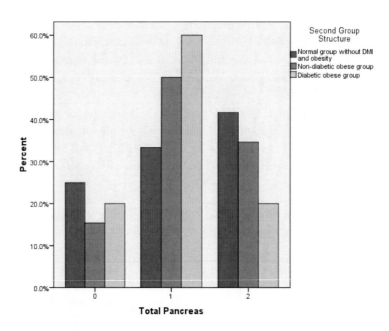

Figure 5. Total pancreatic markers and the *coexisting* status of *obesity* and *diabetes*.

Of the normal group, 33.3 % of individuals had 1 pancreatic marker and 41.7% had 2 pancreatic markers. Of the non-diabetic obese group, 50.0 % of individuals had 1 pancreatic marker and 34.6% had 2 pancreatic markers. Of the diabetic obese group, 60.0% of individuals had 1 pancreatic marker and 20.0% had 2 pancreatic markers.

Table 2. Comparisons Genetic Markers of Diabetes and Obesity Status

Genetic risk factors	Total		Not Overweight		Overweight	
	N	%	N	%	N	%
Pituitary (total)						
0	11	25.6	2	16.7	9	29.0
1	16	37.2	6	50.0	10	32.3
2	16	37.2	4	33.3	12	38.7
Pancreas (total)						
0	8	18.6	3	25.0	5	16.1
1	20	46.5	4	33.3	16	51.6
2	15	34.9	5	41.7	10	32.3

DISCUSSION

The results of the present study indicate that the iris analysis may be a useful tool for understanding the relationships among iris markers, genetic risk, and obesity. Although iridologists are able to identify iris markers which correspond with different organ systems, this study attempts to quantify the relationship between diabetes, obesity, and iris markings in African Americans. The following conclusions are drawn from the research findings.

First, there are significant differences in iris markings among different BMI groups. The results from the first group structure (A) show that the percentage rate for the extremely obese group that had 2 pituitary markers (62.5%) is significantly higher than the normal group (33.3%), the overweight group (22.2%), and the obese group (35.7%). In addition, the percentage rate for the extremely obese group that had 2 pancreatic markers (50.0%) is also higher than the normal group (41.7%), the overweight group (22.2%), and the obese group (28.6%). The extremely obese group has been described as having a stronger constitutional type than the other three groups.

Second, there are differences in iris markings among different diabetic and obese groups. These findings from the second group structure (B) were surprising for two reasons. First were the differences in pituitary signs. It is understandable that more individuals in the diabetic obese group would have pancreatic markers; however, more than half of individuals in the normal group also had 1 pituitary marker. A question to be asked would be "Is there a genetic predisposition for those in the normal group to develop diabetes as well?" In addition, it was not surprising to find that 40% of the diabetic obese subjects had 1 pituitary marker and 60.0% had 2 pituitary markers. However, only 30% of the non-diabetic obese individuals had 1 pituitary marker and 32% had 2 pituitary markers. In this study, we find some significant differences and patterns among groups for the relationships among pancreatic and pituitary markers, obesity, and diabetes. For example, the significant differences existed in the distribution of 2 pituitary makers in which the percentage of 2 pituitary markers (60%) in the diabetic obese group were two times higher than in the normal group and the non-diabetic obese group (30%).

According to these findings, there is a clear indication that the diabetic and obese clients have more genetic characteristics that support part of the original hypothesis, which is to determine if there is a relationship between genetic markers, diabetes, and obesity risk levels. The iris analyses in this study support the results and the hypothesis of the research in determining if there is a significant relationship between genetic markers and diabetes and obesity within the African American population. These findings are important because if an individual who is obese has a marker for pancreas and according to the above results it is established that there is a relationship between pancreatic markers and obesity, it indicates that a person with generic marker is far more susceptible to risk for diabetes than a person without a genetic marker. Therefore, the results herein, could suggest the need for developing prevention and intervention programs to be implemented against obesity and diabetes if a person's color, texture and location of genetic markings on the iris indicate the possibility of developing type 2 diabetes. To reduce deleterious health impacts of genetic markers and imbalances, one might be treated with homeopathic remedies and nutrition, such as vitamins, minerals, herbs, and other products, or with lifestyle change to help with his/her metabolic condition, such as having a well-balanced diet, increasing activity, setting health goals for weight, and having exercise work.

Limitations

Despite these advantages, the results of the current study must be interpreted cautiously because of several limitations. First, as noted earlier, this study used convenience sampling and the subjects were not selected randomly. This sample included only clients who volunteered for the obesity assessment at Dr. Goore's clinical office and may not, therefore, be representative of a more general population of African American obese clients. Second, the relatively small sample size in this study contributes to the uncertain generalizability to the broader population of obesity and diabetic African American clients in the U.S.

As the sample size increases and its associated instruments evolve, the iris analysis of potential diabetics can become more reliable. Additional data collection and control for family history can strengthen the research findings. Comparing iris findings with genetic testing in the future would be also increase reliability of the data.

Policy significance

While the exact nature of the relationship between diabetes and genetic markings remains uncertain, these findings highlight the need for further research as a potential public health strategy for early detection and prevention of diabetes in African American communities. Importantly, because the procedure for iris analysis is non-invasive and easy to implement, there is great potential for allied health professionals to work with iridologists to use this low cost, safe, non-invasive diagnostic tool in promoting health and preventing disease, especially in communities with limited access to health care services.

Moreover, iridology analysis can offer a view of the body that other diagnostic procedures and technologies will not necessarily reveal and it may reveal pre-clinical conditions at a time when intervention may not be effective. Based on the color, texture and location of various markings on the iris, one might be able to identify a potential health issue beforehand. If the imbalances and irregularity are found on/in the iris, some alternative treatment modalities can be developed and the patients can be treated with products such as vitamins, minerals, herbs or other treatment programs such as nutritional programs, lifestyle changes, affirmations, exercise, and meditation. In sum, iridology analysis can be used to understand what 'optimum health' means for an individual person and offer insight into our health potential and disease predispositions.

REFERENCES

[1]   Bressler J, Kao W, Pankow JS, Boerwinkle E. Risk of type 2 diabetes and obesity is differentially associated with variation in FTO in Whites and African-Americans in the ARIC study. PLoS ONE 2010;5(5):e10521.

[2]   Hamman RF, Wing RR, Edelstein SL, Lachin JM, Bray GA. Effect of weight loss with lifestyle intervention on risk of diabetes. Diabetes Care 2006;29:2102-7.

[3]   Hill JO. Understanding and addressing the epidemic of obesity: an energy balance perspective. Endocrine Rev 2006;27:750–61.

[4]   Papas MA, Alberg AJ, Ewing R, Helzlsouer KJ, Gary TL, Klassen AC. The built environment and obesity. Epidemiol Rev2007;29:129-143.

[5]   National Institute of Diabetes and Digestive and Kidney Diseases: Do you know the health risks of being overwright? Internet 2007. Accessed 2011 Aug 05. URL: http://win.niddk.nih.gov/Publications /health_risks.htm.

[6]   Carter JS, Pugh JA, Monterrosa A. Non-insulin dependent diabetes mellitus in minorities in the United States. Ann Intern Med 1996;125(3):221–32.

[7]   Dreeben O. Health status of African Americans. J Health Soc Policy 2001;14(1):1–17.

[8] Gary LT, Gross MS, Browne DC, LaVeist TA. The college health and wellness study: baseline correlates of overweight among African Americans. J Urban Health 2006;83(2):252-4.

[9] Pi-Sunyer FX. Obesity and diabetes in blacks. Diabetes Care 1990;13(11):1144–9.

[10] National Diabetes Information Clearinghouse (NDIC): National Diabetes Statistics [internet]. NIH Publication No. 08-3892, 2007. Accessed 2011 Aug 05. URL: http://diabetes.niddk.nih.gov/ dm/pubs /statistics/.

[11] Mokdad AH, Bowman BA, Ford ES, Vinicor F, Marks JS, Koplan JP. The continuing epidemics of obesity and diabetes in the United States. JAMA 2001;286:1195–200.

[12] Sundquist JM, Winkleby A, Pudaric S. Cardiovascular disease risk factors among older black, mexican-american, and white women and men: an analysis of NHANES III, 1988–1994. J Am Geriatr Soc 2001;49:109–16.

[13] Lanting LC, Joung IM, Mackenbach JP, Lamberts SW, Bootsma AH. Ethnic differences in mortality, end-stage complications, and quality of care among diabetic patients: a review. Diabetes Care 2005;28:2280–8.

[14] Lee JA, Liu CF, Sales AE. Racial and ethnic differences in diabetes care and health care use and costs. Prev Chronic Dis 2006;3(3):1-12.

[15] Smith JP. Economics of health and mortality special feature: nature and causes of trends in male diabetes prevalence, undiagnosed diabetes, and the socioeconomic status health gradient. Proceed Natl Acad Sci United States America 2007;104:13225–31.

[16] Harris MI. Diabetes in America: epidemiology and scope of the problem. Diabetes Care 1998;21(3):11–4.

[17] National Center for Health Statistics Health E-Stats: Prevalence of overweight, obesity and extreme obesity among adults: United States, trends 1976–80 through 2005–2006. Atlanta, GA: Government Printing Office, 2008.

[18] Pietiläinen K, Kaprio J, Borg P, Plasqui G, Yki-Järvinen H. Physical inactivity and obesity: a vicious circle. *Obesity (Silver Spring).2008;*16:409–14.

[19] Flegal KM, Carroll MD, Ogden CL, Curtin LR. Prevalence and trends in obesity among US adults, 1999–2008. JAMA 2010;303(3):235–41.

[20] Sharan F. Iridology: a complete guide to diagnosin g through the iris and to related forms of treatment. Wellingborough, England: Thorsons Publications, 1989.

[21] Andrews J. Endocrinology and iridology. Cape Town, South Africa: Felke Institut, 2006.

[22] Jensen B, Jensone E. Iridology chart. California: International Publishers, 2004.

[23] WIibawa AD, Mulyanto E, Purnomo MH. Early detection on the condition of pancreas organ as the cause of diabetes mellitus by iris image processing and modified SOM Kohonen. IFMBE. 2005;12:1008-10.

[24] Speier S, Nyqvist D, Cabrera O, Yu J, Molano RD, Pileggi A, Moede T, Köhler M, Wilbertz J, Leibiger B, Ricordi C, Leibiger IB, Caicedo A, Berggren PO. Noninvasive in vivo imaging of pancreatic islet cell biology. Nature Med 2008;14(5):574-8.

[25] Chen C, Chuang L, & Wu Y. Clinical measures of physical fitness predict insulin resistance in people at risk for diabetes. J Am Phys Ther Assoc 2008;88(11):1355-64.

[26] Center for Disease Control and Prevention: The Steps Program in Alabama's River Region. Internet, 2009. Accessed 2011 Aug 05. URL: http://www.cdc.gov/steps/steps_communities/states/al/ river_ region.htm.

Submitted: September 05, 2011. *Revised:* November 10, 2011. *Accepted:* November 20, 2011.

In: Public Health Yearbook 2012   ISBN: 978-1-62808-078-0
Editor: Joav Merrick   © 2013 Nova Science Publishers, Inc.

Chapter 31

STRATEGIES FOR FACILITATING THE RECRUITMENT OF LATINAS IN CANCER PREVENTION RESEARCH

Monica Rosales, PhD[*1], *Patricia Gonzalez, PhD*[2] *and Evelinn Borrayo, PhD*[3]

[1]Center of Community Alliance for Research and Education,
City of Hope National Medical Center, Duarte, California, United States of America
[2]Institute for Behavioral and Community Health, San Diego State University, San Diego,
California and [3]Department of Psychology, University of Colorado Denver, Denver,
Colorado, United States of America

ABSTRACT

A pressing need exists to include Latinas in cancer prevention research and to promote the value of early screening to prevent breast cancer. However, several challenges impede engaging Spanish-speaking Latinas in research. Objective: This article focuses on the recruitment process undertaken to secure participants for two breast cancer prevention education studies. Methods: Spanish-speaking Latinas were recruited for both studies. Data collection took place at community-organized events tailored to Latino communities. Emphasis is placed on recruitment strategies used that follow community-based participatory research (CBPR) principles. Results: We report several strategies utilized to contact and motivate Latinas to participate in research seeking to better understand factors that influence their breast cancer screening behaviors. We present recruitment strategies that were tailored to the target population, helped develop participants' trust and engaged the community and that were successful in encouraging and increasing research participation. Conclusions: Factors that challenge the recruitment of ethnic minorities in community settings call for flexible and culturally-sensitive and culturally-appropriate recruitment strategies. By utilizing strategies that follow CBPR principles, we took necessary steps to successfully recruit Latinas into cancer prevention

* Correspondence: Monica Rosales, City of Hope, Center of Community Alliance for Research and Education, City of Hope National Medical Center, 1500 E Duarte Road, Duarte, CA 91010 United States. E-mail: morosales@coh.org

education research studies conducted in community settings. These strategies may serve as a viable solution for addressing barriers to research participation.

Keywords: Participant recruitment, Latinas, community, research, breast cancer

INTRODUCTION

Ethnic minorities are overrepresented in cancer burden, yet underrepresented in research investigating the sources of cancer disparities that affect them so profoundly (1). Despite the existence of a federal mandate to include ethnic minorities in research (2), their underrepresentation in health research persists. Additionally, underrepresentation is, in part, a result of difficulties in recruiting and retaining these groups in research given the multiplicity of social and systemic barriers that hinder their participation (3-4). Ethnic minority representation in research must increase, particularly for Latinos, the fastest growing ethnic group in the United States (5). Increasing the participation of ethnic minorities in cancer research will increase our knowledge of the impact of population-specific factors and behaviors on cancer screening and of disparate cancer screening outcomes.

Latinas have a lower prevalence of breast cancer (BCA), however, they are more likely to be diagnosed at later stages and to have lower survival rates compared to European-Americans (6). A significant gap persists in our knowledge base of factors that impact and influence BCA screening. It is important for healthcare providers to be knowledgeable of the contributing factors associated with disparate outcomes among ethnic minorities and in turn how these factors impact the recruitment of ethnic minorities in cancer research (7). Thus, including Latinas in research intended to eliminate cancer disparities is necessary and of high priority. Social, economic and cultural factors add to the challenge of recruiting ethnic minority participants. Among Latinos, factors that influence research participation include socioeconomic status (SES), healthcare access, health literacy, English language proficiency, and cultural norms, values and beliefs (7).

The purpose of this paper was to describe several strategies that address challenges to the recruitment of Latinas into research (see Table 1).

Table I. Participant Recruitment Strategies

Community Networking
- Initiating contact
o   Contact key community members and identify additional community contacts; disseminate study information and materials
- Involve key community members
o   They can help disseminate study information

Preparing for Participant Recruitment
- Measure Development
o   Pilot test measures prior to study implementation with pilot sample representative of study target sample
- Research team selection and training
o   Research team should have similar characteristics to study sample and should be trained on study purpose and recruitment process

Active Participant Recruitment
- Confidentiality assurance
o Make participants feel comfortable when sharing information by clearly explaining the study purpose and informed consent; provide reassure that participation will be confidential
- Language and literacy
o Have Spanish-speaking research staff ready to assist participants and offer staff assistance as part of research protocol
- Communicating and Establishing Trust
o Culturally appropriate behaviors for rapport building
▪ Engage in pleasant interactions and interact with participants and their family through the use of culturally-appropriate language
o Adapting to extraneous factors
▪ Use snowball techniques when appropriate and necessary
Provision of Resources and Incentives
- Hospitality
- Provide Resources and Incentives

These strategies are aimed to facilitate and increase the successful recruitment of underserved Latinas in health research. We present these strategies by highlighting the recruitment process for two BCA prevention education studies conducted with Spanish-speaking Latinas.

OVERVIEW OF STUDIES

To better understand factors affecting BCA screening, we conducted two studies with Spanish-speaking Latinas in community settings. The first was a 2-phase study designed to develop and test the Latina Breast Cancer Screening (LBCS) scale that measures culturally-shared health beliefs about BCA and BCA screening (8). Items were developed in phase I and scale reliability and validity were assessed in phase II. In the second study, we evaluated the utility of an 8-minute educational video, Where's Maria? (9). This video promotes mammography screening through culturally-sensitive health messages that incorporate culturally-shared beliefs and that are appealing and comprehensible to Latinas. These culturally-shared health beliefs (e.g., feeling healthy, feeling indecent, feeling threatened) influence Latinas' decisions to engage in BCA screening (10-11). Thus, both studies centered on identifying, testing, and understanding Latinas' culturally-shared health beliefs as a means to promote BCA screening and in turn reduce cancer disparities.

Recruitment method

We used strategies that follow community-based participatory research (CBPR) principles to recruit participants. CBPR is a methodological framework that promotes research partnerships between researchers and the community (12). The aims of CBPR are to improve community well-being and to benefit participants by implementing and translating results to inform action for change (12).

Data collection. Data collection took place at community-organized events tailored to Latino communities. Two of these events were annual health fairs, (Día de la Mujer Latina (Day of the Latina Woman) and Family Health and Safety Fair), that promote health awareness through education and preventive care. The third was a cultural event (Mexican Independence Day) which included entertainment, vendors, and community organizations.

Participant characteristics. Both studies included Spanish-speaking Latinas (N = 584) who were 40 years of age and older, and had never been diagnosed with BCA. Most (79%) participants were born outside the U.S. and with a majority (68%) of them born in Mexico. Participants resided in the greater Denver, Colorado area, which has a large Latino population (35% of the population) (13). All study procedures were approved by the university Institutional Review Board and participants signed an informed consent form.

Strategies to facilitate the recruitment of Latinas into research studies

Initiating contact. CBPR emphasizes communication between researchers and community members (12) and the importance of communicating and consulting with community members when conducting research in community settings (4, 12, 14). Through community networking, the researchers can get to know the community and its key members, community organizations, and sources of support (15). Therefore, we contacted members from Latino community agencies (e.g., churches, community clinics/centers) via telephone and met with them in person to explain the purpose of our studies and request assistance in identifying study participants. These contacts helped us identify upcoming community events as data collection sites. To enhance recruitment efforts, we followed a recommended strategy (14) and distributed study announcement flyers at locations frequented by Latinas (e.g., Mexican bakeries, restaurants, and churches).

Involving key community members. Involving key community members in study announcements was another useful strategy. Building relationships in the target communities is important for working with community members in order to devise recruitment strategies and becoming involved and immersed in the community. A CBPR principle is to identify and build on strengths, resources and relationships present in the community, including mediating structures (e.g., churches, organizations) where community members congregate (12). The key community members we contacted were enthusiastic about the studies and willing to facilitate our research efforts. For example, a clergy member (i.e., priest) agreed to announce the study during the Spanish-language mass, an approach previously found to be effective (12). As a result, several women attended the community event with the intent to participate in the study. Involvement in large community organizations provides an outlet for announcing research studies (14,16) and for building trust and credibility within the community (1,17).

Preparing for participant recruitment

Measure Development. The use of culturally-appropriate recruitment and study materials is crucial in research conducted with ethnic minority groups. CBPR suggests involving community members in the development of study materials (12). Thus, during the studies' planning stages, we solicited input on the study questionnaires (i.e., content, format, length, clarity) and cultural appropriateness (i.e., specific use of words and idioms) from women comparable to the study sample (e.g., low income, Spanish-speakers) by following a focus group format with 43 Latinas (20 for the scale study and 23 for the video study) recruited with the help of local community agencies. The primary feedback was that the questionnaires were too lengthy and difficult to comprehend. Consequently, the questionnaires were modified by removing questions and changing Likert scales to a more comprehensible and easy to read format (i.e., no, yes, don't know). Given Latinos unfamiliarity with Likert scales (18) this feedback was important.

Research team. Well-trained research teams are essential to research and crucial for studies conducted with ethnic minority groups. The characteristics of the study staff should be considered when conducting research with ethnic minority groups (17). Furthermore, identifying and including community or institutional staff members who share the same ethnic background and characteristics as the target population is considered a successful strategy for research recruitment (15, 18). In our studies, the research team was primarily of Latino descent, bicultural, and fluent in Spanish. Given our sample, it was important to match the characteristics of the research team to study participants (e.g., sex, Spanish-speaking). Additionally, since several research team staffs were members of the communities where the events took place, we had some knowledge of the locations and of community residents.

Identifying and training the research team is a timely process, yet essential. Ongoing training of the research team should highlight personal characteristics such as sensitivity, flexibility, and adaptability that enhance their work (15). In our studies, prior to each recruitment event the research team was trained on the study protocol, recruitment strategies, obtaining consent, and questionnaire administration. To aid the recruitment process, each research team member received a script consisting of a summary of the study purpose and participant eligibility criteria (e.g., age, cancer history).

Active participant recruitment

Individuals from ethnic minority groups may be hesitant to participate if they are asked to provide personal information without being fully informed of how it will be used (4,14). There is fear of being exploited or experimented on (14). Given these legitimate concerns, researchers must take necessary steps to facilitate understanding and trust of the research process.

Confidentiality. A sense of fear and distrust of research exists among ethnic minority research participants (18). Thus, emphasizing confidentiality is important to ease those fears (17). Through our recruitment process, we explained the informed consent and study in an understandable manner by providing precise details (e.g., meaning of confidentiality, examples of study questions). Participants were informed that they would not be identified in any reports and that their identity and personal information would not be disclosed. Caution has been advised when providing monetary incentives and requesting personal information for providing such incentives (17,18). Thus, when participants expressed apprehension when asked to sign for monetary incentives, concerns were addressed by assuring them of their confidentiality and that their identity would not be disclosed to anyone or linked to their study participation. These confidentiality assurances were fundamental and strengthened our recruitment efforts.

Language and literacy. Many participants were monolingual, Spanish-speakers with low literacy levels; an issue that affects disadvantaged and ethnic minority groups in the US (19). Estimates indicate that approximately 41% of Latinos 25 years of age and older have less than a high school education (20). Therefore, researchers need to be prepared for working with participants with low literacy levels (17,18). In our attempt to address language and literacy barriers, Spanish-speaking research team members were available to help read questions and assist participants in understanding and completing questionnaires. Women with low literacy levels were initially hesitant to participate, however, their apprehension eased when informed that they had the option of being assisted by a member of the research staff. This option was presented as part of the study protocol to help those who needed assistance, feel comfortable. Extra precautions were taken to ensure that participants were allowed to express their opinions and thoughts. Specifically, if participants sought response accuracy or agreement, they were reassured that there was no right or wrong answer, and that we were interested in their personal beliefs and opinions.

Communicating and establishing trust

Culturally-appropriate behaviors for rapport building. Violation of cultural norms such as personalismo, familismo, and respeto, contributes to low research participation. Thus, adapting messages and the recruitment process to fit these cultural norms is important. Most Latinas we encountered possessed little or no research participation experience. For that reason, our strategy of building rapport by engaging in culturally-appropriate behaviors (e.g. respeto, plática, simpatia) was important. We began by engaging in pleasant interactions such as greetings, introductions, handshakes and informal conversation, known as plática (14). Building rapport and interacting with participants' family members (e.g., spouses, sisters, parents, and children) was also beneficial since they often accompanied participants.

We also utilized culturally-appropriate language that emits respeto (respect). Respectful interactions occur within a hierarchical structure mediated by age, gender and status (14,21). Since respeto is displayed by the use of titles (e.g., señor, señora), referring to Latinas as señora (madam) and to their spouses as señor (Mr.) was considerate and helpful. We also addressed participants and adult family members by usted (you), a formal and respectful way of addressing adults in the Latino culture (14,21). Participants and family members appeared to like being greeted in this formal manner and it was an excellent approach to jumpstart rapport. While this type of formal language is not too common in the US, in many Spanish-speaking countries, like Mexico, it is. Using a formal communication style is critical to convey respect and gain trust. Since most participants were born outside the US and likely endorsed traditional cultural values, we used this type of formal language to communicate and interact with them and their families.

Adapting to extraneous factors

Having community-organized events serve as research collection sites presented some challenges that required shifting the original recruitment plan and devising more creative strategies. For example, at some events weather conditions and insufficient event advertisement resulted in low attendance. Therefore, we implemented a snowball technique by asking those who participated in the study if they knew of other eligible women who would be interested in participating. We also visited nearby establishments (e.g., restaurants, grocery stores) where potential participants worked and invited them to participate during their work breaks or at the end of their work shifts. On the event days, we approached vendors and requested permission to leave study flyers with them. These turned out to be successful strategies that enabled us to reach additional participants.

Provision of resources and incentives

Hospitality. Light refreshments (e.g., snacks, water) were provided since eating together is an effective method to generate conversations among participants (17). Family responsibilities such as childcare have been reported to limit study participation (3). Therefore, when participants were accompanied by their children, we offered child care by engaging children with an entertaining activity (e.g., coloring books). Thus, hospitality should be considered another important component of the recruitment process.

Resources and incentives. Spanish health written educational materials consisted of educational pamphlets from ACS (22) and NCI (23) on BCA risk, screening and mammograms. A directory that serves as a guide for support resources (e.g., support and information lines) was also provided (24). Additionally, participants were compensated with a gift (t-shirt and tote bag) and $25. Providing monetary and non-monetary incentives to low-income participants when they are required to disclose personal information is considered appropriate (14,17-18). In our case, the only information our institution required were participants' names and signatures. As mentioned earlier, participants were reassured of their confidentiality when they expressed concerns.

DISCUSSION

Factors such as limited English language proficiency, limited access to healthcare, low SES, and family and cultural factors contribute to health disparities. In order to improve health outcomes and increase ethnic minorities' research participation, more research tailored to ethnic and underserved populations is needed. Factors that challenge the recruitment of ethnic minorities in community settings call for flexibility, a wide range of strategies and the consideration and inclusion of cultural norms. By utilizing strategies that follow CBPR principles, we took necessary steps to successfully recruit Latinas into cancer prevention education research studies conducted in community settings. CBPR helps to strengthen trust and collaboration between community members and researchers and to integrate research results with efforts for community change (12). In an effort to initiate community change, the results from our previous studies (10,11) were utilized to develop two new tools, "Where's Maria?" (9) and the "LBCS" scale (8). These two tools were developed and evaluated with help from the community they were intended to inform and designed to serve.

The variety of strategies implemented and the shifting of the recruitment plan due to unforeseen events make it difficult to clearly identify any single strategy that led to greater success. Regardless, our experiences in recruiting Spanish-speaking Latinas highlight several valuable points. First, it is important and necessary to work with community members and agencies. Key community members helped us build contacts in the community and to identify recruitment sites. Additionally, in studies where participants are primarily monolingual, it is imperative that bilingual and bicultural research assistants be present during data collection to assist in the successful recruitment of these hard-to-reach populations. Being around a familiar other from one's own community or culture engenders trust (25). Thus, culturally and linguistically competent research staff helps facilitate an environment in which participants can gain a sense of trust and consequently be more amenable to partake in research.

Second, communication skills and the ability to relate to participants are crucial factors in successful recruitment (3). In our case, it was essential to interact cordially, engage in relaxed conversations, and address people with formal language since these are Latino cultural norms (14,21). This in turn may increase the likelihood of self-disclosure and improve the quality of the data obtained and of the entire research process. These culturally-appropriate social behaviors helped us build personal contact, a strategy that encourages ethnic minorities' participation in research (16). Third, we recommend expressing genuine gratitude to research participants. Expressing gratitude has been recognized as one of seven relevant principles when conducting research with underrepresented ethnic minorities (1). We expressed gratitude verbally and by offering a small gift including BCA resources.

CONCLUSION

We must first point out that these studies were not designed to empirically evaluate recruitment strategies. Rather, this article describes strategies used to help increase our knowledge of ways to increase ethnic minorities' inclusion in health research. Also, the recruitment strategies presented did not follow all CBPR principles given that we only implemented strategies deemed appropriate to meet the recruitment goals of these studies.

This article highlights the importance of culturally-sensitive and culturally-appropriate research methodologies when conducting research with underserved ethnic minorities. Including ethnic minorities in health related research is essential; however, merely focusing on inclusion is not enough to ensure adequate treatment of ethnic minorities in research (4). Hence, it is important for researchers to incorporate not only new and innovative, but also culturally-appropriate and creative methods for conducting research with ethnic minorities.

Trying to find the "best" methods of ethnic minority recruitment to health education research is challenging. However, our experiences and strategies have proven to be valuable in successfully recruiting Latinas into research studies conducted in community settings and add to the knowledge of "what works" in the research recruitment of this population. However, we must keep in mind that several factors may work together better than one factor alone. Thus, it seems that a recruitment plan consisting of several strategies that allows for flexibility in shifting the original plan by adjusting to "real world" circumstances encountered in community settings may be a good starting point for successful recruitment.

This knowledge can be appraised and built upon by investigators in their research endeavors. It is our hope that the strategies presented serve as a starting point for organizing a plan of action for future research. Research approaches utilizing frameworks that remain consistent with study goals can become effective strategies for addressing and targeting health disparities and health behavior promotion. The value of CBPR principles can be greatly enhanced when researchers make an effort to conduct research in a culturally-sensitive and appropriate manner.

REFERENCES

[1]   Ashing-Giwa K. Can a culturally responsive model for research design bring us closer to addressing participation disparities? Lessons learned from cancer survivorship studies. Ethnicity Dis 2005a;15:130-7.

[2]   National Institute of Health. National Institutes of Health Revitalization Act of 1993. Washington, DC, 1993. Accessed 2011 Sep 01. URL: http://grants.nih.gov/grants/funding/women_min/guidelines_ amended_10_2001.htm.

[3]   Brown BA, Long HL, Gould H, Weitz T, Milliken N. A conceptual model for the recruitment of diverse women into research studies. J Women's Health Gender-Based Med 2000;9(6):625-32.

[4]   Burlew AK. Research with ethnic minorities: Conceptual, methodological, and analytical issues. In: G. Bernal, J.E. Trimble, Burlew AK, Leong FTL, editors. Handbook of racial and ethnic minority psychology. Thousand Oaks, CA: Sage Publications; 2003:179-97.

[5]   U.S. Census Bureau. Detailed tables-American Factfinder; T4-2008. Hispanic or Latino by race-2008 estimates. Accessed 2011 Sep 01. URL: http://wwwfactfindercensusegov. 2008.

[6]   American Cancer Society. Breast cancer facts and figures for Hispanics/Latinos 2009-2011. Atlanta, GA: American Cancer Society, 2009.

[7]   Cabral DN, Napoles-Springer AM, Mike R, McMillan A, Sison JD, Wrensch MR, et al. Population- and community-based recruitment of African Americans and Latinos. Am J Epidemiol 2003;152:272-9.

[8]   Borrayo EA, Gonzalez P, Swaim R, Marcus A, Flores E, Espinoza P. The Latina Breast Cancer Screening scale: Beliefs about breast cancer and breast cancer screening. J Health Psychol 2009;14(7):944-55.

[9]   Borrayo EA. Where's Maria? A video to increase awareness about breast cancer and mammography screening among low-literacy Latinas. Prev Med 2004;39:99-110.

[10]   Borrayo EA, Jenkins SR. Feeling healthy: So why should Mexican-descent women screen for breast cancer? Qual Health Res 2001a;11(6):812-23.

[11]   Borrayo EA, Jenkins SR. Feeling indecent: Breast cancer screening resistance of Mexican-descent women. J Health Psychol 2001b;6(5):537-49.

[12]   Israel BA, Schulz AJ, Parker EA, Becker AB. Review of community-based research: Assessing partnership approaches to improve public health. Annu Rev Public Health 1998;19:173-202.

[13]   U.S. Census Bureau. U.S. Census Bureau, Summary File 1 (SF 1) and Summary File 3 (SF 3). Accessed 2011 Sep 01. URL: http://wwwcensusgov/. 2000.

[14]   Marin G, Marin BV. Research with Hispanic populations. Newbury Park, CA: Sage, 1991.

[15]   Julion W, Gross D, Barclay-McLaughlin G. Recruiting families of color from the inner city: Insights from recruiters. Nurs Outlook 2000;48:230-7.

[16]   Cauce AM, Ryan K, Grove K. Children and adolscents of color, where are you? Participation, selection, recruitment, and retention in developmental research. In: V. McLoyd, Steinberg L, eds. Studying minority adolescents. Mahwah, NJ: Lawrence Erlbaum, 1998:147-66.

[17]   Umana-Taylor AJ, Hamaca MY. Conducting focus groups with Latino populations: Lessons from the field. Fam Relat 2004;53(3):261-72.

[18]   Skaff MM, Chesla CA, Myceu VS, Fisher L. Lessons in cultural competence: Adapting research methodology for Latino participants. J Commun Psychol 2002;30(3):305-23.

[19]   Rosal MC, Goins KV, Carbone ET, Cortes DE. Views and preferences of low-literate Hispanics regarding diabetes education: Results of formative research. Health Educ Behav 2004;31(3):388-405.

[20]   US Census Bureau. U.S. Census Bureau, American Community Survey. Accessed 2011 Sep 01. URL: http://wwwcensusgov/. 2005.

[21] Anez LM, Silva MA, Paris M, Jr., Bedregal LE. Engaging Latinos through the integration of cultural values and motivational interviewing principles. Professional Psychol Res Pract 2008;39(2):153-9.

[22] American Cancer Society. Breast Cancer: Questions and Answers. Atlanta, GA: ACS, 2001.

[23] National Cancer Institute. Mammograms, not just once, bur for a lifetime. Bethesda, MD: NCI, NIH, 1999.

[24] Day of caring for breast cancer awareness. Colorado breast cancer resources directory, 2004-2005, 8th ed. Highlands Ranch, CO: Colorado Cancer Coalition, 2004.

[25] Pasick RJ, Hiatt RA, Paskett EI. Lessons learned from community-based cancer screening intervention research. Cancer 2004;101(S5):1146-64.

Submitted: September 22, 2011. *Revised:* November 26, 2011. *Accepted:* December 07, 2011.

In: Public Health Yearbook 2012
Editor: Joav Merrick

ISBN: 978-1-62808-078-0
© 2013 Nova Science Publishers, Inc.

Chapter 32

PROMOTING YOUTH PHYSICAL ACTIVITY AND HEALTH CAREER AWARENESS IN AN AFRICAN AMERICAN FAITH COMMUNITY

*Judy B Springer, PhD**, *Jeffrey A Morzinski, PhD* *and Melissa DeNomie, MS*

Physical Education Department, Milwaukee Area Technical College, Milwaukee, Wisconsin and Department of Family and Community Medicine, Medical College of Wisconsin, Milwaukee, Wisconsin, United States of America

ABSTRACT

Physical inactivity is prevalent among adolescents. Urban African American youth are especially prone to sedentary lifestyles and may be underexposed to health promotion information. Although many youth are encouraged to pursue post-secondary education, the total number of youth in health career pathways continues to stall, especially youth from underrepresented communities. Objectives: To train adult health advocates and implement a youth physical activity, health knowledge, and health career awareness program in an African American faith community. Methods: Seven adult health advocates (HA) received a six-week training program on promoting youth health. Twenty-four middle- and high-school youth participated in a 10-week program featuring progressive run/walk and didactic sessions with incentives for youth participation in leisure-time physical activity. The OMNI Scale Rating of Perceived Exertion (RPE) instrument assessed cardiorespiratory endurance during activity; survey assessments were completed by HA and youth to rate gains in skills and knowledge, and evaluate satisfaction with program variables.

Results: HA reported increased health knowledge, skills, and confidence (p<.01) to be informational resources for youth. Fourteen (58%) youth attended at least 70% of program sessions, with high satisfaction ratings. Measures of youth RPE showed improved cardiorespiratory endurance (p<.05) from week five to ten. Conclusions: The

* Correspondence: Judy B Springer, PhD, Instructor, Physical Education Department, Milwaukee Area Technical College, 700 West State Street, Milwaukee, WI 53233, United States. E-mail: springej@matc.edu

partnership of healthcare professionals, community-based organizations, and faith community members successfully organized and facilitated a program to improve youth health outcomes. Aligning project activities with partner strengths was important to project success, as was youth recognition.

Keywords: Physical activity, youth, faith community, health advocates

INTRODUCTION

Physical inactivity is a major public health problem in the United States that affects adolescents as well as adults. Three-quarters of teenagers do not meet physical activity recommendations, and their activity levels decline steadily with age, particularly among girls (1). Both education and income are associated with activity levels and obesity (2), and inactivity is exacerbated by living in poor urban areas where reduced funding for physical education programs, lack of enthusiasm/enjoyment for participation, and unsafe environments are more common (3).

In 2009, 82% of 9th to 12th grade students in Milwaukee, Wisconsin, did not participate in recommended levels of physical activity. African American females had the lowest levels, with 86% failing to meet physical activity guidelines (4). The predominantly African American Amani neighborhood in which the present study was conducted has the lowest socioeconomic status in the city, a large high school drop-out rate, and nearly half of the households are in poverty and headed by jobless adults (5).

As well as severe social challenges from violence and crime, the neighborhood has few health services or opportunities for exposure to health careers. Career awareness programs can help students make the transitions from high school to the more demanding secondary education level, and, in the case of health careers, establish positive attitudes toward those careers (6,7). Programs that raise youth awareness of more readily achievable health career options, such as two-year and non-physician track programs, may result in encouraging future health care providers who are more likely to serve in underrepresented communities and work to reduce related health disparities as described in Healthy People 2020 (8,9).

Churches have played an important role in improving health in African American faith communities through promoting physical activity and healthy lifestyle practices for adults (10,11). While well-planned health initiatives may be especially effective in reducing risks of chronic diseases in adult populations, little is known about the effectiveness of faith community health promotion programs that focus on youth or activity levels. Accordingly, when we developed a faith-based community-academic partnership to design and implement a one-year pilot intervention to improve activity in adolescents, we sought to combine physical activity with positive attitudes and knowledge about health and about potential careers in health. The partnership, called Guiding Youth Movement (GYM), included the Milwaukee Area Technical College (MATC), Greater New Birth Church (GNBC), Medical College of Wisconsin (MCW), and the Badgerland Striders (BLS). Objectives of the partnership program were to:

1. Train health advocates to model healthy lifestyle practices and assist in the promotion of health strategies and health career awareness for youth, and

2. Refine, implement, and evaluate a progressive youth physical activity, health promotion, and career awareness program.

PARTNERS AND PROGRAM COMPONENTS

Program partners and responsibilities are described below. The Institutional Review Boards of both the Medical College of Wisconsin and the Milwaukee Area Technical College approved the study.

GYM Steering Committee. Community Partner – JS, MATC and Youth Running Director, BLS, Co-Principal Investigator, co-lead all training activities, directed the curriculum on fitness activities and educational sessions for youth and supervised MATC service-learning students; WD, GNBC, directed the enrollment and retention of project HAs and youth and was the project's liaison to GNBC; Academic Partner – JM, MCW, Principal Investigator, lead project evaluation, co-lead Health Advocate training activities, and co-lead dissemination activities with JS and WD; MD, MCW, managed Institutional Review Board submission, informed consent, and coordinated Steering Committee activities.

GYM Program Staff. Two adult professionals with extensive experience in youth physical activity facilitation carried out the GYM physical activity program including collection of youth running data during activity. Both trainers are seasoned runners; one trainer was a nationally certified personal trainer and the other an advanced practice nurse.

GNBC Nurses' Committee. Nurses' Committee members are health care professionals within the GNBC community. Based on discussions with GYM Steering Committee members, GNBC Nurses' Committee members welcomed GYM youth to their annual Blood Drive and spoke at sessions related to health careers. Nurses' Committee members dialogued with youth about the importance of blood donation, career opportunities in the health care field, and were visible resources within the church for further discussions on health- and career-related topics.

Faith Community. GNBC had 2000 adult and 400 youth members and was located within the Amani Neighborhood at the inception of the program (later moving to accommodate its growing congregation). Key elements of effective church programs for adults used in the GYM intervention included pastoral support for initiatives, organized activities that provide opportunities for engagement, and creative approaches of enlisting parishioners in health promotion to improve the health of youth (12,13). Key to this approach was the use of trained community members, referred to as health advocates (14). Several studies have demonstrated that health advocate-lead education supports healthy behavior changes, including physical activity and nutrition (15,16). Further, these lay leaders may serve as role models of healthy lifestyles, when possible, to reinforce the message to youth and the broader faith community (17). As residents of the community, their sustained engagement may also lead to longer-term effects on prolonging positive health behaviors (14).

MATC service-learning students. At each youth physical activity / education session two MATC service-learning students aided the GYM program. Students were recruited from JS's wellness course and were required to attend. Students aided in the recording of youth accumulated leisure-time minutes, trained alongside youth, and spoke to youth during education sessions about the rigors of returning to school as an adult, opportunities in the health care field, and suggested strategies for academic success.

School and family. Other cues were taken from school- and community-based youth programs: promoting higher perceived physical competence to increase behaviors such as effort and persistence (18); providing positive feedback, transportation to places to be active, and peer support (19); enlisting a family-based approach to health promotion by providing information to parents about healthy nutrition and healthy weight for youth (20); and sustaining an overarching theme of fun or enjoyment (21).

METHODS

Health Advocates (HA): 7 (5 women, 2 men) adult members of Greater New Birth Church in Milwaukee, WI, were selected by their pastor based on previous experience working with GNBC youth and time to attend all HA training at GNBC and most GYM youth-related activities. HAs completed Physical Activity Readiness Questionnaires (ParQ) (22) to determine readiness for physical activity. Upon successful completion of project activities HAs received a $300 stipend. HA ages ranged from 26 to 35 years (mean 30). All had completed high school, four were currently enrolled in post-secondary education programs, and two were college graduates. Two HA had children in the GYM program.

Youth: Of 35 youth recruited, complete data were available for 24 middle- and high-school youth members of GNBC (14 female, 10 male [mean age 13.5 SD=1.98; range 11 to 17]. Based on past attendance and conduct at weekly Bible study sessions determined by the youth pastor and HAs youth were asked to be part of the project. Parents were contacted through a brochure developed by the GYM Steering Committee and distributed at church. Interested persons were instructed to contact the youth minister for registration materials. Pre-intervention Health History Screening Questionnaires (23) were administered by project staff to determine any limitations for physical activity.

Setting: GYM program activities were held during regularly scheduled Wednesday evening Bible study at the Northside YMCA, a site centrally located to the church. Health Occupations classroom tours occurred at MATC, Blood Drive occurred at GNBC, and the 5 km community road race sponsored by the BLS occurred locally.

Instruments

HA: Engagement. Weekly session evaluations were completed by HA and analyzed by GYM program staff for satisfaction, problem solving, and potential program adaptations. A post-training survey was administered to HA to determine their learning and behavior changes. Analysis consisted of descriptive statistics of numerical data.

Youth: Training effect. Cardiorespiratory intensity was self-rated and reported during physical activity using the OMNI Rating of Perceived Exertion. The OMNI scale is a psychophysical estimation method to self-report overall feelings of exertion, or in the case of youth, "tiredness," which correlates strongly with increased heart rate and respiration during physical activity. The RPE scale is used in predicting fitness, clinical and field settings and exercise prescription (24). While standard cardiorespiratory assessments are available for youth (e.g., 20-meter shuttle, 12-minute run) the GYM Steering Committee, under the advice of the lead author, an exercise physiologist, chose the RPE scale to minimize youth feelings of "finishing last," unfit status, etc. yet measure overall effort to assess endurance changes. The OMNI RPE scale may be used to assess ventilatory breakpoint, that is the point during intense exercise at which ventilation increases disproportionately to the amount of oxygen consumed, also understood to be the point at which training effects occur (24). An RPE value of 5 (+1 SD) is recognized to be the ventilatory breakpoint. Changes in RPE over the course of a training program indicate there is an improvement in fitness level (24). Analysis consisted of paired t-tests of collected data.

Engagement: Weekly session evaluations were completed by youth and analyzed by GYM program staff for satisfaction, problem solving, and potential program adaptations. Accumulated minutes of physical activity were self-reported by youth and gathered on a weekly basis by MATC service-learning students and project staff. A post-training survey was administered to youth to determine their learning and behavior changes. Analysis consisted of descriptive statistics of numerical data.

Training and activities

HA training: 6 weekly training sessions (12 hours total) were conducted at GNBC by project staff, with contributions by a physician and two third-year MCW medical students, to cover the basis of HA's own health, the GYM program, factors associated with youth health in high-risk environments, strategies for increasing adherence to healthy behaviors, and safeguards for physical activity.

Each session included a facilitated discussion related to session topics, specifically team building, lecture, discussion, worksheets, and homework activities. A catered meal was also provided each week. During the 10-week GYM program staff sent weekly e-mails to HA advising them of the upcoming activities, suggesting roles for program assistance, ways to meet the expectation of being visible health resources for the youth, and opening lines of communication for feedback. Additionally, staff held bi-weekly debriefing sessions with HA during the GYM program to problem-solve and facilitate suggested program adaptations.

Youth: Youth participants attended ten weekly sessions of 75-90 minutes including didactic sessions plus games (e.g., hula-hoop pass, huddle and dash, relay races), stretching, and progressive run/walk intervals lead by GYM project staff. Alternating run/walk intervals increasing in duration and intensity (e.g., week one included one-minute run followed by one-minute walk, repeated 10 times; week ten included four-minutes run followed by one-minute walk, repeated four times) were performed as a group; youth were encouraged to remain active for the entire run/walk portion. Running-related games such as a ladder run or partner running were used to promote full participation. Project staff participated alongside youth and explained and recorded youth OMNI Scale Rating of Perceived Exertion (24) during the run segments of weeks one, five, seven, and ten.

Educational sessions followed physical activity and included healthy snacks and hydration. Topics focused on improving knowledge of physical activity guidelines, healthy lifestyle practices, exploring the link between spirituality and health, and discovering the strengths/challenges of health careers. Each didactic session was facilitated by GYM project staff, health care professionals, GNBC Nurses' Committee members, and MATC service-learning students and included interactive games and worksheets that reinforced main concepts.

Additionally, based on their training, three HA facilitated the session on nutrition label reading and choosing healthy foods. Project staff developed a one-page synopsis of each session that was sent home to parents to maintain their interest in the program and aid them in establishing healthy habits for their family. Please see Table 2 for a complete listing of activities, facilitators, and handouts.

To promote youth leisure-time physical activity two methods were used: a series of incentives for self-reported accumulated minutes of physical activity was created, and participation in a local 5 km run/walk event was promoted. Youth were provided with a specially designed "GYM Physical Activity Tracker" log and received guidance from project staff and MATC service-learning students on identifying and recording moderate- to vigorous-intensity physical activities. Incentives awarded bi-weekly were based on accumulated minutes (in parentheses) as follows: award ribbon (150); personalized certificate (300); cinch sack (600); personalized medal (1000); three music downloads (1500); $10 gift card (2000); trophy (2500); name, photo, and biography in the BLS newsletter and specialized GYM award pin (3000). To promote engagement with the local community in physical activity, 14 youth, 2 HA, and 4 GYM project staff registered for a local 5 kilometer (3.1 miles) run/walk event organized by the BLS.

HA, Youth, and Families: A Capstone event took place at MATC including a guided interactive tour of health occupation classrooms by MATC administration and program wrap-up elements. Invitations were sent by e-mail and through word-of-mouth to all GYM youth and their families, HA, and GYM project staff.

Table 1. Health Advocate training session topics

Topics	Session Covered
General	
Introduction and facilitator biographies	Session One
Getting to know you interactive games	Sessions One to Six
Health Advocate overview and objectives	Session One
Safeguards for youth as "human subjects" in the GYM[a] program	Session Two
Strategies for advising and motivating youth	Session Five
Health Advocate	
Role of GYM Health Advocate	Session One
Guided self-appraisal of advocates health beliefs and behaviors	Session One
GYM program overview and objectives	Session One
Physical Activity	
Progressive run/walk overview and goal formation	Session Four
Examining the Rating of Perceived Exertion tool	Session Four
Interactive youth game (e.g., huddle and dash, hula hoop pass) exploration	Sessions One to Six
Best practices (e.g., safeguards) in youth physical activity	Session Five
Tour of Northside YMCA location	Session Four
Nutrition Knowledge	
Youth nutrition risk factors	Session Three
Goals for youth in GYM program	Session Three
"How to": food labels, healthy snacks, and beverages	Session Three
Health Careers	
Role of health networks and mentors	Session Six
Service-learning student participation	Session Six

Topics	Session Covered
Nurses' committee role overview	Session Six
Youth Health Outcomes	
Link between spirituality and health for youth	Session Two
Importance of physical activity and nutrition for youth health	Session Five
Physical activity and nutrition in high risk settings: barriers and supports	Session Six

Key: [a]GYM = Guiding Youth Movement.

Table 2. Youth Guiding Youth Movement (GYM) program overview

	Transportation from GNBC[a] to YMCA[b] Walking Warm Up (all) – 5 minutes Games and activities (all) – 15 minutes Stretching (split by gender) – 5 to 7 minutes Progressive Run / Walk Sessions (all) – 20 to 25 minutes Cool Down (all) – 3 to 5 minutes Didactic Sessions (all) – 20 to 25 minutes Transportation from YMCA to GNBC		
Week	Topic for Didactic Session	Facilitator	Take Home Letter to Parent / Guardian
1	Program Overview Importance of Physical Activity for Health	GYM Steering Committee	Fact Sheet: Physical Activity and Obesity
2	Choosing Foods for Fuel as a Runner	GYM Steering Committee	Healthy Foods Runners Need
3	Building a Healthy, Spiritual Foundation / Recipe for a Spiritual Life	GYM Steering Committee	Link Between Spirituality and Health
4	The Process of Choosing a Career in Health Professions	MATC[c] service-learning student	Components of a Health Career Network
5	Components of Proper Running Form	GYM Personal Trainer	Encouraging Lifestyle Physical Activity
6	Team Building / Leadership and Career Paths	GYM Steering Committee and MATC service-learning students	
7	Nutrition Label Reading and Healthy Snacks	GYM Health Advocates	Understanding Nutrition Labels
8	Tips for Success in High School as a Scholar and Athlete	King High School Athletes	Healthy Habit Self-Assessment
9	Various Careers in Health	MATC service-learning students and GYM Personal Trainer	
10	Future Steps for Health and the Importance of Blood Donation	GNBC Nurses' Committee member and GYM Youth	Save the Date: 5 kilometer run/walk
Other Activities	Importance of and Process after Blood Donation	Physician Member of GNBC	
	Observation of Blood Donation / Interview with Nurses' Committee Members	Blood Center of Southeastern Wisconsin and Nurses' Committee Members	

Table 2. (Continued)

Week	Topic for Didactic Session	Facilitator	Take Home Letter to Parent / Guardian
	Community 5 kilometer run/walk event	Badgerland Striders	
	Tour and Interactive Sessions of MATC Health Occupations Classrooms	MATC Faculty and Staff	

Key: [a]GNBC=Greater New Birth Church; [b]YMCA=Young Men's Christian Association; [c]MATC=Milwaukee Area Technical College.

A final awards ceremony was held including the distribution of a specially designed GYM t-shirt for all youth, HA, and project staff; HA testimonials; and future healthy lifestyle directions presented by GNBC Nurses Committee members and GYM project staff.

RESULTS

HA: Based on responses to the ParQ, the one HA with medical conditions requiring physician recommendation for physical activity signed a waiver of medical consultation and agreed to limit participation to low-intensity activities. On average, HA attended five of the six HA training sessions. One HA withdrew after completing the six-week training session due to job relocation and was replaced by a GYM Steering committee member who had resigned from his professional role as a GNBC minister due to continuing his education; as a Steering Committee member he had attended all of the HA training sessions. On average, HA attended 5 of the 10 GYM youth training sessions. All HA attended the GYM Capstone event.

All HA completed weekly surveys assessing their reaction to the program and acquisition of new skills, and all reported that each of the training sessions contributed significantly to their knowledge or understanding of the topics. On a scale from 1 (no contribution to knowledge or understanding) to 7 (a very strong contribution), they rated the sessions strongest for their increased knowledge that focused on Youth Nutrition and Risk Factors / "How to": food labels, snacks and beverages (6.83) and Nutrition and Fitness in High-Risk Settings (6.83). HA also judged their ability to promote healthy lifestyle practices to youth. On a scale (1=low ability; 6=exceptional ability) they rated their post-program ability the highest for displaying positive supportive words and actions toward all GYM youth and their families (6.0), their usefulness / influence as health mentors to GYM youth (5.9), and understanding the spiritual reasons for the recommended nutrition and physical activity practices (5.7), a statistically significant (p<.01) increase from pre-program levels (3.7, 2.3, 3.1, respectively).

The weekly surveys of the most important elements of the training elicited 115 comments centralized around three areas of program content:

1. Health information foundations (44, 38%) "By learning about physical activity and nutrition, we are setting the foundations to help the youth."
2. Environmental influences on health (13, 11%) "Exploring the reality of the influence of unsafe neighborhoods on health."

3. Practicality of program (11, 10%) "The 'hands on' activities like the 2000 steps walked = one mile was very helpful."

Other noted strengths included the importance of their function as role models for the youth, building and maintaining a health career network, the influence the GYM program will have on the GNBC community (including families), and the overall scope of the GYM program. A weakness of the program was having limited time to discuss relevant topics (e.g., the relationship between healthy lifestyle practices and adolescent growth and development).

Youth: For the 14 completers who attended at least 70% of all sessions, average attendance was 8 of 10 sessions; of the 10 at-large youth (i.e. attended at least one session), average attendance was 4 of 10 sessions. Three completers and two at-large youth were children of HA. Based on responses to the Health History Screening Questionnaire, no youth had medical conditions requiring physician permission for physical activity. Pre-existing conditions that may impact physical activity participation included asthma and/or allergies. Please see Table 3 for complete information related to youth characteristics. Ten (71%) completers and five (50%) at-large youth attended the GYM Capstone event.

In the weekly evaluations we asked youth their perception of the session, enjoyment of the activity, and if they were confident to use the healthy ideas presented by the GYM program. Youth rated sessions strongest (1=not at all strong; 4=very strong) that focused on Recipe for a Spiritual Life (3.81), The Importance of Blood Donation (3.69), and The Process of Choosing a Career in the Health Professions (3.63).

Youth rated their enjoyment in physical activity on a similar scale, rating sessions best that included games such as Double Dutch jump rope (3.83), Food Group Hustle (3.47) and jump rope (3.44). Youth also rated their confidence to use healthy ideas from the GYM program in the next week highest (1=no confidence; 4=high confidence) after Tips for Success in High School as a Scholar and Athlete (3.65), The Importance of Blood Donation (3.63), and Importance of Physical Activity for Health (3.6). Please see Table 4 for additional comments by youth related to the program and content.

At regularly scheduled intervals of the run, youth were asked to provide self-rated RPE values. The collected OMNI RPE values indicate two important findings: 1) over time the 14 completer youth experienced a training effect with each conditioning session, meaning the RPE approaching 5 rating during the activity sessions reflected an understood ventilatory breakpoint. Based on collected RPE values, with each progressive run / walk interval the intensity of the workout was high enough to elicit a training effect; 2) the RPE values from pre- to post-test suggest improved cardiorespiratory endurance across time for the youth. From Week Five (run / walk = two minutes / one minute) to Week Ten (run / walk = four / one minutes) RPE value differences were statistically significant (paired t-test, $p<.05$). Please see Figure.

Incentives for youth were based on self-reported minutes yet the amount of minutes reported appeared to be inconsistent. For those recording minutes, average weekly minutes were reported in 65% of the possible cases. Of those registered for the 5 km run/walk, 10 (71%; 8 completer and 2 at-large) youth, 1 (50%) HA, and 4 (100%) GYM project staff participated and completed the event.

Table 3. Guiding Youth Movement (GYM) youth participant characteristics and accumulated minutes of physical activity

	Number	Age in years, average	SD[a]	Body Mass Index	SD	Pre-existing Conditions	Sport or Extracurricular Activities	Accumulated Minutes of Physical Activity, average	SD
Total Enrolled	24	13.5	1.98	26.5	5.94				
Female	14	13.1	1.9	26.1	4.99				
Male	10	14.3	1.95	27	7.32				
Completers[b]	14	14	1.96	25.7	6.68				
Female	5	12.8	2.05	22.6	3.03	Asthma (n=2), Allergies (n=1)	Track and Rugby (n=1); Chorus (n=1)	161 minutes Range 51 to 306	111
Male	9	14.7	1.66	27.3	7.68	Asthma (n=2), Allergies (n=2)	Football (n=2); Track (n=1)	217 minutes Range 41 to 420	119
At-large Youth	10	13	1.94	27.6	4.81				
Female	9	13.22	1.92	28	4.92	Asthma (n=3), Allergies (n=1)	Volleyball (n=1)	138 minutes Range 33 to 279	76
Male	1	11		24				252 minutes	

KEY: [a]SD= standard deviation; [b]Completers=youth who attended at least 7 of 10 GYM sessions.

Table 4. Youth feedback from Guiding Youth Movement (GYM) program, Milwaukee, WI

Question: Name the BEST THING you did or learned today to improve your health.	
Session Number	Youth Response (gender, age)
One – Physical Activity	I began to log my daily physical activities (f, 15)
	Always stay in an activity, keep moving, and stay fit (m, 15)
	I learned that things I do every day are considered exercise (m, 17)
Two – Fuel for Runners	I learned just to keep running, even when I am tired (m, 13)
	Stop eating junk food (f, 15)
	The best thing I did was pushing myself to run the amount of minutes given (f, 16)
Three – Spiritual Link	I liked learning the ingredients [in a cake of spirituality] (f, 15)
	The huddle and dash game was a lot of running and you also had to think (f, 13)
	I liked that I ran and actually kept up (m, 17)
Four – Health Careers	Never give up and push yourself to accomplish your goal (m, 15)
	The ladder run is very fun (f, 15)
Five – Running Form	I learned how to run PROPERLY (f, 17)
	I learned when I run to move my arms (m, 14)
	I liked the relay races (f, 12)
Six – Team Building and Career Choices	I ran for the whole three minutes without stopping (m, 17)
	I need to go to college (m, 13)
	About more professions I knew nothing about (m, 12)
Seven – Nutrition	I learned how to read calorie intake on a food box (m, 16)
	That taco salad is 820 calories so stay away (m, 17)
	Watch what I eat (m, 15)
Eight – Scholar Athletes	What cross country athletes are like (m, 15)
	Learning that we have run 2 miles today (m, 15)
	Running today – I was very, very proud of myself (f, 13)
	I ran the whole time we were supposed to run. I felt great. (f, 15)
Nine – Health Careers	The things it takes to run a job (m, 14)
	Play the games and running (f, 11)
	You can't be a felon if you want a good job (m, 15)
Ten – Blood Donation	You can't give blood for 5 years if you have cancer; how to keep my pace (m, 14)
	I ran for 4 minutes and walked. I tried, and it was fun (f, 15)
	I learned about the value of giving blood (f, 16)
5 km run/walk event	After a lifetime of failure I finally accomplished something…and it was exercise (m, 13)
	I am doing okay as long as I am in the lead [of the GNBC[a] team] (m, 16)
	You are really supposed to throw the water cup on the ground after you get a drink? (f, 14)

Key: [a]GNBC=Greater New Birth Church

Comments from youth centralized around the feelings of accomplishment and satisfaction with reaching an established goal. Please see Table 4 for specific comments related to 5 km run/walk participation.

Nine (64%) of the completers answered surveys assessing their acquisition of new skills and knowledge related to health careers. On a scale (1=no experience or knowledge in this area; 6=exceptional experience or knowledge), their responses were statistically significant (paired t-test, p<0.1) for knowing people in health professions (5.0), developing habits that support health career choices (4.67), and establishing a health network made up of peers, adults and advisors (4.44) from pre- to post-program. Youth evaluation comments centralized around learning about new health career professions, elements of blood donation, and the importance of attending college. Please see Table 4 for additional comments.

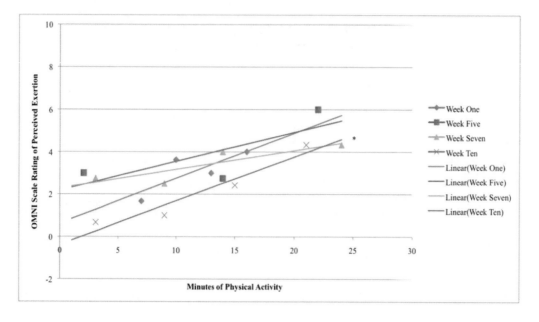

Rating of Perceived Exertion (RPE) for GYM youth (n=14, females=5, males=9) at progressive run / walk intervals. *Significant decreases (paired t-test, p<.05) in RPE occurred for youth from Week Five to Week Ten. For ease of viewing, trend lines have been added.

Figure 1. GYM Youth rating of Perceived Exertion.

DISCUSSION

To our knowledge, this is the first study in the literature of a faith-based community partnership to improve knowledge, activity levels, and attitudes toward health and health careers in middle- and high-school aged youth. This experience in an African American community suggests that the success of faith communities in supporting health initiatives in adults may also hold for promotion of physical activity and increased health awareness for adolescents.

Strengths of the GYM program include 1) a physical activity program that was the right balance between cardiorespiratory intensity (as measured by RPE) for improved endurance and fun (as reflected in the youth comments) for participation; 2) a model that is relatively low cost, accessible, and adaptable to many fitness levels; 3) greater continued youth participation / attendance than other youth extracurricular and non-curricular physical activity programs (25), suggesting the added appeal of the faith community venue for encouraging activity among first-time exercisers; and 4) the promise of the OMNI RPE scale as a cardiorespiratory measurement tool, especially in a group setting with varying fitness levels. Participant satisfaction with the program suggests that this type of program might be successful in other African American churches. Delivering credible, practical information that prompted self-reflection on personal health issues and open dialogue regarding factors associated with youth health was seen as an important factor in the HA training. Self-reported increased confidence and skill suggest that the training content was effective. Youth and HAs participated in a community 5 km run / walk event outside of the regularly scheduled 10-week program, further supporting the potential sustainability of activities. Our findings are preliminary, however, and we were not able to measure the influence of these advocates for role modeling healthy behaviors to youth and other parishioners.

HA attendance was less than expected at the youth sessions. Other peer-supported programs have reported higher attendance rates (16). Our experience highlights the need to consider strategies for improved HA participation in the youth-focused activities as this type of program is developed and refined.

Focusing the program on key objectives with an overarching theme of fun and involvement of all youth appears to have been successful. Alignment between youth interests and facilitated programs may have contributed to the youths' high ratings of satisfaction, improved confidence in healthy lifestyle practices and expanded health career awareness. However, this aspect needs further study.

The youth-reported improved awareness of health careers suggests that the model, similar to those previously suggested (6), is effective in expanding youth health career awareness.

Noteworthy was the valuable contribution of the technical college service-learning students, providing avenues for youth to explore two-year technical degrees through the first-hand accounts of peers (or in this case, near-peers). This was similar to findings of Gonzalez et al. (7) and others (9) who suggested a mentoring program to raise health career awareness for middle school youth.

Much of the success of the program was owing to the support of key GNBC partners including the pastor and volunteers--a concrete reminder to the youth and their parents that the program was valued. Such support has been shown to be a catalyst for successful health initiatives in faith communities (12, 26)

Still, there were no significant increases in leisure-time physical activity of the youth, and only a few reached recommended activity levels. This is consistent with other research that suggests school-based programs must be paired with community-lead initiatives to reach physical activity goals (27). Other limitations include small numbers of HA and youth in this pilot study, which also lacks a control group. Results reported here may be due to chance enrollment of certain types of participants, which may have influenced findings in unpredictable ways. Certain aspects of this evaluation relied on self-reported data. However, the trustworthiness of findings was strengthened by using both quantitative and qualitative data. Future studies might use accelerometers or other measures to track physical activity rather than depending on self-report (10, 28). During the course of the study, the growing GNBC moved from its original location, changed leadership at the youth minister level, and is no longer located in a medically underserved area. We do not know whether this affected the study. Finally, we have limited data regarding the sustainability of the intervention.

CONCLUSION

The one-year pilot project supported a multifaceted approach using parents and other adults in a faith community, outside professionals, and service-learning students to enhance physical activity participation and knowledge and attitudes about health careers. Having a consistent, credible health message conveyed in the home, school, and church reinforces the notion of good health to youth and lays the groundwork for healthy lifestyle practices. Inclusion of parents in the outreach within faith communities needs additional exploration.

ACKNOWLEDGMENTS

Thank you to Pastor Willie Davis for his enthusiasm and commitment to the project; to the Northside YMCA for hosting the youth running and education sessions; to Laure DeMattia, DO for reviewing earlier versions of the manuscript; and to Christine McLaughlin for meaningful edits in later drafts. Funding Support: This research was funded in part by the Healthier Wisconsin Partnership Program, an endowment of the Medical College of Wisconsin.

REFERENCES

[1]   Centers for Disease Control and Prevention. Health behaviors of adults: United States, 2005-2007. Vital and health statistics. Series 10, number 245. (Updated March, 2010) Accessed 2011 August 31. URL: http://www.cdc.gov/nchs/data/series/sr_10/sr10_245.pdf.

[2]   Sallis JF, Zakarian JM, Hovell MF, Hofstetter CR. Ethnic, socioeconomic, and sex differences in physical activity among adolescents. J Clin Epidemiol 1996;49(2):125-34.

[3]   Molnar BE, Gortmaker SL, Bull FC, et al. Unsafe to play? Neighborhood disorder and lack of safety predict reduced physical activity among urban children and adolescents. Am J Health Prom 2004;18(5):378-86.

[4]   Centers for Disease Control and Prevention. Youth Risk Behavior Survey (YRBS) Accessed 2011 August 31. URL: http://www.cdc.gov/yrbss.

[5]   City of Milwaukee. City of Milwaukee Neighborhood Strategic Planning Area Statistics, June 30, 2009 to July 1, 2010. Accessed 2011 August 31 URL: http://itmdapps.ci.mil.wi.us/ publicApplication_SR/neighborhood/neighborhoofm.faces

[6]   Leifer AD, Lesser GS. The development of career awareness in young children. Washington DC: US Department of Health, Education, and Welfare, Education Division. National Institute of Education, Education Work Group, 1996.

[7]   Gonzalez LS, Kearns EH, Lafferty S, Lampignano J, Pappas VM. The middle school mentoring program in allied health: a proposed model. J Allied Health 2000;29(2):114-9.

[8]   Smith SG, Nsiah-Kumi PA, Jones PR, Pamies RJ. Pipeline programs in the health professions, part 1: preserving diversity and reducing disparities. J Natl Med Assoc 2009;101:836-40.

[9]   US Department of Health and Human Service. Healthy People 2020. Accessed 2011 August 31. URL: http://www.healthypeople.gov/2020/

[10]   Whitt-Glover MC, Hogan PE, Lang W, Heil DP. Pilot study of a faith-based physical activity program among sedentary blacks. Prev Chronic Dis 2008;5(2):1-9.

[11]   Durse OK, Sarkisian CA, Leng M, Mangione CM. Sisters in motion: a randomized controlled trial of a faith-based physical activity intervention. J Am Geriatr Soc 2010;58:1863-9.

[12]   Kaplan S, Ruddock C, Golub M, et al. Stirring up the mud: Using a community-based participatory approach to address health disparities through a faith-based initiative. J Health Care Poor Underserved 2009;20:1111-23.

[13]   Baruth M, Wilcox S, Saunders R, Laken M, Condrasky M, Evans RB. The relationship between types of social support and physical activity in African American church members. Med Sci Sports Exerc 2008;40(Suppl 5):S358.

[14]   Brownstein JN, Bone LR, Dennison CR, Hill MN, Miyong KT, Levine DM. Community health workers as interventionalists in the prevention and control of heart disease and stroke. Am J Prev Med 2005;29(5 Suppl 1):128-133.

[15]   Fernandez S, Scales KL, Pineiro JM, Schoenthaler AM, Ogedegbe G. A senior center-based pilot trial of the effect of lifestyle intervention on blood pressure in minority elderly people with hypertension. J Am Geriatri Soc 2008;56(10):1860-6.

[16]   Hayes A, Morzinski J, Ertl K, Wirm C, Patterson L, Wilke N, Whittle J. Preliminary description of the feasibility of using peer leaders to encourage hypertension self-management. WMF 2010;109(2):85-90.

[17]   Anderson N, Wold B. Parental and peer influences on leisure-time physical activity in young adolescents. Res Q Exerc Sport 1992;63:341-8.

[18]   Stuntz CP, Weiss MR. Motivating children and adolescents to sustain a physically active lifestyle: predictors of physical activity motivation and mechanisms of change. Am J Lifestyle Med 2010;4(5):433-44.

[19]   Beets MW, Vogel R, Forlaw L, Pitetti KH, Cardinal BJ. Social support and youth physical activity: the role of provider and type. Am J Health Behav 2006;30(3):278-89.

[20]   Burnet DL, Plaut AJ, Ossowski K, Ahman A, Quinn MT, Radovick S et al. Community and family perspectives on addressing overweight in urban, African-American youth. J Gen Intern Med 2008;23(2):175-9.

[21]   Haverly K, Davison KK. Personal fulfillment motivates adolescents to be physically active. Arch Pediatr Adolesc Med 2005;139:1115-20.

[22]   Public Health Agency of Canada and the Canadian Society for Exercise Physiology. Physical Activity Readiness Questionnaire [Par-Q], 2007.

[23]   Children's Hospital Institute of Sports Medicine. Exercise and physical activity readiness assessment for children and adolescents. 2011, August 31. URL: http://www.chw.edu.au/chism/

[24]   Robertson RJ. Perceived Exertion for Practitioners: Rating Effort with the OMNI Picture System. Champaign, IL: Human Kinetics, 2004.

[25]   Jago R, Baranowski T. Non-curricular approaches for increasing physical activity in youth: a review. Prev Med 2004;39(1):157-63.

[26]   Yanek LR, Becker DM, Moy TF, Gittelson J, Koffman DM. Project Joy: Faith based cardiovascular health promotion for African American women. Public Health Rep 2001;116:68-81.

[27]   Jago R, McMurray RG, Drews KL et al. HEALTHY intervention: Fitness, physical activity, and metabolic syndrome results. Med Sci Sports Exerc 2011;43(8):1513-22.

[28]   Pate RR, Freedson PS, Sallis JF, Taylor WC, Sirard J, Trost SG, Dowda M. Compliance with physical activity guidelines: prevalence in a population of children and youth. Ann Epidemiol 2002;12(5):303-8.

Submitted: October 15, 2011. *Revised:* November 27, 2011. *Accepted:* December 04, 2011.

In: Public Health Yearbook 2012
Editor: Joav Merrick

Chapter 33

SUCCESS OF "PROMOTORES DE SALUD" IN IDENTIFYING IMMIGRANT LATINO SMOKERS AND DEVELOPING QUIT PLANS

Natalia Suarez, MA[*,1,2], *Lisa Sanderson Cox, PhD*[2],
Kimber Richter, PhD[2], *Irazema Mendoza, BA*[2],
Cielo Fernández, MSc[3], *Susan Garrett, BA*[1,2],
Isabel Scarinci, PhD, MPH[4],
Edward F Ellerbeck, MD, PhD[2]
and A Paula Cupertino, PhD[1,2]

[1]Juntos Center for Advancing Latino Health, [2]Department of Preventive Medicine and Public Health, University of Kansas Medical Center, Kansas City, Kansas, [3]El Centro, Inc, Kansas City, Kansas, [4]Minority Health and Health Disparities Research Center, University of Alabama at Birmingham, Birmingham, Alabama, United States of America

ABSTRACT

Many Latino immigrant smokers have demonstrated an interest in quitting. Yet they are hindered in these efforts by a lack of familiarity with and access to evidence-based treatment. Promotores de salud may be a promising approach for addressing this gap. Objective: To identify and recruit promotores, monitor attendance and completion of smoking cessation training, and track the community-based dissemination activities undertaken by promotores. Methods: Our community-academic partnership developed and implemented a 7-session smoking cessation training program for promotores. The training focused on identifying smokers, motivating smokers to develop quit plans, including referral to state-sponsored telephone counseling quitlines (quitline). We

* Correspondence: Natalia Suarez, MA, Research Associate, Juntos Center for Advancing Latino Health, Department of Preventive Medicine and Public Health, University of Kansas Medical Center, 4125 Rainbow Blvd. MS 1056, Kansas City, KS 66160 United States. E-mail: nsuarez@kumc.edu

recorded promotores' activities, total smokers identified by each promotor, cessation plans completed, and referrals to quitlines. We used pre-printed daily activity logs to track outreach activities. Results: A total of 11 promotores completed the 7- session training. Over the course of 4 months, they led 48 community smoking prevention activities, and identified 320 smokers. Promotores identified 5 to 46 smokers each, and referred 167 (52.1%) of all identified smokers to a quitline. Among these, promotores followed-up with 119 (71.2%) and found that 35 (29.4%) smokers developed an assisted quit plan with quitline counselors. Conclusion: Promotores can effectively identify underserved Latino smokers, link them with evidence-based cessation resources, and encourage them to develop quit plans. Promotores may also have a noteworthy impact in the enrollment rates of Latino smokers in quitlines.

Keywords: Promotores de salud, Latinos, smoking cessation, immigrants

INTRODUCTION

Tobacco use remains the leading preventable cause of morbidity and mortality among Latinos in the United States (1-3). Despite the "Clinical Practice Guidelines for Treating Tobacco Use and Dependence" recommendations of counseling and pharmacotherapy to treat smokers, Latinos are significantly less likely than white non-Latinos to receive advice to stop smoking from their healthcare provider or to participate in smoking cessation programs (3-5). Multiple meta-analyses demonstrate support for the efficacy of pharmacotherapy and counseling in increasing abstinence for smokers trying to stop smoking (5). Nationwide state-sponsored telephone counseling quitlines (quitlines) offer smoking cessation counseling in Spanish (6-9) and tailored Spanish-language smoking cessation guides have been developed (10,11).

Despite evidence-based smoking cessation interventions, Latinos report a general lack of knowledge about available smoking cessation resources and perceive a lack of cultural sensitivity within existing Spanish-language resources, particularly immigrants. These variables may contribute to lower use of pharmacotherapy and quitlines (7,12,13). Overall, disadvantageous social conditions (e.g., poverty, education), language barriers, socio-economic factors, healthcare access, and lack of insurance are further obstacles to accessing smoking cessation treatment (14-16). Nonetheless, Latinos have demonstrated a positive attitude toward quitting, and are interested in participating in smoking cessation interventions (13,17,18).

Addressing tobacco related disparities among Latinos require the development of culturally appropriate community-based programs that can increase knowledge and utilization of efficacious smoking cessation treatment resources. Community-based smoking cessation interventions among Latinos have focused on tailored self-help materials, multi-component community interventions, and the use of lay health advisors, also known as promotores de salud (19-24). The broad understanding of promotores is aligned with the notion of natural helpers (25). As described by Israel, natural helpers are trusted people to whom others naturally turn to for advice, emotional support and tangible aid (25). The role of promotores can be particularly important in underserved communities with limited access to health services (26-28). As demonstrated in other studies, promotores can address lack of knowledge by disseminating culturally and linguistically appropriate information on existing appropriate efficacious preventive resources (29,30). Nevertheless, the role of promotores in smoking cessation has not been largely explored.

Smoking cessation interventions incorporating social support for smoking abstinence have been successful in advancing smokers readiness to stop smoking (31). As further explained by Cupertino et al. (32), interventions using promotores are grounded in social cognitive theory (33) wherein health changes occur within a network of social influence. Studies have found that in Latino communities, social support networks serve complementary roles as sources of support, advice, social interaction and role models (25,26,32).

Social networks may be beneficial for impacting tobacco use and promoting healthy behavior change. Therefore, promotores–as community health workers who are simultaneously members of their own community and part of extended social networks- may also serve as a source of active social support and health behavior change (32).

Several promotores trainings have successfully engaged its participants in positive behavior change (e.g., health belief model, stages of change) (34), but the feasibility of connecting Latino smokers to evidence-based cessation treatment using promotores merits further consideration. Our study examined the role of promotores to refer Latino smokers to existing smoking cessation resources rather than implementing the counseling themselves. Our training program was developed to: 1) identify smokers within their communities, 2) help them to develop quit plans, 3) link smokers with a Spanish-language quitline, and 4) assess quit attempts.

METHODS

In 2005, researchers from the Department of Preventive Medicine and Public Health at the University of Kansas Medical Center (KUMC) established a community-based participatory research (CBPR) program with El Centro, Inc, the largest community social services organization in the greater Kansas City area, to reduce cancer-related health disparities among Latinos (please refer to Cupertino et al. (32) for further details about our CBPR partnership).

Our CBPR partnership got awarded a grant in 2006 from Health Care Foundation of Greater Kansas City to implement a promotores program. As a result, together we have implemented the training of promotores to reduce cancer-related disparities (35,36), as detailed in table 1. We developed a 30 hour training program to empower promotores to identify health needs and assets in an area with a high concentration of Latinos. Training included field work accompanied by skills development in leadership, organization, interpersonal relationships, and survey implementation. Upon completion of the training, promotores conducted household surveys designed to identify community health needs (29). Approximately 1 out of 5 households had at least one smoker. Consequently, we decided to focus our intervention on smoking as a key health behavior. Together we developed and received funding to implement a smoking cessation referral program with promotores whose results are reported in this paper.

**Table 1. Community-Academic Partnership Implementing CBPR Principles in
Promotores de Salud Program**

Year	CBPR principles	Implementing CBPR principles in this study
2005	Community-academic partnership established	KUMC and El Centro, Inc. wrote a grant together to train *promotores* de salud and conduct health needs assessments in an area with a high concentration of Latino immigrants.
2006	Community identifies their health concern	Promotores reviewed results from their health needs assessment, considering the high number of household smokers, promotores agreed to focus on cessation.
2007	Community share leadership toguide decision-making	Promotores have participated and continue to participate in all steps of the project. Leadership, budget and decision making is shared in this project.
		We wrote a grant with El Centro to implement a promotores de salud smoking cessation training program in the community.
2008	Community is engaged in research design, including defining research questions	We develop, train, implement and evaluate a promotores de salud program to assess smoking prevalence and promote cessation in the community.
		Promotores de salud, academic and community organization's staff met weekly during the development of this study.
		With 11 promotores de salud, we conducted the first health needs assessment in an area with high concentration of Latinos - 23.8% of households have at least one smoker.
2009	Community guides researchers to effective recruitment strategies	The first generation of promotores de salud recruited the following cohort of promotores. Community Advisory Board (CAB) actively supported recruitment.
	Community collaborates ininterpretation and dissemination of findings	We relied on the results of promotores' health needs assessment to develop this study. We continuously shared the results with promotores de salud, and the community.
2010-Present	Community collaborates in adapting and disseminating models and findings	The CBPR partnership has been co-authoring all publications along with fellow investigators and community members. Together they define dissemination activities in both academic and community settings.
		We are currently writing a grant for promotores to increase awareness about risks of smoking among Latino families.

Table 2. Promotores de Salud Training Curriculum

Topic	Objective	Training Content and Learner Objectives	Feedback & Troubleshoot
1. Pre-Assessment	To demonstrate their knowledge on cigarettes.	Promotores de salud discussed their knowledge on cigarettes and received overall information on the smoking cessation training.	N/A
		1) Articulate the purpose of the program and affirm interest in participating in the program. 2) Identify two personal strengths that will help them be an effective link to the community.	

Topic	Objective	Training Content and Learner Objectives	Feedback & Troubleshoot
2. Communication Skills	To increase their communication skills.	Promotores de salud role played different scenarios as smokers and non-smokers to explore conflict.	As a group, promotores gave their feedback on the scenarios.
		1) Understand what conflict resolution is. 2) Be able to reach an agreement without creating conflict.	
3. Stages of Change	To learn about the different stages smokers go through to quit smoking.	Promotores de salud role played different scenarios demonstrating four stages of changes (pre-contemplation, contemplation, preparation and action).	Promotores were divided into small groups; feedback was provided by research team and promotores within each group.
		1) Understand the different stages of change. 2) To know the appropriate approach depending on the stages of change the smoker is on.	
4. Smoking and Nicotine Dependence	To gain a broad understanding of the addictive nature of tobacco use.	Promotores de salud learned that nicotine is an addictive substance, the properties of nicotine, effects of tobacco use and symptoms of nicotine withdrawal, and the behavioral, pharmacological, and emotional components related to tobacco use.	As a group, promotores discussed each scenario and gave their feedback.
		1) Articulate the difference between tobacco use as a habit and tobacco use as an addiction. 2) Learn the appropriate approach depending on symptoms of nicotine withdrawal. 3) Articulate two primary community resources: quitline, pharmacotherapy assistance.	
5. Smoking cessation medications	To learn about the smoking cessation medication.	Promotores de salud learned about the smoking cessation medication and pharmaceutical assistance programs.	Promotores were divided into small groups; feedback was provided by research team and promotores within each group.
		1) Identify two types of nicotine replacement and two types of non-nicotine medication (Zyban, Chantix). 2) Articulate why medication may aid cessation. 3) Refer to the pharmaceutical assistance programs.	
6. Counseling	To learn about the existing resources in the community, such as counseling.	Promotores de salud learned about telephone counseling quitlines, and behavioral strategies for aiding smoking abstinence. They interacted with counselors to understand the counseling procedures.	Promotores were divided into small groups; feedback was provided by research team and promotores within each group.
		1) Understand the counseling procedure. 2) Give an example of how social factors could influence behavior change. 3) Identify a goal for someone not thinking of quitting, and someone wanting to quit.	

Table 2. (Continued)

Topic	Objective	Training Content and Learner Objectives	Feedback & Troubleshoot
7. Talking to adolescents	To learn how to disseminate information to adolescents.	Promotores de salud learned the appropriate communication skills to approach the adolescents.	Promotores were divided into small groups; feedback was provided by research team and promotores within each group.

Participants

Fourteen trained Spanish-speaking Latino immigrant community members were invited to participate in a smoking cessation community-based training curriculum. Training used an interactive approach focusing on increasing smoking cessation, developing skills to recruit and identify smokers in the community, and motivate them to develop a quit plan with a quitline. Most importantly, promotores were trained to serve as a support for behavior change by increasing awareness, knowledge, and facilitating access to resources. Among the fourteen promotores, eleven completed the smoking cessation training, and implemented community-based smoking cessation outreach and referral activities.

Training curriculum

Our training curriculum, as described in detail in Cupertino et al. (in review) (29), was developed based on the "Empowerment Education - Popular Pedagogy" framework developed by Paulo Freire (37). Within this framework, the individual is encouraged to actively participate and take responsibility for one's own education. The community, through the process of interacting with knowledge, is empowered to improve health in the community (37). As recommended by Freire's model of active learning participation, our curriculum aimed to engage promotores in having a dialogue during training sessions, and included interactive activities to expand their learning.

The training program consisted of 7 sessions of approximately 2 hours each. Sessions were conducted in Spanish. Refreshments and child care were provided to support feasibility of program participation. El Centro, Inc.'s promotores' program director, coordinators, and study staff planned, outlined, and implemented each session, as detailed in Table 2.

Training was divided into three main components: 1) Comprehensive knowledge on tobacco; 2) Nicotine dependence, smoking cessation stages, and smoking cessation medications; 3) Disseminating smoking cessation information in a culturally and linguistically appropriate manner.

In order to enrich the learning experience, each training session included a role-play activity that helped promotores understand the 3 main training components, and develop skills to apply concepts. Minimum reading was required and most sessions relied on visual materials. At the end of each session, promotores were assisted in creating a summary of the objectives and goals reached individually and as a group, as detailed in Table 2. At the final session, promotores signed a confidentiality agreement (pledge), which included a list of outreach preferences (health fairs, home visits, etc.), and time availability for the next 6 months.

Outreach activities

Smoking cessation community outreach activities were an effort carried forward by promotores. They aimed to promote knowledge about smoking cessation resources (such as medications and quitlines), identify Latino smokers, and refer them to a quitline. All smoking cessation community outreach activities were conducted in Spanish. Based on their preferences, promotores conducted these activities at Latino-owned businesses, churches, health fairs, households, and the Consulate of Mexico in the Kansas City area. Promotores set information booths at each visited location, and approached participants with the purpose of disseminating information on the hazards of tobacco consumption and benefits of quitting smoking.

For each outreach activity, promotores were provided with a training summary card featuring the types of smokers, important tobacco facts, and main facts on smoking cessation medications (bupoprion, varenicline, and nicotine replacement therapy (NRT)), a booth sign-in sheet, and educational material about available resources in Spanish.

Individuals who reported being smokers were invited to enroll in the quitline. Upon agreement, promotores helped smokers fill out the quitline enrollment form on site. Promotores were reimbursed for time and transportation for participating in outreach activities and in the smoker identification process.

Measures

Promotores' characteristics
Promotores de Salud completed a socio-demographic survey assessing years lived in the United States (if foreign-born) and in Kansas, race, educational attainment, current employment status, number of household members, current smoking status, household smoking rules (if any), and number of smokers within their social network.

Training and outreach activities

Smoker identification and referral
Promotores received a pre-printed contact diary to prompt them to describe each encounter in terms of: person's name, contact information, referral type (previously known, casual contact, meeting contact, third party referral, self-referred); topic discussed, handout given, perceived efficacy of the encounter, follow-up activities, and overall comments. Our CBPR team was available at weekly meetings to support and troubleshoot the implementation of promotores' activities.

At the end of the training, we mapped promotores' network and monitored activities for 4 months. We observed and recorded promotores' activities and their individual progress towards identifying smokers, developing a quit plan and referring smokers to resources. In ongoing tracking activities meetings, promotores shared experiences and strategies with each other. Those with lower levels of community engagement were encouraged to try strategies identified as successful. At weekly tracking meetings, promotores faxed their referral forms and left a copy of the fax with the promotores group leader.

We closely monitored attendance and completion of smoking cessation activities. Promotores' activities were tracked, as well as each promotor's progress towards identifying smokers and referring them to a quitline.

Trained promotores referred identified smokers to a quitline using fax referral forms. To monitor cessation plans including referral to quitline, we maintained record of the number of participants completing the fax referral forms. Promotores brought fax referral forms to weekly meetings. El Centro, Inc. staff faxed forms to Kansas or Missouri quitlines and tracked the number of fax referral forms sent to the quitline.

Additionally, the quitline sent monthly reports describing call volume for Latinos and identifying who referred them. Smokers that were not ready to quit received mailed educational material but were not enrolled in the quitline. Monthly reports were used to identify participants enrolled in the quitline for an assisted quitting attempt. After 2 months, promotores called participants to further support their quitting process.

RESULTS

Of the 11 promotores de salud who completed training all were female immigrants born in Mexico, had a high school degree or less, were homemakers, and had lived in the state of Kansas for 9 years or less. None of the promotores were current smokers, and all had smoking restrictions in their home. Approximately one third reported having family members who were smokers and reported knowing at least 1 smoker in their social network.

Training and outreach activities

The rate of attendance at the training sessions was 92.2%. Trained promotores implemented a total of 48 culturally and linguistically-tailored smoking awareness outreach activities over a period of 4 months in order to effectively disseminate smoking cessation information. Promotores conducted events at 13 Latino-owned businesses, 6 churches, 7 health fairs, 9 events at the Consulate of Mexico, and 13 home visits with groups of youth and families from the community.

At outreach activities, promotores spoke to community members about the hazards of tobacco consumption and benefits of smoking cessation. Promotores reached a total of 465 individuals: home visits alone reached one third of all participants (32.2%); outreach activities at churches reached 14.8% of participants, and health fairs 10.1%.

Smoker identification and referral

Promotores identified 320 Latino smokers and 167 (52.1%) were referred to the quitline by using a signed fax referral form. Three of the promotores identified 60% of all referred Latino smokers, as highlighted in Figure 1.

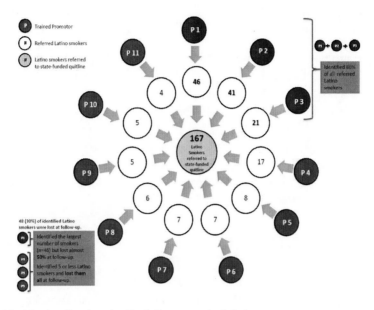

Figure 1. Identified Latino Smokers by Each Promotor de Salud.

Among the 167 Latino smokers referred to a quitline, 119 (71.2%) were successfully reached by promotores for additional follow-up support, while 48 (28.8%) were lost at follow-up due to difficulties in being reached by promotores. Among the 119 Latino smokers reached at follow up by promotores, a total of 35 (29.4%) developed an assisted quit plan by working with quitline counselors, as confirmed by the Kansas and Missouri quitlines month report. The remaining Latino smokers (70.6%) identified by promotores expressed not being ready to develop a quit plan, as shown in Figure 2. Participants who were not ready to quit smoking received educational material from a quitline.

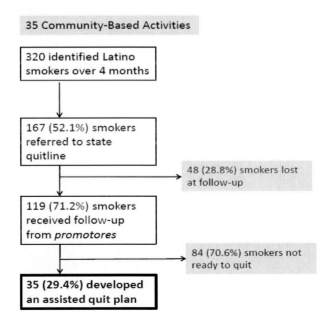

Figure 2. Identified Latino Smokers Referred to a State Quitline by Promotores de Salud.

DISCUSSION

Our community–academic partnership aimed to develop, implement and evaluate a training of Promotores de Salud for the dissemination of smoking cessation resources. In this study, we demonstrated the feasibility of trained promotores to enhance the utilization of evidence-based smoking cessation resources (i.e. state-sponsored telephone counseling quitlines), with the long-term goals of enhancing tobacco use treatment and improving Latino health. This study highlights the engagement of promotores addressing cessation as an opportunity of sustainable community change to address its own health needs (38). Promotores identified the need of disseminating smoking cessation information, and as such, developed activities based on their preferences, and community knowledge.

Training and outreach activities

Findings indicate that promotores had a nearly 100% training attendance rate. Steady participation and engagement in the promotores training was key to the success of the overall promotores dissemination activities. Our high attendance rate indicates that the training program's contents, format, and duration were acceptable to promotores. Most importantly, findings indicate that our training has also contributed to the increased community involvement. Promotores –actively representing the community they serve- contribute to the sustainability and growth of community health worker programs addressing smoking cessation and improving community's overall health.

We found that home visits with adults and youth, as well as outreach activities at churches and community health fairs, were successful venues for reaching Latino smokers, and enrolling them in quitlines. Our findings indicate that trained promotores have skills to effectively reach large numbers of Latino immigrants and recruit smokers in diverse community settings (i.e., health fairs, church congregations, home visits etc). Future studies should further explore the impact of diverse geographical locations of health-focused community-based interventions in reaching, recruiting and treating Latino smokers.

Despite several promotores programs being successful in increasing immunization rates, cancer screening and reaching special populations (21,26), a recent Cochrane review on community health workers showed that few studies have tested the promotores model among Latinos (39) and to our knowledge, only two studies have tested the use of promotores for smoking cessation among Latinos (21,40). Although studies show that promotores play an important role in reaching Latino smokers, the Cochrane review did not connect participants to existing resources and did not use individuals' social networks. In contrast, a community-based intervention using promotores reported an increase in smoking abstinence within Latino communities (21), and showed that promotores can be a culturally appropriate way to facilitate smoking abstinence. In a recent survey of 141 Latino smokers, 76% reported a preference to have smoking cessation programs that included promotores as community health educators (41). Promotores' thriving outreach skills contributed to the feasibility of the overall program.

Smoker identification and referral

Promotores varied significantly in number of outreach activities conducted and number of smokers identified. As indicated in the results, three of the 11 promotores identified 60% of smokers, thus showing that promotores are highly effective in reaching Latino smokers (13,17,18,21). Our findings also highlight that promotores can have a noteworthy impact in the enrollment rates of Latino smokers in quitlines. According to MOQL (Missouri Tobacco Quitline) data collected between July 1, 2005 and June 30, 2009, there were a total of 15,872 tobacco user callers among which only 2% were Latino smokers (42). In other words, during that 4 year period, MOQL received an average of 87 Latino tobacco user callers per year. Yet, in our study, promotores identified and referred 60 Latino smokers to the MOQL in just four months, thus representing 68.9% of MOQL's reported annual Latino tobacco user callers in the 2005-2009 period.

Supporting the literature (13,17,18,21), Latino smokers in our study were interested in getting connected to smoking cessation resources, as promotores referred nearly half of all identified smokers to a quitline. The remaining Latino smokers referred to a quitline by promotores who reported at follow-up not being ready to quit could perhaps have benefited from additional motivational sessions before making the decision to establish a quit plan. These findings indicate the success of promotores de salud in identifying immigrant Latino smokers and developing quit plans. Ultimately, promotores could possibly enhance the utilization of evidence-based smoking cessation resources in the Latino community.

Limitations

This study relied on a small convenience sample. The disadvantage of a small convenience sample is that it may not necessarily be representative of the studied population (i.e., Latino smokers in the studied community). The selection of participants also does not guarantee that the sample was free of bias. Moreover, due to the diversity of the Latino population, these findings should not be compared to other Latino communities in other American cities. Nonetheless, despite the data's limitations, this study does reflect general trends identified by other scholars. Furthermore, our study encountered limitations collecting quitline data. This study found that quitelines had a significant follow-up loss of Latino smokers identified and referred by promotores. Quitlines have a minimum reach in the Latino community; promotores could potentially address this issue by increasing community awareness and use of quitlines.

Further trainings

Although it was not our goal to have promotores serve as smoking cessation counselors, promotores reported a lack of knowledge on smoking cessation medications, motivation skills, or withdrawal symptoms. Future efforts should examine training methods of enhancing promotores' skills and knowledge on smoking cessation treatment. Quitlines have a limited reach in the Latino community; promotores could potentially address this issue by increasing community awareness and use of quitlines. Future studies should closely monitor the loss of motivated smokers after they are referred to state quitline. Our study highlights the sustainability of engaging promotores de salud in the identification and referral of Latino smokers to adequate treatment in order to address tobacco-related disparities and improve the overall health of this underserved community.

ACKNOWLEDGMENTS

This program was supported by a grant awarded to El Centro, Inc. from the Health Care Foundation of Greater Kansas City. We appreciate the efforts of community members, our community partners, and the promotores de salud: Yajaira Arias, Luz Mireya Rios, Aida Apodaca, Catalina Reyes, Erika Suarez, Carolina Delgado, Maria Elena Almanza, Patricia Arias, Amalia Callejas, Alma Rosa Garcia. Special thanks to Mary Lou Jaramillo, Cielo Fernandez and Elizabeth Reynoso from El Centro, Inc. for their ongoing support.

REFERENCES

[1]	ACS. Cancer facts and figures for Hispanics/Latinos 2009-2011. Atlanta, GA: ACS, 2011.
[2]	CDC. REACH surveillance for health status minority communities - United States 2001-2002. MMWR 2004;53(ss6):1-36.
[3]	USDHHS. Tobacco use among US. racial/ethnic minority groups,African Americans, American Indians and Alaska Natives, Asian Americans and Pacific Islanders, and Hispanics: A report of the Surgeon General. Rockville, MD: US Department Health Human Services, 1998.
[4]	Levinson AH, Perez-Stable EJ, Espinoza P, Flores ET, Byers TE. Latinos report less use of pharmaceutical aids when trying to quit smoking. Am J Prev Med 2004;26(2):105-11.
[5]	Fiore M, Jaen, CR, Baker, TB. Treating tobacco use and dependence: 2008 update. Rockville, MD: US Department Health Human Services, 2008.
[6]	Martinez-Bristow Z, Sias JJ, Urquidi UJ, Feng C. Tobacco cessation services through community health workers for Spanish-speaking populations. Am J Public Health 2006;96(2):211-3.
[7]	Bock BC, Niaura RS, Neighbors CJ, Carmona-Barros R, Azam M. Differences between Latino and non-Latino White smokers in cognitive and behavioral characteristics relevant to smoking cessation. Addict Behav 2005;30(4):711-24.
[8]	Perez-Stable EJ, Marin BV, Marin G. A comprehensive smoking cessation program for the San Francisco Bay Area Latino community: Programa Latino Para Dejar de Fumar. Am J Health Promot 1993;7(6):430-42,75.
[9]	Marin G, Perez-Stable EJ. Effectiveness of disseminating culturally appropriate smoking-cessation information: Programa Latino Para Dejar de Fumar. J Natl Cancer Inst Monogr 1995;18:155-63.
[10]	Perez-Stable EJ, Marin G, Posner SF. Ethnic comparison of attitudes and beliefs about cigarette smoking. J Gen Intern Med 1998;13(3):167-74.
[11]	Perez-Stable EJ, Ramirez A, Villareal R, Talavera GA, Trapido E, Suarez L, et al. Cigarette smoking behavior among US Latino men and women from different countries of origin. Am J Public Health 2001;91(9): 1424-30.
[12]	Levinson AH, Borrayo EA, Espinoza P, Flores ET, Perez-Stable EJ. An exploration of Latino smokers and the use of pharmaceutical aids. Am J Prev Med 2006;31(2):167-71.
[13]	Wetter DW, Mazas C, Daza P, Nguyen L, Fouladi RT, Li Y, et al. Reaching and treating Spanish-speaking smokers through the National Cancer Institute's Cancer Information Service. A randomized controlled trial. Cancer 2007;109(2 Suppl):406-13.

[14] Zuniga E, Castaneda X, Averbach A, Wallace SP. Mexican and Central American immigrants in the United State: Health care access. Los Angeles, CA: Regents University California, Mexican Secretariat Health, 2006

[15] Sherrill W, Crew L, Mayo RB, Mayo WF, Rogers BL, Haynes DF. Educational and health services innovation to improve care for rural Hispanic communities in the USA. Rural Remote Health 2005;5(4):402.

[16] Foraker RE, Patten CA, Lopez KN, Croghan IT, Thomas JL. Beliefs and attitudes regarding smoking among young adult Latinos: a pilot study. Prev Med 2005;41(1):126-33.

[17] Serrano VA, Woodruff SI. Smoking-related attitudes and their sociodemographic correlates among Mexican-origin adult smokers. J Commun Health 2003;28(3):209-20.

[18] Cupertino AP, Cox LS, Richter K, Ellerbeck EF. A pilot study of a decision-aid tool for smoking cessation among Latinos. Portland, OR: Society Research Nicotine Tobacco, 2008.

[19] Perez-Stable EJ, Marin BV, Marin G, Brody DJ, Benowitz NL. Apparent underreporting of cigarette consumption among Mexican American smokers. Am J Public Health 1990;80(9):1057-61.

[20] Nevid JS, Javier RA, Moulton JL, 3rd. Factors predicting participant attrition in a community-based, culturally specific smoking-cessation program for Hispanic smokers. Health Psychol 1996;15(3):226-9.

[21] Woodruff SI, Talavera GA, Elder JP. Evaluation of a culturally appropriate smoking cessation intervention for Latinos. Tob Control 2002;11(4):361-7.

[22] Cabral DN, Napoles-Springer AM, Miike R, McMillan A, Sison JD, Wrensch MR, et al. Population- and community-based recruitment of African Americans and Latinos: the San Francisco Bay Area Lung Cancer Study. Am J Epidemiol 2003;158(3):272-9.

[23] Baezconde-Garbanati L, Beebe LA, Perez-Stable EJ. Building capacity to address tobacco-related disparities among American Indian and Hispanic/Latino communities: conceptual and systemic considerations. Addiction 2007;102 Suppl 2:112-22.

[24] Cox L, Okuyemi K, Choi W, Ahluwalia J. A review of tobacco use treatments in U.S. ethnic minority populations. Am J Health Promot 2011;25(5S):S11-S30.

[25] Israel BA. Social networks and social support: implications for natural helper and community level interventions. Health Educ Q 1985;12(1):65-80.

[26] Lewin SA, Dick J, Pond P, Zwarenstein M, Aja G, van Wyk B, et al. Lay health workers in primary and community health care. Cochrane Database Syst Rev 2005;1:CD004015.

[27] Rhodes SD, Foley KL, Zometa CS, Bloom FR. Lay health advisor interventions among Hispanics/Latinos: a qualitative systematic review. Am J Prev Med 2007;33(5):418-27.

[28] Andrews JO, Felton G, Wewers ME, Heath J. Use of community health workers in research with ethnic minority women. J Nurs Scholarsh 2004;36(4):358-65.

[29] Cupertino AP, Suarez N, Sandreson Cox L, Fernandez C, Jaramillo ML, Morgan A, et al. Empowering promotores de salud to engage in community-based participatory research. J Immigr Refugee Stud Rev, in press.

[30] Scarinci IC, Bandura L, Hidalgo B, Cherrington A. Development of a theory-based (PEN-3 and Health Belief Model), culturally relevant intervention on cervical cancer prevention among Latina immigrants using intervention mapping. Health Promot Pract 2011, in press.

[31] Patten C, Offord K., Hurt R, Cox LS, Croghan I, Wolter T, et al. Training persons to intervene with a smoker to promote cessation. Paper presented at the Seventh Annual Meeting of the Society for Research on Nicotine and Tobacco, Seattle, WA, 2001.

[32] Cupertino AP, Berg CJ, Gajewski B, Hui SK, Richter K, Catley D, Ellerbeck E. Change in self-efficacy, autonomous and controlled motivation predicting smoking. J Health Psychol. 2011 Nov 10. [Epub ahead of print]

[33] Bandura A. Self efficacy: The exercise of control. New York: Freeman, 1997.

[34] Scarinci IC, Johnson R, Hardy C, Marron J, Partridge E. Planning and implementation of a participatory evaluation strategy: A viable approach in the evaluation of community-based participatory programs addressing cancer sisparities. Evaluat Program Plann 2009;32(3): 221-8.

[35] Paulette C, Jurado C, Mendoza I. Promotores de Salud. Kansas City, KS: Angeles del Cielo, 2009.

[36] Mendoza I, Cox LS, Fernandez C, Reynoso E, Garrett S, Suarez N, et al. Community-based training curriculum for Promotores de Salud. Baltimore, MD: Society Research Nicotine Tobacco, 2010.

[37] Wallerstein N, Bernstein E. Empowerment education: Freire's ideas adapted to health education. Health Educ Q 1988;15(4):379-94.

[38] Morgan A. Training Promotores de Salud for Door to Door Community Assessments. Kansas Ciy, KS: University Kansas Medical Center, 2009.

[39] Navarro AM, Senn KL, McNicholas LJ, Kaplan RM, Roppe B, Campo MC. Por La Vida model intervention enhances use of cancer screening tests among Latinas. Am J Prev Med 1998;15(1):32-41.

[40] Leischow SJ, Hill A, Cook G. The effects of transdermal nicotine for the treatment of Hispanic smokers. Am J Health Behav 1996;20(5):304-11.

[41] Cox LS, Cupertino AP, Tercyak KP. Interest in Participating in Smoking Cessation Programs among Latino Primary Care Patients. J Clin Psychol Med Settings 2011, in press.

[42] Kayani N, Homan SG, Yun S, Warren VF. Missouri Tobacco Quitline Report, 2010. Jefferson City, MO: Missouri Department Health Senior Services, Division Community Public Health, 2010.

Submitted: October 10, 2011. *Revised:*December 04, 2011. *Accepted:* December 12, 2011.

In: Public Health Yearbook 2012
Editor: Joav Merrick

ISBN: 978-1-62808-078-0
© 2013 Nova Science Publishers, Inc.

Chapter 34

DEVELOPMENTAL DELAY IN CHILDREN WITH BLOOD LEAD LEVELS BETWEEN 5 AND 9 µG/DL

*Edmond A Hooker, MD, DrPH[*1], Marilyn Goldfeder, RN, MPH[2], Jeff Armada, BS[1], Monica Burns, BS[1], Nicholas Lander, BS[1] and Aaron Senich, BS[1]*

[1]Department of Health Administration, Xavier University, Cincinnati, Ohio and
[2]Lead Prevention Program, Cincinnati Health Department, Cincinnati, Ohio,
United States of America

ABSTRACT

It is estimated that 250,000 children in the United States age 1 to 5 years old have blood lead levels (BLL) above 10 micrograms per liter (µg/dl). However, clinical studies indicate that children with BLL between 5-9 µg/dl are at higher risk and also require intervention. The Cincinnati Health Department (CHD) evaluates all children less than 6 years old with BLLs from 5-9 µg/dl using the Denver II Developmental Screening Test (Denver II). Methods: Children aged less than 6 years who had BLLs of 5-9 µg/dl were evaluated by CHD public health nurses and screened for developmental delay using the Denver II. Proportion of patients with an abnormal Denver II was calculated using descriptive statistics and confounding was controlled for using regression analysis. Results: A total of 419 children were identified with BLLs of 5-9 µg/dl. The results of the Denver II included: 203 (48%; 95% CI 43-53%) were normal, 60 (14%; 95% CI 11-18%) were normal with only one caution, 103 (25%; 95% CI 21-29%) were suspect with one or more delays (and any number of cautions), 53 (13%; 95% CI 10-16%) were suspect with more than one caution (no delays). However, there was no evidence for a dose-response relationship between BLLs within the range of 5-9 µg/dl. Conclusion: A significant number of children with BLL of 5-9 µg/dl have evidence of developmental delay, as measured by the Denver II Developmental Screening Test. All children with elevated BLLs should be screened for developmental delay.

---

* Correspondence: Edmond A Hooker, MD, DrPH, Associate Professor, Department of Health Administration, Xavier University, 3800 Victory Parkway, ML 5141, Cincinnati, Ohio 45207-5141 United States. E-mail: ehooker@mac.com

Keywords: Lead poisoning, blood lead level, lead, Denver Developmental Screening Test

INTRODUCTION

Lead poisoning is extremely dangerous and can lead to serious and irreversible damage to humans. Although lead poisoning can damage many different organs, the damage to the central nervous system (CNS) is particularly concerning. Lead is a pervasive neurotoxicant and can lead to permanent neurological impairment and even death (1).

In the United States, the recognition of the dangers of exposure to environmental lead finally resulted in the banning of lead in house paint in 1978 and gasoline for on-road vehicles in 1986 (2). Because of these interventions, mean blood lead levels and percent of children with blood lead levels (BLL) at or above 10 µg/dl have dropped considerably in the United States over the last 20 years (3). Lead is still commonly found in the environment, and in cities with older housing, lead poisoning still occurs frequently. Although there is likely no safe BLL, the Centers for Disease Control and Prevention (CDC) has set the actionable level at 10 µg/dl. Over the last half- century, the CDC has progressively lowered the actionable BLL (4). In 1960, only BLLs of greater than 60 µg/dl were considered actionable. This was lowered many times, and since 1991, BLLs of 10 µg/dl are considered actionable (4). The concern is that this has lead some in public health to consider only individuals with levels of greater than 10 µg/dl to be poisoned (5). However, when the CDC established the BLL of 10 µg/dl at which action was recommended, they recognized that harm may occur at much lower levels (6). In recent years, increasing evidence has indicated that much lower levels may be toxic and require intervention (5,7,8).

The CDC has recommended that, if possible, children with blood lead levels below 10 µg/dl should undergo developmental screening (6). In order to improve the outcomes for children with elevated blood lead levels and to attempt to prevent children from getting BLLs greater than or equal to 10µg/dl, the Cincinnati Health Department (CHD) has developed a special program dedicated to the primary prevention of lead poisoning. This program includes the long term goals of improving outcomes for children with elevated lead levels and attempting to prevent children currently testing in the 5 to 9 µg/dl range from having higher BLLs. In Cincinnati all children with a confirmed (venous blood draw, or two capillary blood draws within 90 days of each other) BLL equal to or greater than 10 µg/dl are referred to the State of Ohio for follow up and intervention. Children under the age of 6 years, who have a confirmed BLL in the 5 to 9 µg/dl range and who live within the city of Cincinnati, can be referred by their clinic or pediatrician to the Lead Primary Prevention Program. This is a home visiting program. During the home visit these children undergo screening for developmental delay using the Denver II Developmental Screening Test (Denver II) (9). Referrals for a suspect screen are as follows. Children who are three years of age or older are referred to the Cincinnati Public School system for more extensive testing by early childhood development specialists. Children under the age of three are usually referred to the Help Me Grow program (HMG), Ohio's birth to age three program. The Ohio Department of Health, Bureau of Early Intervention Services (BEIS) is the lead agency administering the HMG program in Ohio. Occasionally a child's family prefers a referral to another local agency. It is the purpose of this paper to report on the results of developmental screening of children aged 6 years and younger with BLLs of 5 to 9 µg/dl.

METHODS

Children from age 9 months to 72 months, who live in the city of Cincinnati and who were found to have a BLL of 5 to 9 μg/dl, were referred to the Lead Primary Prevention Program of the Cincinnati Health Department (CHD). A reference laboratory, with accuracy to +/- 1 μg/dl, performed all BLLs. The program began in May of 2007, and all children entered into the program from that date until December 2009 were eligible for inclusion in the study.

All children who were referred to the program were screened once using the Denver II. Each screening test was administered a registered nurse at the patient's home. Each registered nurse had been trained to perform the Denver II screening exam. Denver II is a 125 item developmental screening tool for children from birth to 6 years that assesses four domains of development: Personal-Social, Fine Motor-Adaptive, Language, and Gross motor. Each item is scored pass or failure. Each pass or failure is interpreted based on the Denver II normative data. Items that are failed are considered a delay if more than 90% of children of the same age in the normative sample passed the item and a caution if 75-90% of children of the same age in the normative sample passed the item. Results were categorized into four categories: Normal with no cautions or delays, Normal with one caution, Suspect with more than one caution but no delay, and Suspect with one or more delay and any number of caution.

Data collection included patient identification number, age, gender, blood lead levels (BLLs) and the results of the Denver II.

Data analysis

Demographic information was analyzed using descriptive statistics. Means were compared using independent samples t-test, proportions were compared using chi-square, and stepwise regression analysis was utilized to identify significant predictors of an abnormal Denver II test. All test were performed using SPSS version 17.0.0 for Macintosh, August 2008. Chicago: SPSS Inc.

The study was reviewed and approved by the Xavier University Institutional Review Board and the Cincinnati Health Department Institutional Review Board.

RESULTS

During the period between May 2007 and December 2009, a total of 457 children aged 9-72 months were referred to the program and complete records were available for 419. Of the 419 children, 230 (55%) were males and 189 (45%) were females. The results of the Denver II included: 203 (48%; 95% CI 43-53%) were normal, 60 (14%; 95% CI 11-18%) were normal with only one caution, 103 (25%; 95% CI 21-29%) were suspect with one or more delays (and any number of cautions), 53 (13%; 95% CI 10-16%) were suspect with more than one caution (no delays) (see figure 1).

Male gender was associated with a higher percentage of abnormal tests (44% vs. 30% for female gender, p=0.004). This held true even when controlling for BLL and age using regression analysis. Older age (36-72 months) was also associated with more abnormal tests (45% vs. 34% for those aged 9 to 35 months, p=0.036). There was no association between the actual BLL and the percentage of children with an abnormal Denver II (p=0.0493)(see figure 2).

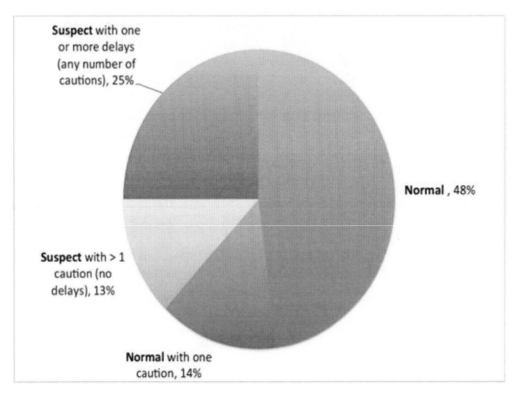

Figure 1. Denver II Developmental Screening Test results in children with Blood Lead Levels between 5 and 9 µg/dl.

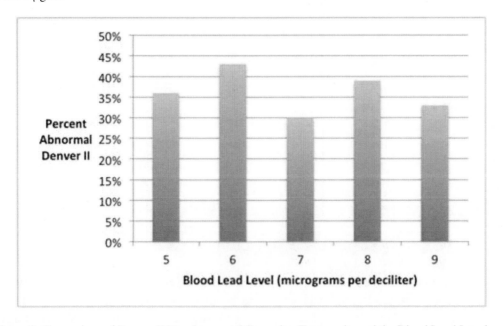

Figure 2. Comparison of Denver II Developmental Screening Test results and the Blood Lead Level.

DISCUSSION

Although the mean BLLs have progressively decreased in the United States over the last 30 years, there are still many children with elevated BLLs (3). Currently, the CDC defines actionable BLL as 10 μg/dl or greater. However, the CDC and many other authors recognize the hazards of levels less than 10 μg/dl (5-8,10). The current research indicates that many children with BLLs between 5 and 9 μg/dl may have developmental delay, as measured by the Denver II Developmental Screening Test. Children with these elevated BLLs were found to have abnormal results on the Denver II in 38% of cases.

The Denver Developmental Screening Test has been used both nationally and internationally since 1967 and was standardized on a group of children without developmental problems (11). The test was subsequently revised in the early 1990s and renamed the Denver II Developmental Screening Test (Denver II). The Denver II was re-standardized on a group of 2096 Colorado children. Although some have questioned the specificity of the Denver II, it is still widely used and respected (12). The advantage of using the test as a screening tool is that it does not require a trained psychologist for administration. The use of the test by the Cincinnati Health Department nurses allows for referral to available resources to help improve developmental outcomes.

The importance of intervention for children with any elevated BLL is highlighted by research into educational attainment. Even levels below 10 μg/dl have been shown to negatively affect later educational attainment and behavior (8,13,14). Muenning, et al. (15) estimate that reducing every child's BLL to less than 1 μg/dl in a single cohort of newborns to 6-years olds would contribute more than a trillion additional dollars to US society during their lifetime. Additionally, children with learning and behavioral problems often are in need of special education, which adds to the financial burden of the public school system (16).

The strength of this study is that shows that a relatively easily administered screening test can be used to identify children with possible developmental delay. Obviously, environmental interventions to mitigate ongoing exposure would also be critical. The program utilizes a well-validated screening tool, and the results are consistent with many other studies indicating that even BLLs of less than 10 μg/dl negatively affect neurodevelopment (8,10,17). However, follow-up formal confirmatory psychological testing results were not available to the researchers. It is possible that some children identified as suspect may have been found to be normal on subsequent testing.

The most recent recommendations from the CDC is that "clinicians should consider referral to developmental programs for children at high risk for exposure to lead and more frequent rescreening of children with blood lead levels approaching 10 μg/dl"(6). The current research shows the feasibility of using the Denver II to screen children at risk for lead poisoning or who have elevated BLLs.

CONCLUSION

A significant number of children less than six years of age with elevated blood lead levels have evidence of developmental delay, as measured by the Denver II Developmental Screening Test. Clinicians need to screen all children with elevated blood lead levels for developmental delay in order to provide early intervention. It is possible that the actionable

BLL might need to be revised to a much lower number than is currently recommended by the CDC.

REFERENCES

[1]   Meyer PA, Brown MJ, Falk H. Global approach to reducing lead exposure and poisoning. Mutat Res 2008;659(1-2):166-75.

[2]   Kovarik W. Ethyl-leaded Gasoline: How. Int J Occup Environ Health 2005;11:384-97.

[3]   Jones RL, Homa DM, Meyer PA, Brody DJ, Caldwell KL, Pirkle JL, et al. Trends in blood lead levels and blood lead testing among US children aged 1 to 5 years, 1988–2004. Pediatrics 2009;123:e376-85.

[4]   Bellinger DC, Bellinger AM. Childhood lead poisoning: the torturous path from science to policy. J Clin Invest 2006;116(4):853-7.

[5]   Gilbert SG, Weiss B. A rationale for lowering the blood lead action level from 10 to 2 [mu] g/dL. Neurotoxicol 2006;27(5):693-701.

[6]   Binns H, Campbell C, Brown M. The Advisory Committee on Childhood Lead Poisoning Prevention. Interpreting and managing blood lead levels of less than 10 µg/dL in children and reducing childhood exposure to lead: Recommendations of the Centers for Disease Control and Prevention Advisory Committee on Childhood Lead Poisoning Prevention. Pediatrics 2007;120:1285-98.

[7]   Jusko TA, Henderson Jr CR, Lanphear BP, Cory-Slechta DA, Parsons PJ, Canfield RL. Blood lead concentrations< 10 µg/dL and child intelligence at 6 years of age. Environ Health Perspect 2008;116(2):243-8.

[8]   Bellinger DC. Very low lead exposures and children's neurodevelopment. Curr Opin Pediatr 2008;20(2):172-7.

[9]   Naar-King S, Ellis DA, Frey MA. Assessing children's well-being: a handbook of measures. Mahwah, NJ: Lawrence Erlbaum, 2004.

[10]   Téllez-Rojo MM, Bellinger DC, Arroyo-Quiroz C, Lamadrid-Figueroa H, Mercado-García A, Schnaas-Arrieta L, et al. Longitudinal associations between blood lead concentrations lower than 10 µg/dL and neurobehavioral development in environmentally exposed children in Mexico City. Pediatrics 2006;118:e323-30.

[11]   Glascoe FP, Byrne KE, Ashford LG, Johnson KL, Chang B, Strickland B. Accuracy of the Denver-II in developmental screening. Pediatrics 1992;89(6):1221-5.

[12]   Glascoe FP. Screening for developmental and behavioral problems. Ment Retard Dev Disabil Res Rev 2005;11(3):173-9.

[13]   Chandramouli K, Steer CD, Ellis M, Emond AM. Effects of early childhood lead exposure on academic performance and behaviour of school age children. Arch Dis Child 2009;94(11):844-8.

[14]   Miranda ML, Kim D, Osgood C, Hastings D. The impact of early childhood lead exposure on educational test performance among Connecticut schoolchildren, Phase 1 Report. Durham, NC: Duke University: Children's Environmental Health Initiative, 2011.

[15]   15   Muennig P. The social costs of childhood lead exposure in the post-lead regulation era. Arch Pediatr Adolesc Med 2009;163(9):844-9.

[16]   Kahn FF. Economic impact of childhood lead poisoning. Oklahoma County Med Soc 2010;83(4):40-3.

[17]   Lanphear BP, Hornung R, Khoury J, Yolton K, Baghurst P, Bellinger DC, et al. Low-level environmental lead exposure and children's intellectual function: an international pooled analysis. Environ Health Perspect 2005;113(7):894-9.

Submitted: November 05, 2011. *Revised:* December 06, 2011. *Accepted:* December 18, 2011.

SECTION FOUR – HIV RESEARCH

In: Public Health Yearbook 2012
Editor: Joav Merrick

Chapter 35

CONDOM USE MEASUREMENT IN ADOLESCENT HIV PREVENTION RESEARCH: IS BRIEFER BETTER?

Christopher D Houck, PhD[1], Angela Stewart, PhD[2], Larry K Brown, MD[1] and the Project SHIELD Study Group*

[1] Bradley/Hasbro Children's Research Center and the Warren Alpert Medical School at Brown University, Providence, Rhode Island and
[2] Bradley Hospital, Providence, Rhode Island, United States of America

ABSTRACT

Self-report measures of condom use are frequently used to determine the efficacy of HIV prevention programs, however, little is known about which condom use formats yield the most reliable data. The current study was conducted to determine how often adolescents respond reliably across three formats of condom use (dichotomous, ordinal, and continuous) and whether participant characteristics are associated with inconsistency. Methods: Survey data were collected from 1,190 adolescents, 15-21 years, participating in a behavioral HIV-prevention trial. Results: Approximately 40% were inconsistent in their reports of condom use. Participant characteristics were not associated with consistency in responding. Conclusion: Single items of condom use may suffice for some purposes, but more precise measurement may require multiple formats.

Keywords: Condom use, measurement, methodology, adolescents

INTRODUCTION

Other than abstinence, correct and consistent condom use is the most effective method for preventing HIV/AIDS. Increasing condom use among adolescents is a target of many HIV prevention interventions, and demonstrating the efficacy of these interventions often relies on

---

* Correspondence: Christopher D Houck, PhD, Bradley/Hasbro Children's Research Center, One Hoppin Street, Suite 204, Providence, RI 02903, United States. Telephone: 401-444-8539. Fax: 401-444-4645. Email: chouck@lifespan.org

establishing condom use behavior change. However, there is no "gold standard" for condom use measurement and all such measures are subject to threats to validity and reliability. A review of the literature identified more than 70 measures of condom use in studies that correlated condom use with sexual risk behavior (1). Among the studies reviewed, the most common formats were ordinal frequency measures asking how often condoms were used (36%), dichotomous formats with yes/no questions about condom use (28%), and proportional measures calculated from the number of protected sexual occasions divided by the total number of sexual occasions (21%).

Little is known about which condom use measurement formats yield the most reliable and valid data among adolescents. One study found that although adolescent reports of sexual behaviors such as engaging in vaginal sex in the last three months (kappa = .72) and number of lifetime sexual partners (intraclass correlation (ICC) = .81) were moderately to highly consistent when test-retest reliability was measured over a two-week period, consistency regarding use of condoms during last sex (kappa = .62) and participant counts of unprotected vaginal sex acts in a three-month period (ICC = .44) were lower, suggesting that condom use measures may be more vulnerable to threats to reliability (2). Another study found significant inconsistencies among college students in their responses on two measures of condom use (3). Sixty-three percent of respondents indicated that using condoms 18-19 out of 20 times represented "always" using a condom; however, one or two unprotected sex acts represents significantly greater risk than zero. Similar results have been found among high-risk heterosexually active adults (4). Together, these studies suggest that condom use measures are also subject to threats to validity.

Little is known about adolescent participant characteristics associated with unreliable reports on measures of condom use. Other literatures provide clues regarding patterns of unreliable responding. From the substance use literature, Farrell and colleagues (5) found that 33% of adolescents provided inconsistent responses between drug use measured dichotomously (yes/no) and continuously (days used in past month). Those who inconsistently responded reported higher rates of nearly half of the drugs measured than those who were consistent, suggesting that inconsistency in response may be associated with more risk behavior. From the adult sexual risk literature, discrepancies in reports of sexual risk behavior based on data collection method are common, such that the average magnitude of combined underreporting and overreporting discrepancies in unprotected sex was 54% when retrospective surveys were compared to a daily diary method (6). Participants, however, tended to underreport with the retrospective measure relative to the daily diary measure, suggesting that responses may vary depending on the type of measure used to collect data. Gender and sexual orientation were related to accuracy of report, such that MSM were more accurate than heterosexual men or women.

Accurate condom use measurement has direct implications for preventing HIV and other STIs and for public health policies. However, researchers often face dilemmas deciding which condom use measures to use with adolescents. The apparent accuracy of partner-by-partner measures of condom use that yield proportion data may be appealing. However, the burden placed on participants, poor recall accuracy for those with many sexual occasions, and participant frustration that may result from being asked many similar questions may be undesirable. Single items that ask respondents to estimate the frequency of condom use may be appealing for their simplicity, yet researchers may be concerned about the accuracy of data collected by this format because of cognitive biases that may influence responses, such as emphasizing recent or salient events or poor estimating skills.

Little information is available regarding the reliability of different formats of condom use assessments with adolescents. Thus, the present study compared congruence of adolescent responses to three formats (dichotomous, ordinal, and continuous) to determine whether these formats yield similar or disparate data. These data are expected to help guide recommendations for researchers in selecting condom use measures for adolescents. This study also examines associations between unreliable responding and participant characteristics (e.g., younger age) to determine whether disparate responses to different condom use formats are associated with greater risk behavior or demographic characteristics of participants. We expected to find congruence for the majority of participants between ordinal and continuous measures, but less agreement between dichotomous assessment (i.e., condom use at last intercourse) and the other formats (e.g., proportion of condom use) because a single protected or unprotected sex act may not be representative of a pattern of sexual behavior. We anticipated no demographic associations with unreliability as there was no literature among adolescents to support such hypotheses, but expected that more sex risk behavior (e.g., having sex with someone the same day they met) and more general risk behavior (e.g., legal arrests) would be related to greater unreliability in responding since greater frequency of risky behaviors may make accurate recall more difficult (5,7,8).

METHODS

Detailed study procedures for Project SHIELD, an HIV prevention program, are described elsewhere (9). Data were collected as part of a multi-site, randomized trial of a brief HIV prevention intervention for adolescents ages 15 to 21 from three US cities (Providence, RI; Atlanta, GA; Miami, FL). Data for the present analyses were available from 1,190 adolescents. Adolescents were recruited for Project SHIELD from primary care clinics and through outreach activities, including posters, flyers, street outreach, and referrals from friends. Adolescents were privately screened to determine whether they were eligible for the study. The inclusion criterion was having engaged in at least one episode of unprotected vaginal or anal sex in the past 90 days. Exclusion criteria were being currently pregnant, attempting to become pregnant, having given birth in the last 90 days, or currently participating in another HIV prevention study. Adolescents were also excluded if they self-reported being HIV-positive, as the aim of the study was primary prevention.

Rhode Island Hospital, Miriam Hospital, University of Miami, and Emory University institutional review boards approved study procedures, and informed consent was obtained from all participants or their guardians. Adolescents completed baseline assessments via audio computer-assisted self-interview (ACASI) to ensure privacy. Assessments were conducted either individually or in a group format with research staff present to answer questions and ensure privacy. Calendars and scripted cues were provided to assist in recall of 90-day time periods. Participants were compensated $50 for their time and effort.

The questionnaire was largely derived from measures used in an HIV prevention trial for high-risk young adults, Project LIGHT, where they demonstrated adequate internal reliability and sensitivity to intervention impact (10). On average, the ACASI took approximately 45 minutes to complete and assessed variables previously shown to be related to HIV risk, including engaging in sex with someone in the past 90 days whom the participant had met the same day, age at first sexual intercourse, a history of previous suicide attempt, and arrest histories (11-14). Questions related to condom use appeared in the first third of the questionnaire, following a series of demographic questions. Urine assays were conducted for three sexually transmitted infections (STIs): gonorrhea, Chlamydia, and trichomoniasis.

Condom use was measured in three formats, in the following order: dichotomous, ordinal, and continuous. 1) For the dichotomous measure, participants were asked to consider their last episode of vaginal or anal sex and respond either "yes" or "no" to the question "The last time you had sex, did you or the other person use a condom?" 2) For the ordinal measure, participants were asked to respond to the question "In the last 90 days, how often did you use a condom when you had vaginal or anal sex?" with five options: "never," "less than half the time," "about half the time," "more than half the time," and "always." The dichotomous and ordinal measures were separated by three questions, on separate screens, related to substance use during sex and recent sexual activity. 3) Finally, for the continuous measure, the proportion of times a condom was used was calculated for each participant. Participants reported the number of partners with whom they had had vaginal or anal sex in the past 90 days. For up to three partners, participants reported the number of vaginal and anal intercourse acts for each partner, followed by the number of times condoms were used during those acts, yielding a proportion of protected sex acts. These partner-specific questions, used to generate a continuous measure of condom use, immediately followed the ordinal assessment.

Data analysis was approached by comparing the responses of the three condom use assessment formats completed by all participants. First, rates of endorsement were compared with the three forms of measurement. The mean proportion of condom use (continuous measurement) was calculated for each response option for the ordinal item "In the last 90 days, how often did you use a condom when you had vaginal or anal sex?" (i.e., "never," "less than half the time," "about half the time," "more than half the time," and "always"; see Table 1, Column A). Similarly, the percentage who reported "yes" to having used a condom at last sex (dichotomous measurement) for each ordinal response option was calculated (see Table 1, Column B).

Table 1. Rates of condom use by response on a brief, ordinal condom use measure

Categories of condom use	n	A Continuous Mean(SD)	B Dichotomous	Consistent between continuous and ordinal measures	Ordinal response greater than continuous measure	Ordinal response less than continuous measure
Never	307	.3 (.13)	3%	85%	NA	15%
Less than half the time	269	.26 (.26)	19%	51%	25%	24%
About half the time	206	.44 (.27)	37%	35%	38%	27%
More than half the time	280	.70 (.27)	66%	58%	26%	15%
Always	128	.91 (.23)	98%	76%	24%	NA

Next, each participant was coded as a "reliable" or "unreliable" reporter based on the match between his/her responses on the continuous and the ordinal measures. Participants were deemed reliable if the proportion of condom use (p) calculated from their partner-specific reports matched the ordinal grouping that they selected using the following ranges: p = 100% and "always"; 100% > p > 60% and "more than half the time"; 60% > p > 40% and "about half the time"; 40% > p > 0% and "less than half the time"; or p = 0% and "never." Then, Pearson Chi-square and t-test analyses were conducted to assess for differences on demographic and behavioral variables between participants who were reliable and those who were not.

RESULTS

The sample was 56% female, with an average age of 18.8 years. The racial/ethnic composition of the sample was representative of the communities where the study was conducted. Fifty-two percent of the sample identified as Black or African American, 23% as Hispanic, 20% as White, and 5% as "Other." Ninety-two percent of the sample identified as heterosexual, 5% as bisexual, 3% as undecided, and 1% as homosexual. Twenty percent reported currently living with a spouse or partner. Approximately 49% of the sample had completed 11th grade or less at the time of the study, 27% had completed the twelfth grade or obtained a GED, and 24% had completed some college or technical school education. Regarding socioeconomic status, 17% indicated that they were currently receiving public assistance.

The sample reported high rates of risk behavior. The mean proportion of condom use in the last 90 days for the total sample was .38. The percentage of participants who used a condom at last intercourse was also 38%. The average number of sex partners was 2.1 (SD = 2.4), with 6.8% reporting more than three partners in the past 90 days. The mean age at sexual debut was 14.5 years (SD = 2.5). Approximately 14% tested positive for an STI on urine screen, and 13.5% indicated that they had had sex in the last 90 days with a partner the same day that they had met him/her. Nineteen percent reported that they had tried to kill themselves at some time during their lifetime, and 35% said that they had been arrested on at least one previous occasion.

Comparing the continuous and dichotomous assessments, the proportion of condom use in the past 90 days was significantly higher among those who used a condom the last time they had sex than among those who did not (0.70 vs. 0.23; t(1,186 df) = -25.5, p < .001). Table 1 shows the relationship between participant responses to the ordinal descriptors and their responses on the continuous and dichotomous formats. Both indicate linear patterns consistent with the ordinal descriptors.

Sixty-one percent of participants reliably responded to the ordinal and continuous assessments for the past 90 days. When participants were unreliable, they more often indicated greater condom use on the ordinal item than they endorsed on questions generating the proportion of condom use (see Table 1).

Bivariate analyses were conducted to examine whether demographic or behavioral differences existed between participants who responded reliably and those who did not. Results suggest that unreliable responders were younger (t(928) = 2.68, p = .007), had fewer instances of unprotected sex (t(1,159) = 5.39, p < .001), were more likely to be African

American (χ^2 (2) = 18.50, p < .001), and were more likely to have an STI on the urine test (χ^2 (1) = 6.07, p = .014). No significant differences emerged related to gender, sexual orientation, number of sexual partners, age at sexual debut, proportion of sex acts with a condom in the last 90 days, sex with someone met the same day, a history of suicide attempt, or a history of legal arrest.

Youth who never used condoms formed the largest group of consistent responders. With this in mind, we considered that this large group of reliable, but particularly risky, adolescents may have strongly influenced the bivariate differences noted above. Because of this potential confounding between consistency and sexual risk (i.e., never using condoms), analyses comparing reliable and unreliable responders on demographic and behavioral variables were conducted again omitting adolescents who endorsed never using condoms. After removing this group, no significant differences remained between reliable and unreliable reporters on age, race, number of unprotected sex acts, or STI results.

DISCUSSION

These data suggest that brief and detailed assessments of condom use in the last 90 days yield consistent responses in approximately 60% of cases, indicating that the majority of adolescents interpret these assessment methods similarly and respond reliably. At a group level, reports of condom use at last sex also corresponded to continuous and ordinal formats. However, 40% of youth were inconsistent in their reporting, which may represent a serious concern for those conducting research or program evaluations.

Rates of reliable responding were highest at the extremes of condom use ("always" and "never"). It would appear that these patterns of use are easiest for adolescents to quantify and lead to the highest rates of reliability. However, some inconsistency emerged even in the extreme ends of the ordinal variable ("always" and "never"). Similar to adults (3), adolescents' interpretation of "always" may include less than 100% of the time and their definition of "never" may include more than 0%. More detail in defining these categories for teens, such as providing corresponding percentages, may be useful in future assessments.

Inconsistency in responding occurred most frequently among adolescents reporting occasional condom use. In fact, the two least reliable groups were those endorsing "less than half the time" and "about half the time." These individuals are often the focus of intervention programs aimed at encouraging the consistent use of condoms among those willing to use them, but doing so sporadically. Research suggests that occasional condom users are at high risk for HIV (15) and therefore should be targeted for intervention. However, accurate condom use measurement among this "occasional" group may be a significant barrier to quantifying behavior change. Multiple measures may be necessary with this population.

When participants were unreliable, they tended to estimate more condom use on the ordinal format than they did on the continuous one. While it is not possible to establish which is the more accurate response, the tendency for adolescents to estimate greater condom use when responding to frequency measures is important when drawing conclusions based on data derived from single ordinal items. Thus, studies using ordinal condom measurement should be aware of possible response biases that underestimate risk behavior when interpreting findings.

There are limitations to this study. Since objective assessment of condom use in the sample is unavailable, none of these measures can be established as a "gold standard." However, computer-assisted survey instruments, like those used in this study, have been shown minimize some of the limitations associated with self-reports of private information and to increase accuracy (6, 16). Also, since all participants were recruited because they had recent unprotected sex, this sample was high risk; how lower-risk adolescents might interpret these items is unknown. However, previous work with adults has suggested that those who report more frequent sexual behavior on (presumably more accurate) daily diaries are less consistent in retrospective reports than those with fewer behaviors (6). Therefore, one might conclude that less risky youth might be more reliable reporters.

Despite recruiting adolescents who endorsed a recent episode of unprotected sex, some participants endorsed consistent condom use during the period of time assessed. Oftentimes, the initial eligibility screening (determining whether adolescents had unprotected sex in the last 90 days) was separated in time from the computer assessment due to arranging appointments for informed consent and assessment procedures. Therefore, an eligible adolescent's last episode of unprotected sex may have fallen outside the window of the last 90 days by the time of the computer assessment. In addition, adolescents may have misunderstood or misled staff during the eligibility screen. However, this may also be to the benefit of the current study, as it provided at least some representation of youth who were consistently using condoms.

Minority participants comprised a greater percentage of the sample than is representative of the United States as a whole. While the racial/ethnic composition was representative of the communities in which the study took place and represents three U.S. cities, these findings may not be generalizable to other populations. For example, African-American youth often report earlier sexual debut than other racial/ethnic groups (17); the impact of how more sexual experience might influence reliability in reporting is unknown. Finally, the order in which these formats were presented may have influenced responding; this study was not designed to assess the impact of the order in which these items were administered. For example, had the partner-by-partner (i.e., continuous) assessment been presented first, rather than last, participants may have been primed to more carefully considered their sexual experiences over the past three months and responded more consistently to the broader, ordinal assessment item.

Social science implications

These findings have significant implications for studies of adolescent risk behavior, as they provide important information regarding the reliability of adolescent reports of condom use. Since there was general agreement across formats, assessment of condom use at last sex may be sufficient for some purposes. Otherwise, adolescents, while often reliable, tended to report more condom use on brief, ordinal measures than detailed, continuous ones, thus the measure of condom use should be taken into account when interpreting research findings. Therefore, precise assessment of changes in condom use rates, the goal of many HIV prevention studies, may require multiple measures.

A large percentage of adolescents (40%) were inconsistent in reporting condom use across different formats, and it was difficult to discern factors associated with inconsistency.

This confirms problematic responding that has been similarly observed with adults, where the rate of disagreement in number of unprotected sex acts by adult reports on daily diaries compared with 3-month retrospective surveys averaged 54% (6). Given that all of the accounts of unprotected sex in the current study were retrospective, it suggests that formatting of the items may influence how adolescents respond. Among adults, McAuliffe and colleagues (6) have found that partner-by-partner assessment techniques have been found to be more reliable than aggregate assessment strategies (asking for total numbers of behaviors summed across partners). While the current study does not allow for conclusions as to which assessment methods were most accurate, researchers may wish to incorporate some partner-by-partner assessment with adolescent samples.

At the same time, the disadvantages of brief methods of condom use assessment must be weighed against the disadvantages of more comprehensive strategies. As noted elsewhere (6), the use of more intensive strategies of collecting accurate data should not lead participants to alter their responses. Among the methods studied here, the potential exists for adolescents to become inattentive or impatient with partner-by-partner questions that involve detailed follow-up questions. As a result, they may reduce the number of partners they endorse or misrepresent their engagement in sexual activity altogether to shorten the time required of the survey. This especially may be a concern in studies with repeated follow-ups, in which adolescents over the duration of the study may grow savvy to the consequences of endorsing sexual activity and the benefits of denying sexual activity. Studies examining patterns of responding over time are needed to answer these important questions.

Initial results suggested that African-American youth and adolescents with a STI-positive urine assay were more likely to be unreliable. Also, inconsistent responders reported fewer unprotected sex acts in the last 90 days. As mentioned, the most inconsistent response options were in the middle of the ordinal scale (i.e., using condoms some, but not all of the time), thus when compared to peers who consistently reported never using condoms, they had fewer unprotected acts. However, after the removal of those who reported "never" using condoms (who also tended to be consistent in their reporting) these differences no longer existed, suggesting that the riskiest youth in the sample were influencing these effects. By eliminating the variability in STIs and unprotected sex associated with this subgroup, these factors were no longer associated with inconsistent responding.

Similarly, analyses of the whole sample suggested that younger participants were less consistent in reporting than older ones, though this difference did not persist when the riskiest adolescents were removed from the analysis. Again, inattentiveness may be associated with this finding. Alternatively, younger adolescents may have been reluctant to acknowledge socially stigmatized behavior and thus underreported lack of condom use when asked repeatedly. These influences of age on reporting cannot be assessed in the present study, but will be important to investigate further.

The social science evidence provided in the current study informs the field regarding strategies for assessing sexual risk behavior and populations for whom special attention might be paid when assessing condom use and looking for change. Adolescents and young adults at the extremes of the behavior, either never using condoms or always using them, appear to be consistent in their reports, and can likely be accurately assessed with either detailed or brief measurement. However, when assessing those in the middle, often of interest in prevention studies, more targeted assessment strategies may be needed.

ACKNOWLEDGMENTS

Project SHIELD Study Group Principal Investigators: Larry Brown, MD, Rhode Island Hospital, Providence, RI; Ralph DiClemente, PhD, Emory University, Atlanta, GA; M Isabel Fernandez, PhD, University of Miami, Miami, FL, Timothy Flanigan, MD, Miriam Hospital, Providence, RI; Deborah Haller, PhD, Virginia Commonwealth University, Richmond, VA; Lori Leonard, ScD, University of Texas, Houston Health Science Center, Houston, TX; Lydia O'Donnell, EdD, Education Development Center, Inc., Newton, MA; William E Schlenger, PhD, Research Triangle Institute, Research Triangle Park, NC; Barbara Silver, PhD, Substance Abuse and Mental Health Services Administration, Rockville, MD. Site Investigators: Richard Crosby, PhD, Emory University, Atlanta, GA; Caryl Gay, PhD, University of Miami, Miami, FL; Janet Knisely, PhD, Virginia Commonwealth University, Richmond, VA; Celia Lescano, PhD, Rhode Island Hospital, Providence, RI; Kevin Lourie, PhD, Rhode Island Hospital, Providence, RI; Louise Masse, PhD, University of Texas, Houston Health Science Center, Houston, TX; Janet O'Connell, MPH, Miriam Hospital, Providence, RI; David Pugatch, MD, Miriam Hospital, Providence, RI; Eve Rose, PhD, Emory University, Atlanta, GA; Ann Stueve, PhD, Columbia School of Public Health, New York, NY; Leah Varga, MA, University of Miami, Miami, FL; Sue Vargo, PhD, Education Development Center, Inc., Newton, MA;

Gina Wingood, ScD, MPH, Emory University, Atlanta, GA. Coordinating Center Investigators, Research Triangle Institute, Research Triangle Park, NC: Jamia L Bacharach, JD, Sylvia Cohn, Courtney Johnson, PhD, Jacquelyn R Murphy, BSc,

Allison Rose, PhD and Scott Royal, PhD, MPH. Consumer Representatives: Christian Aldridge, Beri Hull and Sean Scott.

This research was supported by SAMHSA grant U10 SMS2073 to the cooperating sites: Rhode Island Hospital, Miriam Hospital, Emory University, and University of Miami, and by the Lifespan/Brown/Tufts Center for AIDS Research.

REFERENCES

[1]   Noar SM, Cole C, Carlyle K. Condom use measurement in 56 studies of sexual risk behavior: Review and recommendations. Arch Sex Behav 2006;35:327-45.

[2]   Vanable PA, Carey MP, Brown JL, DiClemente RJ, Salazar LF, Brown LK, Romer D, et al. Test-retest reliability of self-reported HIV/STD-related measures among African-American adolescents in four U.S. cities. J Adolesc Health 2009;44:214-21.

[3]   Cecil H, Zimet GD. Meanings assigned by undergraduates to frequency statements of condom use. Arch Sex Behav 1998;27:493-505.

[4]   White SL, Redding CA, Morokoff PJ, Meier KS, Rossi JS, Gazabon SA, et al. Utility of a 5-point Likert condom frequency scale in at risk sexually active adults. Ann Behav Med 2000;22(Suppl):S075.

[5]   Farrell AD, Danish SJ, Howard CW. Evaluation of data screening methods in surveys of adolescent drug use. Psychol Assess 1991; 3:295-8.

[6]   McAuliffe TL, DiFranceisco W, Reed BR. Effects of question format and collection mode on the accuracy of retrospective surveys of health risk behavior: A comparison with daily sexual activity diaries. Health Psychol 2007;26:60-7.

[7]   Brener ND, Billy JO, Grady WR. Assessment of factors affecting the validity of self-reported health-risk behavior among adolescents: Evidence from the scientific literature. J Adolesc Health 2003; 33:436-57.

[8]   Catania JA, Gibson DR, Chitwood DD, Coates TJ. Methodological problems in AIDS behavioral research: Influences on measurement error and participation bias in studies of sexual behavior. Psychol Bull 1990; 108:339-62.

[9]   Brown LK, DiClemente R, Crosby R, Fernandez MI, Pugatch D, Cohn S, Lescano C, Royal S, Murphy JR, Silver B, Schlenger WE. Condom use among high-risk adolescents: Anticipation of partner disapproval and less pleasure associated with not using condoms. Public Health Rep 2008; 123:601-7.

[10]   NIMH Multisite HIV Prevention Trial Group. The NIMH multisite HIV prevention trial: Reducing HIV sexual risk behavior. Science 1999; 280:1889-94.

[11]   Crosby R, DiClemente RJ, Wingood G, Salazar LF, Rose E, Levine D, et al. Correlates of condom failure among adolescent males: An exploratory study. Prev Med 2005;41:873-6.

[12]   O'Donnell L, O'Donnell CR, Stueve, A. Early sexual initiation and subsequent sex-related risks among urban minority youth: The Reach for Health study. Fam Plann Perspect 2001;33:268-75.

[13]   Houck CD, Hadley W, Lescano CM, Pugatch D, Brown LK, Project SHIELD Study Group. Suicide attempt and sexual risk behavior: Relationship among adolescents. Arch Suicide Res 2008;12:39-49.

[14]   Tolou-Shams M, Brown LK, Gordon G, Fernandez MI. Arrest history as an indicator of adolescent/young adult substance abuse and HIV risk. Drug Alcohol Depend 2007; 88:87-90.

[15]   Weir SS, Roddy RE, Zekeng L, Ryan KA. Association between condom use and HIV infection: A randomised study of self reported condom use measures. J Epidemiol Commun Health 1999;53:417-22.

[16]   Romer D, Hornik RC, Stanton B, Black M, Li X, Ricardo I, Feigelman S. "Talking" computers: A private and reliable method to conduct interviews on sensitive topics with children. J Sex Res 1997;34:3-9.

[17]   Cavazos-Rehg PA, Krauss MJ, Spitznagel EL, Schootman M, Bucholz KK, Peipert JF, Sanders-Thompson V, Cottler LB, Bierut LJ. Age of sexual debut among US adolescents. Contraception 2009;80:158-62.

Submitted: November 01, 2011. *Revised:* January 02, 2012. *Accepted:* January 07, 2012.

In: Public Health Yearbook 2012

Editor: Joav Merrick

ISBN: 978-1-62808-078-0

© 2013 Nova Science Publishers, Inc.

Chapter 36

INTERNET ADVICE ON DISCLOSURE OF HIV STATUS TO SEXUAL PARTNERS IN AN ERA OF CRIMINALIZATION

Bronwen Lichtenstein[*]*, PhD*

Department of Criminal Justice, University of Alabama, Tuscaloosa, Alabama,
United States of America

ABSTRACT

HIV-specific statutes are increasingly popular in the United States and often impose harsh penalties for failure to disclose an HIV diagnosis to sexual partners. The purpose of this study was to examine HIV-related websites for information about non-disclosure as a crime and the relevance of this advice for US audiences. Methods: Internet searches were conducted for HIV-related websites with advice on disclosure to sexual partners. Once identified, these sites were analyzed for content, quality, and type of approach to disclosure and the law. Each site was given a page ranking (P. Score) according to Google's priority listing algorithm, and a value ranking (V. Score) for textual content and quality of advice. Results: Internet advice on disclosure and the law was highly variable. With few exceptions, highly ranked US sites offered less advice than sites in Britain, Canada and Australia. All US sites followed the law by placing the onus of responsibility for disclosure on the HIV-infected individual, but few offered advice on how to disclose or how to obtain proof of disclosure in order to avoid prosecution. None addressed the special risks of African Americans who are most likely to be prosecuted for non-disclosure. Conclusions: HIV advice websites should offer strategies on how to disclose to sexual partners and to document proof in case of prosecution.

Keywords: Internet advice, HIV disclosure, criminalization

[*] Correspondence: Bronwen Lichtenstein, PhD, Department of Criminal Justice, 430 Farrah Hall, University of Alabama, Tuscaloosa, AL 35487-0320 United States. Phone (205) 348 7782; Fax: (205) 348 7178; Email: blichten@ua.edu

INTRODUCTION

HIV-specific statutes are increasingly popular in the United States and often impose harsh penalties for failure to disclose an HIV diagnosis to sexual partners (1). General criminal law is also used to prosecute HIV-related acts involving non-disclosure (1). The precursors to criminalizing HIV non-disclosure arose from moral panics of the 1980s when epidemiologists at the Centers for Disease Control and Prevention (CDC) coined the term "the four H's" to describe homosexuals, heroin users, hookers, and Haitians as risk groups for HIV/AIDS (2).Since marginalized people were viewed as disease bearers from the outset, it is perhaps inevitable that HIV-related behavior was criminalized in the U.S. and that non-disclosure to sexual partners became the lynchpin of efforts to include HIV-specific statutes in the canon of criminal law. The legal requirements for disclosure were embedded in the Ryan White Care Act of 1990, in which states had to agree to prosecute cases of "intentional" HIV exposure in order to receive federal funding for HIV care (3). The 1990s thus became a watershed decade for HIV-specific laws in which non-disclosure was considered to be a criminal act, particularly if an "innocent" partner became infected heterosexually(3,4). The increase in criminalization for HIV-related cases in the U.S. is consistent with trends in other Western countries (5). However, the U.S. has led the way with more prosecutions of HIV-related acts involving non-disclosure or threats to public safety than anywhere else in the world (6).

Evolving law on criminal non-disclosure

US case law on HIV-related crime has evolved over the past 30 years. In the 1980s, non-disclosure of one's HIV serostatus could be prosecuted under existing public health statutes that allowed states to charge people who willfully or knowingly exposed someone to infectious diseases that were a threat to public health. This provision included prosecutions for sexually transmitted infections (STIs) such as syphilis and gonorrhea (7). However, the misdemeanors that could be imposed for breaching public health laws were too lenient for many lawmakers who sought harsher penalties for HIV exposure than public health statutes would allow (8). By 1990, 23 states had enacted HIV-specific laws that were designed to control disease and punish wrongdoers (1,9). A decade later, HIV-specific laws had been enacted in 34 states, and sexual and even non-sexual acts such as spitting, biting, or throwing tainted blood, were being prosecuted under general criminal law (1). In some cases, non-disclosure was being prosecuted even if the accused was unaware of being HIV-infected (10).

General criminal law is widely used to prosecute non-disclosure and non-sexual acts that are perceived to be risky for police officers and other first responders. HIV-infected people have been charged with criminal exposure, aggravated or felonious assault/assault with a deadly weapon, sexual battery, rape, reckless endangerment and murder regardless of whether or not HIV transmission or even sexual activity has taken place. Once convicted, HIV-infected people often receive enhanced penalties because of the perceived seriousness of their crimes (1,11). HIV was criminalized further in the wake of 9/11 when prosecutorial desire to impose penalties for HIV-related behavior received a boost from new laws to combat terrorism. This expansion of law meant that threatening to infect someone with HIV was considered a "terroristic threat" and, in one notable case, was prosecuted as a case of bioterrorism (12).

The upward trend in HIV-related arrests and prosecutions is evident in statistical reports. By 2010, a total of 375 arrests and prosecutions – a low estimate – were documented in the United States (1,11). Almost 30 percent of these cases (n=109) were prosecuted between 2008 and 2011 alone, an increase that is variously attributed to media sensationalism, public outrage, harsher sentencing, and even having to register as a sex offender for life (1,13,14). Public health campaigns that were once popular in promoting shared responsibility by both partners to establish sexual histories, discuss safer sex, and use condoms failed to curtail this trend, perhaps because of the multiplying effects of harsher social attitudes toward sexual crimes, epidemiologic trends in race-gender disparities in HIV/AIDS, and the highly-charged contexts in which most prosecutions occurred.

Public health models for HIV prevention

In the mid-1980s, public health approaches to HIV prevention focused on a particular message: People should enquire about the sexual history of potential partners before having sex (15). This approach to safer sex, termed "the mutual (shared) responsibility" model, recommended seeking information about sexual orientation, drug use, frequency of sexual activity, and STI history as a means of assessing HIV risk (16).The approach was the model of choice for HIV prevention, primarily because of the public health sector's reluctance to place the burden of responsibility solely on HIV-infected people who were already heavily stigmatized as putative AIDS vectors (17). The goals of the campaign were to promote co-equal information sharing, full disclosure of HIV status, and mutual responsibility for initiating condom use. The model assumed that sexual actors would be both self-empowered and self-motivated to engage in safer sex. However, a campaign that was designed primarily for HIV seropositive or at-risk men in the gay community was not always relevant to other actors, especially African Americans and women. Wingood and DiClemente (18) reported that African American women were ill served by public health directives to initiate safer sex with sexual partners. Such women were often accused of sexual cheating and undermining male authority, and, rather than being self-empowered, sometimes faced threats of violence and abandonment as a result of attempts to negotiate condom use.

By the late 1980s, the individual (personal) responsibility model for HIV disclosure, also known as the altruism or "responsibility for the other" approach (19) had gained influence among policymakers (17). According to Bayer (20), many HIV prevention specialists opposed this approach because they believed it would intensify HIV stigma for highly vulnerable groups in society. Nevertheless, ethics concerns over the special responsibilities of HIV-infected persons in a deadly epidemic, and the potential for HIV transmission in the absence of disclosure, provided the impetus for widespread acceptance of the personal responsibility approach to HIV prevention (20). The model posited that HIV-infected people must disclose their seropositive status prior to sexual activity, and also to assume responsibility for both disclosure and safer sex. Mutual exchange of information between sexual partners, and shared responsibility for safer sex were no longer a public health priority. The CDC formalized the individual responsibility model in a report titled "Advancing HIV prevention: New strategies for a changing epidemic – United States 2003" (17). The link between the individualistic approach to HIV prevention and legal enforcement of this approach was underwritten in expectations of "contractual responsibility," in which recipients of HIV care were fully responsible for HIV disclosure (19). As noted, this change in public health policy meant that U.S. citizens who received public HIV care could be prosecuted if they failed to disclose their HIV seropositive status to sexual partners (3).

The law versus medicine

The law enforcement approach to HIV non-disclosure to sexual partners is at odds with recent medical advances in HIV care. First, the advent of antiretroviral medicines (ARVs) meant that HIV-infected people were able to lead longer and healthier lives (21) in which the chances of HIV transmission were greatly reduced when ARVs were taken as prescribed (22). On the basis of these advances, the CDC promoted routine HIV testing in the belief that early diagnosis and treatment would save lives and prevent transmission to sexual partners (23). This recommendation took account of the life-saving benefits of the new HIV drugs, but did not reduce the burden of disclosure for HIV-infected people. If anything, the policy meant that people who heeded the CDC's recommendation for early testing and were then diagnosed with HIV suddenly faced the prospect of legally prescribed sexual activity on a permanent basis. Second, rather than recognize the changing medical landscape for HIV transmission, lawmakers increased their efforts to impose stiff penalties on HIV-infected people who were assumed to place others at risk by failing to disclose their HIV status. What accounts for this divergence between medicine and the law? Critics have charged that stigma rather than medical evidence drove the zeal to criminalize non-disclosure, particularly in cases involving heterosexuals (4). As a case in point, HIV is often compared to infectious diseases such as Hepatitis B or C, also acquired through injection drug use or unprotected sex. After HIV emerged as a public health threat in the 1980s, these less sensationalized conditions did not attract the same stigma despite high rates of morbidity and even mortality (24,25). Unlike HIV, exposure to Hepatitis B and C is rarely prosecuted under public health statutes and even more rarely under general criminal law (26).

Broad social trends and epidemiologic changes can help to explain recent trends in criminalization. Poverty (27), drug use (27), minority ethnic status (28), and mental illness (29) are all indicators of HIV risk in the United States. African Americans are 10 times more likely than Whites to acquire HIV/AIDS, a disparity that has widened over time (28). Furthermore, today's criminal cases are driven mostly by heterosexual rather than same-sex acts, particularly if they involve Black men (4,29,30,31). This racial patterning suggests that social factors and, perhaps, racial stereotyping are at work in re-stigmatizing HIV. The hardening public attitudes toward acts that classify as sexual offenses (32) have also contributed to harsher attitudes toward HIV non-disclosure. These attitudes were driven, in part, by media sensationalism over sex crimes (33), so that people who fail to disclose an HIV-positive diagnosis were likely to be perceived as sexual predators, especially if they were male (11). History has shown that public attitudes toward issues of race/ethnicity, gender, and sexuality are particularly potent when it comes to the law (34).

Criminalization leads to fear of being tested for HIV (35,36), and to erroneous beliefs that non-disclosure of seropositive HIV status to sexual partners is driving the epidemic, despite evidence that the lack of HIV testing and treatment is a greater problem (37). The success of HIV criminalization as an HIV prevention tool is certainly in question; new HIV cases in the U.S. have remained stubbornly high, at around 56,000 annually over the past decade (38).

Persson and Newman (4) wrote that the law enforcement approach to HIV non-disclosure is counterproductive, and involves blame motifs involving perpetrators and victims (4) "in a revival and reframing of the old familiar discourse of 'innocent victims' and 'guilty others' so prevalent in early news reporting" (p. 633).

This polarization is at the heart of high-profile cases in which HIV-infected men (e.g. Nushawn Williams, an African American man who infected mostly White women) have been prosecuted for non-disclosure. Scholars argue that the refocus on individual responsibility represents a victim-perpetrator antagonism which, in the words of Galletly and Pinkerton (39): "Reinforces the 'them versus us' dichotomy that is central to prevailing theories of stigma" (p. 457). Indeed, fears over this type of stigmatization were the original impetus for formulating the mutual responsibility model when moral panics over HIV were at their peak in the 1980s. The transition to the individual responsibility model signals a maturing epidemic, as well as a law and order approach to infection control after HIV was associated with sexual crime and, not incoincidentally, communities of color.

The disclosure dilemma

Legal enforcement of an HIV-positive status ignores the difficulties of disclosing to sexual partners. Serovich and Mosack (40) reported that perhaps 50% of HIV-infected people do not disclose to sexual partners for fear of being rejected, abandoned, or even assaulted.

The criminalization of non-disclosure therefore presents a new wrinkle among HIV-infected people: Risk rejection or even violence if you disclose and prosecution if you do not. Being liable for prosecution begins even before deciding whether or not to disclose to sexual partners. Few people are aware that HIV-specific statutes override confidentiality laws when someone is charged with an HIV-related crime and how medical records can be subpoenaed as evidence for the prosecution (41). In other words, an HIV-positive diagnosis can be used against the accused in a court of law.

Most HIV-infected people are counseled about their rights and responsibilities at time of diagnosis, including about legal requirements for disclosure to sexual partners. In the Internet age, HIV-infected people are also likely to consult relevant websites on how to disclose to sexual partners, especially if they fear rejection, seek anonymity, or wish to be protected from legal jeopardy. The purpose of the present study was to examine the relevance of advice on HIV disclosure and the law for Internet users in the United States.

The specific goals were to: 1) Identify websites that offer information on HIV disclosure and the law, 2) Identify the intended audience for U.S. websites, 3) Conduct a content analysis on quality of the advice, 4) Compare the search engine rankings with the quality of advice, and 5) Describe the approaches to such advice according to the Mutual Responsibility and Individual Responsibility models as described above.

METHODS

Ethics approval was obtained from the Institutional Review Board at the University of Alabama, which was followed by multiple Google searches using search terms such as "HIV disclosure," "Telling/Partner/HIV," and "How do I disclose HIV?" The searches were conducted on four different computers at home, work, and a computer laboratory in order to circumvent a process known as personalization, the method by which Google uses personal search histories and a page-rank algorithm to filter results (42). This reiterative search produced more than 300 pages of results, mostly news items, legal documents, or scientific articles (they were discarded) as well as duplicated results for HIV-related websites. All duplicates of relevant items were counted only once in the final tally. In the second stage of the research, a Priority Score (P. Score) was assigned to the remaining 113 items on HIV disclosure, that is, the page ranking assigned by the search engine itself. The most-highly ranked item was assigned a score of 1 ("highest accessibility") with other items ranked sequentially, ending with the 113th item on the list ("lowest accessibility").

The content analysis consisted of a detailed review of relevant websites for information on HIV disclosure and the law. Only 50 (44%) of the 113 websites on HIV disclosure had information or advice about disclosure and the law. A value ranking (V. Score) was assigned to these sites, as calculated from the amount of text and quality of advice. The amount and quality of information were related closely. This content was then ranked from 1 to 5, with the least helpful (one to two sentences) receiving a score of 1, moderately helpful (several paragraphs to one page) receiving scores of 2 and 3 respectively, and very helpful (multiple pages with links) receiving a score of 4. Only one website received the top score of 5 because it was entirely dedicated to HIV disclosure and the law.

Once the ranking was complete, the author identified sites that offered peer-to-peer advice (informal), doctor-patient or institutional-legal advice (formal), or some other type of approach to disclosure and the law. The research also assessed whether or not each website addressed disclosure according to evolving legal standards for public health policy and the law. Then, the study examined the type of approach ("shared responsibility" versus "individual responsibility") to see if the advice was tailored to client advocacy (the shared responsibility model), the law (the individual responsibility model), or some other approach. Finally, the target audience for each website was identified to determine if the advice was generic or crafted for a particular demographic or community.

RESULTS

The results are organized into four sub-sections according to the specific research questions for the study. The first section describes the priority rankings that were generated by the search engine, and the relevance of these results for U.S. Internet users. This section is followed by an assessment of the quality of the advice on the most highly ranked sites, and approach to advice on HIV disclosure and the law. The third section analyses the usefulness of advice on the 10 top ranked websites for US Internet users. Finally, the question of: "whose responsibility?" is discussed in relation to website advice on disclosing to sexual partners within the framework of U.S. law.

Priority rankings

Only 44% of websites with advice on HIV disclosure provided information about the legal aspects of disclosing to sexual partners. Moreover, while 13 (65%) of the top 20 sites, as ranked by Google, addressed disclosure and the law – a reasonable showing - the percentage declined steadily thereafter. Table 1 presents a list of 21 U.S. and international sites that offered information on disclosure and the law (space limitations preclude listing all results in this category). These highly placed sites stood a reasonable chance of being read because they appeared in the top half of the rankings. Since the top five of these websites originated in the United States, the legal advice was relevant contextually to U.S. users. However, sites in the United Kingdom, Canada, and Australia ranked higher overall and were slightly more numerous as well.

Table 1. HIV sites citing legal reasons for disclosure by Priority and Value Scores (N=21)

P. Score[1]	Website	Audience	Tag line	V. Score[2]	Location
1.	AIDSmeds.com	HIV+	To tell or not to tell	2	US
2.	Thewellproject.org	HIV+ women	HIV & disclosure	2	US
3.	Thebody.com	HIV+	Should you disclose . . . ?	4	US
4.	Webmd.com	General	Telling others	1	US
5.	Mdjunction.com	General	To tell or not to tell	2	US
6.	IPPF.org	Youth	Some countries have laws	3	UK
9.	Gmfa.org.uk	HIV+ men	Sexual transmission & law	4	UK
10.	Catie.ca	HIV+	HIV, disclosure & the law	3	Canada
11.	Aidslex.org (law)	HIV+	Disclosing your HIV status	5	Australia
12.	Friendsofaids.org	HIV+	Ready to disclose?	1	US
13.	Positivewomensnetwork	HIV+ women	Sex, HIV, and the law	3	Canada
14.	Methedoctor.com	General	Some things to consider . . .	2	Indonesia
20.	Poz.com	HIV+	Daring to disclose	2	US
24.	Pozitude.co.uk	HIV+	HIV, sex & the law	4	UK
26.	Ehow.com	General	HIV disclosure laws	4	US, UK
30.	Doh.state.fl.us	HIV+	Why is disclosure important?	3	US

Table 1. (Continued)

P. Score[1]	Website	Audience	Tag line	V. Score[2]	Location
39.	Positivelypositive.ca	HIV+ men	Why is disclosure important?	3	Canada
40.	Wdxcyber.com	Women	Relationships and HIV	1	US
41.	HIVsa.org.au	HIV+	Know your rights!	3	Australia
47.	*AIDSlondon.com*	HIV+	Disclosure	4	UK
50.	Avert.org	HIV-related	Criminal transmission	4	UK

[1]. Numbers for the P. Score reflect the Internet rankings and are not in consecutive order.

[2]. Scores: One to two sentences =1; One or two short paragraphs =2; Half to one page=3; Multi-page or link=4; Entire report=5.

Compared to no-frills advice in four of the top U.S. websites, these foreign sites had detailed, friendly advice and even referrals to legal advisors if needed.

The top ranked U.S. websites offered multiple pages in the form of homepage, sections, designer graphics and videos, and links to other sites. Advertisements appeared for treatments and services within the site or on the page of Google results. The highest ranking (1/113) went to AIDSmeds.com, a New York-based advocacy network for people seeking advice on HIV treatment and clinical trials. The site was visually appealing, highly interactive, had news about HIV drugs and clinical trials, and provided ready access to affiliated sites for further information. Unlike other top ranked sites, AIDSmeds.com offered advice on disclosure and the law, which referred users to government services (e.g., "The Department of Public Health in your state is a good source of information about what the legal procedure is in your state and how it might apply to you"). Photographs, video clips, and graphics on the homepage suggested that the website catered to a cross-section of the HIV-infected community, although White men were typically depicted on the main page and links. The superior ranking of this site reflected its popularity in providing information on treatment advances and new developments in clinical care and, of course, advertising links to expensive, name brand HIV drugs. The site offered a link to RealHealth, a health website for African Americans, but the absence of an exclusive or even primary focus on HIV/AIDS on RealHealth suggests that the site lacked relevance for HIV-infected African Americans seeking information on how to disclose to sexual partners.

The lowest ranked US site (103/113) was the Florida-based dabtheaidsbearproject.com ("An American journey of hope"), a grassroots, multi-media website with photographs of AIDS bears ("Angel Bears") and their human friends. The graphics were accompanied by a description of the bears' origin as symbols of comfort during a time when HIV was a certain death sentence. On the homepage, messages of hope and self-empowerment offered a warm welcome to HIV-infected people and friends. However, this friendliness was offset by a stern warning about non-disclosure being both immoral and a felony in most states and a 3,500-word legal section which threatened search engines with legal action if they used algorithms, spyware, and other tracking devices for commercial or other purposes. Although Google's search-and-store method of classifying data probably determined the website's Internet ranking, the threatening tone of the legal section might also have contributed to the low priority score in Table 1.

Value rankings

Table One lists the V. Score on quality of advice. The V. Scores ranged from 1 (least helpful) to 5 (most helpful) and bore little relation to Google's priority rankings. For instance, the top ranked U.S. site (AIDSmeds.com) provided a cursory 10 lines of information for a score of 2. The second-ranked site (Thewellproject.com, a women's resource network) also earned a score of 2 for 10 lines of grimly worded text on the legal consequences of non-disclosure. The third ranked site (Thebody.com) provided comprehensive and up-to-date information for a score of 4, but the fourth ranked site (Webmed.com) offered a meager two lines for a score of 1(the advice was less helpful than in the lowest-ranked U.S. site). Most remaining websites did not originate in the United States.

Foreign websites earned higher quality scores than U.S. websites. Sites in the United Kingdom, Canada, and Australia provided detailed legal information (e.g., explanations about the difference between reckless and intentional transmission in U.K. law), as well as advice on how to disclose to sexual partners in keeping with the law. These sites were often affiliated with government agencies and had benefited from the expertise that agency personnel provided to community-based organizations as a public service. Most of these sites catered to particular audiences or communities.

To illustrate, Gmfa.org.uk (Gay Men Fight AIDS in the United Kingdom) offered expert advice on HIV disclosure and the law in accessible language ending with the gentle reminder to "take responsibility for your own health and safety when having sex." In keeping with its mission for advocacy and self-empowerment, the website lamented the trend toward criminalization (which it deemed ineffective) and provided a link to an affiliate that advocated for legal change. In contrast to the U.S. sites, Black men were depicted in almost every image on the homepage and links, suggesting that the writers took account of HIV statistics involving men of color and had tailored their message accordingly.

The Body.com (a site for HIV-infected people) offered high quality advice for HIV-infected people, which helped to support the site's self-proclaimed position as "the largest HIV/AIDS resource on the net." Webpage authors offered friendly advice, which occasionally challenged the criminalization of HIV. For example, in a column titled "Sex While HIV Positive: The New Criminals," the writer offered advice on how to obtain proof of disclosure and expressed doubt about the wisdom of criminalization by stating: "[T]he more I have learned about the criminalization of HIV non-disclosure, the more I am convinced these laws are applied badly and actually do more harm than good. If I don't get tested, I can't be prosecuted for not disclosing my status, right?" An accompanying video blog discussed the fear of people being tested because of criminalization, which led to forgoing life-saving drugs that would also prevent HIV transmission. By contrast, few of the other U.S. websites went into such detail, with most advice consisting of simple directives to disclose to sexual partners as a moral and legal necessity.

How useful is the US advice?

Narratives on HIV disclosure and the law can help Internet users to resolve the legal aspects of safer-sex, that is, sexual activity within the law. Table Two summarizes advice on HIV disclosure and the law in top ranked U.S. websites; that is, the 10 sites that were most likely to be read by Internet users seeking advice on disclosure.

Table 2. Disclosure + law content in top 10 U.S. websites

No 1. Aidsmeds.com, No. 5, Mdjunction.com (10 lines)

"It's important for you to be aware of what the laws are in your state with regard to contract tracing and partner notification. Contact tracing refers to the efforts of government agencies to identify any and all persons who might be at risk of contracting HIV from an infected person. Partner notification refers to information conveyed to spouses, sexual partners, needle sharers and others who might be at risk for HIV infection. The laws regarding this vary from state to state. In many states, partner notification can be done anonymously through the state's Department of Health. The Department of Health in your state is a good source of information about what the legal procedure is in your state and how it might apply to you."

No 2. Thewellproject.com (10 lines)

"In most cases, sharing your HIV status is a personal choice, but in the case of sexual relationships, it can be a legal requirement. It is best if you disclose your status prior to having sex with anyone new. Non-disclosure of HIV status in a sexual relationship can lead to criminal charges whether or not your partner becomes infected with HIV. In most states, the law requires that you disclose your HIV status before knowingly exposing or transmitting HIV to someone else. Penalties vary from state to state. In many states, you can be found guilty of a felony for not telling a sexual partner you are HIV+ before having intimate contact."

No 3. TheBody.Com (43 lines, multiple links, e-card: 15 lines of text excerpted below)

"Currently about 27 [sic] states have established criminal penalties for knowingly exposing or transmitting HIV to someone else. In California, the "Willful Exposure" law (although narrowly written and difficult to prosecute) makes exposing someone else to HIV (whether they become infected or not) a felony punishable by up to eight years in prison. In Alabama, you can be prosecuted for "Conducting yourself in manner likely to transmit the disease." (Just the thought of that is scary) . . . If you tell the other person that you have HIV before insertion, you cannot be prosecuted criminally. It would have to be proven in court that you had "specific intent" to infect the other person in order to be prosecuted criminally. In a civil case, the specifics to which you could be found guilty are much more flexible -- so be careful. Check with your local ASO (AIDS Service Organization) or legal services to find out what the laws are in your area."

No 4. WebmMD.com, No. 6, Friendsofaids.org (2 lines, e-card)

"State laws make it illegal to knowingly infect others. If you have unprotected sex without telling others, you're putting yourself at legal risk, as well as endangering the health of your partners."

No 7. Poz.Com (7 lines, multiple links, e-card)

"Bear in mind that sometimes you are legally required to disclose to a sexual partner. Many states have laws that make it illegal to transmit HIV or to have unprotected sex without telling your partner your status. Don't panic: Prosecutions are relatively rare because prosecutors usually have to prove that the person with HIV intended to infect his or her partner, which isn't easy. To find out if your state has a criminalization law on the books, visit www.lambdalegal.org."

No 8. Ehow.com (32 lines, e-card: 10 lines of text excerpted below)

"There are some circumstances in which it is legal for others to disclose [your HIV status], but this is only in very specific circumstances. 1. ***Willful Exposure:*** Willful exposure happens when someone knows she has HIV and does not disclose to sex partners and is not mindful of the possible transmission. Several states have passed laws to treat willful exposure as a criminal offense. 2. ***Criminalization:*** Many states have laws in place to criminalize willful exposure, and in the history of the disease, at least 300 people have been criminally prosecuted for knowingly infecting others. Depending on the state, the crime can be as severe as manslaughter or attempted manslaughter charge."

No 9. Doh.state.fl.org (13 lines, e-card)

"Discussing and disclosing HIV status is a two-way street. Be it right or wrong, most people feel that when a person knows that he/she is HIV+ then he/she has an obligation to tell the other person, and counselors are encouraged to help people with this process. Also, laws in some areas require disclosure of HIV+ status prior to sex.However, both partners should be responsible for knowing their own status, disclosing their own status when it seems important, and asking their partner about their status if they want to know. There is debate around whether partners have a right to know if their partner is HIV+, in order to be able to make a fully informed decision about what sexual behavior to engage in. Some HIV+ persons believe that if they only have protected sex, there is no need for disclosure, especially with casual partners, and that encouraging disclosure only serves to further stigmatize HIV+ persons. These issues can be complicated by complex gender role norms and local laws—23 [sic] states have laws that make it a crime for a person to engage in certain risk behaviors without disclosing their HIV status."

No 10. Wdxcyber.com (2 lines)

"It is important to note that you are obliged to tell your partner about your status before any sexual activity occurs. In some US states, this is the law."

All ten sites emphasized the basic importance of complying with the law. Once again, the amount of advice varied widely with the most complete information appearing on Thebody.com. A webpage titled: "Should you disclose?" sounded a cautionary note, followed by statements such as: "Many of these laws were written early in the epidemic, and were fear driven. . . Deciding who should be punished, and for what offense, often lies in the hands of politicians and court systems that base their decisions on old data and personal prejudices." The site defined willful exposure according to California law, explained how non-disclosure could lead to both criminal and civil penalties, and urged readers to disclose their HIV status in order to avoid the risk of prosecution. Links to other web pages led to advice on how to obtain proof of disclosure, including this nugget of wisdom: "You can share your status before you meet your date in person, such as over the Internet, or in a print personal ad, after a few preliminary dates when you know you'd like to pursue the relationship further." Personal anecdotes helped to frame the importance of disclosure. For example: "For Tracy Johnson, 22 and HIV-positive, romance often begins at a karaoke bar. There's music, conversation and innocent touching. He's at ease until it's time for the first kiss -- that's when he leans in, pulls out the document and asks the object of his affection to sign, indicating he's shared that he has HIV. That piece of paper, he believes, could save him from years behind bars if a partner ever alleges that he didn't disclose his status. He carries it everywhere." A photograph of an African American man accompanied the text - the first such image to appear on any of the top U.S. sites in relation to HIV disclosure.

The middle ground for advice was occupied by websites such as the Florida Department of Health's Dohfla.org, the HIV advocacy website Poz.com, and eHow.com, a general advice website. These sites offered formal advice on HIV disclosure and the law as well as a link to inSpot.org for partner notification. InSpot is a sexual health site that allows people with STIs to notify partners by sending an anonymous e-card to the recipient's address. The site has a variety of messages to suit the sender's style, gender, or type of sexual encounter. Two of these messages read: "I got diagnosed with an STD and you might have been exposed. Get checked out" and more explicitly, "I got screwed while screwing, you might have too." The e-card option guaranteed anonymity for the sender but lacked hardcopies that could be printed out for proof of disclosure.

With ten lines of primary text, eHow.com was the most informative of the intermediate sites in defining willful exposure as a crime, discussing state laws, and providing a link to inSpot. Two intermediate sites (Aidsmeds.com and Mdjunction.com) offered identical advice, which consisted of advising users to contact their respective health departments. With ten lines of advice, Thewellproject.com advised readers that disclosure of a positive HIV diagnosis to sexual partners was a legal requirement, and that non-disclosure was a felony crime in many states. Despite being a California-based health resource for women, the site did not have advice on legal issues facing California women, such as mandatory HIV testing of sex workers, laws that target female sex workers for criminal non-disclosure, and prosecutions that frame HIV-infected women as prostitutes.

The least helpful sites also provided few lines of text. For example, with only two lines on HIV disclosure and the law apiece, the women's resource siteWdxcyber.com, the HIV advocacy site Friendsofaids.org, and the general medical website Webmd.com were the least explanatory of all websites in the sample. These forums issued a formal warning about the risks of prosecution without useful tips on how to disclose in order to avoid legal trouble. Elaboration would have helped Internet users to understand the legal complexities of non-disclosure, especially on questions such as: Is "knowingly" the same as "intentionally?" Does kissing or oral sex count as sex for legal purposes? How do I avoid being rejected, injured, or "outed" if I disclose?

It is worth reiterating that the highly ranked US websites were not always the best sources for information on disclosure and the law. Some lower-ranked sites were more informative but were too far down the list to be read by most Internet users. Some overseas sites were excellent purveyors of advice even if their legal sections were too parochial for U.S. use. For example, the Canadian website Positiveside.ca advised users about obtaining proof of disclosure by inviting a friend, medical provider, or counselor to be present during the act of disclosure (e.g., by taking the disclosee to a doctor's appointment) or by keeping written evidence of disclosure from the Internet or in a personal diary in order to prevent any he said/he said scenarios in court. The text was accompanied by an image of a naked man in handcuffs and a warning that: "Even if you told a person before sex that you are HIV positive, the person might lie and say that you did not. Judges and juries have decided many of the legal cases about HIV, sex and disclosure based on credibility – whom they believed or didn't believe. In a court case, it is important to have evidence to show that you disclosed and that the other person knew your HIV status."

Whose responsibility?

Advice on U.S. websites was often brief and legalistic (e.g., "State laws make it illegal to knowingly infect others") with an explicit emphasis on individual responsibility. Some advocacy sites had conflicting advice on whether or not to follow U.S. law for disclosing a positive HIV diagnosis to sexual partners. For example, ambivalence toward the law was evident in this text from Aidsmeds.com: "For those who are single and are HIV positive, if and when to disclose can be addressed in different ways. Some people prefer to get the issue out into the open immediately. Others prefer to wait and see if the relationship is going to develop beyond a first date or casual dating. Still others feel that as long they're having safer sex, the risk is minimal to the other person, so why even bring the subject up?" The site offered a stepwise process to calculate the risk of rejection but fell short on offering helpful tips about how to disclose, obtain proof of disclosure, and avoid "he said/she said" scenarios that could end in litigation.

Conflicting advice sometimes appeared on web pages and links that were authored by different people over a period of years. Taking Thebody.com as an example, a 2002 item titled "Should you disclose your HIV status to a potential sexual partner?" offered timely warnings about criminalization while also stating: "Disclosure is not easy for everyone, and in certain situations is not an option (such as where disclosing could cause physical injury to yourself)." By 2011, sites such as Poz.com and Thebody.com had abandoned this position, adopted a defensive tone over the proliferation of HIV-specific laws, and urged members to watch out for potential legal problems. This stance appeared in statements such as:"I guess we should all start making any sexual partners [use a condom] or sign a consent form saying they understand the risks" (Poz.com), and: "Most of us are caring, law-abiding human beings who want to be good citizens. So we're stuck in that rock and hard place where we have to figure out, 'How do I prove I didn't break that law?' . . . It really is bizarre what we have to go through to protect ourselves" (Thebody.com).The legal mandate of individual responsibility was certainly irksome to some people who had shouldered the burden of disclosure from the outset. An advocate protested: "Given this new reality [the effectiveness of ARV drugs in reducing HIV transmission], I am reconsidering my options. [F]or once it would be nice if my prospective partners took responsibility for their own health and asked me if I had HIV so that I wouldn't have to carry the burden of telling them first" (Vanessa Johnson, Thebody.com). This defiance was tempered by surrender to U.S. law and regret that the mutual responsibility model had never appeared to be a viable option.

Websites that advocated mutual responsibility were fewer in number. The U.K site International Planned Parenthood Fund (IPPF.org) was a notable exception. In the 2010 report Happy, Healthy and Hot, the IPPF (43) took a bold stand by stating: "Young people living with HIV have the right to decide if, when, and how to disclose their HIV status" (p. 3), and further, "Some countries have laws that violate the right of young people living with HIV to decide whether to disclose or face the possibility of criminal charges" (p. 6). These statements provoked outrage from conservative websites such as Concerned Women for America (CWFA.org) and Red State (Redstate.com), which complained of radical extremism and hippy sensibilities from the 1970s. On Poz.com, the opening salvo of a U.S-European forum also hinted at opposition to the individual responsibility model for disclosure. Here, the convener challenged the panel by asking: "Who's responsible for new infections? Criminalization says it's the [Person with AIDS]. Prevention says both partners. Right now, criminalization is winning." The cultural divide between Europeans and the U.S. was revealed in vigorous discussions about the rights and wrongs of criminalization for non-disclosure, especially in prosecuting Black men "for having sex with white women . . . The case of Nushawn Williams is like a dark cloud hanging over this whole discussion." This flashpoint was evident in statements about criminalization being punitive and "useless" for HIV prevention (Europe) compared to being "inevitable" or "just retribution" for a wronged partner (U.S.). Even among advocates on the panel, the shared responsibility model was being debated in relation to disclosure and U.S. law.

DISCUSSION

The results of this study indicate that highly ranked websites (i.e., medical or HIV sites that attract large audiences) are more likely to be consulted than sites that appear lower in the ranking hierarchy. This finding has implications for the accessibility of Internet advice on HIV disclosure and the law. First, information on the legal aspects of disclosure was missing from one third of the top ranked websites, suggesting that Internet users might be poorly served when they seek critical advice on disclosure in an era of HIV criminalization. Second, the quality of advice from these websites did not match their priority rankings. For example, the well-known U.S. POZ.com (an advocacy website), which offered advice from a friendly, consumer-oriented perspective, earned a lower Google ranking than suggested by the popularity of POZ magazine, a waiting room staple in HIV clinics in the United States. The discrepancy between quality of information and ranking score highlights a growing problem for Internet searches in the age of personalization. Unless users enter a web address themselves, then they are beholden to search engines that prioritize sites according to popularity (the highest number of hits) and commercial value (advertising links), and also to websites that use metatags to increase their visibility (42). Google's ranking algorithm tailors

Internet results according to a user's search history so that retrievals can vary greatly from one person or computer to another. Another complicating factor is that Internet searches produce an abundance of media stories, scientific articles, legal caches, blogs, and sundry posts on HIV disclosure and the law; in other words, a surfeit of information that has to be sifted through in order to reach the desired destination. However, this abundance is not only eye opening but also instructive about the risks of prosecution for HIV-related offenses. For example, the present author's searches for websites on HIV disclosure produced media headlines such as "Man charged with failing to disclose HIV status to partner," "Man charged with murder for spreading HIV," and "Iowa man sentenced to 25 years in prison for failure to disclose." These results were as ubiquitous as they were alarming and served as a clarion call to Internet users about the risks of non-disclosure.

The lack of information on HIV disclosure and the law on many U.S. websites can be compared to the comprehensive information on sites in the U.K., Australia, and Canada. The brevity of U.S. advice on the legal aspects of HIV disclosure was also at odds with amount of advice on other HIV-related topics on the U.S. sites, including when and how to disclose to family members. One explanation for the deficit of legal information relates to the practical difficulties of addressing the legal background of 50 states that have diverse criminal codes and statutes for non-disclosure as a crime. (There are no federal laws in the U.S.). Although the problem could easily be remedied by providing a link to each state's HIV laws, most U.S. sites avoided the issue by referring users to state health departments or by making brief statements about non-disclosure as a crime. Websites from countries with a single legal system (e.g., England, Canada, Australia) did not encounter this problem, most likely because of greater access to official information and expertise that was provided specifically for HIV-related websites. However, the issue of quality is a vexed one for the Internet regardless of mitigating factors such as a country's system of laws or funding support. Purcell, Wilson, and Delamothe (44) noted that many popular websites fail to satisfy the informational needs of users who seek advice for health problems, a troubling finding when health consumers are expected to be both proactive and self-empowered in the Internet age (45).

The ideal of self-empowerment can be especially difficult to achieve when it comes to eliciting information about a partner's STI history (46). Although the proactive approach to information seeking was the basis for the mutual responsibility model for HIV prevention in the 1980s, the present study found that present models of information-sharing went one way – from HIV-infected people to their sexual partners, as required by U.S. law. One caveat to this finding was that advocacy-minded U.S. websites tended to advise HIV-infected people to obtain proof of disclosure to guard against prosecution in contested cases. The fact that most websites in the present study fully endorsed the individual responsibility model for HIV-infected users suggests a natural evolution of events in terms of public sentiment and the law - a trend recently bolstered by CDC policies to ensure that HIV-infected people disclose to sexual partners (47). Despite this evolution, the ambivalence of some websites suggests that advocates have not endorsed fully the flight from mutual responsibility or accepted the legal premise that non-disclosure is responsible for spreading HIV.

The present study found one-size-fits-all advice on many U.S. sites. This uniformity neglected the special risks of prosecution for African Americans who are HIV-infected in disproportionate numbers compared to other citizens. Research by Stein et al. (48) found that Black men were over three times less likely to disclose to sexual partners than Whites and Hispanics and were twice as reluctant as Black women to do so. In the United Kingdom,

Elford et al. (49) reported that Africans were significantly less likely than gay men to disclose to sexual partners about being HIV-infected. The Serovich et al. (40) study of HIV disclosure patterns found that non-disclosure rates were high (<50%) regardless of racial differences, and that the act of disclosure is difficult and socially fraught for many people. African American men's avoidance of disclosure may account, in part, for racial disparities in criminal prosecutions for HIV-related crimes although the reverse might also be true: Black men, who are historically portrayed in terms of a "monstrous masculinity" (3) might be reluctant to disclose if they fear being targeted for prosecution by health officials and the police. Such men need tailored advice on how to disclose, why they should disclose, and how to obtain proof of disclosure in order to avoid prosecution. It is possible that such advice is being delivered at time of diagnosis or in informal or community forums. However, the men's reluctance to disclose as identified by Stein et al. (48) and even greater reluctance to be tested for HIV as evident from "take the test, risk arrest" warnings that circulate among African American men (50), suggest that the anonymity of the Internet could be useful for reaching this audience, and for providing life-saving information that is also an "insurance policy" against prosecution.

Finally, there is the question of where HIV-infected people are likely to seek advice for disclosure. As noted, HIV-infected people are usually counseled in a health setting at the time of their initial diagnosis. This counseling might be followed up by additional advice on HIV disclosure at the same site at a later date. However, it is difficult to remember advice being delivered in emotionally highly charged situations, and a significant proportion of HIV-infected people are lost to follow-up care after being diagnosed (51). It is here that the Internet can fill an important role in providing supplementary information on HIV disclosure and the law, and it is imperative that excellent, post-diagnosis advice is available for people who seek anonymity while coming to terms with a life-changing condition. The advice should, at a minimum, provide a confidential helpline for Internet users who fear being prosecuted for non-disclosure, links to information on relevant laws of their state, and also offer e-referrals to legal professionals or local AIDS service agency employees who could then explain these laws in detail.

The findings of this study should be interpreted with caution. It is possible that the Internet searches yielded data that would be different if performed at a different time and place. The search engine's personalized algorithm guarantees that Internet results always will be somewhat idiosyncratic, although the results presented here were generated from four different computers in an effort to avoid this problem. Second, the searches generated hundreds of pages of results that had to be culled carefully, sorted, labeled, and then cross-identified. It is unlikely that a typical individual would take the same trouble to identify relevant advice on HIV disclosure and the law. Third, there is the danger of subjective judgments about the quality of advice, especially in a sole-rater content analysis. In order to avoid this problem, the present author compared the data in each category in a reiterative, line-by-line basis until satisfied that the scores were distributed fairly. However, it should be acknowledged that the sole-rater content analysis is a limitation of the study, and that an inter-rater system would have enhanced the reliability of the results.

The social science implications of the present study are threefold. First, racial differences and race-based stereotyping, especially as they pertain to stigma and HIV serostatus disclosure, present a challenge for public health goals to expand HIV testing (52).The results presented here suggest that African American men, who are often targeted for prosecution, have little access to culturally-relevant information on the why, where, when, and how of disclosure, or to dedicated websites that promote their legal rights while also advocating HIV testing to protect their own and their partners' health. This deficit should be addressed as a matter of urgency. Second, the lack of culturally relevant information, together with media hyperbole about cases involving African American men, are likely to stymie national goals for expanded HIV testing. If Internet users are exposed to sensationalized media reports, and if website information is lacking or consists mainly of terse "it's the law" declarations, then users likely to become more fearful than informed about the topic. U.S. websites should address disclosure and the law in friendly, personalized terms in order to empower people to disclose to sexual partners while ensuring their own safety in potentially awkward, perhaps dangerous situations. Following the Canadian, U.K., and Australian models, this information could come from a central clearing house that provides accurate, consistent, and well written material as a public service. Third, the present study highlighted how HIV stigma drove U.S. legal policy, more recently in relation to minority ethnic status. Since multiple stigmas affect the most vulnerable populations, and HIV criminalization has gathered pace in recent years, community websites could make a better effort at offering tailored advice for at-risk populations, and could also engage in legal advocacy to help reduce the stigma of being HIV-infected as presently conceived in U.S. law.

REFERENCES

[1]   Bennett-Carlson R, Faria D, Hanssens C. Positive Justice Project: Ending and defending against HIV criminalization. A manual for advocates. Volume 1. New York, NY: Center HIV Law Policy, 2010. Accessed 2011 June 12. URL: http://www.hivlawandpolicy.org/resources/view/564

[2]   Treichler PA. How to have theory in an epidemic: Cultural chronicles of AIDS. Durham, NC: Duke University Press,1999.

[3]   Strub S. Prevention vs. prosecution: Creating a viral underclass, 2011. Accessed 2011 Oct 28. URL: http://blogs.poz.com/sean/archives/2011/10/prevention_vs_prosec.html

[4]   Persson A, Newman C. Making monsters: Crime and race in recent Western media coverage of HIV. Soc Health Illness 2008;30:632-46.

[5]   Bernard E. Prosecutions for HIV exposure and transmission on the rise throughout Europe. Accessed 2011 Jul 27.URL: http://www.aidsmap.com/en/news9/9FFE7E7EA6-2E16-4376-8FC4-A8E82B6325 A2.asp

[6]   Pebody R. North America and Western Europe lead the world in criminalising HIV transmission and exposure. XVIII International AIDS Conference, Vienna, Austria, 2010. Accessed 2011 Jul 22. URL: http://www.aidsmap.com/North-America-and-Western-Europe-lead-the-world-in-criminalising-HIV-transmission-and-exposure/page/1447653/

[7]   Lahey KE. The new line of defense: Criminal HIV transmission laws. Syracuse J Legis Pol 1995;1:85-95.

[8]   Lazzarini Z, Bray S, Burris, S. Evaluating the impact of criminal laws on HIV risk behavior. J Laws Med Ethics 2002;30(2):239-53.

[9]   Krom D. HIV-specific knowing transmission statutes: A proposal to help fight an epidemic. St John's J Leg Comm1999;14:253-78.

[10]   Canadian HIV/AIDS Legal Network, 2011. Criminal law and HIV. Accessed 2011 Jul 30. URL: http://library.catie.ca/PDF/ATI-10000s/18149.pdf

[11]   Bennett-Carlson R, Faria D, Hanssens C. Positive Justice Project: Prosecutions and arrests for HIV exposure in the United States, 2008-2011. New York, NY: The Center for HIV Law & Policy, 2011. Accessed 2011 Aug 20. URL: http://www.hivlawandpolicy.org/resources/view/456

[12]   Homeland Security Newswire. HIV positive Michigan man fights bioterrorism charge after allegedly
        biting neighbor, 2010. Accessed 2011 Jul 12. URL: http://homelandsecuritynewswire.com/hiv-
        positive-michigan-man-fights-bioterrorism-charge-after-allegedly-biting-neighbor

[13]   Bickerstaff E. HIV and the media in the US. Impact:12 (February). UK: National AIDS Trust, 2007.

[14]   Del Amo J, Carol AM, Martinez C, Field V, Broring, G. HIV/AIDS and migration in European
        printed media: An analysis of daily newspapers. Brussels, Belgium: AIDS & Mobility Working
        Group, 2006. Accessed 2011 May 7. URL: http://ws5.evision.nl/systeem3/images/final%20
        report%20version%207%20november.pdf

[15]   Koop CE. Surgeon General's report on acquired immune deficiency syndrome. Washington DC:
        Public Health Service, 1986.

[16]   Cochran SE, Mays VM. Sex, lies, and HIV. N Engl J Med 1990;322:774-775.

[17]   Offer C, Grinstead O, Goldstein E, Mamary E, Alvarado N, Euren J, et al. Responsibility for HIV
        prevention: Patterns of attribution among HIV-seropositive gay and bisexual men. AIDS Educ Prev
        2007;19(1):24-35.

[18]   Wingood GM, DiClemente RJ. The effects of an abusive primary partner on the condom use and
        sexual negotiation practices of African-American women. Am J Pub Health 1997;87(6):1016-8.

[19]   Duffin R. Serostatus, risk and responsibility. New South Wales Department of Health, 2004. Accessed
        2011 November 7. URL: http://www.sprc.unsw.edu.au/media/File/SRB06.pdf

[20]   Bayer R. AIDS prevention – Sexual ethics and responsibility. N Engl J Med 1996;334:1540-2.

[21]   National Institute of Allergy and Infectious Diseases. HIV/AIDS: Treatment of HIV infection.
        Washington, DC: U.S. Dept Health Human Serv, 2009. Accessed 2011 Aug 1.
        URL:http://www.niaid.nih.gov/topics/hivaids/understanding/treatment/pages/default.aspx

[22]   Donnell D, Baeten JM, Kiarie J, Thomas KK, Stevens W, Cohen CR et al. Heterosexual HIV-1
        transmission after initiation of antiretroviral therapy: A prospective cohort analysis. Lancet
        2010;375(9731):2092-8.

[23]   Centers for Disease Control and Prevention. Advancing HIV Prevention: Progress Summary, 2003-
        2005. Atlanta, GA: Nat Cent HIV/AIDS Vir Hep STDTB Prev, 2005.Accessed 2011 Jun 19. URL:
        http://www.cdc.gov/hiv/topics/prev_prog/AHP/resources/factsheets/pdf/Progress_2005.pdf

[24]   Centers for Disease Control and Prevention. Hepatitis C information for the public. Atlanta, GA: Nat
        Cent HIV/AIDS, Vir Hep STD TB Prevention, 2008. Accessed 2011 Jul 10: URL:
        http://www.cdc.gov/hepatitis/C/cFAQ.htm

[25]   Hepatitis B Foundation. General Information. Accessed 2011 Jun 30. URL:
        http://www.hepb.org/patients/general_information.htm

[26]   James R. A review of HIV transmission and exposure cases in Australia, the United Kingdom,
        Sweden and Switzerland. Int AIDS Soc Conf, Vienna, Austria, 2010. Accessed 2011 Oct 26. URL:
        http://birkbeck.academia.edu/MatthewWeait/Papers/219944/Who_Gets_Prosecuted

[27]   Karon JM, Fleming, PL, Steketee RW, De Cock KM. HIV in the United States at the turn of the
        century: An epidemic in transition. Am J Pub Health 2001;91(7):1060-8.

[28]   The Henry J. Kaiser Family Foundation. Black Americans and AIDS, 2007. Accessed 2011 Oct 28.
        URL:http://www.kff.org/hivaids/upload/6089-04.pdf

[29]   Rosenberg SD, Goodman, LA, Osher, FC, Swarz MS, Essock SM, Butterfield MI et al. Prevalence of
        HIV, hepatitis B, and hepatitis C in people with severe mental illness. Am J Pub Health
        2001;91(1):31-37.

[30]   Mykhalovskiy E, Betteridge G, McLay D. HIV non-disclosure and the criminal law: Establishing
        policy options for Ontario, Toronto. Toronto, CA: Canada's AIDS Treatment Information Exchange,
        2010. Accessed 2011 Aug 1. URL: http://www.catie.ca/pdf/Brochures/HIV-non-disclosure-criminal-
        law.pdf

[31]   Worth H, Patton C, Goldstein D. Reckless vectors: The infecting 'Other' in HIV/AIDS law. Sex Res
        Soc Pol 2005;2(2):3-14.

[32]   Wnuk D, Chapman JE, Jeglic EL. Development and refinement of a measure of attitudes toward sex
        offender treatment. J Off Rehab 2006;43(3):35-47.

[33]   Heath L. Mass media and fear of crime. Am Behav Sci 1996;39(4):379-386.

[34] Lichtenstein B. Social stigma in the sexual epidemics: Dangerous Dynamics. CO: Lynne Reiner Publishers, 2012.

[35] Kenney SV. Criminalizing HIV transmission: Lessons learned from history and a model for the future. J Cont Law Pol 1992;8:245-73.

[36] Merminod A. The deterrence rationale in the criminalization of HIV/AIDS. Lex Electr, 2009;13:3. Accessed 2011 Jul 10. URL: http://www.lexelectronica.org/docs/articles_226.pdf

[37] Shouse RL,Kajese T, Hall HI,Valleroy LA.Late HIV Testing – 34 states,

[38] 1996-2005. Morb Mort Week Rep, 2009;58(24):661-65.

[39] Galletly CL, Pinkerton SD. Conflicting messages: How criminal HIV disclosure laws undermine public health efforts to control the spread of HIV. AIDS Behav 2006;10:451-61.

[40] Serovich JE, Mosack KE. Reasons for HIV disclosure or nondisclosure to casual sexual partners. AIDS Educ Prev 2003;15(1):70-80.

[41] Grossman HP, Guillory AK. Law trends and news. Washington, DC: AmBar Assoc, 2004. Accessed 2011 Jul 7. URL: http://www.americanbar.org/content/newsletter/publications/law_trends_news_practice_area_e_newsletter_home/hipaa.html

[42] Pariser, E. The filter bubble: What the internet is hiding from you. New York, NY: Penguin, 2011.

[43] International Planned Parenthood Federation. Healthy, happy, and hot: A young person's guide to their rights, sexuality and living with HIV. Accessed 2011 July 21. URL:http://www.ippf.org /NR/rdonlyres/B4462DDE-487D-4194-B0E0-193A04095819/0/HappyHealthyHot.pdf

[44] Purcell GP, Wilson P, Delamothe T. The quality of health information on the internet: As for any other medium it varies widely: Regulation is not the answer. BMJ 2002;324(7337):557-8.

[45] Lewis, T. Seeking health information on the internet: Lifestyle choice or bad attack of cyberchrondria? Med Cult Soc 2006;28(4):521-39.

[46] Wolitski RJ, Bailey CJ, O'Leary A, Gomez CA, Parsons JT. Self-perceived responsibility of HIV-seropositive men who have sex with men for preventing HIV transmission. AIDS Behav 2003;7(4):363-72.

[47] Gorbach PM, Galea JT, Amani B, Shin A, Celum C, Golden MR. Don't ask, don't tell: Patterns of HIV disclosure among HIV positive men who have sex with men with recent STI practising high risk behaviour in Los Angeles and Seattle. Sex Trans Dis 2004;80: 512-7.

[48] Stein MD, Freedberg KA, Sullivan LM, Savetsky J, Levenson SM, Hingson R, et al. Disclosure of HIV status to sexual partners. Arch Int Med 1998;158:253-57.

[49] Elford J, Ibrahim F, Bukutu C, Anderson J. Disclosure of HIV status: The role of ethnicity among people living with HIV in London. J Acquir Immune Defic Syndr 2008;47:514-21.

[50] Lichtenstein B. Overcoming Stigma. National Harbor, MD: NatSummit HIV Diag Prev Access Care, 2010.

[51] Cairns G. London patient surveys find widely different rates of patients referred to care and lost to follow-up, 2009. Accessed 2011 Jul 12. URL: http://www.aidsmap.com/London-patient-surveys-find-widely-different-rates-of-patients-referred-to-care-and-lost-to-follow-up/page/1434061/

[52] The White House Office of National AIDS Policy. National HIV/AIDS Strategy for the United States, 2010. Accessed 2011 Nov 1. URL: http://www.whitehouse.gov/sites/default/files/uploads/NHAS.pdf

Submitted: November 01, 2011. *Revised:* January 02, 2012. *Accepted:* January 07, 2012.

In: Public Health Yearbook 2012
Editor: Joav Merrick

ISBN: 978-1-62808-078-0
© 2013 Nova Science Publishers, Inc.

Chapter 37

UNDERSTANDING THE AGREEMENTS AND BEHAVIORS OF MEN WHO HAVE SEX WITH MEN WHO ARE DATING OR MARRIED TO WOMEN: UNEXPECTED IMPLICATIONS FOR A UNIVERSAL HIV/STI TESTING PROTOCOL

Jason W Mitchell, MPH, PhD[1],
David A Moskowitz*, PhD[2]
and David W Seal, PhD[3]

[1]Division of Health Promotion & Risk Reduction,
University of Michigan School of Nursing, Ann Arbor, Michigan
[2]Department of Epidemiology & Community Health,
New York Medical College, Valhalla, New York
[3]Department of Global Community Health and Behavioral Sciences,
School of Public Health and Tropical Medicine, Tulane University,
New Orleans, Louisiana, United States

ABSTRACT

Men with a female partner who also have sex with men (MSMW) have been identified as a bridge population for possible HIV transmission to heterosexual women. Social science research that examines how relational and social aspects of MSMW partnered with women is needed to better understand the possible mechanisms that may contribute to HIV/STI risk among MSMW, their female relationship partners, and secondary male sex partners. Methods: The present study assessed whether self-reported accounts of sexual agreements and relationship behaviors of MSMW with a current female partner corresponded to their sexual risk behaviors with secondary male sex partners. A cross-

* Correspondence: David A Moskowitz, PhD, New York Medical College, School of Health Sciences & Practice, Rm. 213, Dept. of Epidemiology & Community Health, Valhalla, New York 10595 United States. E-mail: david_moskowitz@nymc.edu

sectional study design was used to collect anonymous data from a convenience sample of 145 MSMW who had a current female partner and also sought to engage in sex with men. Results: The data indicated that the majority of MSMW engaged in oral and/or anal sex with another male without their female partner knowing. Of men reporting strictly monogamous heterosexual relationships, only 14.5% reported actually only having sex with their female relational partner. The men's average last tests for HIV and STIs were 87.5 and 181.9 months prior, respectively; and most men self-reported low condom use during oral sex and inconsistent condom use during anal intercourse. Conclusions: Universal HIV/STI testing is urgently needed to improve testing rates among MSMW who are unlikely to admit risk-behaviors. Additionally, tailored HIV prevention strategies such as couples-based sexuality and HIV/STI counseling may be beneficial for MSMW.

Keywords: HIV, STIs, MSMW, sexual risk behaviors, agreements, relational factors, bridge population, universal HIV/STI testing

INTRODUCTION

Although men who have sex with men (MSM) are estimated to represent two to five percent of the population, more than half of all new HIV infections each year are among MSM in the United States (1). The primary sexual risk factor for HIV transmission between MSM is unprotected anal intercourse (UAI) (2), yet, not all MSM solely engage in male-to-male sex. Additionally, heterosexual women account for almost one-third of individuals infected by HIV and are more susceptible to HIV infection through unprotected vaginal intercourse than are heterosexual men (3,4). Hypothetically, men who have UAI with other men and unprotected vaginal intercourse or UAI with women may increase new HIV infections among heterosexual women, and help sustain the disproportionate impact of HIV/AIDS among MSM. Prior research has supported this notion that men who engage in sexual risk behaviors with both men and women (MSMW) may serve as a bridge population for HIV transmission (5-11). Because many of these specific men are partnered, social aspects that help to create and maintain their relationships ultimately might be the key predictors of protective or, alternatively, risky sexual health behaviors.

In response to how HIV may be transmitted through bridge populations, a growing body of research has emerged to examine the social and relational characteristics and dynamics of men in concurrent sexual partnerships. Research with MSMW, either labeled as non-gay identified or behaviorally bisexual men, has examined sexual risk behaviors to determine the likelihood of HIV and STI transmission to female sex partners. Published data on MSMW indicated several individual characteristics that are associated with an increase in sexual risk behaviors, including: 1) having sex with both men and women, 2) a non-gay identity, and 3) concealment of same-sex behavior from female partners (9, 12-19). Other research has examined correlates and reasons for why MSMW use condoms and test for HIV less frequently (19-22).

However, gaps in the HIV prevention literature, which deal specifically with the social/relational aspects of MSMW, remain understudied. Few studies have collected and described self-reported sexual risk behavior and relationship data, including agreements of MSMW who actively placed advertisements on the Internet (i.e., www.craigslist.org) for same-sex encounters. Moreover, little is known about the association between self-reported data on relationship behaviors and relationship agreements among MSMW with their female partners and the sexual risk behaviors in which MSMW engage with male secondary sex partners. Research that examines the intersection of these important social aspects (specifically, the concordance/discordance of sexual behaviors and agreements with relationship partners among MSMW) is needed in order to design suitable HIV/STI prevention interventions.

The present study sought to assess whether self-reported accounts of sexual agreements and relationship behaviors of MSMW with a steady female partner corresponded to their sexual risk behaviors with secondary male sex partners. The overall aim of the present research was to expand our understanding of the contributing factors, including relationship agreements, to HIV and STI risk transmission among MSMW, their female relationship partners, and any secondary male sex partners they may have. Specifically, this study has three objectives: 1) to describe the distribution of relationship types, agreements, and self-reported sexual behaviors (including condom use) among female partnered MSMW who actively sought out and engaged in sexual behaviors with men; 2) to examine the degree to which agreements match with behaviors among MSMW; and 3) to assess the differences and similarities of self-reported relationship agreements and sexual risk behaviors among the sample.

METHODS

Men, regardless of sexual identity, who placed an advertisement to engage in sex with other men on each Craigslist.org mirror website where English was the primary language, were invited to take a brief online survey. Various cities and locations throughout the US (and internationally) have a Craigslist.org website assigned to their respective location (i.e., a mirror website). Each Craigslist.org location where English was the predominant language was used to recruit for the present study. The first one hundred men's sexual advertisements at each of the Craigslist websites were selected to receive a block message that informed them of our research study. A link embedded in the email took them directly to the anonymous survey. The first page contained a consent form. Participants could not advance to the actual survey without first consenting. Participants were not compensated for their time. After excluding men who did not complete all of the necessary information to answer our research questions (n = 193) and those who were either single (n = 328) or partnered with a male (n = 157), a sample of 145 men was left for our analysis. We purposely excluded men who reported being single and those who were partnered with a male due to our research interest in the dynamics of concurrent sexual partnerships among female-partnered men who were seeking male-to-male sexual behaviors. Data from 145 men with current female partners who also sought sex with males were used to examine our objectives.

Measures used

Basic demographic data were elicited: sexual identity, age, city size, race/ethnicity, income, education, self-reported HIV serostatus, and number of months since last reported HIV and STI test. Participants were asked to categorize their sexual identity as 'heterosexual', 'homosexual', 'bisexual', or 'will not label'. City size options included, '< 10,000 persons', '10,000 – 50,000 persons', '51,000 – 100,000 persons', '101,000 – 500,000 persons', '501,000 – 1 million persons', and 'over 1 million persons'. Education level was obtained through the following categories: 'finished some high school', 'graduated high school', 'graduated high school and finished some college, 'graduated college, 'graduated college and finished some graduate work', and 'received a graduate degree'.

Relationship type and length

To assess relationship type, we asked participants to check one of the following categories: 1) 'I'm single, not involved in a relationship'; 2) 'I'm in a non-cohabitating relationship with a woman (you're not living together)'; 3) 'I'm in a cohabitating relationship with a woman (you're living together)'; and 4) 'I'm legally married to, or have a civil union with, a woman'. As previously mentioned, men who chose category one (i.e., who were single) were excluded from our analyses. The men indicated the length of their current relationship in months.

Relationship agreement

To capture the diversity in relationship agreements that participants may have had with their female partners, we asked which category best described the sort of agreement they had with their current main partner. These were: 1) 'implicitly monogamous (without talking about it, you and your partner just know you are monogamous)'; 2) 'explicitly monogamous (you and your partner have actually discussed that you both will be monogamous)'; 3) 'non-monogamous, but you tell your main partner when you have fooled around with other individuals'; 4) 'non-monogamous, but you do not tell your main partner when you have fooled around with other individuals'; and 5) 'non-monogamous, but only when both you and your partner fool around with another person together (you only have threesomes with you, your partner, and a third person)'.

Male-to-male sexual behaviors with or without female partner

Participants were asked to select the statement that best described the sort of same-sex sexual behaviors enacted while being in their current relationship. These statements were: 1) 'I have only ever fooled around or had sex with my partner'; 2) 'I have fooled around with other men WITHOUT my partner being there and have had oral intercourse but HAVE NOT had anal Intercourse'; 3) 'I have fooled around with other men WITHOUT my partner being there and have had oral AND anal intercourse'; 4) 'I have fooled around with other men WITH my partner being there and have had oral intercourse but HAVE NOT anal intercourse'; and 5) 'I have fooled around with other men WITH my partner being there and have had oral and anal intercourse'.

Because not all sexual behaviors that men engage in were addressed with this measure, one potential limitation is the assessment of men who had anal sex, but not oral sex, with or without the female partner being there.

Relationship partner's awareness of male-to-male sexual behaviors

Married men (who comprised the overwhelming majority of the sample) were asked whether their female partners were aware of their same-sex behaviors.

Participants responded to the following statement, "I am currently married to my wife, and she DOES know about my hooking up with other men", by selecting either 'yes' or 'no'.

Number of male sex partners

Men were asked to indicate the number of male sex partners they had accrued over the previous 12 months for oral intercourse. An additional question was asked to obtain data on how many male sex partners the men had for anal intercourse in the previous 12 months.

Condom use

Men were asked the following two questions, "In the past 12 months, what percent of the time did you use condoms during oral intercourse when having sex with men?" and "In the past 12 months, what percent of the time did you use condoms during anal intercourse when having sex with men?"

For each measure regarding condom use, participants were given eight possible responses: 1) 'I never had this sort of sexual partner'; 2) 'I never used a condom'; 3) 'I practically never used a condom'; 4) 'I rarely used a condom'; 5) 'I sometimes used a condom'; 6) 'I usually used a condom'; 7) 'I practically always used a condom'; and 8) 'I always used a condom'.

These categories were collapsed into 'always', 'sometimes', and 'never' wears a condom for both oral and anal sex behaviors (where "sometimes" was comprised of individuals who selected answers three through seven). MSMW selecting, "I never had this sort of partner," were excluded from the individual analyses.

Analysis

Stata/SE Version 11 (StataCorp LP, College Station, TX) for Mac was used to conduct all analyses. Descriptive statistics were calculated to describe the study sample's demographics, relationship characteristics, sexual behaviors, and lack of condom use for oral and anal sex with males.

Pearson's chi-square test was then used to assess the degree to which participants' relationship agreements and relationship sexual behaviors were concordant or discordant. The independent t-test was used to assess differences among participants' self-reported relationship agreements, relationship sexual behaviors, and agreement-behavior discordance for their last reported HIV and STI tests, and condom use.

Missing data were present in the measures for relationship duration, sexual risk behaviors with males, and condom use with males. Most notably, forty percent of the men did not report how long they have been in their current relationship with their female partner.

It remains unclear as to why so many men did not report how long they have been in their current relationship with their female partner. Future research must take into account this limitation and possible, significant bias. Missing data on other measures were minimal and are noted when the results are presented.

RESULTS

Demographic and relationship characteristics for the sample are presented in table 1. The mean age for participants was 44.7 years (SD = 12.1); men as young as 19 and as old as 79 years participated in the study. The majority of the sample self-identified as: white (88%); bisexual (75%); and married to their female partner (79%). Most men also had completed some college or attained a bachelor's degree (66.7%); earned at least $50,000 (63.9%); and lived in locales with a population of 100,000 persons or less (51.4%). The proportion of men from small- to medium-sized towns was due to our sampling technique of selecting craigslist.org mirror-sites for cities and towns that varied in population size (e.g., NYC.craigslist.org, Asheville.craigslist.org, Anchorage.craigslist.org, etc.).

Table 1. Demographic and relationship characteristics of 145 MSMW study participants

Characteristic	% (N)
Race	
White	88.3% (128)
Latino	6.2% (9)
African American	1.4% (2)
Indian	1.4% (2)
Other	2.7% (4)
Sexuality	
Heterosexual	12.4% (18)
Homosexual	6.2% (9)
Bisexual	73.8% (107)
Chose no label	7.6% (11)
Self-reported HIV serostatus	
Negative	93.8% (136)
Positive	1.4% (2)
Unknown	4.8% (7)
Relationship status	
Dating a female partner	10.3% (15)
Living with female partner	11.0% (16)
Married to a female partner	78.6% (114)
Relationship agreement	
Implicit monogamy	22.1% (32)
Explicit monogamy	15.9% (23)
Non-monogamous: Disclose when unfaithful	8.3% (12)
Non-monogamous: Does not disclose when unfaithful	51.0% (74)
Non-monogamous: Threesomes or partner knows	2.8% (4)

Characteristic	% (N)
Self-reported sexual behaviors with or without female partner	
Only had sex with female partner	5.5% (8)
Had oral and/or anal sex; female partner not present	89.0% (129)
Had oral and/or anal sex; female partner present	5.5% (8)
Female partner knows about sexual behaviors with men[c]	10.3% (15)
	Mean (SD), [Range]
Age (years)	44.7 (12.1), [19 − 79]
Relationship duration (months)[a]	211.3 (142.9), [9 − 562]
Last HIV test (months)[b]	87.5 (125.0), [0 − 289]
Last STD test (months)[b]	181.9 (225.1), [0 − 481]

Notes: [a] Approximately 40% of the sample did not respond to this measure (i.e., 58 missing cases).
[b] Twenty-four men did not respond to these measures.
[c] Applicable to married men only

Findings

Approximately one-half of the men indicated that their current relationship was non-monogamous without disclosing to their current female partner when they were unfaithful. Furthermore, 89% of the men self-reported that they had oral and/or anal sex with another male without their female partner being present. However, 10% of men did report that their female partners knew about their sexual behaviors with men.

Table 1 shows the distribution of relationship types, agreements, and extra-relationship behaviors. In terms of how well the agreements correspond to actual and allowed behaviors, there were key differences in concordance and discordance ($X^2(6, 137) = 58.27$, $\Phi^2 = .40$, p < .001).

Of men reporting strictly monogamous heterosexual relationships, only 14.5% actually reported having sex with only their relational partner. Most monogamous men (80.0%) reported having sex with others without their partner present. A few monogamous men (5.5%) reported have sex with others with their partner present. Although these men reported being in a strictly monogamous heterosexual relationship, the data indicated that, in reality, sex was occurring outside of their relationship and without their partner being there.

Of men reporting non-monogamous relationships in which they disclose extra-relationship sexual encounters, 0.0% reported only having sex with their relational partner, 83.3% reported sex without their partner present, and 16.7% reported sex with their partner present.

Of men reporting non-monogamous relationships in which they do not disclose extra-relationship sexual encounters, 0.0% reported only having sex with their relational partner, 100.0% reported sex without their partner present, and 0.0% reported sex with their partner present. Finally, of men only engaging in threesomes, 0.0% reported only having sex with their relational partner, 25.0% reported sex without their partner present, and 75.0% reported sex with their partner present.

Table 2 provides data on participants' self-reported sexual risk behaviors and condom use with male partners. Over the previous 12 months, men reported an average of 15 male partners for oral sex and 5 male partners for anal sex. Not all men with a female partner reported having oral or anal sex with another male in the previous 12 months.

Of the men who did (n = 121, 83%), some had oral and/or anal sex with another male without using a condom. About two-thirds of those reporting never used a condom for oral sex with a male. Approximately 14% of MSMW 'never' used a condom for anal sex with a male; 59% reported 'sometimes' or inconsistently used condoms for anal sex with a male; and 27% of men stated that they 'always' used a condom for anal sex with another male.

Most surprisingly, the average times since last HIV and STI test were approximately 7 years, 4 months and 15 years, 2 months, respectively. That is, considering the number of partners accrued each year and the lapse in HIV/STI testing, the average MSMW in our sample could not possibly be certain of his HIV/STI status.

No significant statistical differences were found between men's reported last HIV and STI test by relationship agreement or relationship sexual behaviors. Further, neither number of oral/anal sex partners nor condom use statistically differed by participants' relationship agreement type, relationship sexual behaviors, or agreement-behavior discordance.

Table 2. MSMW self-reported sexual risk behaviors and condom use with male secondary sex partners

Sexual risk behavior[a]	*Mean* (SD), [Range]
Oral sex with male	15.4 (26.8), [0 – 200]
Anal sex with male	5.1 (14.5), [0 – 100]
Condom use: Never[b]	% (*n*)
Oral sex with male	67.3% (74)
Anal sex with male	13.7% (10)
Condom use: Sometimes[b]	% (*n*)
Oral sex with male	28.2% (31)
Anal sex with male	58.9% (43)
Condom use: Always[b]	% (*n*)
Oral sex with male	4.5% (5)
Anal sex with male	27.4% (20)

Notes: [a] Minimal missing data occurred for MSMW's self-reported sexual risk behaviors with males (9 cases). Not all MSMW had oral and/or anal sex with another male. Thirteen MSMW self-reported no oral sex with a male. Sixty-three MSMW self-reported no anal sex with a male.

[b] Missing data occurred for MSMW's self-reported condom use with males (24 cases). Regarding condom use with males, eleven MSMW self-reported no oral sex with a male. Forty-eight MSMW self-reported no anal sex with a male.

DISCUSSION

Behavioral and structural HIV and STI prevention interventions that focus on improving the HIV/STI testing behaviors of MSMW, sexual health, and related communication within relationships are urgently needed for behaviorally bisexual individuals, including MSMW who currently have a female relationship partner. Findings from the present study highlight the disconnect that exists between men's reported relationship agreements, relationship behaviors regarding sex with or without their current female partner, and sexual risk behaviors (e.g., inconsistent condom use) in which they engage with secondary male sex partners. Simply put, most MSMW in this sample were not talking with their female relationship partners about their engagements in sexual behaviors with men, were using condoms inconsistently during anal intercourse, and were not getting HIV/STI tested. In many instances, the men were actively breaking their expressed monogamous agreements.

The lack of HIV and STI testing and inconsistent rates of condom use during oral and anal intercourse with male partners is of concern. These trends highlight the potential for the unknowing transmission of STIs and HIV to female relationship partners of MSMW. For example, the average time since last HIV/STI test was more than seven years. Given this lapse, it is likely that the men might have contracted one of the less manifest STIs (e.g., HIV, HPV, Chlamydia) and potentially, may have transmitted such infections to partners. To speculate on these low testing rates: MSMW may not consider themselves at risk for STIs and HIV because they do not consider themselves "gay." Generally, there may be a disconnect between the behaviors practiced by MSMW and their perceptions of the risks associated with these behaviors—a disconnect that MSM and gay men may not make. Our findings of lapsed HIV and STI testing and infrequent use of condoms among MSMW further contribute and support what previous research has found with bisexual men in the U.S. [19, 20, 22]. Our results are also quantitative, represent MSMW throughout the U.S., and further highlight the lack of disclosure about male-to-male sexual behaviors to their steady female partners.

The present research provides strong evidence for the need for universal STI and HIV testing by healthcare providers. Simply, all men and women should be tested. The low testing rates coupled with the men not mentioning their male-to-male sexual behaviors to their female partners, is worrisome for preventing STIs and the transmission of HIV. Hypothetically, some women partnered to these men might not recognize their inadvertent risk for STIs and HIV and the need to get tested. They unknowingly may be providing their primary healthcare provider or gynecologist with misinformation about their relationship and related sexual behaviors. Additionally, a similar trend might be occurring when MSMW visit their primary care physicians. Stigma, shame, guilt, or perceptions of being judged may act as obstacles towards truthful and full patient-provider communication. To circumvent these two possible scenarios, universal testing, regardless of an admission of risk, is necessary. In addition to universal testing, programs that encourage both partners within the couple to communicate about their relationship and sexual health are urgently needed, essential, and necessary for preventing HIV and other STIs.

Condom use was not particularly consistent during anal intercourse, with seven out of ten men reporting inconsistent or absent condom use. This trend did not vary between different groups of MSMW, or between those with concordant or discordant relationship agreements and behaviors. While the number of anal male partners was relatively low compared with number of oral intercourse partners (about 10 fewer per year on average), the risk of infection of STIs and HIV significantly increases for unprotected anal intercourse [23]. It only takes one unprotected experience to transmit disease. Ultimately, many of these men are making sexual health decisions for their female partners, who may be operating under the assumption of monogamy. Tailored intervention programs that help MSMW come out of the proverbial closet and address their same-sex sexual encounters with their partners are needed.

However, this is no small task. Shame, alienation, guilt, and the likelihood of divorce all may act as disincentives to truthful communication. MSMW alternatively may prefer to engage in sex with other men without disclosing such acts to their steady female partners because of the thrill that they experience. In the final analysis, and considering the average man in this sample was in his mid-forties, coming to terms with an unconventional sexuality may be too difficult and disruptive for MSMW.

A structural intervention (e.g., a universal HIV/STI testing protocol) may be an optimal way to circumvent the difficulties of interpersonal disclosures. Such a protocol would allow healthcare providers to identify men who may have contracted diseases before they transmit it to their female partner or secondary male partners.

Limitations

Despite these key findings, our research did have limitations related to missing data (i.e. overall condom use and relationship duration), lack of data to conclude the degree to which the MSMW also were sexually active specifically with their current female partner, recall bias, and the inability to determine causality or temporal associations among the various relationship factors and sexual risk behaviors. Our research also did not collect data on every possible sexual encounter of MSMW's male-to-male sexual behaviors with or without their female partner (i.e., men who had anal sex, but not oral sex, with or without the female partner being there). A halo effect may have been present, with MSMW reporting an agreement type other than what was actually true in order to rationalize their sexual risk behaviors with other men outside of their relationship (i.e., reporting non-monogamous agreements with their partners, even though no such agreements were made). However, we purposely used an anonymous survey design to help decrease measurement error and participant bias [24].

In addition, individual-level data were collected only from the men in each relationship. Dyadic data would be much more informative. Such data would show how both partners understand their agreements and whether both partners operate under the same precise agreement. A final limitation might have been the demographic makeup of the sample itself. The men were predominately White, well educated, and relatively wealthy.

Ironically, this sample actually may provide more novel data than if the sample had been more diverse racially. Previous research with MSMW has almost exclusively focused on sexual risk behaviors among minority populations, particularly African Americans [9, 19, 20, 25, 26]. Largely White populations have been studied far less.

Future social science research should be conducted to correct these limitations. Additionally, future research that focuses on dyadic data (e.g., information from both partners) is needed to measure the level of awareness that relational partners of MSMW have of their same-sex behaviors. Research that examines how relational and societal factors may inhibit or facilitate an individual's ability to discuss his or her sexual needs, including the preferred type of relationship and establishment of a sexual agreement, is urgently needed among MSMW relationships. Finally, the push for universal HIV testing in the United States and abroad may enhance awareness and provide a structural mechanism to instigate sexual health communication between couples.

Implications for social science

This research was merely one instance showing how a social science perspective can provide different insights into public health. Where more traditional epidemiologic studies focus on deficit-based models regarding at-risk populations (e.g., drug use leading to HIV risk in gay men), social science tests innovative social interaction- and relationship-based predictors that help to more precisely define and understand the intricacies of populations.

As shown by the research, investigating aspects of the relationship can help illuminate the unique dynamics that may exist between partners and how public health programs can intervene to address these issues. For example, our main goal was to explore the sexual risk behaviors and relationship characteristics among MSMW; however, our study revealed inconsistent testing behaviors, inconsistent condom use, and the disconnect between what MSMW reported about their same-sex behaviors and what they reported about their agreements formed with their steady female partners.

Another positive aspect of using a social science research perspective (and shown by the present research) is the encouragement of more nuanced groupings within populations. Public health and epidemiological studies often focus on race/ethnicity, age, occupations, geographic areas, socioeconomic status, gender, and sexual orientation to indicate differences between individuals.

In contrast, social science offers categorizations within populations that group men and women by their social identities, social networks, individual differences on social variables, and, as exemplified by the current study, subtypes of relationships. In short, a social frame placed on health research increases the external validity of studies' findings. Arguably, it is more likely that individuals would, in reality, self-categorize under such social categories rather than the more rigid, demographic ones suggested by epidemiology.

As a concluding point, social science research into health problems can help provide support for public health programs and interventions. Universal HIV/STI testing has been hotly debated over the past few years. The encouragement of primary care physicians to test everyone, regardless of obvious risk factors, remains controversial; however, social-based research studies, such as the present research, provide evidence for why such a change in protocol may be necessary.

The sample of MSMW described in this study happens to be in dire need of a structural intervention, such as universal HIV/STI testing. As previously mentioned, it may be too stigmatizing or deleterious for the relationship for the men to communicate to their female partners either their extra-dyadic sexual encounters or their need to be HIV/STI tested. It is certain that future social science research studies will continue to provide evidence for the most efficacious interventions for at-risk groups, such as MSMW and their female partners.

ACKNOWLEDGMENTS

This manuscript was supported by the center (P30-MH52776) and NRSA (T32-MH19985) grants from the National Institute of Mental Health. Special thanks are extended to the participants for their time and effort.

REFERENCES

[1]   CDC Prevalence and awareness of HIV infection among men who have sex with men, 21 Cities, United States, 2008. MMWR 2010; 59(37):1201-7.

[2]   Coates TJ. What is to be done? AIDS 2008;22:1079–80.

[3]   CDC. HIV in the United States, 2010. Accessed 2011 Oct 27. URL: http://www.cdc.gov/hiv/resources/factsheets/us.htm

[4]   CDC. HIV/AIDS and Women, 2007. Accessed 2011 Oct 27. URL: http://www.cdc.gov /hiv/topics/women/overview_partner.htm

[5]   Chu SY, Peterman TA, Doll LS, Buehler JW, Curran JW. AIDS in bisexual men in the United States: Epidemiology and transmission in women. Am J Public Health 1992;82:220-4.

[6]   Kahn JG, Gurvey J, Pollack LM, Binson D, Catania JA. How many HIV infections cross the bisexual bridge? An estimate from the United States. AIDS 1997;11:1031-7.

[7]   O'Leary A, Jones KT. Bisexual men and heterosexual women: How big is the bridge? How can we know? Sex Transm Dis 2006;33:594-5.

[8]   Prabhu R, Owen CL, Folger K, McFarland W. The bisexual bridge revisited: Sexual risk behavior among men who have sex with men and women, San Francisco, 1998-2003. AIDS 2004;18:1604-6.

[9]   Siegel K, Schrimshaw EW, Lekas H, Parsons JT. Sexual behaviors of non-gay identified non-disclosing men who have sex with men and women. Arch Sex Behav 2008;37:720-35.

[10]   Wood RW, Krueger LE, Pearlman TC, Goldbaum G. HIV transmission: Women's risk from bisexual men. Am J Public Health 1993;83:1757-9.

[11]   Zule WA, Bobashev GV, Wechsberg WM, Costenbader EC, Coomes CM. Behaviorally bisexual men and their risk behaviors with men and women. J Urban Health 2009;86(1):S48-S62.

[12]   Agronick G, O'Donnell L, Stueve A, Doval AS, Duran R, Vargo S. Sexual behaviors and risks among bisexually and gay-identified young Latino men. AIDS Behav 2004;8:185-97.

[13]   CDC. HIV/STD risks in young men who have sex with men who do not disclose their sexual orientation-Six U.S. cities, 1994-2000. MMWR 2003;52:81-5.

[14]   Doll LS, Peterson LR, White CR, Johnson ES, Ward JW, The Blood Donor Study Group. Homosexuality and nonhomosexuality identified men who have sex with men: A behavioral comparison. J Sex Res 1992;29:1-14.

[15]   Goldbaum G, Perdue T, Wolitski R, Rietmeijer C, Hedrich A, Wood R, et al. Differences in risk behavior and sources of AIDS information among gay, bisexual, and straight-identified men who have sex with men. AIDS Care 1998;12:13-21.

[16]   Stokes JP, Vanable P, McKirnan DJ. Comparing gay and bisexual men on sexual behavior, condom use, and psychosocial variables related to HIV/AIDS. Arch Sex Behav 1997;26:383-97.

[17]   Wold C, Seage GR, Lenderking WR, Mayer KH, Cai B, Heeren T, et al. Unsafe sex in men who have sex with both men and women. J Acquir Immune Defic Syndr 1998;17:361-7.

[18]   Jeffries WL. Sociodemographic, sexual, and HIV and other sexually transmitted disease risk profiles of nonhomosexual-identified men who have sex with men. Am J Public Health 2009;99:1042-5.

[19]   Dodge B, Jeffries WL, Sandfort TGM. Beyond the down low: Sexual risk, protection, and disclosure among at-risk black men who have sex with both men and women (MSMW). Arch Sex Behav 2008;37:683-96.

[20]   Washington TA, Wang Y, Browne D. Difference in condom use among sexually active males at historically black colleges and universities. J Am Coll Health 2009;57:411-8.

[21]   Jeffries WL, Dodge B. Male bisexuality and condom use at last sexual encounter: Results from a national survey. J Sex Res 2007;44:278-89.

[22]   Jeffries WL. HIV testing among bisexual men in the United States. AIDS Educ Prev 2010;22;356-370.

[23]   Vittinghoff E, Douglas J, Judson F, McKirnan D, MacQueen K, Buchbinder SP. Per-contact risk of human immunodeficiency virus transmission between male sexual partners. Am J Epidemiol 1999;150:306-11.

[24]   Catania JA, Gibson DR, Chitwood DD, Coates TJ. Methodological problems in AIDS behavioral research: Influences on measurement error and participation bias in studies of sexual behavior. Psychol Bull 1990;108:339-62.

[25] Millet G, Malebranche D, Mason B, Spikes P. Focusing "down low": bisexual black men, HIV risk and heterosexual transmission. J Natl Med Assoc 2005;97(Suppl 7):52S-9.

[26] Reback CJ, Larkins S. Maintaining a heterosexual identity: Sexual meanings among a sample of heterosexually identified men who have sex with men. Arch Sex Behav 2010;39:766-73.

Submitted: November 03, 2011. *Revised:* January 03, 2012. *Accepted:* January 07, 2012.

In: Public Health Yearbook 2012
Editor: Joav Merrick

ISBN: 978-1-62808-078-0
© 2013 Nova Science Publishers, Inc.

Chapter 38

REFASHIONING STIGMA: EXPERIENCING AND MANAGING HIV/AIDS IN THE BIOMEDICAL ERA

Yordanos Mequanint Tiruneh[*]

Department of Sociology, Northwestern University, Evanston,
Illinois, United States of America

ABSTRACT

This paper explores the stigma experiences of people living with HIV/AIDS (PLWHA) and evaluates the impact of antiretroviral treatment (ART) on their (a) lived experiences and (b) illness management. Qualitative research for this study is based on 105 in-depth interviews and ethnographic observation conducted between May and October of 2008 at an urban HIV clinic in a teaching hospital in Addis Ababa, Ethiopia. A phenomenological approach to data analysis isolated socio-cultural meanings underlying empirical variations of stigma experiences and examined how the availability of treatment alters the experience of living with chronic stigmatized diseases. The study reveals that ART can effect a physical and social rebirth with a renewed sense of self-worth that, together, improve the negative self-concept people develop following an HIV diagnosis. The study also demonstrates that stigma attached to HIV/AIDS remains pervasive in the era of ART. Indeed, ART creates new stigma concerns related to healthcare practices that arise when patients refill prescriptions and follow up on their treatment. This refashioned nature of stigma demands that we identify patterns of change in the perception, experience, and management of the illness. Identifying and analyzing sources of stigma for PLWHA allows us to isolate stigma triggers and devise structural changes that can reform elements of healthcare institutions that intensify HIV stigma. Such research is particularly important in resource-poor settings where the AIDS crisis lingers and the socio-cultural factors that influence the outcomes of intervention strategies require attention.

Keywords: Stigma, HIV/AIDS, Antiretroviral therapy (ART), illness management, lived experience, Ethiopia

---

[*] Correspondence: Yordanos M. Tiruneh, Department of Sociology, Northwestern University, 1810 Chicago Avenue, Evanston, IL 60208 United States. E-mail: yordanos@u.northwestern.edu or yordanosnu@gmail.com

INTRODUCTION

AIDS is one of the leading causes of morbidity and mortality among adults in Ethiopia. In 2005, the cumulative number of AIDS deaths was 1,267,000 with a projection to reach 1.9 million in 2010 (1). AIDS accounted for 34% of young adult deaths, of which 66.3% occurred in urban areas (1). It is estimated that, from 2000 to 2015, AIDS will increase mortality by 6% and reduce the population by 16% compared with what would have occurred in the absence of the disease (2). Likewise, the average life expectancy in Ethiopia is 45.5 years, a figure that is estimated to decrease by 15% due to AIDS from 2010 to 2015 (2). The anticipated universal coverage of ART, however, is assumed to reduce AIDS mortality by 41% compared to a projection without treatment and decrease the reduction in life expectancy due to HIV/AIDS (1). Stigma is one of the major social drivers of the epidemic in Ethiopia, hindering early diagnosis and disclosure of one's HIV serostatus (3). Stigma is rooted in the ignorance, cultural and religious beliefs, poverty, and fear that surround the disease (4). This fear imposes a huge burden on efforts to contain the epidemic and care for PLWHA (4).

Since January 2005, Highly Active Antiretroviral Therapy (HAART) has been available to PLWHA in Ethiopia, free of charge, through the national ART program, which is supported by various national and international initiatives (5). Across the country, 45,595 people had started treatment by the end of July, 2006, of which 47% were adult males and 48% were adult females (5). The availability of ART in resource-poor settings generates a significant hope to reconstruct HIV as a chronic manageable condition and reduce the stigma that has been associated with HIV (6, 7). ART's capacity to relieve or improve many symptoms of HIV infection, thereby restoring health and productivity and facilitating social integration (6), allows PLWHA to escape detection and the accompanying stigma that others associate with those who have the disease.

However, few studies have explored the lived experiences of those following biomedical management of the disease since HIV treatments have become available in such resource-poor settings (1, 2). The relationship between stigma concerns of PLWHA and ART is among the lived experiences that require attention. HIV/AIDS is a disease that is often identified with "immoral" behavior and is perceived as contagious and threatening to the public. Furthermore, its contraction is often viewed as having been brought on by the diseased individual (8, 9). For these reasons, HIV/AIDS is more highly stigmatized than other illnesses such as cancer (10), SARS, or tuberculosis (11). Studying HIV stigma in a range of socio-cultural and political settings is imperative if we hope to understand the differential experiences of PLWHA (7, 12). Ethiopia represents such a setting, as it exhibits all the above-mentioned stigma concerns associated with socio-cultural and political environments. Indeed, because HIV is transmitted by socially produced behaviors that occur in specific social contexts, the experience and management of the disease is similarly context specific (13). Therefore, although almost everyone living with HIV faces some form of stigma, the lived experiences and illness management practices of PLWHA in disparate socio-cultural contexts are affected differentially precisely because socio-cultural context affects the particular forms and triggers of stigma that occur.

In his classical work on stigma, which now forms the basis of most stigma studies, Erving Goffman defines stigma as a powerfully discrediting attribute that changes individuals' perception of the self and how they are viewed by others (14). Although

Goffman did not have AIDS in mind when he defined stigma, scholars agree that HIV involves all three types of Goffman's stigmatized attributes: physical imperfection caused by progressive opportunistic infections, behavioral flaws characterized by moral transgression, and affliction through membership in a social group considered a "risk group" (e.g., commercial sex workers, IV drug users, and people with socially devalued sexual behaviors) (15). Based on this classic definition, Alonzo et al. defined stigma as the construction of a deviation from the "normal" due to undesirable or distinguishing attributes that impose a risk of isolation from the self as well as society (8). HIV stigma is a social construct that is rooted in the far larger conceptualizations of gender, sexuality, race, class, and culture. Its salience rises and falls throughout the illness trajectory because the attributes that trigger stigma can be concealed at some stages of the illness but not in others. Moreover, the targets of stigma vary across cultures, and are uniquely experienced by each person depending on the social environment and the nature of the stigmatizing condition (8, 10). Holzemer et al. point to the cyclic nature of HIV stigma. Stigma begins with a trigger (HIV testing, illness symptoms, or filling a prescription) that leads to negative health outcomes (such as suboptimal treatment adherence and disease progression), that, in turn, become triggers in their own right (16).

Extant research concerning stigma in the context of HIV yields several observations: First, HIV is an extraordinarily unique illness with universal, multi-dimensional stigmatization that can arise immediately following a diagnosis, at the appearance of symptoms, and even because it is still considered untreatable by many people (8, 10). Second, PLWHA often experience social rejection, isolation, economic discrimination, blame, and a negative self-concept (10, 17). Third, HIV stigma is persistent in spite of our better understanding of the disease and the advent of successful treatment options (18), and efforts to reduce stigma have met with only moderate success (19). Few studies afford provisional support to the link between stigma reduction and ART provision (20, 21) while others challenge the argument that availability of treatment reduces stigma (22, 23). Fourth, stigma negatively affects the success of effective HIV prevention and care efforts (including adherence to prescribed medical regimens). Most studies indicate that the greater the stigma the more consistently it is associated with missed doses of prescribed medications, medication non-adherence, and poor health outcomes (24–28).

A review of the relevant literature exposes two gaps. First, not many studies have examined stigma from the sufferers' perspectives using their lived experiences to anchor the analysis (7, 15). Second, only a few studies have been conducted to examine how HIV treatment has reshaped the public conceptualization of HIV/AIDS and how stigma affects illness management on the part of PLWHA (20-23). By examining the lived experiences and illness management of PLWHA, this qualitative study examines the dynamic relationship between HIV treatment and stigma, three years after free provision of ART in an urban setting in Ethiopia. It is both important and timely to examine how ART has refashioned HIV stigma, particularly in resource-poor settings like Ethiopia where the AIDS crisis is still rampant and the impacts of ART remain recent and, largely, unknown.

METHODS

This paper is part of a larger project that explores the lived experiences and illness management of PLWHA in Ethiopia. The overall goal of the study was to understand how

PLWHA in Ethiopia perceive, experience, and manage their illness in the era of effective HIV treatment. The study was conducted in an urban HIV/AIDS clinic at a teaching hospital in Addis Ababa, Ethiopia. Consistent with trends seen in most metropolitan areas in developing countries, Addis is characterized by extreme socio-economic and cultural contrasts, with a few modern sectors that are relatively technologically advanced by Western standards and many others that remain culturally traditional. The city is further characterized by extreme socioeconomic polarization, with huge income disparities between a few millionaires and most others, who struggle for daily survival. It is the most diverse city in Ethiopia, attracting people representing a range of cultures and ethnicities from all over the country, including a recently urbanized rural population that has migrated to the big city in search of jobs. This rural-urban exodus coupled with the continuously growing population in such a limited economy escalates unemployment, overburdens the city's poorly developed infrastructure, and engenders widespread ghettos that exhibit all the vices associated with urban poverty.

This urban setting was chosen as the research site for several epidemiological and social reasons. First, HIV is highly prevalent in and inflicts considerable social and economic impacts on urban areas. For instance, two-thirds (66.3%) of all urban deaths of people between the ages of 15 and 49 are due to AIDS (4). Second, Addis exhibits a relatively high rate of people living with HIV (11.5%), and houses several HIV treatment sites (4). Third, as already noted, Addis is characterized by a great diversity of ethnicities, socioeconomic statuses, religions, and worldviews. And, fourth, in Addis traditionalism and modernism simultaneously inform all aspects of life. All of these societal factors shape the contexts in which PLWHA construct their social identities and their choices of illness-management strategies. This complex admixture of societal factors facilitated the selection of a diverse participant sample, revealing the realities of life for PLWHA as anything but monolithic.

Since the literature contains no sociological studies of the illness experiences of people living with HIV in the study area, the present research employs a qualitative approach suited to the examination of phenomena that otherwise are inaccessible through comprehensive scientific investigation. Between May and October of 2008, six months of ethnographic observation and interviews were conducted at St. Michael's hospital, which facilitated obtaining a rich, exploratory account of individual experiences and actual practices that would be unattainable through quantitative investigation. In-depth interviews were conducted with 105 PLWHA who were selected randomly during their clinic visits. To form the sample, clinic nurses chose every other or every third patient (depending on the total number of patients on a given day) to inform potential participants about the research. The researcher then approached those who agreed to participate in the study to explain its purpose and procedures in detail. The researcher obtained informed consent from the participants after a thorough explanation and clarification of the study's nature, purpose, and potential risk.

To take part in the study, participants had to satisfy the following criteria: being 18 years of age or older, having begun antiretroviral therapy at least six months prior to the study, and experiencing no acute/serious symptoms of illness at the time of the interview. Acute illness was added as a criterion of exclusion because interviewing sick people potentially raised two ethical issues: First, information given by sick participants might be unreliable and incomplete, simply because of the strain of being interviewed, threatening the study's scientific rigor. Second, approaching potential research subjects who were acutely ill would be inconsiderate and might increase their suffering. Such exclusion of potential participants might introduce bias in the data insofar as acutely sick people might view their illness and illness management differently from those whose symptoms are milder or no longer present. However, over the course of the interviews, several accounts of participants' experiences with acute symptoms of the illness were elicited by probing relatively healthier subjects to reflect on times when they had been very sick. Consequently, applying acute illness as an exclusion criterion did not significantly compromise the study.

All of the interviews were conducted in one of the examination rooms in the clinic, which provided a private space for a confidential exchange. Each interview was completed with collection of socio-demographic information. To protect confidentiality, case numbers were assigned to each participant. Ethical approvals were obtained from the Northwestern University Institutional Review Board, Addis Ababa University, Medical Faculty, Institutional Review Board, and the Ethiopian Science and Technology Agency.

The interviews averaged 75 minutes in length, with none running beyond two hours, and were conducted in Amharic by the researcher, a native speaker. The interview guide supported the gathering of information on typical days in their lives; their relationships with families, friends, and neighbors; what it means to them to spend time with people in their social networks; their social lives before and after an HIV-positive diagnosis; and how they navigate their relationships with and responsibilities for others while undergoing HIV treatment. After providing unprompted descriptions of their experiences of stigma in response to the aforementioned questions, participants were asked a direct question about whether or not they had experienced stigma due to their HIV serostatus. The majority of the stigma data were obtained through the former, unprompted questions, rather than from the one specifically about stigma. The direct question on stigma yielded minimal data, usually related to external experiences of stigma, mostly enacted. Then the stigma experiences of PLWHA were examined using an interpretive phenomenological approach in order to understand how the social world inhabited by individuals living with HIV contributes to similarities and differences in their stigma experiences. With this approach, it was possible to elicit more than subjective descriptions of experiences, revealing meanings embedded in the lived experiences of PLWHA that in some cases are not apparent to the participants themselves (29). Moreover, phenomenology makes it possible to explore stigma experiences from the individual perspectives of PLWHAs based on their lived experiences.

All of the interviews were recorded and translated into English, and then analyzed using phenomenological methods to explore the meanings of peoples' experiences (29). Investigating interviewees' phenomenology entailed probing their perceptions of their experiences as ART recipients to elicit from them the meanings they attach to their subjective experiences of "living with HIV." This entailed asking them to express their feelings about and reactions to taking their medications as well as following their medical regimens and the associated recommendations (such as dose schedules and dietary prescriptions). Participants were also asked to share their perceptions of the outcomes of treatment and of their overall experience with managing their medications in their respective social worlds in their daily lives. This method is intended to capture the meanings of participants' lived experiences based on reflective description of those experiences on the part of the people themselves within their familiar social contexts. In this way the researcher was able to explore the participants' social worlds as perceived in their narratives and understand how these perceived meanings shape and organize peoples' experiences as they live with HIV/AIDS. Interview transcripts and field notes were coded carefully using HyperResearch qualitative software. Perspectives identified by similar codes were compared and categorized into groups. Emergent themes were identified and related to people's socio-cultural perception and experiences of living with HIV in the era of biomedical treatment and its impact on illness management. The results of these analyses are reported below.

RESULTS

The study site served a diverse population at the time the research was conducted (see Table 1). Among the total of 105 study participants, 62 (59%) were women. The mean age of the participants was 37.7 years; their ages ranged from 21 to 58 years. The length of time since participants had started ART ranged from 6 to 76 months (mean=31.6 months). Thirty-nine (37.1%) were single, whereas 31 (29.5%) were married, 18 (17.1%) were widowed, and 17 (16.2%) were separated/divorced. Only 15 (14.3%) of the participants had studied at the college level, whereas 47 (44.7%) had elementary education or had also attended but did not graduate from high school. Thirteen (12.4%) of the participants were illiterate (could not read or write). Sixty-six (62.9%) were Orthodox Christians. There were 18 Protestants (17.1%) and 13 Muslims (12.4 %).

Table 1. Sociodemographic characteristics of PLWHA (n=105)

Characteristics	Number
Sex	
Female	62
Age	
18–29	21
30–39	41
40–49	12
50 and above	31
Marital Status	
Married	31
Never married	39
Divorced	7
Separated	10
Widowed	18
Have Children	
Yes	64
Educational Status	
Illiterate	13
Elementary	31
High School	16
High school/voc. school graduate	30
College education	15
Employment Status	
Employed in the formal sector	30
Self-employed	43
Unemployed	32
Monthly Income	
No income	18
No regular income	23
Under 500 birr (under $50)	33
500–1499 birr ($50–$150)	19
1500 birr and above (above $150)	12

Characteristics	Number
Religion	
Orthodox Christian	66
Muslim	13
Protestant	18
Jehovah's Witness	3
ND Christian	3
No religion	2
Months on ART	
6–24	40
25–48	58
49 and above	7

Over two-thirds of the participants (74, comprising 70.4%) had no income or led a very impoverished life with marginal incomes of less than 500 birr per month (equivalent to $50).

More than ninety percent (91.4%) of the 105 participants mentioned having experienced stigma. These experiences varied widely in both type and degree. The degree of stigma experienced was greater among people who admitted that they contracted the disease due to their own risk-taking behavior than it was among those who felt they had no control over the acquisition of the disease (e.g., it was contracted following a medical procedure or while being confined in prison or a refugee camp). In either case, the stigma attached to HIV/AIDS is still pervasive in the era of effective treatment. Since the HIV epidemic in Ethiopia is not associated with homosexuality or IV drug use, social identity did not stand out in explaining differential stigma experiences at the macro level. At the micro level, however, HIV is associated closely with morality and evil (8), and most of the stigma concerns are rooted in the dominant moral discourses surrounding HIV. In particular, these discourses characterize HIV as being a product of deviations from sexual moralities (30) and, in the context of this study set in Ethiopia, this means having multiple sexual partners or being adulterous.

The lived experiences of PLWHA taking ART in Ethiopia was characterized by a complex ongoing struggle of, on the one hand, managing stigma and, on the other, following HIV treatment as prescribed. This study illustrates how ART lessens certain types of stigma while augmenting others and creates new stigma triggers that PLWHA had never had to negotiate before the medication's roll-out. By identifying these associations between ART and stigma, both positive and negative, the remainder of this section provides more detailed evidence of the lived experiences of PLWHA in the biomedical era.

Concealing difference

ART is beneficial in concealing discreditable attributes associated with HIV/AIDS by improving biomedical conditions and combating stereotypical bodily symptoms associated with the disease. Many PLWHA using ART mentioned feeling healthy, being able to resume functional daily living, and needing less frequent clinic visits as countervailing factors that reduce the sense of "differentness" and negative self-concept that typically accompany an HIV-positive diagnosis. The following quotes emphasize several respects in which normalcy is restored following improved health conditions:

Everybody expected me to die. After I started the medicine and as I got well physically, I guess people started to even doubt whether we [my wife and I] have the virus or not for certain (Male, 47).

Now, there is nothing that I worry about. I am happy, as people who didn't shake hands with me before embrace me today. People have started to give me the right treatment . . . Before I started the treatment, I had stopped going to social gatherings, but now I go to weddings, funerals, and I am active in social life (Female, 58)

I am working, doing what everybody else is doing. If I were inferior to other healthy people, say if I were bedridden, I would have been scared. But now I am not worried. I am healthy now, and I got all my confidence back (Female, 29)

As these quotes suggest, a second way in which medical treatments restore normalcy is through bringing back functional competence and helping people regain social and economic liberation, vital quality-of-life interests that once were threatened by the illness. Opportunistic illnesses that prevented PLWHA from working were major stigma triggers that were often intensified by corresponding stigma associated with being economically dependent. Perceived HIV stigma was reduced for PLWHA by improved functional status (expressed in terms of functional activity and the ability to participate in the labor force), as many interviewees had been bedridden or seriously ill before treatment. Consequently, some PLWHA reported having built a strong positive relationship with their medication (calling it a friend, a lover, a supporter, or a partner), which enables them to fight against impending physical as well as social death (stigma) and promises better health and social rebirth.

Creating support

Pill taking also resulted in the creation of substitute social networks with promising social capital that were helpful in supporting illness management and coping with stigma. Such networks were created naturally when PLWHA met at HIV clinics for follow-up appointments or to refill their prescriptions, or artificially through support groups created by civic organizations (non-governmental organizations and patient organizations). Such relationships persisted beyond the settings in which they were formed and naturally created networks often last longer than do those created in artificially organized support groups. These new relationships facilitated the exchange of material resources (money, food, shelter) as well as non-material resources (information, encouragement) and acceptance of health status among people undergoing medical treatment. Additionally, they helped PLWHA develop a sense of belongingness, and construct a collective identity borne of HIV-tainted blood. This sense of collective identity is illustrated by one participant as follows:

The medication has earned me a lot of friends. People who come from different Kifle Ketemas [the lowest administrative unit in Ethiopia, equivalent to a county] meet here. A person who takes ART and a prisoner is the same. We take care of each other . . . like prisoners take care of each other. The same is true with people who take the medication . . . . We help each other. (Male, 40)

Such anecdotes highlight the unintended positive consequences of ART that tended to ameliorate the effects of disease stigmatization. That they were facilitated by institutions and circumstances that would not exist in the absence of ART suggests how beneficial outcomes might materialize from otherwise bad situations.

Medication as stigma trigger

Although ART is perceived as enabling PLWHA to conceal differences and create social ties, the regimen management it entails often generates external stigma by publicizing what Goffman (14) characterized as discreditable attributes (HIV status per se, and the physical changes associated with treatment, bring discredit to the sufferer). In some cases undergoing ART actually reinforces stigma by reminding PLWHA that they are possessors of these discredited attributes. HIV treatment imposes stigma concerns at various levels of regimen management. The most frequently mentioned stigma trigger is the location and configuration of health care facilities, as PLWHA often wished not to be associated with the clinics from which they obtained services. Most of the participants in this study, for example, were not comfortable with the location of the HIV clinic they had to use. Their HIV clinic was segregated from other infectious disease clinics and made it difficult for patients to maintain their privacy. Service notices that were commonly posted on doors, walls, and notice boards indicated the clinic's purpose. By Western standards of privacy for PLWHA, the HIV clinics in Ethiopia are far less equipped to maintain the privacy of individuals. The following quotes demonstrate how the PLWHA in this study feared exposure due to the physical structure of ART clinics:

> This has been repeatedly said; the location of the HIV clinic is very embarrassing. One time, I met a friend around the waiting area, and while I was talking with him, it was my turn and my name was called. He then knew about my status (Male, 37)

> I mean, you see everybody who is attending this clinic; it is kind of out in the open and people obviously know what this clinic is for. I do not believe the clinic is doing a great job in serving us confidentially given the location (Female, 29)

Long wait times at the clinic and certain procedures that PLWHA needed to follow to refill their prescriptions were reported as stigma triggers, potentially threatening regimen recommendations. After all, PLWHA in Ethiopia know that being HIV-positive is a sufficient source of stigma once one's HIV status is known, so being exposed as such in public triggers that stigma. Another participant described his clinic experience in these terms:

> Sometimes, it is difficult to come here, line up with other people, and take the medication. Recently, it is getting better. [Before], there was a need to line up for three or four hours to take the medication. People do not want to be seen by other people who come to get treatments for other sicknesses; people might be afraid. These things push many people living with the virus to stop taking the medication (Male, 38)

Some even argued that the "differentness" and deviancy identified with HIV was reinforced by the medical profession itself, because, generally, HIV clinics were segregated from other infectious disease clinics and involve special paperwork and procedures of operation: "I would have been very happy if HIV is treated like other illnesses. I do not see the reason to have a separate clinic for HIV if we are seen like any other patient" (Female, 29). Many participants mentioned their concerns about stigma resulting from following routine clinical procedures, such as taking their charts to the pharmacy. A patient explained:

> The [HIV-positive patient's] chart has a unique cover that makes it different from other patients' charts. That difference by itself makes you liable to peoples' gossip. I often see people hiding their charts under their shirts or putting them in a plastic bag when they take them to the pharmacy. I sometimes offer to take other peoples' charts along with mine when I see their discomfort (Female, 25)

Outside of the clinic setting, stigma concerns extended to the handling of pills—transporting medication, storing medication at home, and discarding empty pill bottles. Public familiarity with ART heightened the disclosure concerns of PLWHA. As one patient explained,

> People recognize the medication. It is better these days. Earlier it[pill bottle] even had a logo on it, you know, the red ribbon, the HIV logo. It [ART] can be identified. Now the bottle doesn't have such a mark, but people have already associated that particular bottle with HIV medicine, even if it is not . . . (Male, 29)

In some cases, internalized fear of disclosure escalated to a remarkable degree of obsession and paranoia. The following excerpt demonstrates the magnitude of such fear and the conflicting pressures that some PLWHA experienced in an effort to normalize and conceal their situation:

> The great majority of the public is informed about ART. People know and could identify the ART tablet. If you are once noticed taking ART, you will be automatically labeled as "HIV" . . . . I am not even comfortable leaving my pills at home. I put on a big jacket and I keep all my pills in my pocket . . . . No one can tell what is inside my pocket. For this reason I refill my prescription strictly on a monthly basis. This is because I do not feel safe to leave my pills at home . . . . If something unexpected happens, for instance, if a fire breaks out in a nearby house and extends to other houses in the neighborhood, people might end up seeing my pills in an effort to control the fire. Also, the door of my house is made of a corrugated iron sheet. The space in between the joints of the door provides easy access to look into what is in the room (Male, 47)

This example demonstrates the diversity of lived experiences of PLWHA in contrasting socio-cultural settings. Here, the patient is explicitly concerned with the stigma he will suffer, whereas in a wealthy country the discovery of pills is most commonly associated with the fear that others might find them, take them, and harm themselves.

People with HIV who traveled frequently and were obliged to take their doses outside their homes also cited packaging and the number of pills to be taken per dose/day as a stigma concern:

> If only one tablet was taken, it would be easy to just carry one in a small container or something, but taking three different tablets makes it difficult to be discreet. It is packed in a big bottle, and it is noisy, too. Some people drop the whole container when they try to hide it. And for people who travel a lot it is even more difficult (Male, 40)

Another woman also mentioned her stigma concern related to packaging:

> My pills have a huge potential to stigmatize me. That is why, for instance, every time I refill my prescription, I transfer all the pills in another container as I don't want people to see the original package, which is also cumbersome and noisy (Female, 50)

The second way in which pill taking augmented an internalized negative self-concept lies in the visible physical changes that were observed after a severe illness, which, in the case of PLWHA, was felt as an indirect confirmation of their HIV status. Such physical changes can either be positive (improving an individual's appearance) or negative (creating visible symptoms of medication side effects that further served as stigma triggers by highlighting physical imperfections). The following quote illustrates how negative physical changes after treatment became a visual cue to stigma:

> I lost everything. I became slim and looked like a man. No curves at all. I went to my doctor and cried because I was so upset that I was not told about the side effects. The doctor said that the side effect was only alteration of a body shape, which is not life threatening and she did not think it is important to inform me. Imagine how it could be psychologically traumatic for a single young woman like me to live with this new physique. It is better to die. What is bad about dying? It is much better than living with this body shape. It is really disgusting to have your body shape disproportioned all of a sudden. To make the situation worse, everybody that I know asks me what happened to me as the change was so noticeable (Female, 29)

The final way in which pill taking augmented negative self-concept was by reminding PLWHA of their status as HIV-positive, and devaluing them as inferior and dependent on medication for normal functioning. The following quote illustrates how some people internalize a negative self-concept from being dependent on pills:

> When I think of the two tablets that keep me alive, I hate myself and I feel that I am dead. Sometimes I get furious to see myself like a walking corpse, and other times I see myself as a doll that functions with a battery. I would say, without these batteries [pills], I am nothing (Male, 50)

In some cases, pills triggered a sense of internalized blame for contracting the disease. For people who assumed total personal responsibility for contracting the virus, pill taking was the price that they had to pay for their unfortunate mistakes. "When I take my medication, I always think of the moment I made a mistake [had casual sex]," one participant explained (Female, 30). Pill taking may also play a symbolic role in lowered expectations, perceptions of vulnerability, and dependence on others, even among people who know of their HIV serostatus.

Management of medication-induced stigma

The interview data revealed that PLWHA were engaged on a constant basis in concealment work to assert normalcy and conceal discreditable attributes or indicators that serve as stigma triggers, such as pill taking. The following quote shows the engagement with both impression and information management that is typical of PLWHA:

> The reason why many people, especially those who live in a house rented from private owners, stop their medication is that they are afraid of being identified with the medicine. Even when they go to the hospital regularly, people are careful not to set a noticeable pattern and be suspected that their visit was to refill their ART. Most people hate to take their medication from a nearby hospital or health center, as people living in the same locality go to the same health institutions and chances of being identified is high. For example, PLWHA living in my surroundings don't want to get their HIV treatment from St. John [hospital pseudonym] for the hospital serves people from our neighborhood. A person who runs into someone from his neighborhood won't show up to the hospital again and will discontinue taking the medication . . . . For all these reasons, many discontinue their medication (Female, 41)

Concealment work included silence, hiding/passing as "normal," lying, skipping a dose, and even stopping medication entirely. Most PLWHA emphasized that they literally lied about or hid their medication from most people in their social network. As one man explained,

> I am keeping it secret because of the stigma. Otherwise, if it were diabetes, I would have said I have diabetes. If it was diabetes pills, I would definitely have taken it differently. I am talking to you now because you are a professional. Otherwise, I do not want anybody to know that I am HIV-positive. If people ask me about my pills, I would say I am diabetic or hypertensive. I will never say that I have HIV. The stigma is still strong (Male, 49)

PLWHA also strived constantly to conceal their status and diverted suspicion by passing as "normal" or doing things that they used to do before becoming ill, such as consuming alcohol or using drugs. Often, medication management was compromised when PLWHA were at work, engaged in leisure time, or were amid others in a social setting. In such instances, they avoided exposure, simply lied about diagnosis and treatment, or diverted attention from themselves while taking the medication. A woman described her effort to conceal her HIV status as follows:

> It is hard to keep this thing [HIV] under wraps, especially if you are seen at the clinic [HIV]. Thank goodness I haven't encountered anyone in a place where they can be sure of my diagnosis. If anyone sees me at any time, I will say that I came for a diabetes checkup. People only know that I am diabetic. I once ran into my cousin, and when she asked me why I came here, I told her that I had my diabetic follow-up here [at the hospital]. I am always cautious. For fear of being noticed, I cover myself with my wraps all year long, wear sunglasses even if it is raining [laughter] . . . . It is hard. (Female, 50)

In the case of HIV, concealment work was frequently complicated by complex medication regimens. PLWHA's routines were dictated by their dose schedules. A woman described the demanding nature of managing stigma triggers as follows:

> When I have social commitments, or if I go to places where there is nothing to drink, I take my medication just with my saliva to be sure I take it on time. Now I am getting

used to taking the drug without water. But whenever I plan to go somewhere, I always think about the people that I will be seeing; sometimes I will go after 10 o'clock, which is after taking my morning pills. The medication has taken spontaneity out of my life. This is such a depressing life. Sometimes I say to myself, for how long can I keep up with this hide-and-seek? But then again I fear . . . (Female, 30)

Frequently, self-exclusion, as a strategy to manage stigma, was intensified in an effort to manage internalized fears of disclosure. PLWHA avoided stigma triggers by voluntarily excluding themselves from available services or otherwise denying themselves opportunities for less-stigmatizing treatment alternatives. To minimize stigma triggers, PLWHA sometimes bought medication directly from a pharmacy, on the black market, or from poor patients who were desperate for money even if it meant risking their lives. Such behaviors persisted even while free treatment was offered at designated HIV clinics. The following quote illustrates this:

A very rich man in my neighborhood came to my house, as everybody knows my status, and asked me to sell him my medication because he did not want to go to the clinic and get his treatment. This is because of fear of disclosure. Then I told him, "Listen, my CD4 count and yours may not be the same. Why don't you go to the clinic and get proper service? Also, I do not want to sell my medication and die. My life is as worthy as yours." He said, "You get three months' worth of supply, so please sell two months of supply to me." I said no way. I told him that the medication is free, and he can go get it from the clinic. He mentioned his worries about being seen at the HIV clinic, and I reassured him that unless he discloses, no one would know about him just because he went to the clinic. He refused and said he would rather try the Holy water, and went to his hometown, only to die after a short while (Female, 49)

This case indicates that, although experiencing "layered stigma" (stigma related to both poverty and HIV/AIDS) usually adds difficulty to the lives of PLWHA, HIV stigma also affects affluent people who are perhaps even more desperate to protect their privacy.

Self-exclusion based on access to medication affected the willingness not only to seek health services but also economic opportunities. Some PLWHA refrained from taking job offers that might make it difficult to avoid signaling their HIV status. As one participant explained,

I love to work, and I don't even mind working as a daily laborer. But I don't want anyone to see my medication. For instance, I had an opportunity to be employed in a hair salon as stylist, but the owner told me that I would have to start work at 6:00 in the morning. That would have meant I couldn't take my medication at 8:00 because she would be around. So I declined the job offer (Female, 31)

Social withdrawal was another common stigma management strategy that was employed within networks comprised of people who did not know their HIV serostatus. The rationale for social withdrawal was based on both disclosure concerns and health concerns. Existing networks may engage in certain normative activities (such as drinking alcohol) that may not be compatible with living with the virus. Yet withdrawal potentially intensified an internalized negative self-concept for the possessor, as she or he continued to be aware of being different (8). As one participant explained,

It is just confusing even for me. You know how it is. My inner self tells me to stay away. I don't know why but my personality has changed. I am easily irritable now. I became a complainer. I easily get upset. I was not like that, but now I have a short temper. When people chat with me, I get bored; I don't have much interest (Male, 39)

Regardless of the various stigma management strategies used, there were times when stigma triggers were unavoidable. In such instances, PLWHA followed one of two schemata. First, they might compromise their prescribed medication practices by skipping a dose or discontinuing treatment. Second, they might abandon information and impression management efforts and, instead, actively resist stigma through public HIV education and activism. Some adopted a more passive approach, simply learning to be less concerned about stigma. People who were economically independent, had supportive networks in which others accepted them and made them feel normal, or had experienced deteriorated health while attempting to manage stigma, were most likely to adopt passive stigma resistance. Alternatively, people who lacked supportive networks, had no reliable means of subsistence, or experienced discrimination from people in their close network often engaged in active stigma resistance such as public advocacy or willful self-acceptance. Together, then, these findings reveal how the advent of ART has changed the landscape of HIV stigmatization and how people variably managed stigma experiences in an era of effective treatment.

DISCUSSION

Based on its findings that ART both helps and hinders stigma experiences and management of PLWHA, this study proposes an alternate directional pathway between stigma and disease/illness management. Unlike most previous studies that have focused on a single element of disease experience, the present study uniquely presents the lived experiences of PLWHA as they relate to both stigma and normalization. Integrating these two aspects of HIV experiences helps broaden the understanding of the complex experiences of people coping with HIV/AIDS, which, according to empirical studies (10,11) as well as general theoretical formulations of stigma (13), qualifies as the most stigmatized disease across many cultures. The findings depict the various ways in which individuals suffer from stigma, including those that are attached to taking ART. The study also evinces ways in which ART enables individuals to achieve normalcy despite dealing with a chronic illness.

More specifically, the present study's findings indicate that ART restores a sense of normalcy in three ways. Primarily, as other research has found (8,15, 23), ART improves a patient's biophysical trajectory directly or indirectly, which decreases stigma because physical imperfections (especially those stereotypically associated with the "HIV body") are minimized dramatically. Second, functional health status plays an important role in determining the degree to which people feel rejected socially (10). In this way, ART targets the "layered stigma" (17) that PLWHA experience, not simply because of the immorality to which the acquisition of the disease is often attributed, but also because of its implicit association with other forms of negative social representations (such as nonproductive/dysfunctional status). In the face of massive poverty, PLWHA in Ethiopia have to navigate a socio-economic and political environment in which such factors, based largely on dependence, determines a community's response to HIV/AIDS. Indeed, rather than assuming that stigma leads patients to default on their medical treatment, this study demonstrates the opposite outcome in many cases, in which stigma leads to increased dedication to treatment, highlighting the necessity of examining stigma experiences within the broader social context.

A third way in which normalization through ART was observed in this study is coincidental to the treatment but rather is due to the role of clinics. PLWHA who must visit clinics in the course of treatment form networks outside of their existing social networks with other PLWHA. Relationships forged in this way, through a shared sense of differentness and vulnerability, soften and diffuse negative impacts of stigma experiences. Moreover, the organic nature of support groups formed naturally through clinical encounters may be even more instrumental in equipping patients with "tricks of the trade" (8) for concealing HIV status, coping with stigma, navigating resources, and (in some cases) coming out and resisting HIV-related stigma.

However, outside of ART's normalizing influence, other findings of this study are consistent with those of other studies in both developing and developed countries, suggesting that stigma partly explains poor adherence to ART (24–28, 31–34). This study also supports stigma models in Africa (16) that demonstrate that HIV-related stigma among people undergoing ART sustain a vicious circle of illness for PLWHA. For a considerable number of participants in this study, internalized fear of disclosure was the main reason for treatment default and dose irregularity. This often led to worsening health conditions and, thereby, stimulated additional stigma concerns. This underscores the dilemma faced by PLWHA, whose health status is caught between the need to follow a treatment regimen as prescribed and the desire to conceal an HIV-positive status and pass as "normal." While it has been established that information-based awareness does not result in widespread reduction of stigma (35), the present study takes the argument one step further, asserting that factual information about stigmatized health conditions might lead to public identification of sufferers and subsequent stigmatization. Today, public awareness of the pills that are administered in ART has become a liability to individuals undergoing treatment.

This study has also provided evidence regarding attitudes toward pills in Ethiopian society, demonstrating that the salient association between pill taking and illness in Ethiopia results in particularly low expectations for positive outcomes that might result from taking pills. This finding confirms the argument in Alonzo et al. (8) that lowered expectations formed out of sympathy (mostly within intimate networks) and extraordinary support are sometimes taken as expressions of stigma and vulnerability. In particular, in the context of the study area, pill taking is associated with being sick, unlike in the West, where pill taking is a relatively normal practice as people regularly consume vitamins, nutritional supplements, and common over-the-counter pain medications such as aspirin and ibuprofen. In Ethiopia, people who take pills regularly are presumed vulnerable to some debilitating condition, and often stigmatized for it. That is, most people in the study area believe that if you are taking pills something must be wrong with you.

The introduction of ART in resource-poor settings both increases and reduces HIV stigma at various junctures of the treatment process. This study echoes the views of other studies in poor settings that find that ART lessens stigma experiences that emanate from physical imperfections and socio-economic dependence (21,23); yet, it also increases the psychosocial vulnerability that PLWHA encounter at health facilities, augments other stigma experiences, and even creates new stigma triggers that stem from the process of following medical regimens. In this regard, health institutions in social settings like Ethiopia provide distinct social spaces for diverse cultural systems that interact to frame and shape illness management strategies of PLWHA. On the one hand, health facilities in resource poor Africa are entering the age of "normalization" of HIV and as per conventional medicine treatment should follow the model of other chronic illnesses such as diabetes or cancer. On the other hand, they must acknowledge the complex social realities of AIDS and the unique pressures of HIV stigma in the African context, which deter/delay the shift in the social construction of HIV/AIDS from a death sentence to a chronic manageable condition. The differing nature of such findings indicates that in order to understand the dynamic and evolving illness management experiences of PLWHA, it is imperative to account for aspects of stigma and normalization as well as how people navigate and reconcile the two schemata.

In areas of high HIV prevalence, where stigma is still rampant and unintended disclosure is a serious issue, adherence to a prescribed regimen is a considerable challenge in spite of the treatment's capacity to restore self-worth. To overcome this challenge, HIV clinics should adopt policies and reconfigure facilities to provide due consideration for privacy. Measures to address challenges involved in accessing treatment and thereby reduce treatment default or lapses might include fewer personally identifying procedures, waiting areas that reduce public exposure, decreased wait times, considerate and understanding health professionals who are attentive to the social context of PLWHA, and well-integrated care including mental health services. Similarly, concerns with frequency of dosage, pill size, and pill packaging undermine effective incorporation of medication into the daily lives of PLWHA. Accordingly, dosage simplification and easy-to-handle packaging would facilitate the practicalities of following up on treatment in the face of a serious social risk of stigma.

In spite of these challenges, there are reasons for optimism independently of the opportunity to improve clinical facilities and engagement. The interview data collected in this study show that ideological resistance to the notion of "differentness" is expanding in the wake of ART's roll-out. PLWHA often abandon efforts related to information and impression management and start resisting stigma when they grow tired of the "hide and seek" drama of concealing their HIV status. Indeed, many who pervasively experience stigma are nevertheless encouraged by the outcomes of the medication and truly question the "discredit" attached to the disease when they consider that they are able to do whatever others are doing. Some such people depart from the vicious circle of stigma and decide to fight back against stigma triggers through actively teaching the public about HIV or, passively, by willfully reducing their stigma concerns. This finding reveals wide variation in stigma experiences, which can be affected by PLWHA's general economic, identity, or social status. Considering how recently the scale-up of ART in Ethiopia began, the positive outcomes realized through the treatment might triumph over the stigma attached to HIV in the long run. However, much remains to be learned about the complex interplay between disease stigmatization and effective treatment in the context of poverty.

Overall, the findings of this study underscore the need to study such experiences at the individual level. Nonetheless, it also suggests the importance of extrapolating from individual experiences in order to seek more context-specific, comprehensive solutions (e.g., reconfiguring the structure of particular medical clinics or catering outreach to religious or prevailing cultural beliefs in localized areas). Many of these solutions might be structural in nature, demonstrating the benefits of such evidence-based studies that identify the social and structural drivers of poor health management by addressing underlying social conditions that interfere with proper prevention and treatment intervention approaches. Additionally, public health initiatives aimed at educating people about HIV/AIDS might address the stigma associated with the disease by encouraging patients to combat their negative and exhausting attempts at concealment by emphasizing how diligent adherence to ART can foster positive bonding and advocacy.

It must be acknowledged, of course, that some of the aforementioned recommendations might be site-specific. Despite the wide variety of stigma experiences this study details, the generalizability of the research is limited by the setting in which it took place. Although the specialty teaching hospital in which the research was conducted attracts a hybrid population, it is also a very particular urban setting. Additionally, the results of this clinic-based research may be subject to sample bias by excluding the views and experiences of clinic non-attendees, especially in light of the myriad healing choices that people with HIV/AIDS navigate. The views of people who opt not to visit a clinic or who decided not to use ART were not captured in this study, as the primary objective was to assess the lived experiences of PLWHA in relation to their use of ART. Further studies in community settings as opposed to clinics are recommended to capture data regarding people who opt out of biomedical treatment. Yet, while these limitations might restrict the generalizability of and bias this study, they do not detract from the depth and richness of the experiences it captures and analyzes. Indeed, the study provides evidence pertaining to structural conditions (the physical layout, culture, and exigencies of clinic settings) that influence stigma and the positive outcomes that such settings engender by facilitating the formation of substitute support networks and the increased exchange of information.

SOCIAL SCIENCE IMPLICATIONS

This study implies that social science has much to offer in the study of HIV/AIDS and PLWHA. Our understanding of the disease and its effects on both individuals and society will benefit by continuing to follow the shift from an individual-based approach to one that examines the long-term, structural response to HIV by examining the social factors and cultural practices that hinder efficient prevention and treatment efforts (13). In particular, this study further demonstrates the utility of highlighting structural and cultural factors that might undermine response measures at the individual level. It provides evidence that stigma remains a major social driver of the HIV epidemic in resource-poor settings, compromising effective illness management as well as optimal adherence to treatment.

Theoretically, stigma has generally been considered a negative factor in disease treatment; however, this study showcases that it does not have the same negative effects on everybody. Indeed, it has positive effects on some individuals and serves as a source of empowerment depending on their status in other social domains. By exploring the social dimensions of stigma, it is possible to identify the specific ways in which stigma operates within the larger socioeconomic and cultural dynamics in particular social contexts. Identification of how stigma affects illness management, in what circumstances it affects people, who it affects, and what other social factors synergize with it to shape illness management and lived experiences in the Ethiopian context contributes to our understanding of the ways in which social factors influence medical compliance or non-compliance. This in turn represents a contribution of medical sociology to health practices research that seeks to identify factors in the development and implementation of intervention strategies than can improve the lived experiences and illness management of PLWHA and others suffering from chronic, stigmatized diseases.

ACKNOWLEDGMENTS

The author extends her sincere thanks and appreciation to the people living with HIV/AIDS for their participation in this study and the clinic staff for their cooperation during fieldwork. The author also wishes to express her thanks to Professors Carol Heimer, Wendy Griswold, and Celeste Watkins- Hayes at Northwestern University for their support at all stages of this research and to Elizabeth Lenaghan for reading and commenting on this work. Finally, thanks are due to the author's loving family for their unwavering support throughout this project.

REFERENCES

[1]   Federal Ministry of Health. AIDS in Ethiopia: Sixth report. Addis Ababa, Ethiopia: Ministry Health, 2006.

[2]   Garbus L. HIV/AIDS in Ethiopia: Country profile. San Francisco, CA: AIDS Policy Research Center, University California, 2003.

[3]   Federal Ministry of Health. Ethiopian national behavioral surveillance survey BSS [serial on the Internet], 2005.

[4]   Banteyerga H, Kidanu A, Nyblade L, MacQuarrie K, Pande R. Exploring HIV and AIDS stigma and related discrimination in Ethiopia: Causes, manifestations, consequences and coping mechanisms. Addis Ababa: Miz-Hasab Research Center, 2003.

[5]   Federal Ministry of Health. Health and Health Related Indicators 2005/2006. Addis Ababa, Ethiopia, 2006.

[6]   World Health Organization. Progress on global access to HIV antiretroviral therapy: An update on 3 by 5. Geneva, Switzerland: WHO, 2005.

[7]   Bernays S, Rhodes T, Terzic KJ. "You should be grateful to have medicines": Continued dependence, altering stigma and the HIV treatment experience in Serbia. Aids Care-Psychological and Socio-Medical Aspects of AIDS/HIV [proceedings paper]. 2010;22:14-20.

[8]   Alonzo AA, Reynolds NR. Stigma, HIV and AIDS: An exploration and elaboration of a stigma trajectory. Soc Sci Med 1995;41(3):303-15.

[9]   Herek GM. Thinking about AIDS and stigma: A psychologist's perspective. J Law Med Ethics 2002;30:594-607.

[10]   Fife BL, Wright ER. The dimensionality of stigma: A comparison of its impact on the self of persons with HIV/AIDS and cancer. J Health Soc Behav 2000;41(1):50-67.

[11]   Mak WS, Mo PKH, Cheung RYM, Woo J, Cheung FM, Lee D. Comparative stigma of HIV/AIDS, SARS, and tuberculosis in Hong Kong. Soc Sci Med 2006;63:1912-22.

[12]   Parker R, Aggleton P. HIV and AIDS-related stigma and discrimination: A conceptual framework and implications for action. Soc Sci Med 2003;57:13-24.

[13]   Auerbach J D, Parkhurst JO, Cáceres CF. Addressing social drivers of HIV/AIDS for the long-term response: Conceptual and methodological considerations. Glob Publ Health 2011;1-17.

[14]   Goffman E. Stigma: Notes on the management of spoiled identity. Englewood Cliffs, NJ: Prentice-Hall, 1963.

[15]   Gilbert L. 'My biggest fear was that people would reject me once they knew my status . . .': Stigma as experienced by patients in an HIV/AIDS clinic in Johannesburg, South Africa. Health Soc Care Comm 2010;18(2):139-46.

[16]   Holzemer WL, Uys L, Makoae L, Stewart A, Phetlhu R, Dlamini PS, et al. A conceptual model of HIV/AIDS stigma from five African countries. J Adv Nurs 2007;58(6):541-51.

[17]   Deacon H. Towards a sustainable theory of health-related stigma: Lessons from the HIV/AIDS literature. J Comm Appl Soc Psychol 2006;16:418-25

[18]   Stein J. HIV/AIDS stigma: The latest dirty secret. Afr J AIDS Res 2003;2(2):95-101.

[19]   Colbert AM, Kim KH, Sereika SM, Erlen JA. An examination of the relationships among gender, health status, social support, and HIV-related stigma. J Assoc Nurs AIDS Care 2010;21:302-13.

[20]   Castro A, Farmer P. Understanding and addressing AIDS-related stigma: From anthropological theory to clinical practice in Haiti. Am J Public Health 2005;95(1):53-9.

[21]   Wolfe WR, Weiser SD, Leiter K, Steward WT, Percy-de Korte F, Phaladze N, et al. The impact of universal access to antiretroviral therapy on HIV stigma in Botswana. Am J Public Health 2008;98(10):1865-71.

[22]   Roura M, Urassa M, Busza J, Mbata D, Wringe A, Zaba B. Scaling up stigma? The effects of antiretroviral roll-out on stigma and HIV testing. Early evidence from rural Tanzania. Sex Transm Infect 2009;85(4):308-12.

[23]   Campbell C, Skovdal M, Madanhire C, Mugurungi O, Gregson S, Nyamukapa C. "We, the AIDS people. . .": How antiretroviral therapy enables Zimbabweans living with HIV/AIDS to cope with stigma. Am J Public Health 2011;101(6):1004-10.

[24]   Dlamini PS, Wantland D, Makoae LN, Chirwa M, Kohi TW, Greeff M, et al. HIV stigma and missed medications in HIV-positive people in five African countries. Aids Patient Care Stds 2009;23(5):377-87.

[25]   Rintamaki LS, Davis TC, Skripkauskas S, Bennett CL, Wolf MS. Social stigma concerns and HIV medication adherence. AIDS Patient Care Stds 2006;20(5):359-68.

[26]   Bogart LM, Wagner GJ, Galvan FH, Klein DJ. Longitudinal relationships between antiretroviral treatment adherence and discrimination due to HIV-serostatus, race, and sexual orientation among African–American men with HIV. Ann Behav Med 2010;40:184-90.

[27]   Weiser S, Wolfe W, Bangsberg D, Thior I, Gilbert P, Makhema J, et al. Barriers to antiretroviral adherence for patients living with HIV infection and AIDS in Botswana. J Acquir Immune Defic Syndr 2003; 34(3):281-8.

[28]   Gebremariam MK, Bjune GA, Frich JC. Barriers and facilitators of adherence to TB treatment in patients on concomitant TB and HIV treatment: A qualitative study. BMC Public Health 2010;10:651.

[29]   Lopez KA, Willis DG. Descriptive Versus Interpretive Phenomenology: Their Contributions to Nursing Knowledge. Qual Health Res 2004;14(5):726-35.

[30]   Conrad P. The social meaning of AIDS. Soc Policy 1986;17(51).

[31]   Siegel K, Schrimshaw EW, Raveis VH. Accounts for non-adherence to antiviral combination therapies among older HIV-infected adults. Psych, Health Med 2000;5(1):29-42.

[32]   Vanable PA, Carey MP, Blair DC, Littlewood RA. Impact of HIV-related stigma on health behaviors and psychological adjustment among HIV-positive men and women. AIDS Behav 2006;10:473.

[33]   Zhou YR. "If you get AIDS . . . you have to endure it alone": Understanding the social constructions of HIV/AIDS in China. Soc Sci Med 2007;65(2):284-95.

[34]   Carr RL, Gramling LF. Stigma: A health barrier for women with HIV/AIDS. J Assoc Nurs AIDS Care 2004;15:30-9.

[35]   Campbell C, Nair Y, Maimane S, Nicholson J. 'Dying twice': A multi-level model of the roots of AIDS stigma in two South African communities. J Health Psychol 2007;12(3):403-16.

Submitted: November 05, 2011. *Revised:* January 04, 2012. *Accepted:* January 08, 2012.

In: Public Health Yearbook 2012
Editor: Joav Merrick

ISBN: 978-1-62808-078-0
© 2013 Nova Science Publishers, Inc.

Chapter 39

CONDOM USE ATTITUDES AND HIV RISK AMONG AMERICAN MSM SEEKING PARTNERS FOR UNPROTECTED SEX VIA THE INTERNET

Hugh Klein*, PhD[1] and Rachel L Kaplan, PhD, MPH[2]*
[1] Kensington Research Institute, Silver Spring, Maryland
[2] Mack Center on Mental Health and Social Conflict, School of Social Welfare,
University of California–Berkeley, Berkeley, California

ABSTRACT

This study examines attitudes toward condom use in a national random sample of 332 MSM who use the Internet to seek men with whom they can engage in unprotected sex. Data collection was conducted via telephone interviews between January 2008 and May 2009. The following three research questions were addressed: 1) How do these men feel about using condoms, both ideologically and personally? 2) How do condom use attitudes relate to actual HIV risk behavior practices? 3) What factors underlie men's attitudes toward condom use? The findings indicated that men held weakly-positive attitudes toward condom use overall, but were noticeably more negative in their attitudes regarding the personal use of condoms. Condom use attitudes were related consistently and inversely to involvement in HIV risk practices. In both multivariate and structural equation analyses, men's condom-related attitudes were the single strongest factor associated with their involvement in risky sex. A number of factors were found to be correlated with more favorable attitudes toward condom use. These were: caring about potential sex partners' HIV serostatus, experiencing fewer drug-related problems, having a lower level of educational attainment, not preferring to have "wild" or "uninhibited" sex, higher self-esteem, being African American, and not perceiving great accuracy in the information that sex partners supply verbally about their HIV serostatus.

Keywords: Condom, attitudes, men who have sex with other men, MSM, HIV, risk, Internet

---

* Correspondence: Hugh Klein, PhD, 401 Schuyler Road, Silver Spring, Maryland 20910 United States. E-mail: hughk@aol.com (primary) and hughkhughk@yahoo.com (secondary)

INTRODUCTION

Men who have sex with men (MSM) represent one of the groups considered most at risk for the sexual transmission of HIV, at least in part due to their comparatively high risk per exposure via anal sex. The risk per exposure is estimated to be 1.00% for receptive anal sex and 0.06% for insertive anal sex as compared to 0.01-0.32% for receptive vaginal sex and 0.01-0.10% for insertive vaginal sex (1). As condoms represent an effective method of HIV prevention, extensive efforts have been made by researchers to understand condom use attitudes in a variety of populations and to promote consistent condom use. In the United States, recent research shows that among MSM, increases in safer sex fatigue are associated with increases in the number of partners with whom they reported engaging in unprotected sex (2). Surprisingly, there has been limited research addressing condom-related attitudes among MSM in the United States. A few studies, however, have examined condom attitudes and behavior in subpopulations of MSM, such as African American MSM (3,4), Latino MSM (5), and methamphetamine-using HIV-positive MSM (6). These studies have shown that, among African American MSM, stronger peer condom use norms were associated with a lower frequency of risk behavior involvement (3); and lesser involvement in HIV risk behavior was associated with the perception of social norms that support condom use (4). In a sample of Latino MSM, participants most commonly cited pleasure as the reason for a lack of condom use (5). In a sample of methamphetamine-using HIV-positive MSM, researchers found that among men with negative attitudes about condoms, there was an association between methamphetamine use frequency and unprotected sex (6).

Although condoms are highly effective for HIV prevention when used correctly, research has shown that most individuals do not use condoms consistently (7), and others intentionally seek partners for unprotected sex. Previous research indicates a variety of factors associated with the motivation among MSM for barebacking (that is, the intentional practice of engaging in unprotected anal intercourse) (8). These factors include the desire to: cope with psychosocial vulnerabilities (9), create intimacy with partners (9), exchange semen (10), maximize physical and/or emotional pleasure (11), and overcome social isolation (12). Research efforts are underway to develop alternative methods of HIV prevention that are acceptable among MSM (13). Condoms are currently the best known strategy for HIV prevention during sexual contact. Therefore, understanding the condom-related attitudes and behavior of men who seek other men for unprotected sexual contact is an important part of strategizing ways in which this subpopulation of MSM can increase safety and health by preventing HIV infection. As we previously noted, though, little has been written about condom-related attitudes among MSM, especially with regard to specific attitudes about particular aspects of condom use (e.g., perceived inconvenience, embarrassment regarding use, discomfort, etc.). Most of the published studies have reported, simply, that negative attitudes toward condoms are associated with greater involvement in risky practices (14).

Recent research has examined the use of the Internet among MSM for meeting potential sex partners, typically finding that this practice is associated with a variety of HIV risk behaviors. For example, one recent study (15) showed that 40% of MSM Internet users acknowledged engaging in unprotected anal sex. Similarly, in a study comparing self-identified barebackers and non-barebackers, barebackers were more likely to spend more time on the Internet looking for potential sex partners [16]. Furthermore, researchers have found that men who seek sex online report more unprotected sex and sexually transmitted infections compared to their peers who do not use the Internet to identify sex partners (17,18). In a study that examined online ads and profiles on MSM-oriented unprotected sex-focused websites, the rates of advertised high-risk sexual behaviors were very high, including oral sex with ejaculation in the mouth (88.0% receptive, 77.4% insertive), anal sex with ejaculation in the anus (79.7% insertive, 69.4% receptive), multiple partner sex (77.9%), and felching (16.5%) (19). Evidence shows increasing numbers of young MSM who meet their first sexual partner online (20). In another sample of MSM who use the Internet, guessing the HIV serostatus of the sexual partner, as compared to checking the online profile and pre- and post-sex discussions, was associated with higher levels of unprotected anal sex (21).

In the present paper, a structural approach is used to develop a better understanding of how attitudes toward condom use are related to HIV risk taking in a sample of men who use the Internet specifically to find other men with whom they can engage in unprotected sex. Based on previously published studies, the following conceptual model was examined (see Figure 1):

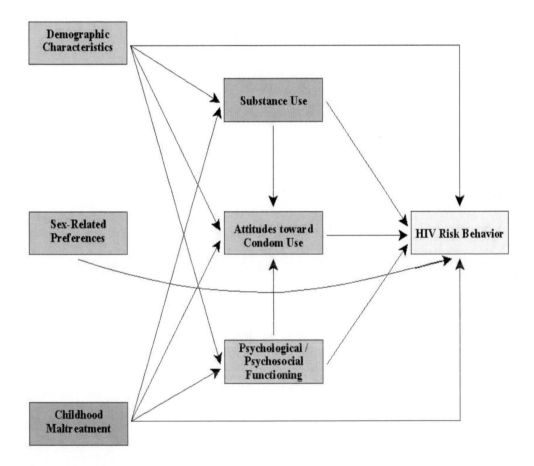

Figure 1. Conceptual Model.

In this model, attitudes toward condom use are conceptualized as an endogenous measure–that is, both as an independent variable, contributing to the understanding of men's involvement in risky behaviors, *and* as a dependent variable, varying based upon the effects of numerous other types of measures. As the conceptual model shows, condom-related attitudes are one of six types of influences hypothesized to affect men's HIV risk practices. The others are demographic variables (e.g., race/ethnicity, age, HIV serostatus), sex-related behavioral preferences (e.g., self-identification as a sexual "top" versus a "bottom," preferring to have sex that is "wild" or "uninhibited"), substance use/abuse, childhood maltreatment experiences, and psychological/psychosocial functioning (e.g., depression, self-esteem, impulsivity).

To a great extent, this conceptual model owes its intellectual origins to the notion of syndemic and to Syndemics Theory. "Syndemic" refers to the tendency for multiple epidemics to co-occur and, in the process of affecting some of the same people, for the various maladies to interact with one another, with each one worsening the effects of the others (22,23).

Walkup et al. (24) noted that health problems may be construed as syndemic when two or more conditions/afflictions are linked in such a manner that they interact synergistically, with each contributing to an excess burden of disease in a particular population. It is noteworthy that their work addresses the syndemic of HIV, substance abuse, and mental illness. A good example of how conditions may become syndemic is offered by Romero-Daza et al (25) in their study of sex work. The authors wrote:

> Streetwalkers' continuous exposure to violence, both as victims and as witnesses, often leaves them suffering from major emotional trauma. In the absence of adequate support services, women who have been victimized may turn to drug use in an attempt to deal with the harsh realities of their daily lives. In turn, the need for drugs, coupled with a lack of educational and employment opportunities, may lead women into prostitution. Life on the street increases women's risk for physical, emotional, and sexual abuse as well as their risk for HIV/AIDS. Exposure to traumatic experiences deepens the dependence on drugs, completing a vicious cycle of violence, substance abuse, and AIDS risk (pp. 233-234)

A number of authors, particularly during the past few years, have written about syndemics and Syndemics Theory as they apply to the HIV epidemic (23,25-27), including specific mention of the applicability of the concept and theory to men who have sex with men (27).

Using the conceptual model shown above in the present study, we examine a population of MSM who used the Internet specifically to find partners for unprotected sex. Our focus in this paper is to examine attitudes toward condom use among men in this population. Specifically, we address the following research questions: 1) How do members of this population feel about condom use–both condom use in general and condom use as it applies to the men themselves? 2) How, if at all, do condom-related attitudes relate to men's involvement in HIV risk practices? 3) What factors are associated with having more favorable attitudes regarding condom use?

METHODS

This paper draws from data that were collected between January 2008 and May 2009 for The Bareback Project, a study funded by the National Institute on Drug Abuse. The study sample consisted of men who use the Internet specifically to find other men with whom they can engage in unprotected sex. Some of the 16 websites from which the sample of 332 men were recruited catered exclusively to unprotected sex (e.g., Bareback.com, RawLoads.com). Other websites used did not cater to unprotected sex exclusively but did make it possible for site users to identify which individuals were looking for unprotected sex (e.g., Men4SexNow.com, Squirt.org). Using the 16 websites, a national random sample of men was derived.

Random selection was based on a combination of the first letter of the person's online username, his race/ethnicity (as listed in his profile), and the day of recruitment. Men of color were oversampled, to ensure good representation of men belonging to racial minority groups and to facilitate the examination of racial differences in risk behaviors and risk-related preferences. Recruitment took place seven days a week, during all hours of the day and nighttime, variable from week to week throughout the project, to maximize the representativeness of the research sample, in recognition of the fact that different people use the Internet at different times.

Initially, men were approached for participation either via instant message or email (much more commonly via email), depending upon the website used. Potential participants were provided with a brief overview of the study and informed consent-related information, and they were given the opportunity to ask questions about the study before deciding whether or not to participate. Potential participants were also provided with a website link to the project's online home page, to offer additional information about the project and to help them feel secure in the legitimacy of the research endeavor.

Interested men were scheduled for an interview soon after they expressed an interest in taking part in the study, typically within a few days. To maximize convenience for participants, interviews were conducted during all hours of the day and night, seven days a week, based on interviewer availability and participants' preferences. All of the study's interviewers were gay or lesbian, to engender credibility with the target population and to enhance participants' comfort during the interviews.

Participants in the study completed a one-time, confidential telephone interview addressing a wide array of topics. The questionnaire that was used was developed specifically for The Bareback Project. Many parts of the survey instrument were derived from standardized scales previously used and validated by other researchers. The interview covered such subjects as: degree of "outness," perceived discrimination based on sexual orientation, general health practices, HIV testing history and serostatus, sexual practices (protected and unprotected) with partners met online and offline, risk-related preferences, risk-related hypothetical situations, substance use, drug-related problems, Internet usage, psychological and psychosocial functioning, childhood maltreatment experiences, HIV/AIDS knowledge, and some basic demographic information. The interviews lasted an average of 69 minutes (median = 63, s.d. = 20.1, range = 30–210). Participants who completed the interview were offered $35.

Approval of the research protocol was given by the institutional review boards at Morgan State University (approval number 07/12-0145), where the principal investigator and one of the research assistants were affiliated, and George Mason University (approval number 5659), where the other research assistant was located.

Measures used

The principal variable of interest in this research is a 17-item scale pertaining to men's attitudes toward condom use. Individual items were scored on a five-point Likert scale, and higher scores on the scale corresponded with more conducive attitudes toward condom use. The scale was derived from the work of Brown (28) and it was found to be highly reliable (Cronbach's alpha = 0.91). Only items that were relevant to MSM and their sexual practices were used, so that the scale would be applicable to the study population.

For the second part of the analysis, examining the relationship between condom attitudes and risk practices, several HIV risk practice measures were examined, all using a past-30-day time frame of reference. These included: overall proportion of sex acts involving the use of condoms (a continuous measure based on responses to separate items inquiring about oral, anal, and vaginal sex), proportion of anal sex acts involving the use of condoms (a continuous measure derived from the variables just described), overall proportion of sex acts involving internal ejaculation (a continuous measure based on responses to separate items inquiring about where ejaculation occurred during oral, anal, and vaginal sex), proportion of anal sex acts involving internal ejaculation (a continuous measure derived from the items just described), having any sexual relations while under the influence of alcohol and/or other drugs (yes/no), number of male sex partners (continuous), number of times having "wild" or "uninhibited" sex (self-assessed, continuous measure), and number of times having sex of any kind in a gay bath house or sex club (continuous). Men's estimated total number of lifetime sex partners was also examined (continuous).

For the third part of the analysis, focusing on identifying the factors associated with better/worse attitudes toward condom use, a variety of factors in several domains were considered. The first consisted of *demographic and background variables*. These were: age (continuous), race/ethnicity (categorical), sexual orientation (gay versus bisexual), relationship status (involved versus not involved), educational attainment (continuous), and sexual role identity (top, versatile top, versatile, versatile bottom, bottom). The second consisted of several *HIV-related measures*. These included: HIV serostatus (positive, negative, unknown), knowing anyone currently living with HIV or AIDS (two separate yes/no measures), the number of people known who died from AIDS (continuous), preferred HIV serostatus of sex partners (positive, negative, does not matter), perceived accuracy of HIV serostatus information provided verbally by sex partners (ordinal), and perceived accuracy of online HIV serostatus information (ordinal). The third domain pertained to men's *risk-related preferences for sexual practices*, including how rough they preferred their sex to be (continuous), how long they most liked their sexual sessions to last (continuous), how much they liked having sex in public venues (continuous), how much they liked having sex that was "wild" or "uninhibited" (continuous), and liking to have anonymous sex (yes/no). The fourth domain pertained to *substance use/abuse* and included the following measures: currently a user of illegal drugs (yes/no), number of drug problems experienced (continuous), and total amount of illegal drug use (continuous measure of quantity × frequency of recent use, summed across nine drug types). The final domain assessed *psychological and psychosocial functioning*. Measures examined were: self-esteem (using the Rosenberg self-esteem scale [29]; Cronbach's alpha = 0.89), impulsivity (derived from the Barratt Impulsiveness Scale [30]; Cronbach's alpha = 0.76), depression (using the CES-D [31]; Cronbach's alpha = 0.93), optimism about the future (using the Life Orientation Test–Revised [32]; Cronbach's alpha =

0.78), current life satisfaction (adapted from the Satisfaction with Life scale [33]; Cronbach's alpha = 0.83), HIV/AIDS information burnout (derived from HIV Knowledge Questionnaire [34]; Cronbach's alpha = 0.76), and childhood maltreatment experiences (separate measures for sexual abuse, physical abuse, emotional abuse, and neglect, taken from the Childhood Trauma Questionnaire [35]; Cronbach's alpha = 0.94).

Analysis

Part 1 of the analysis, focusing on identifying men's attitudes toward condom use, relied upon descriptive statistics. Part 2, examining the relationship between condom attitudes and involvement in risk practices, primarily used simple regression as the analytical strategy, as the independent variable and all but one of the dependent variables examined were continuous in nature. The one exception–whether or not the person had engaged in any recent sex while under the influence of alcohol and/or other drugs–was dichotomous, thereby making logistic regression the appropriate analytical tool.

Part 3, focusing on the factors associated with men's condom-related attitudes, was undertaken in two steps. First, bivariate relationships were assessed for each of the independent variables outlined above and condom attitudes, using the latter as the dependent variable. Whenever the independent measure was dichotomous (e.g., sexual orientation, HIV-positive serostatus), Student's *t* tests were used. Whenever the independent variable was continuous (e.g., educational attainment, self-esteem level), simple regression was used. Then, all items found to be related either significantly (p<.05) or marginally (.10>p>.05) to condom-related attitudes were entered into a multivariate equation, and then removed in stepwise fashion until a best fit model containing only statistically-significant measures remained.

In Part 4, the relationships depicted in Figure 2 (which were the result of the Part 2 and Part 3 analysis) were subjected to a structural equation analysis to determine whether the way the relationships depicted there is an appropriate and effective representation of the study data. SAS's PROC CALIS procedure was used to assess the overall fit of the model to the data. When we use this type of structural equation analysis, we look for several specific outcomes: (1) a goodness-of-fit index as close to 1.00 as possible, but no less than 0.90, (2) a Bentler-Bonett normed fit index value as close to 1.00 as possible, but no less than 0.90, (3) an overall chi-square value for the model that is statistically nonsignificant, preferably as far from attaining statistical significance as possible, and (4) a root mean square error approximation value as close to 0.00 as possible, but no greater than 0.05. If these conditions are met, then the relationships depicted are considered to indicate a good fit with the data.

Throughout all of the analyses, results are reported as statistically significant whenever p<.05.

RESULTS

In total, 332 men participated in the study. They ranged in age from 18 to 72 (mean = 43.7, s.d. = 11.2, median = 43.2). Racially, the sample is a fairly close approximation of the American population, with 74.1% being Caucasian, 9.0% each being African American and

Latino, 5.1% self-identifying as biracial or multiracial, 2.4% being Asian, and 0.3% being Native American. The large majority of the men (89.5%) considered themselves to be gay and almost all of the rest (10.2%) said they were bisexual. On balance, men participating in The Bareback Project were fairly well-educated. About 1 man in 7 (14.5%) had completed no more than high school; 34.3% had some college experience without earning a college degree; 28.9% had a bachelor's degree; and 22.3% were educated beyond the bachelor's level. Slightly more than one-half of the men (59.0%) reported being HIV-positive; almost all of the rest (38.6%) reported being HIV-negative.

Attitudes toward condom use

Overall, men's attitudes toward condom use were rather ambivalent, averaging 2.96 on a 1–5 scale (see Table 1). On the positive side, most study participants felt that men should not be embarrassed to suggest a condom (93.0%), that using a condom was not a reason for feeling embarrassment (83.0%), and that they would not object if one of their partners asked them to use a condom (61.8%). But on the negative side, most study participants felt that condoms were unreliable (64.5%), that they were not pleasant to use (74.6%), that their use could not enhance sexual pleasure (63.9%), that they looked ridiculous (63.6%), and that putting on a condom was a sexual turn-off (63.9%). Nearly two-thirds of the men studied said that they simply do not like the idea of using condoms (65.5%) and even more of the men said that they would avoid using condoms if at all possible (70.6%).

Table 1. Attitudes toward Condom Use

Attitude Item	Percentage Disagreeing	Percentage Neutral	Percentage Agreeing
☼☼ In your opinion, condoms are too much trouble.	31.8	19.4	48.8
Condoms are unreliable.	16.7	18.8	64.5
☼☼ Condoms are pleasant to use	74.6	15.2	10.3
There is no reason why a man should be embarrassed to suggest a condom.	3.3	3.6	93.0
☼☼ You think that proper use of condoms can enhance sexual pleasure.	63.9	16.7	19.4
Many people make using condoms an erotic part of foreplay.	35.5	27.6	37.0
☼☼ You just don't like the idea of using condoms.	65.5	13.0	21.5
☼☼ You think condoms look ridiculous.	18.2	18.2	63.6
Condoms are inconvenient.	55.2	14.8	30.0
You see no reason to be embarrassed by the use of condoms.	8.2	8.8	83.0
☼☼ Putting a condom on an erect penis can be a real sexual turn-on.	63.9	15.2	20.9
☼☼ Condoms are uncomfortable.	57.3	13.9	28.8
☼☼ Using a condom makes sex unenjoyable.	47.0	18.5	34.5
☼☼You would avoid using condoms if at all possible.	70.6	9.7	19.7
Putting on a condom is an interruption of foreplay.	50.6	16.1	33.3

Attitude Item	Percentage Disagreeing	Percentage Neutral	Percentage Agreeing
☼☼ There is no way that using a condom can be pleasant.	25.5	18.2	56.4
☼☼ You would have no objection if your partner suggested that you use a condom.	29.1	9.1	61.8

☼☼ attitude toward personal condom use.

As Table 1 also shows, if a differentiation is made between men's attitudes toward condom use in general (that is, condom use as a concept, not applied to their specific behaviors) and their attitudes toward using condoms themselves (that is, attitudes toward personal condom use), a rather different picture emerges. Whereas men's attitudes toward *condom use in general* were positive overall (mean score = 3.38), their attitudes toward *personal condom use* were noticeably more negative (mean score = 2.73).

Condom-related attitudes and behavioral risk

As expected, men's attitudes toward condom use were related closely to their involvement in sexual risk practices (see Table 2). This was true for the global measure of condom-related attitudes and for the component measure of attitudes toward personal condom use. In every instance, better attitudes toward condom use were associated with lesser involvement in risky sex. This was true for the overall proportion of all sex acts involving the use of condoms (p<.0001), the proportion of anal sex acts involving the use of condoms (p<.0001), the proportion of all sex acts involving internal ejaculation (p<.0001), the proportion of anal sex acts involving internal ejaculation (p<.0001), the likelihood that the person recently had engaged in any sex acts while under the influence of alcohol and/or other drugs (p=.0003), the number of sex partners that the person reported having had recently and during his lifetime (both p<.0001), the number of times recently having engaged in sex adjudged to be "wild" or "uninhibited" by the man himself (p=.0005), and the number of times recently having had sex in a place like a gay bath house or a sex club (p=.036).

When examined in a multivariate manner, condom-related attitudes are the single strongest factor associated with men's involvement in risky sex. One specific example demonstrating this is presented in Figure 2, where the outcome measure is proportion of all sex acts involving the use of condoms. Six variables were found to contribute uniquely to the dependent variable. First, knowing people who are currently living with AIDS was associated with greater condom use when compared to people who knew no one currently living with AIDS (ß=.11, p=.034). Coinciding with this, knowing people who died from AIDS was associated with protecting oneself with condoms (ß=.12, p=.032). Third, men who were HIV-positive used condoms less than one-half as much as their HIV-negative and serostatus-unknown counterparts (ß=.17, p=.002). Fourth, Caucasian men engaged in about one-third as much protected sex as their nonwhite counterparts (ß=.17, p=.002). Fifth, the more confident men were in the truthfulness of HIV serostatus information supplied to them by their sex partners, the less they tended to use condoms (ß=.15, p=.006). Finally, the more positive men's attitudes toward using condoms were, the more they tended to practice protected sex (ß=.29, p<.0001). Together, these items explained 23.8% of the total variance.

Factors associated with condom-related attitudes

As Figure 2 shows, seven items contributed uniquely to the overall understanding of men's attitudes toward condom use once the effects of the other measures were taken into account.[1] The first factor was race/ethnicity. African American men had more favorable attitudes toward condom use overall than their counterparts of other racial groups did (ß=.13, p=.008). The second factor was educational attainment, with higher education tending to be linked with greater opposition to condom use (ß=.13, p=.010). The third factor was not caring about potential sex partners' HIV serostatus. Men who said that they did not care about the HIV serostatus of potential sex partners had more negative attitudes toward condom use than did men who specifically wanted their partners to be HIV-positive or HIV-negative (ß=.15, p=.004). The fourth contributing measure was liking to have sex that is "wild" or "uninhibited."

Table 2. Attitudes toward Condom Use and Involvement in Risky Sex

Risk Behavior Measure	Overall Condom-Related Attitudes	Attitudes toward Personal Condom Use
% of protected sex acts	*p*<.0001	*p*=.0005
% of protected anal sex	*p*<.0001	*p*<.0001
% of sex acts with internal ejaculation	*p*<.0001	*p*=.0014
% of anal sex acts with internal ejaculation	*p*<.0001	*p*=.0004
had any sex while "under the influence"	*p*=.0003	*p*=.0009
number of recent sex partners	*p*<.0001	*p*<.0001
number of lifetime sex partners	*p*<.0001	*p*=.0011
number of times recently having "wild" or "uninhibited" sex	*p*=.0005	*p*=.0006
number of times recently having sex in a gay bath house or a sex club	*p*=.0356	*p*=.0334

The more that men wanted their sex to be "wild" or "uninhibited," the more negative their attitudes toward condoms were (ß=.24, p<.0001). The fifth factor was the number of drug problems that men experienced, with a greater number of drug-related problems (i.e., abuse/dependency symptoms) being associated with more negative attitudes toward condom use (ß=.13, p=.009). The sixth measure retained in the multivariate equation was the perceived accuracy of information provided by sex partners about their HIV serostatus. The more that men believed in the accuracy of what their sex partners told them about their HIV serostatus, the less favorably disposed they tended to be regarding condom use (ß=.15, p=.004). Finally, level of self-esteem was found to be associated with men's attitudes toward condom use, with higher self-esteem corresponding to more favorable condom-related attitudes (ß=.17, p=.001). Together, in the multivariate analysis, these items explained 21.9% of the total variance.

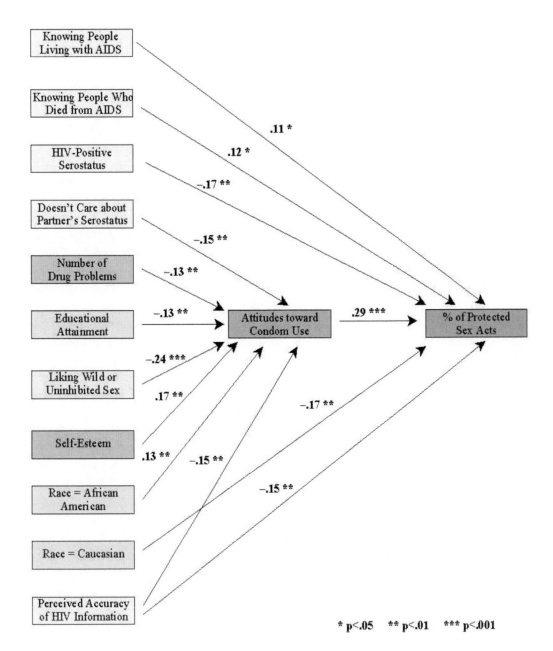

Figure 2. Condom-Related Attitudes and protected Sex.

The overall role of condom-related attitudes

Figure 2 portrays the specific role played by men's attitudes toward condom use when it comes to their involvement in protected sex. The structural equation analysis revealed that this way of depicting the data is an excellent representation of the interrelationships amongst the variables. The goodness-of-fit index for this model is 0.995, which is supported by the Bentler-Bonett normed fit index value of 0.977, indicating a strong overall "fit" for the data. The model's chi-square value is 9.52 (10df), which is not statistically significant (p=.484) and does not approach attaining statistical significance. Finally, the root mean square error approximation has a value of 0.000.

POTENTIAL LIMITATIONS

As with any research study, the present study has a few potential limitations. First, the response/participation rate was low (<10%), which could raise concern of selection bias and, therefore, the representativeness of the sample. Although it is difficult to be certain that the men who participated represent the men who did not, there is compelling evidence to suggest that differences between the two groups are minimal. Before The Bareback Project was started, the principal investigator conducted a large-scale content analysis with a random national sample of one of the main websites used by some men in the present study to meet other men seeking unprotected sex partners (19,36,37). The demographic composition of that sample and the one obtained in The Bareback Project closely match one another in terms of age representation, racial group composition, sexual orientation, and rural/suburban/urban location of residence. The two samples also resemble one another closely in terms of the types of sexual practices that men sought. The similarity of the two samples suggests that men who chose to participate in the present study represent those who did not, in terms of identifiable characteristics that are likely to be the best indicators of selection bias. Despite these similarities, the participation rate remains on the low side and thus represents a potential limitation for generalizability.

Second, as with most research data on sexual behaviors, the data in this study are based on uncorroborated self-reports. Therefore, it is unknown whether participants underreported or overreported their involvement in risky behaviors. The self-reported data probably can be trusted, however, as noted by other authors of previous studies with similar populations (38). This is particularly relevant for self-reported measures that involve relatively small occurrences (e.g., number of times having a particular kind of sex during the previous 30 days), which characterize the substantial majority of the data collected in this study (39). Other researchers have also commented favorably on the reliability of self-reported information in their studies regarding topics such as condom use (40).

A third potential limitation is the possibility of recall bias. For most of the measures used, respondents were asked about their beliefs, attitudes, and behaviors during the past 30 days. This time frames was chosen specifically: 1) to incorporate a large enough time frame in order to facilitate meaningful variability from person to person, and 2) to minimize recall bias. Although the authors cannot determine the exact extent to which recall bias affected the data, other researchers who have used similar measures have reported that recall bias is sufficiently minimal that its impact upon study findings is likely to be negligible (41). This seems to be especially true when the recall period is small (42,43), as was the case for the main measures used in the present study.

CONCLUSION

Despite these potential limitations, the present authors believe that the current study has much to offer. As hypothesized, condom-related attitudes were associated (consistently and inversely) with men's sexual risk practices. They were, in fact, the single strongest factor related to HIV risk identified in the structural equation modeled in Figure 2. Reducing HIV risk in this population will depend heavily on finding ways to change how men feel about using condoms. The data indicate an important difference between men's attitudes about condoms in general and their attitudes about using them personally. Although men in the sample had weakly-positive attitudes about condoms overall, their attitudes about using condoms themselves were considerably more negative. In other words, the men were not opposed to condoms ideologically; they simply preferred not to use condoms themselves.

Thus, intervention strategies must consider the question of how to make condoms more appealing and less unpleasant to men who prefer intentional condomless sex. Previous research suggests that highlighting the sexual/sensory aspects of condoms and eroticizing safer sex might help increase condom use among MSM (7). Indeed, when asked in the present study how they felt about the statement, "Many people make using condoms an erotic part of foreplay," men's responses were very divided (see Table 1), suggesting the possibility of progress in this area. Specific strategies to eroticize safer sex for members of this target population need to be developed, implemented, and subsequently tested for effectiveness. A number of community-based HIV prevention, education, and intervention programs around the United States have offered workshops about eroticizing safer sex, in an effort to teach members of the MSM community about specific strategies that can be undertaken to make condom use and other safer sex strategies more palatable. Programs such as those offered by Gay Men's Health Crisis in New York City [44], the Howard Brown Health Center in Chicago, and Project ARK in St. Louis are to be applauded, as are community-specific approaches such as AIDS Project Los Angeles' Red Circle Project (targeting safer sex among Native Americans) and Bockting, Rosser, and Scheltema's (45) program targeting safer sex among transgendered persons. Likewise, in recent years, websites dedicated to promoting erotic safer sex have begun to appear on the Internet, and we believe that they offer great promise in combating HIV risk-taking among MSM. An excellent example of this may be found on the Washington, DC-based group's DCFukit website, at www.dcfukit.org. Finding innovative ways to eroticize safer sex may be an important approach to changing how MSM think about condom use, and that, in turn, is likely to be an effective way of reducing their involvement in risky sexual practices.

One approach to accomplishing this may be to develop Internet-based prevention and intervention programs targeting the MSM community, as recent evidence has suggested that this approach may be effective in decreasing risk in this population. For example, Bowen and colleagues (46,47) tested the feasibility, acceptability, and efficacy of an Internet-based HIV prevention intervention targeting MSM in rural communities. Their preliminary findings indicated community support for such an intervention, with MSM in the study reporting reduced anal sex and increased condom usage. Likewise, another Internet-based prevention intervention among MSM demonstrated reductions in sexual contact with partners who were HIV-positive or HIV-serostatus-unknown (48). Internet-based prevention/intervention approaches may be particularly apropos with populations similar to that involved in the present study because these men actively used the Internet to find partners for unsafe sex.

The present study also identified several specific factors that were associated with men's attitudes toward condom use. We wish to discuss the implications of some of these findings. First, we discovered that men who said that they did not care whether their sex partners were HIV-positive or HIV-negative had more negative attitudes toward condom use overall than their counterparts who did care about their sex partners' HIV serostatus. In other research as well, a partner's indication of HIV serostatus has been shown to be linked to condom use attitudes and behaviors among MSM (5,49). Intervention programs working with MSM need to emphasize the importance of considering one's partners' HIV serostatus as one makes decisions regarding the types of sexual behaviors in which one is/not willing to engage. Intervention messages need to emphasize the importance of considering condom use and other safer sex strategies for men who engage in sex with serodiscordant partners.

Along the same lines, the present study found that the more accurate that men perceived HIV information supplied by would-be sex partners to be, the more negative their condom-related attitudes tended to be. This finding suggests that men who ask their partners about their HIV serostatus prior to having sex are apt to rely upon that information, supplanting it for their general feelings about using condoms. If their partners tell them that they are HIV-negative, then our findings suggest that the men accept this verbal information and act accordingly. Although we believe that it is important to discuss sexual partners' HIV serostatus, this strategy does not ensure protection from HIV transmission. HIV prevention strategies targeting MSM should, therefore, emphasize the importance of making decisions on the basis of personal safety and protection without relying primarily upon a partner's word.

This study also found that attitudes toward condom use were more positive among African American men than they were among men belonging to other racial/ethnic groups. This finding, coupled with the lower overall rates of condom use practiced by Caucasian men (see Figure 2), suggests a need to target Caucasian men in future prevention, education, and risk reduction intervention efforts. A number of published studies have reported on racial differences in HIV risk taking among MSM (50–52), leading some authors to advocate culturally-specific targeted interventions. Our own research findings suggest a need to target Caucasian MSM, particularly those using the Internet to identify partners for unprotected sex, and to develop strategies that can be effective at modifying how these men feel about using condoms.

In conclusion, the present study found that attitudes toward condom use among MSM seeking partners for unprotected sex via the Internet are the single strongest factor associated with men's involvement in risky sex. HIV risk reduction efforts need to find ways to change the way that men feel about using condoms.

They need to change the prevalent notions that condoms are unpleasant to use, that they reduce sexual pleasure, that they interrupt foreplay, and that putting them on a sex partner cannot be an erotic act–all notions that were commonplace in the men participating in this study. It is important to bear in mind that condom use attitudes do not exist or develop in isolation. The factors that help shape them (which the present study's findings suggest may be race/ethnicity, caring about sex partners' HIV serostatus, educational attainment, substance use/abuse problems, and level of self-esteem) can lead researchers toward the development of successful prevention intervention strategies.

Social science implications

Sexual behavior and sexual risk are social and/or interpersonal by nature and cannot be examined in a contextual vacuum. Although MSM were asked individually about their sexual behaviors and attitudes, sexual behaviors themselves take place in a complex social environment. Public health strategies can appear to be at odds with an individual's choices when making personal decisions about sexual behavior. Social scientists strive to understand the social determinants of health in an effort to mitigate the impact of HIV/AIDS. However, the importance of psychosocial functioning can, inadvertently, become secondary to disease prevention. Social scientists must seek ways to balance individuals' sexual and psychosocial needs with the larger public's health and safety concerns. Understanding condom use attitudes and other psychosocial measures of functioning simultaneously can improve our ability to enhance individual-level and societal-level health and to address the needs of individuals more adequately.

Condom use attitudes can offer clues about individuals' choices according to their social, emotional, psychological, and sexual needs. These ways to examine risk behavior and the prevention of HIV transmission are not applicable exclusively to MSM seeking unprotected anal intercourse (UAI). Rather, they apply across populations and are particularly relevant for discussions about decision-making processes and models such as Empowerment Theory, the Theory of Reasoned Action, and the Health Belief Model. For MSM seeking UAI, the perceived benefits of having UAI outweigh the perceived risks.

Actively seeking unprotected sex indicates a tipping in the perceived risk / perceived benefit scales in favor of more risk, according to health researchers and prevention specialists (53). However, 'safe' and 'risk' are subjective terms that are defined relatively, according to individuals' needs, desires, and preferences. As social scientists, our goal is not to pathologize behaviors, such as actively seeking unprotected sex, as was the case in this study of MSM. Instead, our efforts should include psychosocial factors and the social determinants of health that correlate with condom use and attitudes toward using condoms. Failing to do so would be a failure to understand individuals and groups comprehensively, particularly from a social science perspective on behavior that is social and/or interpersonal in nature.

The findings of this study support the Health Belief Model in that MSM in the sample held beliefs about condom use that directly corresponded to their sexual risk practices. As noted, in order to promote health by reducing HIV transmission in this high-risk population, it is essential for men to change the way they view personal condom use. This, however, must be approached within the broader context of an individual's needs and psychosocial health.

ENDNOTES

[1]In the interest of conserving space, the specific outcomes of the bivariate analyses undertaken prior to this multivariate analysis have been omitted. Readers wishing additional information about the bivariate analysis findings are invited to contact the first author for additional information/details.

ACKNOWLEDGMENTS

This research was supported by a grant from the National Institute on Drug Abuse (5R24DA019805). The authors wish to acknowledge, with gratitude, the contributions made to this study's data collection and data entry/cleaning functions by Thomas P Lambing.

REFERENCES

[1]   Levy JA. HIV and the pathogenesis of AIDS, 3rd ed. Washington, DC: ASM Press, 2007.

[2]   Ostrow DG, Silverberg MJ, Cook RL, Chmiel JS, Johnson L, Li X, Jacobson LP. Prospective study of attitudinal and relationship predictors of sexual risk in the Multicenter AIDS Cohort Study. AIDS Behav 2008;12:127-38.

[3]   Bakeman R, Peterson JL, Community Intervention Trial for Youth Study Team. Do beliefs about HIV treatments affect peer norms and risky sexual behaviour among African-American men who have sex with men? Int J STD AIDS 2007;18:105-8.

[4]   Peterson JL, Rothenberg R, Kraft JM, Beeker C, Trotter R. Perceived condom norms and HIV risks among social and sexual networks of young African American men who have sex with men. Health Educ Res 2009;24:119-27.

[5]   Carballo-Diéguez A, Miner M, Dolezal C, Rosser BR, Jacoby S. Sexual negotiation, HIV-status disclosure, and sexual risk behavior among Latino men who use the Internet to seek sex with other men. Arch Sex Behav 2006;35:473-81.

[6]   Nakamura N, Mausbach BT, Ulibarri MD, Semple SJ, Patterson TL. Methamphetamine use, attitudes about condoms, and sexual risk behavior among HIV positive men who have sex with men. Arch Sex Behav 2011;40:267-72.

[7]   Scott-Sheldon LA, Marsh KL, Johnson BT, Glasford DE. Condoms + pleasure = safer sex? A missing addend in the safer sex message. AIDS Care 2006;18:750-4.

[8]   Neville S, Adams J. Condom use in men who have sex with men: A literature review. Contemp Nurse 2009;33:130-9.

[9]   Bauermeister JA, Carballo-Diéguez A, Ventuneac A, Dolezal C. Assessing motivations to engage in intentional condomless anal intercourse in HIV risk contexts ("Bareback Sex") among men who have sex with men. AIDS Educ Prev 2009;21:156-68.

[10]   Holmes D, Warner D. The anatomy of a forbidden desire: men, penetration and semen exchange. Nurs Inq 2005;12:10-20.

[11]   Balán IC, Carballo-Diéguez A, Ventuneac A, Remien RH. Intentional condomless anal intercourse among Latino MSM who meet sexual partners on the Internet. AIDS Educ Prev 2009;21:14-24.

[12]   Carballo-Diéguez A, Bauermeister J. "Barebacking": intentional condomless anal sex in HIV-risk contexts. Reasons for and against it. J Homosex 2004;47:1-16.

[13]   Nodin N, Carballo-Diéguez A, Ventuneac AM, Balan IC, Remien R. Knowledge and acceptability of alternative HIV prevention bio-medical products among MSM who bareback. AIDS Care 2008;20:106-15.

[14]   Whittier DK, St. Lawrence J, Seeley S. Sexual risk behavior of men who have sex with men: Comparison of behavior at home and at a gay resort. Arch Sex Behav 2005;34:95-102.

[15]   Berg RC. Barebacking among MSM Internet users. AIDS Behav 2008;12:822-33.

[16]   Grov C, DeBusk JA, Bimbi DS, Golub SA, Nanin JE, Parsons JT. Barebacking, the Internet, and harm reduction: an intercept survey with gay and bisexual men in Los Angeles and New York City. AIDS Behav 2007;11:527-36.

[17]   Liau A, Millett G, Marks G. Meta-analytic examination of online sex-seeking and sexual risk behavior among men who have sex with men. Sex Transm Dis 2006;33:576-84.

[18]   McKirnan D, Houston E, Tolou-Shams M. Is the web the culprit? Cognitive escape and Internet sexual risk among gay and bisexual men. AIDS Behav 2007;11:151-60.

[19]   Klein H. HIV risk practices sought by men who have sex with other men, and who use Internet websites to identify potential sexual partners. Sex Health 2008;5:243-50.

[20]   Bolding G, Davis M, Hart G, Sherr L, Elford J. Where young MSM meet their first sexual partner: The role of the Internet. AIDS Behav 2007;11:522-6.

[21]   Horvath KJ, Nygaard K, Rosser BRS. Ascertaining partner HIV status and its association with sexual risk behavior among Internet-using men who have sex with men. AIDS Behav 2010;14:1376-83.

[22]   Singer M. Introduction to syndemics: A systems approach to public and community health. San Francisco, CA: Jossey-Bass, 2009.

[23]   Singer MC, Erickson PI, Badiane L, Diaz R, Ortiz D, Abraham T, Nicolaysen AM. Syndemics, sex and the city: Understanding sexually transmitted diseases in social and cultural context. Soc Sci Med 2006;63:2010-21.

[24]   Walkup J, Blank MB, Gonzales JS, Safren S, Schwartz R, Brown L, Wilson I, Knowlton A, Lombard F, Grossman C, Lyda K, Schumacher JE. The impact of mental health and substance abuse factors on HIV prevention and treatment. J Acquir Immune Defic Syndr 2008;47:S15-9.

[25]   Romero-Daza N, Weeks M, Singer M. "Nobody gives a damn if I live or die": Violence, drugs, and street-level prostitution in inner-city Hartford, Connecticut. Med Anthropol 2003;22:233-59.

[26]   Gielen AC, Ghandour RM, Burke JG, Mahoney P, McDonnell KA, O'Campo P. HIV/AIDS and intimate partner violence: Intersecting women's health issues in the United States. Trauma Violence Abuse 2007;8: 178-98.

[27]   Mustanski B, Garofalo R, Herrick A, Donenberg G. Psychosocial health problems increase risk for HIV among urban young men who have sex with men: Preliminary evidence of a syndemic in need of attention. Ann Behav Med 2007;34:37-45.

[28]   Brown IS. Development of a scale to measure attitude toward the condom as a method of birth control. J Sex Res 1984;20:255-63.

[29]   Rosenberg M. Society and the adolescent self-image. Princeton, NJ: Princeton University Press, 1965.

[30]   Von Diemen L, Szobot CM, Kessler F, Pechansky F. Adaptation and construction of the Barratt Impulsiveness Scale BIS 11 to Brazilian Portuguese for use in adolescents. Rev Bras Psiquiatr 2007;29:153-6.

[31]   Radloff LS. The CES-D scale: A self-report depression scale for research in the general population. Appl Psychol Meas 1977;1:385-401.

[32]   Scheier MF, Carver CS. Optimism, coping, and health: Assessment and implications of generalized outcome expectancies. Health Psychol 1985;4:219-47.

[33]   Diener E, Emmons RA, Larsen RJ, Griffin S. The satisfaction with life scale. J Pers Assess,1985;49:71-5.

[34]   Carey MP, Morrison-Beedy D, Johnson B. The HIV-Knowledge Questionnaire: Development and evaluation of a reliable, valid, and practical self-administered questionnaire. AIDS Behav 1997;1:61-74.

[35]   Bernstein DP, Fink L. Childhood Trauma Questionnaire: A retrospective self-report manual. San Antonio, TX: Psychological Corporation, 1998.

[36]   Klein H. Differences in HIV risk practices sought by self-identified gay and bisexual men who use Internet websites to identify potential sexual partners. J Bisex 2008;9:125-40.

[37]   Klein H. Sexual orientation, drug use preference during sex, and HIV risk practices and preferences among men who specifically seek unprotected sex partners via the Internet. Int J Environ Res Publ Health 2009;6:1620-35.

[38]   Schrimshaw EW, Rosario M, Meyer-Bahlburg HFL, Scharf-Matlick AA. Test-retest reliability of self-reported sexual behavior, sexual orientation, and psychosexual milestones among gay, lesbian, and bisexual youths. Arch Sex Behav 2006;35:225-34.

[39]   Bogart LM, Walt LC, Pavlovic JD, Ober AJ, Brown N, Kalichman SC. Cognitive strategies affecting recall of sexual behavior among high-risk men and women. Health Psychol 2007;26:787-93.

[40]   Morisky DE, Ang A, Sneed CD. Validating the effects of social desirability on self-reported condom use behavior among commercial sex workers. AIDS Educ Prev 2002;14:351-60.

[41] Kauth MR, St. Lawrence JS, Kelly JA. Reliability of retrospective assessments of sexual HIV risk behavior: A comparison of biweekly, three-month, and twelve-month self-reports. AIDS Educ Prev 1991;3:207-14.

[42] Fenton KA, Johnson AM, McManus S, Erens B. Measuring sexual behaviour: Methodological challenges in survey research. Sex Transm Infect 2001;77:84-92.

[43] Weir SS, Roddy RE, Zekeng L, Ryan KA. Association between condom use and HIV infection: A randomised study of self reported condom use measures. J Epidemiol Community Health,1999;53:417-22.

[44] Palacios-Jimenez L, Shernoff M. Facilitator's guide to eroticizing safer sex: A psychoeducational workshop approach to safer sex education. New York: Gay Men's Health Crisis, 1986.

[45] Bockting WO, Rosser BRS, Scheltema K. Transgender HIV prevention: Implementation and evaluation of a workshop. Health Educ Res 1999;14:177-83.

[46] Bowen AM, Horvath K, Williams ML. A randomized control trial of Internet-delivered HIV prevention targeting rural MSM. Health Educ Res 2007;22:120-7.

[47] Bowen AM, Williams ML, Daniel CM, Clayton S. Internet based HIV prevention research targeting rural MSM: Feasibility, acceptability, and preliminary efficacy. J Behav Med 2008;31:463-77.

[48] Carpenter KM, Stoner SA, Mikko AN, Dhanak LP, Parsons JT. Efficacy of a web-based intervention to reduce sexual risk in men who have sex with men. AIDS Behav 2010;14:549-57.

[49] Horvath KJ, Oakes JM, Rosser BR. Sexual negotiation and HIV serodisclosure among men who have sex with men with their online and offline partners. J Urban Health 2008;85:744-58.

[50] Millett GA, Flores SA, Peterson JL, Bakeman R. Explaining disparities in HIV infection among black and white men who have sex with men: A meta-analysis of HIV risk behaviors. AIDS 2007;21:2083-91.

[51] Mutchler MG, Bogart LM, Elliott MN, McKay T, Suttorp MJ, Schuster MA. Psychosocial correlates of unprotected sex without disclosure of HIV-positivity among African-American, Latino, and White men who have sex with men and women. Arch Sex Behav 2008;37:736-47.

[52] Rhodes SD, Yee LJ, Hergenrather KC. A community-based rapid assessment of HIV behavioural risk disparities within a large sample of gay men in southeastern USA: A comparison of African American, Latino, and white men. AIDS Care 2006;18:1018-24.

[53] Adam PC, Murphy DA, de Wit JB. When do online sexual fantasies become reality? The contribution of erotic chatting via the Internet to sexual risk-taking in gay and other men who have sex with men. Health Educ Res 2011;26:506-15.

Submitted: November 05, 2011. *Revised:* January 06, 2012. *Accepted:* January 09, 2012.

In: Public Health Yearbook 2012
Editor: Joav Merrick

ISBN: 978-1-62808-078-0
© 2013 Nova Science Publishers, Inc.

Chapter 40

BEYOND SEXUAL PARTNERSHIPS: THE LACK OF CONDOM USE DURING VAGINAL SEX WITH STEADY PARTNERS

Lara DePadilla, PhD, Kirk W Elifson, PhD
and Claire E Sterk*, PhD

Department of Behavioral Sciences and Health Education, Rollins School of Public Health, Emory University, Atlanta, Georgia, Unites States of America

ABSTRACT

The purpose of this paper is to identify independent correlates of the lack of condom use when engaging in vaginal sex with steady partners among HIV-negative African American adults. The conceptual model includes proximal as well as more distal domains. Methods: Cross-sectional data were collected between May 2009 and August 2011. Recruitment involved active and passive recruitment strategies. Computer-assisted, individual interviews were conducted with 1,050 African American adults. Multivariate logistic regression was used to identify independent predictors of a lack of condom use with steady partners in the past 30 days. Results: In multivariate analysis, being older than 35, being partnered, perceiving having a steady partner as important, and ever having been homeless were associated positively with the odds of a lack of condom use during vaginal sex with steady partners in the past 30 days. On the other hand, reporting more than one steady partner in the past 30 days, having health insurance during the past 12 months, and perceived neighborhood social cohesion were negatively associated. Conclusions: These findings highlight the need for HIV risk-reduction prevention and intervention efforts that consider distal as well as proximal domains. Such a perspective allows for a broader sociological inquiry into health disparities that moves beyond epidemiological factors that commonly guide public health research.

Keywords: Condom, steady partner, socioeconomic status, African American

---

* Correspondence: Claire E. Sterk, Emory University, Rollins School of Public Health, 1518 Clifton Road NE, Atlanta, GA 30322. E-mail: csterk@sph.emory.edu

INTRODUCTION

African Americans, specifically those belonging to the lower socioeconomic strata and who typically live in disadvantaged urban neighborhoods, have been impacted disproportionately by HIV (1). In 2009, African Americans comprised 14% of the United States population, but 44% of new HIV infections occurred among them (2). Between 2005 and 2008, African Americans experienced the largest increase in rate of HIV diagnoses as compared to members of other racial groups (2). In addition, African Americans were found to have the highest lifetime risk for a diagnosis of HIV infection of all racial/ethnic groups. Specifically, the rate among African Americans was one in 22 as compared to a rate of one in 170 among whites, and one in 52 among Hispanics/Latinos (3). These data also show that, by region in the U.S., African Americans accounted for the majority of HIV cases in the South (55.7%) (3).

Since the 1990s, social scientists have called for a "syndemic" approach to the HIV epidemic and associated disparities (4-7). In the public health community, the increasing need for recognizing such an approach is reflected in the emerging body of literature on multi-level approaches to the HIV/AIDS epidemic, including an emphasis on the social determinants of health and health disparities (8-10). By placing individual behaviors in the larger context of poverty, unequal access to health care, uneven criminal justice involvement, and residence in crumbling neighborhoods with limited social capital, tailored prevention and intervention efforts may be more likely to be effective in curtailing the devastating impact of the HIV/AIDS epidemic on African Americans. As one of its main goals, the National HIV/AIDS Strategy calls for prioritizing the reduction of HIV-related health disparities (11). Given that condom use as a safer sex strategy remains one of the most effective risk-reduction strategies among African Americans, especially in the U.S. South where much of the epidemic is driven by heterosexual transmission (3), in this paper, we focus on condom use during vaginal sex with steady partners. Specifically, we aim to gain a better understanding of distal and proximal factors that influence the use of condoms during vaginal sex with steady partners. Examples of proximal factors include relationships and sexual partnerships and in the more distal domain, socioeconomic status and neighborhood social capital.

Partner type and condom use

The way in which a person categorizes a sex partner may determine condom use behavior. In this inquiry, we limit the focus to male condoms because the use of female condoms is relatively low in the United States (12). Among women, researchers have found condom use with new or casual partners to be more common than condom use with regular partners (13). In addition, study findings show condom use to be least consistent with steady partners and explanations given for this include the notion that a steady partnership, beyond a sexual engagement, also involves emotional connectedness and trust (14, 15). The identification of the nature of a partner type (e.g., steady and casual) typically is left to study participants. Consequently, researchers as well as prevention and intervention experts may be applying definitions that do not capture everyday complexities of steady and casual partnerships, with the latter including transactional sex for which one partner is paid and the other pays. Having sex with a steady partner has been associated with a decrease in the odds of protected vaginal sex among women (16,17), while having sex with a casual partner has been associated with an increased likelihood of condom use among women as well as men (18). Among the barriers to condom use identified in the context of sex with steady partners are the perceived distraction from sexual intimacy and a possible reduction of sexual pleasure, its association with distrust in a partner and the assumption of unfaithfulness, and inadequate communication and negotiation skills (14,19,20). Foregoing condom use with a steady partner may serve as a means of establishing trust (21). When examining gender, some researchers found that women generally are more communicative about condom use and safer sex than men (22,23), although others found no gender differences (24,25).

Much of the research on condom use and sex partner type has focused on at-risk individuals, which include vulnerable African American men and women (26) who live in a social context characterized by distress that is triggered by negative social conditions such as poverty, easy access to alcohol and other drugs, and limited social cohesion. Several researchers found such macro-level factors to lead to partner concurrency (27,28). Partner concurrency refers to having multiple sex partners during the same time period, possibly including steady and non-steady partners. Partner concurrency has been associated with a higher number of unprotected vaginal sex acts with all types of sex partners, including steady and non-steady partners alike, but not specifically with steady partners (29). The impact of having more than one partner and how the partners are categorized may be important to consider when examining partner types and condom use.

Socioeconomic status, social capital, and condom use

Recognizing the influence of the larger socioeconomic context on condom use, it seems important to consider factors such as employment, income, and economic stability when exploring reasons for using or not using condoms. Economic hardship has been shown to have a negative association with condom use in a national sample of young adults (30). Perhaps as an example of extreme economic difficulties, being homeless has been found to be associated with unprotected sex among women as their homeless status resulted in more immediate challenges for daily survival and might overshadow the long-term HIV risk due to unprotected sex (17).

Finally, being in an economically motivated sexual relationship was associated with reduced condom use among African American women (31). The authors hypothesize that this is because the women's limited financial and material resources results in a reliance on sex partners and cultural norms in the women's social and sexual networks may be more accepting of economically motivated sexual relationships. It may also be that women in such relationships who do not use condoms seek to emulate primary relationships where sexual intimacy is driven by mutual trust as opposed to financial support (14).

Social capital has emerged in the literature as a valuable concept to understanding inequality, including health disparities (32-34). It has been used to examine the unequal distribution of social resources available to individuals within their communities and across social networks (35-37). In recent years, social capital has been joined with the concept of "community" in an effort to promote "community as the site where responsibility for ameliorating social problems lies" (38).

In this paper, we define social capital as the resources of individuals in social relationships as well as the resources within their social networks and community (39). Two key dimensions of social capital are perceived social cohesion and perceived social disorder. Social capital, specifically perceived social cohesion, has been associated negatively with gonorrhea rates (40, 41) and increased odds of condom use at last sex among African American youth (42). However, a qualitative investigation that highlighted the presence of positive role models as a form of social capital found that the lack of such role models was perceived to increase HIV risk-taking (43). Similarly, a study on gang membership also found it to reduce HIV protective behaviors (41). Whereas gang membership likely results in social capital, especially perceived social cohesion, it also may encourage behaviors that place a person at risk for HIV (e.g., social norms unsupportive of condom use result in unsafe sex). Yet others found that women who ceased using drugs and no longer engaged in transactional sex to pay for their habit increasingly became alienated from their social and sexual networks (44). Hence, as their HIV risk-taking decreased, their social capital did so as well.

Perceived social disorder, our second dimension of social capital, has also been associated with sexual risk-taking. For example, findings from recent studies show a link between social disorder (e.g., public drinking and visible drug sales and use) and increased rates of sexually transmitted infections (STIs) (41, 45). Additionally, perception of violence and homicide rates have also been associated with increased STI rates (41).

Substance use and condom use

Substance use as a risk factor for unprotected sex arises in the context of relationships and sexual partnerships, as a correlate of socioeconomic status and as a characteristic of the social environment, making it an important situational construct to consider. The use of alcohol and other drugs has been associated with unprotected sex (46,47). However, interesting gender differences emerge and it seems that the interaction of alcohol use by partner type and unsafe sex holds for women but to a more limited extent for men as men may have more direct control over condom use than women (48). For example, binge drinking has been associated with increased STI incidence among women seeking treatment at a clinic although the association was not found for men (46).

Similar dynamics may come into play when drugs other than alcohol are being used. Female drug users tend to be more stigmatized by their male counterparts as well as by society-at- large (7). Others have challenged the link between the use of alcohol and other drugs and the lack of condom use, especially when exploring this at the event level (18). Among users of illicit drugs, recent findings show unsafe sex to be related to the use of certain types of drugs (e.g., cocaine, methamphetamine and amphetamine) but not other drugs (e.g., marijuana and heroin) among drug-offending males (47).

Finally, researchers found that the setting in which drugs are being used and in which sex occurs influences condom use (49). For example, use in a crack house in which the norms allow for the exchange of sex for crack tends not to involve condom use. This may account for why recent crack use has demonstrated an association with reduced odds of condom use among low-income women (17).

The multi-domain approach of this study, including proximate and more distal factors, guides our inquiry to assess independent correlates of the lack of condom use during vaginal sex with steady partners, while controlling for substance use. We consider relationships and sexual partnerships as a key proximal domain and socio-economic status and social capital as more distal domains. By adding to the current knowledge about the dynamics regarding the lack of condom use with steady partners, we hope to contribute to ongoing efforts to reduce the health disparities, specifically those related to HIV/AIDS, faced by poor African Americans who reside in inner-city neighborhoods with limited social capital.

METHODS

Data for this study were collected as part of People and Places, a cross-sectional study of people and their perceptions of how their neighborhood impacted their daily lives and actions. Data were collected between May 2009 and August 2011 in Atlanta, Georgia. Participants (n=1,050) were recruited from 77 census block groups, using active community outreach strategies (e.g., recruiting directly in neighborhoods or via key respondents) and passive methods, specifically by posting flyers. The sampling frame was designed to ensure sufficient variability by gender, age, and drug use.

Eligible respondents self-identified as African American, were at least age 18, and had lived in the same neighborhood for the past year. Additional eligibility criteria for this paper were having had vaginal sex with a steady partner in the past 30 days and self-reporting as HIV- negative. The sexual activity criterion was added to ensure that we would be able to explore condom use behaviors in the context of vaginal sex in the past 30 days. A negative HIV status was included as a means of recognizing that condom use among HIV negative individuals serves as a main means to protect against HIV acquisition.

The survey included demographics, psychosocial characteristics, licit and illicit drug use history, sexual activity history, criminal justice involvement, and neighborhood perceptions. The Emory University Institutional Review Board approved the study protocol. Interviews lasted approximately 90 minutes and were conducted in a private office at the study site, which was located in one of the neighborhoods. Participants were compensated $30 for their time.

Measures

Outcome measure: Lack of Condom Use during Vaginal Sex with Steady Partners was derived from two questions. Participants were asked the number of times they engaged in any type of sex with steady partners in the past 30 days prior to the interview and then the question: "Of the [insert number of times] that you had vaginal sex with a steady partner or partners in the past 30 days, how many times did you or your partner use a male condom?" The responses were dichotomized as no condom use (1) and having used condoms at least once (0).

Demographics: Gender was self-identified as "male" (0) and "female" (1). Age (in years) was calculated using the participant's date of birth and the date of the interview.

Use of alcohol and other drugs: Alcohol use, crack/cocaine use and marijuana use in the past 30 days were dichotomized with 0=No and 1=Yes. Crack/cocaine and marijuana were selected in addition to alcohol due their prevalence in the Atlanta area (50).

Relationship and sexual partnership: Partnered was coded as not having a partner (0) or being with a partner, regardless of the living situation (1). The importance of a relationship with a steady partner was dichotomized into it being important (1) versus it not being important (0). Participants were asked about number of sexual partners by type of partner (steady, casual, and paid or paying) during the last 30 days. For this study, multiple partners was conceptualized as a three-level variable: having one steady partner, having more than one steady partner and possibly other types of partners, or only one steady partner with other types of partners. Given the focus on condom use with steady partners, which is least likely to be the case as compared with other partner types, each response option includes steady partners.

Socioeconomic status: Income was measured through a series of questions about the amount of income received in the past 30 days from a variety of sources including legal employment, "under the table" income, public assistance, retirement benefits, unemployment benefits, family sources, illegal income, and other sources. A total was calculated and the participant was asked to confirm the amount. For the purposes of this study, the square root of income was computed to make the variable conform to a normal distribution. The square root was applied as it resulted in a less skewed and less kurtotic transformed variable then taking the natural log. Employed reflected the respondent's current employment status and was dichotomized as not being employed (0) and being employed, either full or part-time (1). Homelessness was dichotomized as never having been homeless (0) to ever having been homeless (1). Educational attainment was captured by dichotomizing the responses between less than a high school education (0) and a high school education (including GED) or greater (1). Having health insurance was measured as no or inconsistent health insurance coverage in the past 12 months (0) versus having had health insurance coverage for all of the last 12 months (1). Current living situation was assessed as residing in your own house, condominium, townhome, or apartment (1) versus not having your own residence (0).

Social capital: Perceived social cohesion was measured using a 5-item scale (51) with questions such as "How often do you and people in your neighborhood do favors for each other?" and "How often do you and other people in the neighborhood ask each other for advice about personal things, such as child-rearing or job-openings?" (Cronbach's alpha = .78). Item responses ranged from 0=Never to 3=Often and scores were summed such that higher scores corresponded to greater perception of social cohesion. Perceived neighborhood disorder was assessed with a 7-item scale (52) that included statements such as "In my neighborhood, people watch out for each other" and "Police protection in my neighborhood is adequate" (alpha=.81). One item from the original scale was removed due to its similarity to perceived social cohesion. Response options ranged from 0=Strongly Disagree to 4=Strongly Agree. Higher scores corresponded to greater perceived disorder. Knowledge of crime in the neighborhood was measured by asking if the respondent knew if any of a series of violent events (e.g., shooting, sexual assault, robbery, or mugging) occurred in their neighborhood during the past 6 months, with responses ranged from never (0) to often (3) (alpha=. 71). Observed violence in the neighborhood was measured with seven questions from the Community Experiences Questionnaire (53). The items addressed having observed in the neighborhood during the past year events such as "somebody got hit, punched, or slapped" and "somebody got arrested or taken away by the police". Response options ranged from never (0) to often (3). Higher scores corresponded to greater levels of having observed violence (alpha=. 87).

Analysis

Generalized estimating equations (GEE) applying a logit link were used to conduct logistic regression with the software package SPSS Statistics 19.

The respondents were sampled by census block group and GEE was used because it provides a means of accounting for the correlation between people within these groups. GEE calculates the standard errors of parameter estimates based upon the within-cluster similarity of the residuals (54) thereby providing more accurate confidence intervals. Crude odds ratios were calculated and variables found to be significant at the level of $p < .10$ were included in the multivariate analysis. Missing data were minimal (2.6%) and any cases lacking a variable included in the multivariate model were dropped for that analysis.

A sensitivity analysis was also conducted with respect to the outcome variable of a lack of condom use. It has been asserted that grouping the "sometimes users" of condoms with the "always" users of condoms or "never" users of condoms can lead to inaccurate assessment of statistical associations (55). To avoid such errors, the alternate proportion of always using condoms versus sometimes or never using condoms was tested as the outcome in multivariate analysis and the analysis revealed that the results did not alter the basic conclusions of the study.

RESULTS

Descriptive statistics are displayed in table 1. The study sample included nearly equal proportions of men and women (49% and 51%) and 51% were over the age of 35. The age of 35 is used as a cut-off because we are interested in exploring the impact of drug use. Drug researchers tend to refer to those over 35 as older (56).

Being over 35 was associated with increases in the odds of the lack of condom use when engaging in vaginal sex in the past 30 days with steady partners (hereafter referred to as "lack of condom use"). Alcohol use demonstrated a trend toward a positive association with a lack of condom use, whereas crack cocaine or marijuana use was not associated with lack of condom use.

The relationship and sexual partnership characteristics demonstrated significant associations with the lack of condom use: having a partner and considering a steady relationship to be important were associated positively with a lack of condom use, while having more than one steady partner (but not having other types of partners in addition to a single steady partner) was associated negatively with a lack of condom use compared to having only one steady partner.

In the domain of socioeconomic status, having ever been homeless was associated with an increase in the odds of a lack of condom use, while having health insurance was associated with a decrease in the odds of a lack of condom use. Among the social capital indicators, perceived social cohesion was associated with a decrease in the odds of a lack of condom use, but perceived neighborhood disorder was associated with an increase the odds of a lack of condom use.

Table 2 includes the variables that were associated significantly with a lack of condom use at the level of $p < .10$ in bivariate analysis. In multivariate analysis, being older than 35 was associated with an increase in the odds of a lack of condom use.

The relationship variables were associated significantly with the outcome variable also. Both being partnered (OR=2.64; CI: 1.96, 3.54) and considering having a steady partner to be important (OR=1.35; CI: 1.02, 1.81) were associated positively with a lack of condom use. Having more than one steady partner and possibly other types of partners compared to having only one steady partner in the past 30 days was protective against a lack of condom use (OR=0.22; CI: 0.13, 0.36). However, having only one steady partner and other types of partners compared to having only one steady partner was not associated with a lack of condom use. The domains of socioeconomic status and social capital also revealed significant associations with a lack of condom use. Ever having been homeless was associated positively (OR: 1.38, CI: 1.06, 1.81) with the outcome variable, while having health insurance consistently over the past 12 months was associated negatively (OR: 0.71, CI: 0.52, 0.96) with the outcome variable. An increase in perceived social cohesion was associated with reduced odds of lack of condom use with a steady partner (OR: 0.96; CI: 0.92, 0.99).

DISCUSSION

In this study, we examine the impact of relationship and sexual partnership factors as well as more distal social factors on a lack of condom use when engaging in vaginal sex with steady partners among African American men and women. A majority of the sample (57%) reported not having used a condom when having vaginal sex with a steady partner in the past 30 days prior to the interview.

Table 1. Descriptive statistics and crude odds ratios (n=1050)

Variable	Mean (SD)/ Number (%)	Lack of Condoms Past 30 Days with Steady Partners	
		OR	95% CI
Never Use of Condoms Steady Partners	.57		
Demographics			
Gender	.51	1.09	(0.88, 1.35)
Age (>35)	.51	2.12	(1.70, 2.65)***
Use of Alcohol and Other Drugs			
Alcohol Past 30 Days	.71	1.27	(0.96, 1.68)†
Crack/Cocaine Past 30 Days	.27	1.17	(0.91, 1.52)
Marijuana Past 30 Days	.52	0.96	(0.75, 1.23)
Relationship and Sexual Partnerships			
Partnered	.74	2.82	(2.12, 3.74)***
Steady Partner Important	.78	1.86	(1.39, 2.48)***
Multiple Partners[a]			
At least two steady partners	.10	0.20	(0.12, 0.34)***
Only one steady partner with other partners	.10	0.99	(0.62, 1.56)
Socioeconomic Status			
Income[b]	25.75 (13.72)	1.00	(0.99, 1.01)
Employed	.23	0.89	(0.67, 1.18)
Homeless	.37	1.63	(1.27, 2.08)***
High school	.60	1.09	(0.83, 1.44)
Health Insurance[c]	.36	0.73	(0.56, 0.95)*
Own Home	.10	0.93	(0.61, 1.41)

Variable	Mean (SD)/ Number (%)	Lack of Condoms Past 30 Days with Steady Partners	
		OR	95% CI
Social Capital			
Perceived Social Cohesion	9.08 (3.91)	0.96	(0.93, 0.99)*
Perceived Neighborhood Disorder	16.11 (5.57)	1.03	(1.00, 1.05)*
Knowledge of Crime	3.79 (2.53)	1.00	(0.95, 1.06)
Observed Crime	11.37 (5.88)	1.00	(0.98, 1.02)

† p < .10, * p < .05, ** p < .01, *** p < .001.
[a]Reference category is having only one steady partner.
[b]Square root transformed.
[c]Reference category is not having health insurance consistently over the past 12 months.

A lack of condom use with steady partners commonly is reported in the literature (29,57), due to a partner's negative attitude toward condoms (57) and the association of condom use with a lack of trust and love (21). Our findings show that being partnered and perceiving having a steady partner as important were associated positively with a lack of condom use, the latter independent of relationship status. Considering having a steady partner as important may result in unsafe behaviors, without considering the potential HIV status of the partner or recognizing that many individuals are unaware of their HIV status (58). A second concern is that the decision not to use condoms may be based on the assumption that a steady partner is not having sex with other people (59). In the literature, concurrent sexual partnerships have been highlighted as contributing to the HIV epidemic, especially among African American men and women (60). It has been asserted that examining not only the individual but also the nature of the partnership is necessary to improve the understanding of HIV acquisition, particularly as it relates to concurrent partnerships (57).

In this study, one-fifth of the participants reported having more than one partner in the past 30 days. Among those who reported more than one steady partner (compared to having only one steady partner) in the past 30 days a negative association was found in the odds of a lack of condom use with steady partners.

Table 2. Adjusted odds ratios

	Lack of Condoms Past 30 Days with Steady Partners (n=1023)	
Variable	OR	95% CI[a]
Demographics		
Age (>35)	2.12	(1.61, 2.79)***
Use of Alcohol and Other Drugs		
Alcohol Past 30 Days	1.12	(0.80, 1.55)
Relationship and Sexual Partnerships		
Partnered	2.64	(1.96, 3.54)***
Steady Partner Important	1.35	(1.02, 1.81)*
Multiple Partners[a]		
At least two steady partners	0.22	(0.13, 0.36)***
Only one steady partner with other partners	1.08	(0.66, 1.78)

Table 2. (Continued)

	Lack of Condoms Past 30 Days with Steady Partners (n=1023)	
Socioeconomic Status		
Homeless	1.38	(1.06, 1.81)*
Health Insurance[b]	0.71	(0.52, 0.96)*
Social Capital		
Perceived Social Cohesion	0.96	(0.92, 0.99)*
Perceived Neighborhood Disorder	1.02	(1.00, 1.05)†

† $p < .10$, * $p < .05$, ** $p < .01$, *** $p < .001$.
[a] Reference category is having only one steady partner.
[b] Reference category is not having health insurance consistently over the past 12 months.

However, for study participants who indicated having had at least one steady and additional non-steady partner (e.g., casual or transactional partners) compared to having only one steady partner, no association was found with the lack of condom use with steady partners. Past qualitative research findings also showed the importance of differentiating between the patterns of concurrent relationships (61).

That study showed that people in multiple partnerships used condoms only with partners other than their "primary" or steady partners in most situations. The failure to show an association between having only one steady partner in addition other types of partners and a lack of condom use with steady partners is consistent with those findings. Condom use within the steady partnership would not be impacted by additional partners. However, the results of the current study also imply that if more than one person is considered steady that demarcation may not preclude condom use with steady partners.

Beyond the relationship and sexual partnerships, we found condom use to be impacted by dimensions from more distal domains. The socioeconomic factor of ever having been homeless was associated positively with a lack of condom use. Experiencing homelessness may represent acute economic deprivation and reduce concerns about future HIV acquisition due to a lack of condom use (17). Having health insurance during the past 12 months also was associated negatively with a lack of condom use. It may be that those who have health insurance are more likely to seek regular health checks and exhibit healthy behaviors more generally. For example, a study of a national sample of women found that women who had health insurance were more likely to have received health checks such as a pap smear (62).

The domain of social capital revealed an association between perceived social cohesion and a reduction in the odds of a lack of condom use. This finding is consistent with previous research that has found that social cohesion exhibited a protective effect against HIV risk behaviors (40,42). Other dimensions of social capital were not associated with a lack of condom use, possibly because these are too distal for our inquiry.

Substance use was not associated with a lack of condom use. This is not unexpected given that drinking in particular is more often associated with condom use with non-steady partners (18,63). It may also be that situational factors do not impact condom use with steady partners because condom use is not prevalent with steady or regular partners in general (29,57).

Limitations

This study has a number of limitations. The sampling approach is not a random sampling strategy and there may be an inherent bias in who was enrolled in People and Places (64). All interviews were conducted in the Atlanta, Georgia metropolitan area. There may very well be local or regional influences or subcultural differences between these participants and those residing elsewhere that could affect the generalizability of the data.

Sexual behavior represents a sensitive topic that may be subject to respondent social desirability bias. Given the fact that sexual behavior was assessed based on self-report, the extent to which respondents under or over-reported their behaviors is unknown. Nevertheless, others have shown information on (e.g., sexual behaviors, alcohol consumption, and drug use) to be valid (65-68). Another potential limitation of the self-reported information is recall bias. We focused mainly on the time frame of the "past 30 days" as a means to minimize recall bias. Although we are unable to determine the extent to which recall bias affected the data, others who conducted research on similar topics reported that bias is sufficiently nominal that its impact upon study findings is likely to be minimal (69).

The cross-sectional design precludes any causal inferences. Among the measures, the non-steady partners included both casual and paid or paying partners; and these two alternatives to steady partners may be qualitatively different. Overall, there is a need for more refined research on partner types. The analysis also did not account for same sex partnerships, as the focus was heterosexual vaginal sex given the salience of this behavior for the HIV/AIDS rates among African Americans. Finally, we only examined the concurrency status of the participants. It would be useful to include a measure of their perception of whether their partners also have additional partners to understand better the nature of the relationship and how it relates to a lack of condom use with steady partners.

Social science implications

Given that a lack of condom use when engaging in vaginal sex with steady partners during the past 30 days is prevalent, factors beyond the individual and outside the interpersonal domain become more important. Much attention has been paid to the economic disparities among African Americans in the United States; this study accounts for the importance of socioeconomic status when assessing the lack of condom use in this specific type of partnership. Patterns of deprivation have been linked to concurrency among African Americans (60) and increase the importance of identifying specific aspects of disparities that are associated with a lack of condom use with steady partners. The results of this study suggest that it is not only extreme indicators such as the experience of homelessness, but also access to health resources such as health insurance, that influence whether one will consider using condoms with a steady partner. These findings also indicate that not only personal but also collective resources, such as perceived social cohesion, impact a lack of condom use with steady partners. Trust and reciprocity within social networks have been associated with health and psychological well-being more generally (70), and may contribute to health-related decision making involving condom use. Factors outside the partnership (e.g., social and sexual network norms) provide potential pathways to increasing the use of condoms even in steady partnerships where a lack of condom use is the norm (13,29).

The multi-domain approach to understanding why people do or do not use condoms with certain partners is typical of sociological inquiry. In addressing our research question, we aimed to provide an epistemology of the HIV-related health disparities experienced by African Americans. We show how factors beyond the individual impact actions, in this case, the influence of socioeconomic characteristics and social capital. These tap into the position of the individual in society (e.g., homelessness and having health insurance) as well as the conditions of the neighborhood in which one resides. Recently, public health has gained an appreciation for the importance of social capital, specifically social cohesion and our findings support this path of inquiry. It is through this type of epistemology that social science may make contributions; it shows the importance of considering epidemiological information in the larger socio-political and ecological context.

ACKNOWLEDGMENTS

This research was supported by funding from the National Institute on Drug Abuse RO1DA025607) and the Center for AIDS Research at Emory University (P30AI050409). The views presented are those of the authors.

REFERENCES

[1]   CDC. Acquired immunodeficiency syndrome (AIDS) among blacks and Hispanics--United States. MMWR, 1986;35(42):655-8,663-6.

[2]   CDC. HIV among African Americans. 2010. Retrieved from http://www.cdc.gov/hiv/topics/aa/pdf /aa.pdf.

[3]   CDC. Estimated lifetime risk for diagnosis of HIV infection among Hispanics/Latinos--37 states and Puerto Rico, 2007. MMWR 2010;59(40):1297-301.

[4]   Marshall P, Singer M, Clatts M. Integrating cultural, observational, and epidemiological approaches in the prevention of drug abuse and HIV/AIDS. NIDA Monograph. Washington, DC: Government Printing Office, 1999:97-115.

[5]   Singer M. AIDS and the health crisis of the US urban poor: The perspective of critical medical anthropology. Soc Sci Med 1994;39:931-48.

[6]   Singer M. Introduction to syndemics: A systems approach to public and community health. San Francisco, CA: Jossey-Bass, 2009.

[7]   Sterk C. Fast lives: Women who use crack cocaine. Philadelphia, PA: Temple University Press, 1999.

[8]   Aral SO, Adimora AA, Fenton KA. Understanding and responding to disparities in HIV and other sexually transmitted infections in African Americans. Lancet, 2008;372(9635):337-40.

[9]   CDC. Estimates of new HIV infections in the United States, 2006-2009. 2011. Retrieved from http://www.cdc.gov/hiv/topics/surveillance/factsheets.htm

[10]   Harrison KM, Dean HD. Use of data systems to address social determinants of health: A need to do more. Public Health Rep, 2011;126(Suppl 3):1-5.

[11]   White House Office of National AIDS Policy. National HIV/AIDS strategy. 2010. Retrieved from http://aids.gov/federal-resources/policies/national-hiv-aids-strategy/nhas.pdf.

[12]   Dancy BL, Berbaum ML. Condom use predictors for low-income African American women. West J Nurs Res 2005;27(1):28-44.

[13]   Macaluso M, Demand MJ, Artz LM, Hook EWI. Partner type and condom use. AIDS 2000;14(5):537-46.

[14]   Catania J, Coates TJ, Kegeles S. A test of the AIDS Risk Reduction Model: Psychosocial correlates of condom use in the AMEN cohort survey. Health Psychol 1994;13(6):548-55.

[15] Wingood G, DiClemente R. Partner influences and gender-related factors associated with noncondom use among young adult African American women. Am J Community Psychol 1998;26:29-51.

[16] Lichtenstein B, Desmond RA, Schwebke JR. Partnership concurrency status and condom use among women diagnosed with trichomonas vaginalis. Womens Health Issues 2008;18(5):369-74.

[17] Ober A, Iguchi M, Weiss R, Gorbach P, Heimer R, Ouellet L, et al. The relative role of perceived partner risks in promoting condom use in a three-city sample of high-risk, low-income women. AIDS Behav 2011;15(7):1347-58.

[18] Scott-Sheldon L, Carey M, Vanable P, Senn T, Coury-Doniger P, Urban M. Alcohol consumption, drug use, and condom use among STD clinic patients. J Stud Alcohol 2009;70(5):762-70.

[19] Schilling R, El-Bassel N, Schinke S, Gordon K, Nichols S. Building skills of recovering women drug users to reduce heterosexual AIDS transmission. Public Health Rep 1991;106:297-304.

[20] Theall KP, Sterk CE, Elifson KW. Male condom use by type of relationships following an HIV intervention among women who use illegal drugs. J Drug Issues 2003;33:1-28.

[21] Corbett AM, Dickson-Gómez J, Hilario H, Weeks MR. A little thing called love: Condom use in high-risk primary heterosexual relationships. Perspect Sex Reprod Health 2009;41(4):218-24.

[22] Allen M, Emmers-Sommer TM, Crowell TL. Couples negotiating safer sex behaviors: A meta-analysis of the impact of conversation and gender. In: Allen M, Preiss RW, Gayle BM, Burrell NA, editors. Interpersonal communication research: Advances through meta-analysis. Mahwah, NJ: Lawrence Erlbaum, 2002:263-79.

[23] Noar SM, Morokoff PJ, Harlow LL. Condom negotiation in heterosexually active men and women: Development and validation of a condom influence strategy questionnaire. Psychol Health 2002;17:711-35.

[24] Aida Y, Falbo T. Relationships between marital satisfaction, resources, and power strategies. Sex Roles 1991;24(1/2):43-56.

[25] Noar SM, Zimmerman RS, Atwood KA. Safer sex and sexually transmitted infections from a relationship perspective. In: Harvey JH, Wenzel A, Sprecher S, editors. Handbook of sexuality in close relationships. Mahwah, NJ: Lawrence Erlbaum, 2004:519-44.

[26] Ickovics J, Yoshikawa H. Preventive interventions to reduce heterosexual HIV risk for women: Current perspectives, future directions. AIDS 1998;12:S197-208.

[27] Adimora AA, Schoenbach VJ. Social context, sexual networks, and racial disparities in rates of sexually transmitted infections. J Infect Dis 2005;191(Suppl 1):S115-S22.

[28] Magnus M, Kuo I, Shelley K, Rawls A, Peterson J, Montanez L, et al. Risk factors driving the emergence of a generalized heterosexual HIV epidemic in Washington, District of Columbia networks at risk. AIDS 2009;23(10):1277-84.

[29] Senn TE, Carey MP, Vanable PA, Coury-Doniger P, Urban M. Sexual partner concurrency among STI clinic patients with a steady partner: Correlates and associations with condom use. Sex Transm Dis 2009;85(5):343-7.

[30] Ford JL, Browning CR. Neighborhood social disorganization and the acquisition of trichomoniasis among young adults in the United States. Am J Public Health 2011;101(9):1696-703.

[31] Dunkle K, Wingood G, Camp C, DiClemente R. Economically motivated relationships and transactional sex among unmarried African American and white women: Results from a U.S. national telephone survey. Public Health Rep 2010;125(S4):90-125.

[32] Schuller T. Reflections of the use of social capital. Rev Soc Econ 2007;65(1):11-28.

[33] Lockhart WH. Building bridges and bonds: Generating social capital in secular and faith based poverty-to-work programs. Sociol Relig 2005;66(1):45-60.

[34] Putnam RD. Bowling alone: The collapse and revival of american community. New York, NY: Simon Schuster, 2000.

[35] Bourdieu P. Distinction: A social critique of the judgement of taste. Cambridge, MA: Harvard University Press, 1984.

[36] Coleman JS. Social capital in the creation of human capital. Am J Sociol 1988;94:95-121.

[37] Lin N. Social capital: A theory of social structure and action. Cambridge, MA: University Press, 2001.

[38] Bryson L, Mowbray M. More spray on solution: Community, social capital and evidence based policy. Aust J Soc Issues 2005;40(1):91-106.

[39]   Thomas-Slayter BP, Fisher WF. Social capital and AIDS-resilient communities: Strengthening the AIDS response. Glob Public Health 2011:1-21.

[40]   Ellen JM, Jennings JM, Meyers T, Chung S-E, Taylor R. Perceived social cohesion and prevalence of sexually transmitted diseases. Sex Transm Dis 2004;31(2):117-22.

[41]   Thomas J, Torrone E, Browning C. Neighborhood factors affecting rates of sexually transmitted diseases in Chicago. J Urban Health 2010;87(1):102-12.

[42]   Kerrigan D, Witt S, Glass B, Chung S-e, Ellen J. Perceived neighborhood social cohesion and condom use among adolescents vulnerable to HIV/STI. AIDS Behav 2006;10(6):723-9.

[43]   Cené C, Akers A, Lloyd S, Albritton T, Powell Hammond W, Corbie-Smith G. Understanding social capital and HIV risk in rural African American communities. J Gen Intern Med 2011;26(7):737-44.

[44]   Sterk C, Elifson K, Theall K. Individual action and community context: The health intervention project. Am J Prev Med 2007;32(Suppl 6):S177-S81.

[45]   Lang D, Salazar L, Crosby R, DiClemente R, Brown L, Donenberg G. Neighborhood environment, sexual risk behaviors and acquisition of sexually transmitted infections among adolescents diagnosed with psychological disorders. Am J Community Psychol 2010;46(3):303-11.

[46]   Hutton HE, McCaul ME, Santora PB, Erbelding EJ. The relationship between recent alcohol use and sexual behaviors: Gender differences among sexually transmitted disease clinic patients. Alcohol Clin Exp Res 2008;32(11):2008-15.

[47]   Leigh B, Stall R. Substance use and risky sexual behavior for exposure to HIV: Issues in methodology, interpretation, and prevention. Am Psychol 1993;48:1035-45.

[48]   Pulerwitz J, Amaro H, Jong WD, Gortmaker SL, Rudd R. Relationship power, condom use and HIV risk among women in the USA. AIDS Care 2002;14(6):789-800.

[49]   Kopetz CE, Reynolds EK, Hart CL, Kruglanski AW, Lejuez CW. Social context and perceived effects of drugs on sexual behavior among individuals who use both heroin and cocaine. Exp Clin Psychopharmacol 2010;18(3):214-20.

[50]   DePadilla L, Wolfe M. Drug abuse patterns and trends in Atlanta--Update: June 2010. Epidemiologic Trends in Drug Abuse: Proceedings of the Community Epidemiology Work Group. Bethesda, MD: US Department Health Human Services, 2010.

[51]   Sampson RJ, Morenoff JD, Felton E. Beyond social capital: Spatial dynamics of collective efficacy for children. Am Sociol Rev 1999;64(5):633-60.

[52]   Ross CE, Mirowsky J. Disorder and decay. Urban Aff Rev, 1999;34(3):412-32.

[53]   Schwartz D, Proctor LJ. Community violence exposure and children's social adjustment in the school peer group: The mediating roles of emotion regulation and social cognition. J Consult Clin Psychol 2000;68(4):670-83.

[54]   Hanley JA, Negassa A, Edwardes MDd, Forrester JE. Statistical analysis of correlated data using generalized estimating equations: An orientation. Am J Epidemiol 2003;157(4):364-75.

[55]   Crosby R, DiClemente RJ, Holtgrave DR, Wingood GM. Design, measurement, and analytical considerations for testing hypotheses relative to condom effectiveness against non-viral STIs. Sex Transm Infect 2002;78(4):228-31.

[56]   Gfroerer J, Penne M, Pembertin M, Folsom R. Substance abuse treatment need among older adults in 2020: The impact of the aging baby-boom cohort. Drug Alcohol Depend 2003;69:127-35.

[57]   Gorbach P, Holmes KK. Transmission of STIs/HIV at the partnership level: Beyond individual-level analyses. J Urban Health 2003;80(0):iii15-iii25.

[58]   Campsmith ML, Rhodes PH, Hall I, Green TA. Undiagnosed HIV prevalence among adults and adolescents in the United States at the end of 2006. J Acquir Immune Defic Syndr 2010;53(5):619-24.

[59]   Drumright LN, Gorbach PM, Holmes KK. Do people really know their sex partners?: Concurrency, knowledge of partner behavior, and sexually transmitted infections within partnerships. Sex Transm Dis 2004;31(7):437-42.

[60]   Adimora AA, Schoenbach VJ, Doherty IA. HIV and African Americans in the southern United States: Sexual networks and social context. Sex Transm Dis 2006;33(7):S39-S45.

[61]   Gorbach P, Stoner BP, Aral SO, H. Whittington WL, Holmes K. "It takes a village": Understanding concurrent sexual partnerships in Seattle, Washington. Sex Transm Dis 2002;29(8):453-62.

[62] Coughlin SS, Leadbetter S, Richards T, Sabatino SA. Contextual analysis of breast and cervical cancer screening and factors associated with health care access among United States women, 2002. Soc Sci Med 2008;66(2):260-75.

[63] Raj A, Reed E, Santana MC, Walley AY, Welles SL, Horsburgh CR, et al. The associations of binge alcohol use with HIV/STI risk and diagnosis among heterosexual African American men. Drug Alcohol Depend 2009;101(1-2):101-6.

[64] Heckathorn DD. Respondent-Driven Sampling: A New Approach to the Study of Hidden Populations. Soc Problems 1997;44(2):174-99.

[65] Anglin M, Hser Y, Chou C. Reliability and validity of retrospective behavioral self-report by narcotics addicts. Evaluation Rev 1993;17:91-103.

[66] Higgins ST, Budney AJ, Bickel WK, Badger GJ, Foerg FE, Ogden D. Outpatient behavioral treatment for cocaine dependence: One-year outcome. Exp Clin Psychopharmacol 1995;3(2):205-12.

[67] Miller M, Paone D. Social network characteristics as mediators in the relationship between sexual abuse and HIV risk. Soc Sci Med 1998;47(6):765-77.

[68] Nurco DN. A discussion of validity: Self-report methods of estimating drug use. Washinfgton, DC: NIDA Res Monogr 57, US Government Printing Office, 1985:4-11.

[69] Jaccard J, Wan CK. A paradigm for studying the accuracy of self-reports of risk behavior relevant to AIDS: Empirical perspectives on stability, recall bias, and transitory influences. J Appl Soc Psychol 1995;25:1831-58.

[70] Nieminen T, Martelin T, Koskinen S, Aro H, Alanen E, Hyyppä M. Social capital as a determinant of self-rated health and psychological well-being. Int J Public Health, 2010;55(6):531-42.

Submitted: December 15, 2011. *Revised:* January 19, 2012. *Accepted:* January 29, 2012.

SECTION FIVE – ACKNOWLEDGMENTS

In: Public Health Yearbook 2012
Editor: Joav Merrick

ISBN: 978-1-62808-078-0
© 2013 Nova Science Publishers, Inc.

Chapter 41

ABOUT THE EDITOR

Joav Merrick, MD, MMedSci, DMSc, is professor of pediatrics, child health and human development affiliated with Kentucky Children's Hospital, University of Kentucky, Lexington, United States and the Department of Pediatrics, Hadassah-Hebrew University Medical Center, Mount Scopus Campus, Jerusalem, Israel, the medical director of Health Services, Division for Intellectual and Developmental Disabilities, Ministry of Social Affairs and Social Services, Jerusalem, the founder and director of the National Institute of Child Health and Human Development. Numerous publications in the field of pediatrics, child health and human development, rehabilitation, intellectual disability, disability, health, welfare, abuse, advocacy, quality of life and prevention. Received the Peter Sabroe Child Award for outstanding work on behalf of Danish Children in 1985 and the International LEGO-Prize ("The Children's Nobel Prize") for an extraordinary contribution towards improvement in child welfare and well-being in 1987.

Contact:

Office of the Medical Director, Division for Mental Retardation, Ministry of Social Affairs, POBox 1260, IL-91012 Jerusalem, Israel.

E-mail: jmerrick@zahav.net.il
Home-page: http://jmerrick50.googlepages.com/home

In: Public Health Yearbook 2012
Editor: Joav Merrick
ISBN: 978-1-62808-078-0
© 2013 Nova Science Publishers, Inc.

Chapter 42

ABOUT THE NATIONAL INSTITUTE OF CHILD HEALTH AND HUMAN DEVELOPMENT IN ISRAEL

The National Institute of Child Health and Human Development (NICHD) in Israel was established in 1998 as a virtual institute under the auspicies of the Medical Director, Ministry of Social Affairs and Social Services in order to function as the research arm for the Office of the Medical Director. In 1998 the National Council for Child Health and Pediatrics, Ministry of Health and in 1999 the Director General and Deputy Director General of the Ministry of Health endorsed the establishment of the NICHD.

MISSION

The mission of a National Institute for Child Health and Human Development in Israel is to provide an academic focal point for the scholarly interdisciplinary study of child life, health, public health, welfare, disability, rehabilitation, intellectual disability and related aspects of human development. This mission includes research, teaching, clinical work, information and public service activities in the field of child health and human development.

SERVICE AND ACADEMIC ACTIVITIES

Over the years many activities became focused in the south of Israel due to collaboration with various professionals at the Faculty of Health Sciences (FOHS) at the Ben Gurion University of the Negev (BGU). Since 2000 an affiliation with the Zusman Child Development Center at the Pediatric Division of Soroka University Medical Center has resulted in collaboration around the establishment of the Down Syndrome Clinic at that center. In 2002 a full course on "Disability" was established at the Recanati School for Allied Professions in the Community, FOHS, BGU and in 2005 collaboration was started with the Primary Care Unit of the faculty and disability became part of the master of public health course on "Children and society". In the academic year 2005-2006 a one semester course on "Aging with disability" was started as part of the master of science program in gerontology in our collaboration with the Center for Multidisciplinary Research in Aging. From 2011 teaching medical second, fourth and six year medical students at Hadassah-Hebrew University Medical Center, Jerusalem.

RESEARCH ACTIVITIES

The affiliated staff have over the years published work from projects and research activities in this national and international collaboration. In the year 2000 the International Journal of Adolescent Medicine and Health and in 2005 the International Journal on Disability and Human development of Freund Publishing House (London and Tel Aviv), in the year 2003 the TSW-Child Health and Human Development and in 2006 the TSW-Holistic Health and Medicine of the Scientific World Journal (New York and Kirkkonummi, Finland), all peer-reviewed international journals were affiliated with the National Institute of Child Health and Human Development. From 2008 also the International Journal of Child Health and Human Development (Nova Science, New York), the International Journal of Child and Adolescent Health (Nova Science) and the Journal of Pain Management (Nova Science) affiliated and from 2009 the International Public Health Journal (Nova Science) and Journal of Alternative Medicine Research (Nova Science).

NATIONAL COLLABORATION

Nationally the NICHD works in collaboration with the Faculty of Health Sciences, Ben Gurion University of the Negev; Department of Physical Therapy, Sackler School of Medicine, Tel Aviv University; Autism Center, Assaf HaRofeh Medical Center; National Rett and PKU Centers at Chaim Sheba Medical Center, Tel HaShomer; Department of Physiotherapy, Haifa University; Department of Education, Bar Ilan University, Ramat Gan, Faculty of Social Sciences and Health Sciences; College of Judea and Samaria in Ariel and in 2011 affiliation with Center for Pediatric Chronic Illness and Center for Down Syndrome, Department of Pediatrics, Hadassah-Hebrew University Medical Center, Mount Scopus Campus, Jerusalem.

INTERNATIONAL COLLABORATION

Internationally with the Department of Disability and Human Development, College of Applied Health Sciences, University of Illinois at Chicago; Strong Center for Developmental Disabilities, Golisano Children's Hospital at Strong, University of Rochester School of Medicine and Dentistry, New York; Centre on Intellectual Disabilities, University of Albany, New York; Centre for Chronic Disease Prevention and Control, Health Canada, Ottawa; Chandler Medical Center and Children's Hospital, Kentucky Children's Hospital, Section of Adolescent Medicine, University of Kentucky, Lexington; Chronic Disease Prevention and Control Research Center, Baylor College of Medicine, Houston, Texas; Division of Neuroscience, Department of Psychiatry, Columbia University, New York; Institute for the Study of Disadvantage and Disability, Atlanta; Center for Autism and Related Disorders,

Department Psychiatry, Children's Hospital Boston, Boston; Department of Paediatrics, Child Health and Adolescent Medicine, Children's Hospital at Westmead, Westmead, Australia; International Centre for the Study of Occupational and Mental Health, Düsseldorf, Germany; Centre for Advanced Studies in Nursing, Department of General Practice and Primary Care, University of Aberdeen, Aberdeen, United Kingdom; Quality of Life Research Center, Copenhagen, Denmark; Nordic School of Public Health, Gottenburg, Sweden, Scandinavian Institute of Quality of Working Life, Oslo, Norway; Centre for Quality of Life of the Hong Kong Institute of Asia-Pacific Studies and School of Social Work, Chinese University, Hong Kong.

TARGETS

Our focus is on research, international collaborations, clinical work, teaching and policy in health, disability and human development and to establish the NICHD as a permanent institute in Israel in order to conduct model research and together with the four university schools of public health/medicine in Israel establish a national master and doctoral program in disability and human development at the institute to secure the next generation of professionals working in this often non-prestigious/low-status field of work. For this project we need your support. We are looking for all kinds of support and eventually an endowment.

SUPPORT FOR OUR WORK

In The United States

In the United States the Israel Foundation for Human Development was created in order to support the work of the National Institute of Child Health and Human Development in Israel. It is possible to send donations to the Israel Foundation for Human Development Inc, which is a recognized tax-exempt organization in the United States (charitable non-for-prifit organization with 501c (3) tax exempt number 56-230-6116). Checks for the Foundation in the United States can be send to Israel Foundation for Human Development Inc., President Arlene Feldman, 2 Lawrence Street, New Hyde Park, New York 11040. Phone: 516-352-3596. E-mail: AFeldman@FarrellFritz.com

Contact in Israel

Professor Joav Merrick, MD, MMedSci, DMSc
Medical Director, Division for Mental Retardation
Ministry of Social Affairs, POBox 1260
IL-91012 Jerusalem, Israel
E-mail: jmerrick@zahav.net.il

SECTION SIX - INDEX

INDEX

C

D

F

H

I

J

K

L

M

N

S

T

U

V

W

X

Y

Z